Surgery: Issues, Challenges and Clinical Perspectives

Surgery: Issues, Challenges and Clinical Perspectives

Editor: Thomas Harvey

FOSTER ACADEMICS
www.fosteracademics.com

www.fosteracademics.com

FOSTER ACADEMICS

Cataloging-in-Publication Data

Surgery : issues, challenges and clinical perspectives / edited by Thomas Harvey.
p. cm.
Includes bibliographical references and index.
ISBN 978-1-64646-553-8
1. Surgery. 2. Surgery--Case studies. 3. Medicine. I. Harvey, Thomas.
RD31.5 .S87 2023
617--dc23

Foster Academics,
118-35 Queens Blvd., Suite 400,
Forest Hills, NY 11375, USA

ISBN 978-1-64646-553-8 (Hardback)

Contents

Preface

This book aims to highlight the current researches and provides a platform to further the scope of innovations in this area. This book is a product of the combined efforts of many researchers and scientists, after going through thorough studies and analysis from different parts of the world. The objective of this book is to provide the readers with the latest information of the field.

Surgery refers to a branch of medicine that deals with the manual and mechanical treatment of wounds, illnesses and other disorders. Several techniques can be utilized depending on the type of surgery. The two most common types of surgical techniques include minimally invasive surgery and open surgery. There are several challenges associated with surgery such as bleeding problems during surgery, death due to surgery, difficulty breathing after surgery, injury during surgery, bruising and swelling after surgery, anesthesia complications during surgery, etc. There are various subspecialties of surgery such as breast surgery, craniofacial surgery, podiatric surgery, genitourinary surgery, endocrine surgery and dental surgery. This book aims to shed light on the issues, challenges and clinical perspectives in surgery. It presents researches and studies performed by experts across the globe. This book will serve as a reference to a broad spectrum of readers.

I would like to express my sincere thanks to the authors for their dedicated efforts in the completion of this book. I acknowledge the efforts of the publisher for providing constant support. Lastly, I would like to thank my family for their support in all academic endeavors.

Editor

1

The Road to Technical Proficiency in Cytoreductive Surgery for Peritoneal Carcinomatosis: Risk-Adjusted Cumulative Summation Analysis

Francesco Santullo[1], Carlo Abatini[1], Miriam Attalla El Halabieh[1], Federica Ferracci[3], Claudio Lodoli[1], Lorenzo Barberis[3], Francesco Giovinazzo[2], Andrea Di Giorgio[1] and Fabio Pacelli[1,3]*

[1]Surgical Unit of Peritoneum and Retroperitoneum, Fondazione Policlinico Universitario A. Gemelli IRCCS, Rome, Italy, [2]General Surgery and Liver Transplant Unit, Fondazione Policlinico Universitario A. Gemelli IRCCS, Rome, Italy, [3]Dipartimento di Medicina e Chirurgia Traslazionale, Università Cattolica del Sacro Cuore, Rome, Italy

*Correspondence: Carlo Abatini carlo.abatini@guest.policlinicogemelli.it

Background: Cytoreductive surgery (CRS) is a technically demanding procedure, and there is considerable debate about its safe application. This study investigated the learning curve for CRS and the clinical outcomes of consecutive patients treated by a single surgeon at a single institution.

Methods: We collected 251 consecutive patients who underwent CRS for peritoneal metastases by a single surgeon at Fondazione Policlinico Universitario A. Gemelli IRCCS, between January 2016 and December 2020. The learning curve was estimated using the cumulative summation analysis (CUSUM) for operative time (OT). Risk-adjusted CUSUM (RA-CUSUM) charts were developed using a composite variable (surgical failure), defined as the occurrence of at least one of the following events: major postoperative complications (Clavien–Dindo grade ≥3), blood loss ≥500 mL, incomplete cytoreduction. Three learning phases were thus derived from the RA-CUSUM analysis, and were compared in terms of perioperative outcomes.

Results: CUSUM-OT showed that the operation time improved significantly after the 161th case. RA-CUSUM analysis allowed to break the CRS learning curve into three different phases: phase 1, “the learning phase” (cases 1–99), phase 2 “the experienced phase” (cases 100–188), and phase 3, “the mastership phase” (cases 189–251). The rate of major postoperative complications decreased significantly over the three phases ($p = 0.019$). Operative time decreased significantly as well ($p = 0.031$) and was significantly shorter in phase 3 with respect to the other two phases (phase 3 vs phase 2: 420 min vs 500 min, $p = 0.017$; phase 3 vs phase 1: 420 min vs 503 min, $p = 0.021$). Blood loss consistently decreased throughout the three phases ($p = 0.001$). The rate of incomplete cytoreduction was significantly lower in phase 3 than in phase 2 (4.8% vs 14.6%, $p = 0.043$).

Conclusion: The CRS failure rate stabilized after the first 99 cases, and the complete surgical proficiency was achieved after 189 cases. A standardised and mentored learning model is a safer strategy to shorten the learning process, to reduce morbidity and mortality, to improve oncologic outcomes.

Keywords: peritoneal metastases, cytoreductive surgery (CRS), hyperthermic intraperitoneal chemotherapy (hipec), peritonectomy, learning curve, CUSUM, RA-CUSUM

INTRODUCTION

The peritoneal of gastrointestinal and gynaecological malignancies is usually associated with poor prognosis (1). Also, peritoneal carcinomatosis (PC) has been marginally affected by systemic chemotherapy and previously considered by the oncologists as an end-of-life condition, not amenable for surgery (2–4). Nowadays, the treatment of PC is radically changing thanks to a better understanding of tumours biology and their dissemination pattern. Therefore, PC is considered a form of loco-regional disease that could benefit from a multimodal approach combining aggressive surgery and chemotherapy (5).

Cytoreductive surgery (CRS) followed by hyperthermic intraperitoneal chemotherapy (HIPEC) is currently the standard of care in selected patients with PC from various abdominal malignancies (6, 7). CRS aims to remove every macroscopically visible tumour implant within the peritoneal cavity, and then a heated chemotherapy local infusion eradicates any residual microscopic disease (8). Therefore, CRS plus HIPEC results in a highly complex and lengthy surgical procedure involving multi-visceral resection, burdened by high morbidity due to the synergistic effect of cytoreduction, hyperthermia, and local chemotherapy cytotoxicity (9).

Over the years, CRS and HIPEC have improved the selection of more suitable patients and is now considered safe and comparable to other high-risk surgical oncology procedures in terms of complications rate (9).

In spite of this, the learning curve for CRS plus HIPEC is not standardised yet, because the surgical procedures required to clear the peritoneal metastasis are often complex and heterogenous, and the caseload is limited, even in high-volume cancer centres (10).

In our tertiary referral hospital, the surgical treatment of PC from colorectal cancer (CRC) (11) and pseudomyxoma peritonei (PMP) (12) has reached an acceptable perioperative outcome and long-term survival, with respectively a 3-year OS of 43% for CRC and a 5-year OS of 91% for PMP.

This study aimed to generate learning curves for CRS based on the performance of a single surgeon at a single institution performing cytoreductive surgery for PC from various abdominal malignancies.

METHODS

Study design

We retrieved clinical data for 251 consecutive patients who underwent CRS for peritoneal carcinomatosis (regardless of the origin) by a single surgeon at Fondazione Policlinico Universitario A. Gemelli IRCCS between January 2016 and December 2020. All CRS were performed by a single experienced general surgeon (AD) with no previous experience in cytoreductive surgery for carcinomatosis. AD completed the European School of Peritoneal Surface Oncology (ESPO) training during the study time-period. He was mentored along the process by another experienced general surgeon (FP), who also had already experience with peritoneal surgery and HIPEC.

We analysed the learning curve for CRS using the cumulative summation (CUSUM) and the risk-adjusted cumulative summation (RA-CUSUM) methods (13). The operation time was assessed with the CUSUM method. The RA-CUSUM was calculated using a composite variable (surgical failure) that merges all the variables presumably involved into the learning process and creates a curve plotting change in the success rate over an increasing number of cases. Surgical failure was defined as the occurrence of at least one of the following events: major post-operative complications (Clavien–Dindo grade ≥3), blood loss ≥500 mL, incomplete cytoreduction. Three learning phases were thus derived from the RA-CUSUM analysis, and were compared in terms of perioperative outcomes.

All patients provided written informed consent and entered a follow-up program. Data were collected and stored in a prospectively maintained database. The study was approved by the local Institutional Review Board (IRB). We use the STROBE statement checklist (v 4.0) for our research.

Preoperative evaluation

After a complete preoperative workup, all patients were reviewed at our institutional peritoneal disease multidisciplinary team (MDT). The extent of peritoneal disease was subsequently assessed by diagnostic laparoscopy, and the peritoneal carcinomatosis index (PCI) scoring system was recorded for each patient. The decision of the multidisciplinary team in offering cytoreductive surgery depends on the primary oncological disease:

- *Pseudomixoma Peritoneii:* CRS and HIPEC were offered to all medically fit patients with PMP. The main goal was to achieve a complete cytoreduction; however, if this was not possible due to the extension of the disease, maximal tumour debulking was performed.
- *Colorectal and gastric peritoneal metastasis:* CRS and HIPEC was offered in case of potentially complete cytoreduction of peritoneal disease without extra-abdominal metastases.

Patients not eligible for cytoreductive surgery were referred for systemic chemotherapy.

- *Ovarian cancer, mesothelioma, and other less common histology:* before progressing to CRS and HIPEC, these cases were discussed by the institutional MDT.

Cytoreductive surgery with HIPEC

Following the laparotomy, a revaluation of PCI was performed. The surgical intent was to obtain a maximal cytoreduction and perform the HIPEC. Patients who could not achieve a complete cytoreduction, generally due to the extent of disease or their general conditions, underwent a maximal tumour debulking without HIPEC. Cytoreductive surgery was performed using the Sugarbaker technique (10). When the disease was limited, patients underwent selective peritonectomy. The surgical purpose was to remove all visible peritoneal metastases through diaphragmatic, parietal anterior, and pelvic peritonectomy with greater and lesser omentectomy. In addition, multiple organ resections were performed depending on disease involvement if an CC-0/1 resection could be achieved. Organ resections included segmental colectomy, proctectomy, small bowel resections, gastrectomy (partial or rarely total), segmental liver resection, cholecystectomy, splenectomy, and hysterectomy with bilateral salpingo-oophorectomy in females. The HIPEC procedure was then performed using the closed technique. In 8 cases, the HIPEC procedure was performed using CO_2 technology (14).

HIPEC regimens varied according to histology: oxaliplatin were used for colorectal cancer, mitomycin for colorectal cancer, pseudomixoma peritoneii and gastric cancer, whereas cisplatin for gastric cancer, ovarian cancer and mesothelioma. The target temperature, likewise, was set between 40–42 °C and the time duration was 60 or 90 min. Glucose 5% solution was used for oxaliplatin and physiologic solution 0.9% for other drugs. An adequate intra-abdominal patient filling volume was 2–2.5 L/mq.

Data

The clinical and pathological variables for each patient were retrospectively reviewed. The following clinical variables were recorded: age, sex, body mass index (BMI), Eastern Cooperative Oncology Group (ECOG) performance status (PS), primary tumour location, operative time, PCI score, completeness of cytoreduction (CC score), blood loss and post-operative complications, which were divided into minor (Clavien-Dindo I-II), and major (Clavien-Dindo ≥III3) (15).

Intraoperative blood loss was calculated, at the end of the procedure, by the combination of absorbent materials (number of used gauzes) and volume of blood in canisters. The 500 mL cut-off was choice considering previous literature data (16) and present NICE guidelines (17, 18). The completeness of the cytoreduction (CC) score was determined at the end of each procedure. CC-0 reflected no remaining visible disease. CC-1, 2, and 3 implied remaining diseases less than 2.5 mm, 2.5 to 2.5 cm, and greater than 2.5 cm. The procedures were divided into "complete cytoreduction" and "incomplete cytoreduction" based on the primary tumour histology. Colon cancer, gastric cancer, and mesothelioma CC-0 were deemed complete cytoreduction, while CC-1/2/3 cases were considered incomplete (19). CC-0/1 were considered a complete cytoreduction in PMP and mesothelioma (20, 21).

Statistics

Descriptive statistics were used to describe the patients' surgical and pathological characteristics. Continuous variables are reported as medians and ranges, and categorical variables are reported as numbers and percentages of the overall group.

We examined the learning curve for CRS using CUSUM and RA-CUSUM analyses. The patients were ordered chronologically. The CUSUM analysis for operation time (CUSUMOT) was defined as:

$$CUSUM_{OT} = \sum_{i=1}^{n} (x_i - \mu)$$

where x_i is the single patient's operation time, and μ is the mean operation time. The RA-CUSUM analysis was defined as

$$RACUSUM = \sum_{i=1}^{n} (x_i - \tau) + (-1)^{xi} P_i$$

where $x_i = 1$ indicates the presence of surgical failure, otherwise, $x_i = 0$; τ represents the event rate, and P_i is the expected surgical failure rate derived from a logistic regression model with a backward stepwise selection of the variable procedure. The entire series is plotted from left to right on the horizontal axis. The curve moves down for each success and up for each failure. We delineated the end of the learning process as the point where the curve reached the steady state (13, 22).

Based on the trend displayed by the curve, the whole sample was divided into three phases: phase 1, "the learning phase", phase 2, "the experienced phase", and phase 3, "the mastership phase". The different phases were compared using the χ^2 test and Student t-tests for parametric estimations and Wilcoxon Mann-Whitney U test for nonparametric estimations. $p \leq 0.050$ was considered statistically significant. Statistical analyses were performed using SPSS version 24.0 (IBM, Armonk, New York, USA) software for Windows.

RESULTS

Two hundred fifty-one patients underwent CRS for peritoneal carcinosis from various origins during the study period. Patient characteristics are shown in **Table 1**. The median age was 59 years (range: 26–86 years). One hundred and forty-five patients were females (57.8%), and 106 were males (42.2%). Considering the primary cancer sites, 115 (45.8%) were colorectal cancer, 19 (7.6%) were gastric cancer, 48 (19.1%) were PMP, 16 (6.4%) were mesothelioma, 42 (16.7%) were ovarian cancer, and 11 were from various origin (pancreatic, biliary) and were grouped as other. The median PCI score calculated after laparotomy was 12 (range 3–30). Two hundred and twenty-three (88.8%) patients received a complete cytoreduction, while 28 (11.2%) received an incomplete cytoreduction. The median operating time was 502 (140–900) min. The complete operative details are shown in **Table 2**.

TABLE 1 | Baseline characteristics and operative details.

Variable	*N* (%)
Gender	
Female	145 (57.8)
Male	106 (42.2)
Age, years [median (range)]	59 (26–86)
BMI [median (range)]	24.2 (17–41.7)
ECOG PS	
0	139 (55.4)
≥1	112 (44.6)
Primary tumor histotype	
Colorectal	115 (45.8)
Gastric	19 (7.6)
PMP	48 (19.1)
Mesothelioma	16 (6.4)
Ovarian	42 (16.7)
Other	11 (4.4)
Operative time, min [median (range)]	500 (140–900)
PCI [median (range)]	12 (3–30)
Surgical Procedures	
Right colectomy	91 (36.3)
Left colectomy	18 (7.2)
Rectal resection	122 (48.6)
Pelvic peritonectomy	163 (64.9)
Hysterectomy/oophorectomy	122 (48.6)
Diaphragmatic peritonectomy	134 (53.4)
Mesenteric cytoreduction	54 (21.5)
Omentectomy	181 (72.1)
Gastric resection	19 (7.6)
Small bowel resection	65 (25.9)
Segmental liver resection	6 (2.4)
Splenectomy	65 (25.9)
Ostomy	93 (37.1)
Completeness of Cytoreduction (CCR)	
Complete	223 (88.8)
Incomplete	28 (11.2)
HIPEC	
No	41 (16.3)
Yes	210 (83.7)
Blood loss >500 mL	
No	182 (72.5)
Yes	69 (27.5)

All patients were managed in the intensive care unit for at least one night in the post-operative period. No major intraoperative complications occurred. There were 3 (1.2%) post-operative in-hospital deaths.

One-hundred and six (42.2%) patients developed post-operative complications: grade I/II complications occurred in 64 (25.5%) patients, and grade III/IV complications occurred in 42 (16.7%) patients. Considering major complications, 9 (3.5%) patients experience post-operative bleeding, 20 (7.9%) abdominal collections, and 13 (3.9%) anastomotic leaks (AL). Among the 9 patients with post-operative bleeding, 7 needed surgeries with relaparotomy and surgical hemostasis, while the remaining 2 patients were treated with angioembolisation.

The percentage of AL was analysed considering all the 334 anastomoses. Two (15.4%) ALs were from an ileocolic anastomosis, 1 (7.7%) from a colo-colic anastomosis and 10 (76.9%) from a colorectal anastomosis. Seven (53.8%) of the 13 patients with AL received a protective ileostomy during the first surgery. Among all the ALs, 3 of them were treated conservatively (percutaneous drainage plus broad-spectrum antibiotic therapy), while 10 patients underwent re-operation with resection of the anastomotic complex and colostomy or ileostomy, depending on the leak. The leading cause of abdominal collection was pancreatic fistula (10 patients; 3.9%). Among the 20 patients with abdominal collections, 12 were treated with percutaneous drainage plus antibiotic therapy, while the rest (8 patients) underwent relaparotomy and surgical drainage. The complete description of post-operative complications is shown in **Table 2**.

The learning curve for CRS was assessed using the CUSUM and RA-CUSUM methods. The CUSUM-OT curve shows an initial long plateau, with the first downward slope only after 161 cases (**Figure 1**). Afterwards, the reduction appears slow and inconstant, as documented by the multiple peaks and throughs in the plot (**Figure 1**). In the RA-CUSUM graph,

TABLE 2 | Postoperative complications.

Variable	*N* (%)
Complications	
No	145 (57.8)
Yes	106 (42.2)
Complication grade (Clavien-Dindo)	
Grade I–II	64 (25.5)
Grade III–IV	42 (16.7)
Postoperative mortality	3 (1.2)
Postoperative ileus	10 (3.9)
Pulmonary complications	21 (8.4)
Postoperative bleeding	9 (3.5)
Abdominal collection	20 (7.9)
Genitourinary infection	11 (4.4)
Anastomotic leak[a]	13 (3.9)[a]
Surgical site infection	18 (7.2)
Renal failure	4 (1.6)

[a]*Analyzed considering all the 334 anastomosis.*

the curve moved upwards for surgical failure and downwards for surgical success. The RA-CUSUM analysis revealed that the surgical failure rate was significant in the initial phase until case 99. Next, the slope remained stable until case 198 and then gradually decreased (**Figure 2**). Consequently, according to the RA-CUSUM curve, the CRS learning curve breaks into three different phases: phase 1, "the learning phase" (cases 1–99), phase 2 "the experienced phase" (cases 100–188), and phase 3, "the mastership phase" (cases 189–251).

Perioperative outcomes throughout the three learning phases are shown in **Table 3**. There were no significant differences in age, sex, BMI, ECOG grade, and primary tumour histotype among the three phases.

PCI constantly increased over the different phases and was significantly higher in phase 3 than in the other two phases (phase 3 vs phase 2: 16 vs 12, $p = 0.029$; phase 3 vs phase 1: 16 vs 10, $p = 0.001$).

Concerning the completeness of cytoreduction, even though there was no consistently significant reduction among all three phases, the rate of incomplete CCR was significantly lower in phase 3 with respect to phase 2 (4.8% vs 14.6%, $p = 0.043$). Moreover, a trend of lower incomplete CCR was observed in phase 3 than in phase 1, though not significant (4.8% vs 12.1%, $p = 0.094$). Consequently, the HIPEC administration rate increased across the three phases ($p = 0.001$) but was significantly higher in phase 3 than in the other two phases

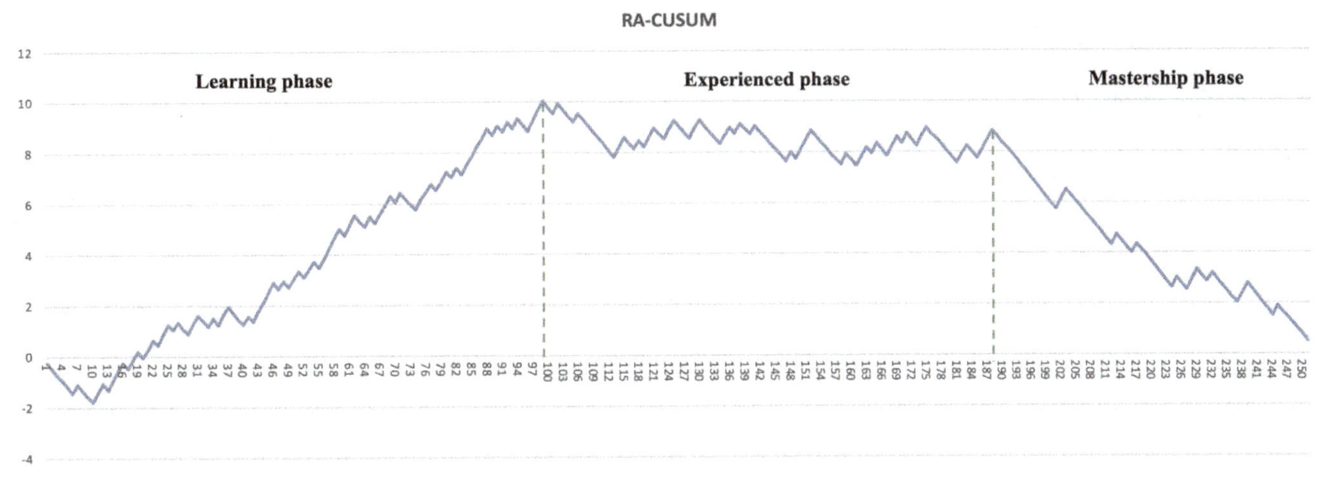

FIGURE 1 | CUSUM curve of operation time (CUSUMOT).

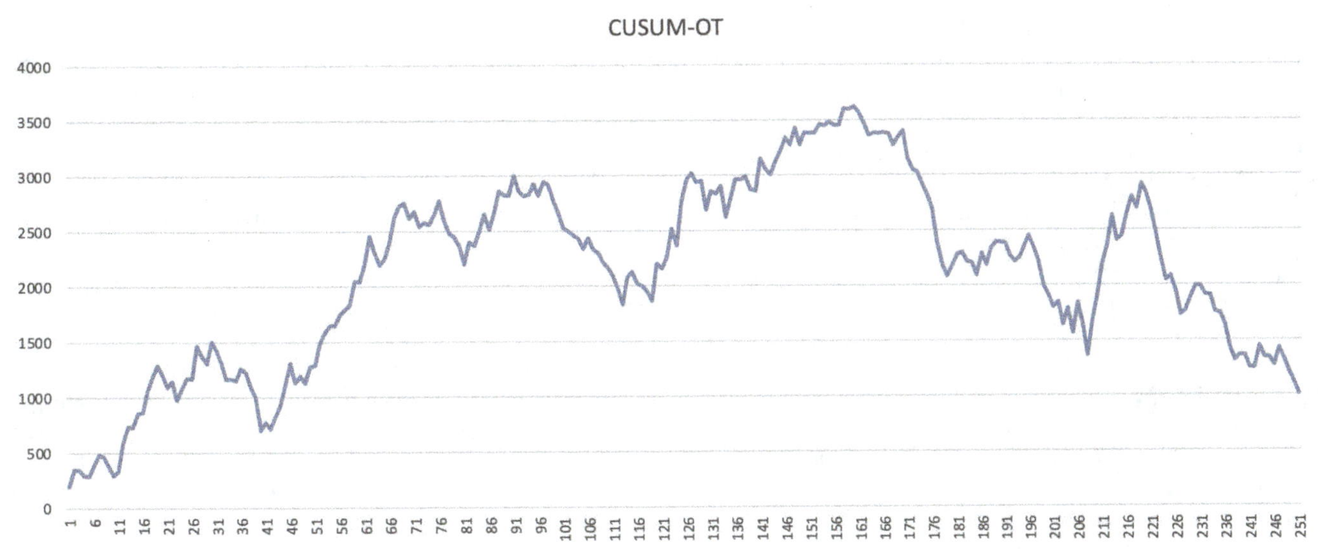

FIGURE 2 | Risk-adjusted CUSUM curve (RA-CUSUM).

TABLE 3 | Comparison of baseline characteristics and perioperative outcomes among the three phases defined by the RA-CUSUM analysis.

Parameters	Phase 1 (*n* = 99)	Phase 2 (*n* = 89)	Phase 3 (*n* = 63)	*p*-value	Phase 1 vs 2	Phase 2 vs 3	Phase 1 vs 3
Age (years)	55 (26–80)	60 (35–86)	61 (34–79)	0.138	0.178	0.382	0.068
Gender							
Male	39 (39.4)	45 (50.6)	22 (34.9)	0.120	0.082	0.056	0.567
BMI (Kg/m^2)	23.9 (17–34.6)	24.7 (17–31.3)	24.6 (18–41.7)	0.080	0.469	0.101	0.031
ECOG							
≥1	47 (47.5)	36 (40.4)	29 (46)	0.605	0.333	0.493	0.858
PCI	10 (3–27)	12 (3–30)	16 (3–27)	0.001	0.096	0.029	0.001
Primary tumor histotype							
Colon	44 (44.4)	41 (46.1)	30 (47.6)	0.894	0.689	0.963	0.689
Gastric	9 (9.1)	7 (7.9)	3 (4.8)				
PMP	17 (17.2)	17 (19.1)	14 (22.2)				
Mesotelioma	5 (5.1)	7 (7.9)	4 (6.3)				
Ovarian	17 (17.2)	15 (16.9)	10 (15.9)				
Other	7 (7.1)	2 (2.2)	2 (3.2)				
Completeness of cytoreduction							
Incomplete	12 (12.1)	13 (14.6)	3 (4.8)	0.152	0.616	0.043	0.094
HIPEC							
Yes	78 (78.8)	70 (78.7)	62 (98.4)	0.001	0.561	0.001	0.001
Operative time (min)	503 (140–800)	500 (200–900)	420 (200–808)	0.031	0.963	0.017	0.021
Major complications							
Clavien-Dindo 3–5	22 (22.2)	15 (16.9)	5 (7.9)	0.019	0.230	0.085	0.013
Blood loss							
>500 mL	43 (43.4)	21 (23.6)	5 (7.9)	0.001	0.002	0.012	0.001

(phase 3 vs. phase 2: 98% vs. 78.8%, $p = 0.001$; phase 3 vs. phase 1: 98% vs. 78.8%, $p = 0.001$).

The rates of major post-operative complications decreased significantly over the three phases ($p = 0.019$). Despite the rates of post-operative complications not being significantly different among phases 1 and 2 and phases 2 and 3, there was a significant reduction in complication rates in phase 3 compared to phase 1 (phase 3 vs phase 1: 7.9% vs 22.2%, $p = 0.013$).

Operative time decreased significantly over the three phases ($p = 0.031$) and was significantly lower in phase 3 than in the other two phases (phase 3 vs phase 2: 420 min vs 500 min, $p = 0.017$; phase 3 vs phase 1: 420 min vs 503 min, $p = 0.021$). Blood loss constantly and significantly decreased among the three phases ($p = 0.001$).

DISCUSSION

Considering the results of the case series published in the literature, the number of operations necessary to overcome the learning curve varies from 130 to 220 cases (23–26). The first report was in 2007 when Smeenk et al. (23) showed a significant increase in complete cytoreduction from 35.6% to 65.1% after 130 cases. A similar learning curve of 140 cases based on completeness of cytoreduction and severe morbidity was reported by Kusamura et al. in 2012 (24). In two other series, the operative outcomes are improved following 220 (25) and 180 (26) cases, respectively.

In our understanding, such heterogeneity could be due to the use of different analytical methods and outcomes to evaluate surgical proficiency in CRS. In other complex surgical procedures, such as pancreaticoduodenectomy (22), the operation time is frequently used as a primary outcome to measure the surgical skill improvement and it decreases with the surgeons' experience. However, especially in CRS, operation time is affected by several factors, such as PCI, location of PM, primary disease, regardless of the surgeon's skill and experience. In addition, the relationship between operative time and post-operative complications is not well defined yet. Furthermore, CUSUMOT plot shows a rather steady trend in our paper, and only after 161 cases a late and slow reduction is visible. Additionally, several inconstant peaks were visible in the late period after the 161 cases (**Figure 1**), suggesting an inconsistent reduction in the operative time.

To overcome this limitation, we outline a composite variable (surgical failure) that merges all the parameters supposedly entailing the learning process.

Among the three phases defined by the RA-CUSUM curve, we found no difference in the rate of incomplete cytoreduction, but there was a significant reduction in the rate of severe postoperative complications.

During the first 99 cases, we found a complication rate of 22.2%, comparable with the one reported in the literature (27). Moreover, this value is higher than 16.7%, which is the median value of the major complication rate of our whole series (**Table 3**). Furthermore, the rate of incomplete cytoreduction in this phase is 12%, comparable with the value reported by other papers (24, 27, 28).

This means that our results are within acceptable limits (i.e. minimal level of proficiency) in terms of morbidity, mortality, and completeness of cytoreduction, also during the initial phase, when surgeries are performed without having gained the highest level of expertise.

After the 99th case, the RA-CUSUM curve reaches a steady-state until the 188th case (i.e. the experienced phase). A possible explanation for this "deadlock period" without any apparent improvement in surgical skills could be that we implemented our surgical indications after gaining experience and autonomy, including patients with a higher disease burden. As a matter of fact, in our series, the PCI and the consequent surgical challenge gradually increases during the study period (**Table 3**). Hence, the improved skills acquired in this phase were partially hidden by the significant surgical abilities required to manage a more significant disease load. Moreover, the results obtained in this phase (major complication rate 16.9%, incomplete cytoreduction rate of 14.6%) are acceptable and widely comparable with other data reported from other series (27, 29). Hence, a relatively long period is necessary to improve these results considering the advanced technical skills needed to face a more extensive disease.

Following a relatively long period of stability, the RA-CUSUM slope takes a gradual decrease after the 189th case (i.e. the mastership phase), with a clear improvement of all the surgical outcomes. In this phase, the achieved surgical abilities allow dealing with a more extensive and challenging disease (median PCI = 16), achieving a remarkably low rate of incomplete cytoreduction (4.8%) and complication rate (7.9%). Moreover, our major complication rate is lower than other series reported in the literature (27–31). The improvement of the rate of incomplete cytoreduction accounts for the significantly higher rate of HIPEC administration in the last phase compared with the other two (**Table 3**).

Additionally, to highlight further the surgical proficiency acquired in the mastership phase, we found a significant reduction in operative time compared with the learning phase ($p = 0.021$) and the experienced phase ($p = 0.017$).

Pondering on our results, the achievement of the technical proficiency required 189 cases, which is comparable with the 130–220 cases reported in the literature. Before achieving the complete proficiency and after the first 99 cases, the surgeon could safely perform CRS in patients with a moderate extension of the disease, obtaining a complication rate and an incomplete cytoreduction rate widely comparable to other series in the literature.

In this study of an experienced surgeon without prior experience of CRS and HIPEC, the incidence of major post-operative complications and the rate of incomplete cytoreduction, even in phase 1, were comparable with the incidence in prior studies (24, 27, 28). The reason for these results could be the accurate and targeted selection of patients with a low tumour burden in the early phase, performed under the direct supervision of the mentor and in a multidisciplinary context. In this way, the surgeon could deal with the type of disease most suited to his surgical skills at every stage of his learning process. Therefore, the mentorship by another experienced general surgeon with previous experience with peritoneal surgery and HIPEC and a well-defined multidisciplinary team is crucial to expedite an otherwise long and steep learning curve, decrease its untoward outcomes in the early period, and ameliorate oncological outcomes.

As shown in this study and earlier studies, the long and insidious learning curve before achieving surgical proficiency is the main obstacle to the safe diffusion of CRS and HIPEC. Estimating that the average amount of CRS and HIPEC at reference high-volume centres varies from 24 to 123 cases per year, achieving technical competency can take several years (32).

This study has some limitations. First, our analyses did not investigate whether the initial training period has some impact on oncological outcomes. However, the incomplete cytoreduction rate, which represents a surrogate marker for oncologic outcomes, was not inferior to the historical data from previous reports (27–31). And secondly, it is unclear which technical aspect of CRS or HIPEC provided the most outstanding contribution to the long learning curve. Identifying the crucial steps in the learning process could shorten the achievement of surgical proficiency.

In conclusion, a long learning curve was necessary even for an experienced general surgeon to achieve technical proficiency. Moreover, the technical aspect of CRS is relatively unfamiliar to most general surgeons. Hence, a mentorship model in high-volume centres by surgeons with experience and knowledge of this disease should be paramount to reduce the learning curve. Therefore, considering a possible future direction, it is crucial to develop standardised training programs to shorten the learning process reduce morbidity and mortality, and improve oncologic outcomes.

ETHICS STATEMENT

Ethical review and approval was not required for the study on human participants in accordance with the local legislation and institutional requirements. Written informed consent for participation was not required for this study in accordance with the national legislation and the institutional requirements.

AUTHOR CONTRIBUTIONS

FS, FF, AD and CA contributed to study conception and design. CA, MAEH, and LB contributed to the acquisition of data. FS, CA, and FG contributed to writing the manuscript. FP, FG, and CL contributed to the drafting of the manuscript. FS, AD, and FP contributed to critical revision. All authors contributed to the article and approved the submitted version.

REFERENCES

1. Franko J, Shi Q, Goldman CD, Pockaj BA, Nelson GD, Goldberg RM, et al. Treatment of colorectal peritoneal carcinomatosis with systemic chemotherapy: A pooled analysis of North Central Cancer Treatment Group phase III trials N9741 and N9841. *J Clin Oncol.* (2012) 30:263–7. doi: 10.1200/JCO.2011.37.1039
2. Zani S, Papalezova K, Stinnett S, Tyler D, Hsu D, Blazer 3rd DG Modest advances in survival for patients with colorectal-associated peritoneal carcinomatosis in the era of modern chemotherapy. *J Surg Oncol.* (2013) 107:307–11. doi: 10.1002/jso.23222
3. Sun T, Li K, Xu G, Zhu K, Wang Q, Dang C, et al. Postoperative oxaliplatin-based hyperthermic intraperitoneal chemotherapy: an effective and safe palliative treatment option for colorectal cancer with peritoneal metastasis. *World J Surg Oncol.* (2021) 19(1):200. doi: 10.1186/s12957-021-02320-4
4. Wisselink DD, Braakhuis LLF, Gallo G, van Grevenstein WMU, van Dieren S, Kok NFM, et al. Systematic review of published literature on oxaliplatin and mitomycin C as chemotherapeutic agents for hyperthermic intraperitoneal chemotherapy in patients with peritoneal metastases from colorectal cancer. *Crit Rev Oncol Hematol.* (2019) 142:119–29. doi: 10. 1016/j.critrevonc.2019.06.014
5. Coccolini F, Gheza F, Lotti M, Virzì S, Iusco D, Ghermandi C, et al. Peritoneal carcinomatosis. *World J Gastroenterol.* (2013) 19:6979–94. doi: 10.3748/wjg.v19.i41.6979
6. Quenet F, Elias D, Roca L, Goéré D, Ghouti L, Pocard M, et al. A UNICANCER phase III trial of hyperthermic intra-peritoneal Chemotherapy (HIPEC) for colorectal peritoneal carcinomatosis. PRODIGE 7. *Eur J Surg Oncol.* (2019) 45:e17. doi: 10.1016/j.ejso.2018.10.086
7. van Driel WJ, Koole SN, Sikorska K, Schagen van Leeuwen JH, Schreuder HWR, Hermans RHM, et al. Hyperthermic intraperitoneal chemotherapy in ovarian cancer. *N Engl J Med.* (2018) 378:230–40. doi: 10.1056/nejmoa1708618
8. Sugarbaker PH. Peritonectomy procedures. *Peritoneal Carcinomatosis: A Multidisciplinary Approach.* (2007) 221:247–64. doi: 10.1007/978-0-387-48993-3_15
9. Foster JM, Sleightholm R, Patel A, Shostrom V, Hall B, Neilsen B, et al. Morbidity and mortality rates following cytoreductive surgery combined with hyperthermic intraperitoneal chemotherapy compared with other high-risk surgical oncology procedures. *JAMA Netw Open.* (2019) 2: e186847. doi: 10.1001/jamanetworkopen.2018.6847
10. Vining CC, Izquierdo F, Eng OS, Turaga KK. Cytoreductive surgery and hyperthermic intraperitoneal chemotherapy: Technical considerations and the learning curve. *J Surg Oncol.* (2020) 122:85–95. doi: 10.1002/jso.25939
11. Di Giorgio A, Santullo F, Attalla El Halabieh M, Lodoli C, Abatini C, Calegari MA, et al. Clinical and molecular features in patients undergoing cytoreductive surgery and hyperthermic intraperitoneal chemotherapy for peritoneal carcinosis from colorectal cancer. *J. Gastrointest Surg.* (2021) 25(10):2649–59. doi: 10.1007/s11605-021-05073-3
12. Santullo F, Pacelli F, Abatini C, Attalla El Halabieh M, Fortunato G, Lodoli C, et al. Cytoreduction and hyperthermic intraperitoneal chemotherapy for pseudomyxoma peritonei of appendiceal origin: A single center experience. *Front Surg.* (2021) 8:715119. doi: 10.3389/fsurg.2021.715119
13. Steiner SH. Monitoring surgical performance using risk-adjusted cumulative sum charts. *Biostatistics.* (2000) 1:441–52. doi: 10.1093/biostatistics/1.4.441
14. Rotolo S, Di Giorgio A, Santullo F, Attalla El Halabieh M, Lodoli C, Abatini C, et al. Cytoreductive surgery and mitomycin C hyperthermic intraperitoneal chemotherapy with CO2 recirculation (HIPEC-CO2) for colorectal cancer peritoneal metastases: analysis of short-term outcomes. *Updates Surg.* (2021) 73(4):1443–48. doi: 10.1007/s13304-021-01034-2
15. Clavien PA, Barkun J, De Oliveira ML, Vauthey JN, Dindo D, Schulick RD, et al. The clavien-dindo classification of surgical complications: Five-year experience. *Ann Surg.* (2009) 250:187–96. doi: 10.1097/SLA. 0b013e3181b13ca2
16. Kubi B, Nudotor R, Fackche N, Nizam W, Cloyd JM, Grotz TE, et al. Impact of perioperative blood transfusions on outcomes after hyperthermic intraperitoneal chemotherapy: A propensity-matched analysis. *Ann Surg Oncol.* (2021) 28:4499–507. doi: 10.1245/s10434-020-09501-7
17. Klein AA, Bailey CR, Charlton AJ, Evans E, Guckian-Fisher M, McCrossan R, et al. Association of anaesthetists guidelines: cell salvage for peri-operative blood conservation 2018. *Anaesthesia.* (2018) 73:1141–50. doi: 10.1111/ anae.14331
18. Klein AA, Arnold P, Bingham RM, Brohi K, Clark R, Collis R, et al. AAGBI guidelines: the use of blood components and their alternatives 2016. *Anaesthesia.* (2016) 71:829–42. doi: 10.1111/anae.13489
19. Elias D. Peritoneal colorectal carcinomatosis treated with surgery and perioperative intraperitoneal chemotherapy: Retrospective analysis of 523 patients from a multicentric french study. *J Clin Oncol.* (2010) 28:63–8. doi: 10.1200/JCO.2009.23.9285
20. Govaerts K, Lurvink RJ, de Hingh IHJT, van der Speeten K, Villeneuve L, Kusamura S, et al. Appendiceal tumours and pseudomyxoma peritonei: Literature review with PSOGI/EURACAN clinical practice guidelines for diagnosis and treatment. *Eur J Surg Oncol.* (2021) 47(1):11–35. doi: 10. 1016/j.ejso.2020.02.012
21. Kusamura S, Kepenekian V, Villeneuve L, Lurvink RJ, Govaerts K, de Hingh IHJT, et al. Peritoneal mesothelioma: PSOGI/EURACAN clinical practice guidelines for diagnosis, treatment and follow-up. *Eur J Surg Oncol.* (2021) 47:36–59. doi: 10.1016/j.ejso.2020.02.011
22. Kim S, Yoon YS, Han HS, Cho JY, Choi YR, Lee B. Evaluation of a single surgeon's learning curve of laparoscopic pancreaticoduodenectomy: risk-adjusted cumulative summation analysis. *Surg Endosc.* (2021) 35:2870–8. doi: 10.1007/s00464-020-07724-z
23. Smeenk RM, Verwaal VJ, Zoetmulder FAN. Learning curve of combined modality treatment in peritoneal surface disease. *Br J Surg.* (2007) 94:1408–14. doi: 10.1002/bjs.5863
24. Kusamura S, Baratti D, Deraco M. Multidimensional analysis of the learning curve for cytoreductive surgery and hyperthermic intraperitoneal chemotherapy in peritoneal surface malignancies. *Ann Surg.* (2012) 255:348–56. doi: 10.1097/SLA.0b013e3182436c28
25. Andréasson H, Lorant T, Påhlman L, Graf W, Mahteme H. Cytoreductive surgery plus perioperative intraperitoneal chemotherapy in pseudomyxoma peritonei: aspects of the learning curve. *Eur J Surg Oncol.* (2014) 40:930–6. doi: 10.1016/j.ejso.2014.03.001
26. Polanco PM, Ding Y, Knox JM, Ramalingam L, Jones H, Hogg ME, et al. Institutional learning curve of cytoreductive surgery and hyperthermic intraperitoneal chemoperfusion for peritoneal malignancies. *Ann Surg Oncol.* (2015) 22:1673–9. doi: 10.1245/s10434-014-4111-x
27. Piso P, Nedelcut SD, Rau B, Königsrainer A, Glockzin G, Ströhlein MA, et al. Morbidity and mortality following cytoreductive surgery and hyperthermic intraperitoneal chemotherapy: Data from the DGAV StuDoQ registry with 2149 consecutive patients. *Ann Surg Oncol.* (2019) 26:148–54. doi: 10.1245/ s10434-018-6992-6
28. Narasimhan V, Das A, Warrier S, Lynch C, McCormick J, Tie J, et al. Evaluation of cytoreductive surgery and HIPEC for peritoneal surface malignancies: analysis of 384 consecutive cases. *Langenbeck's Arch Surg.* (2019) 404:527–39. doi: 10.1007/s00423-019-01805-x
29. Kusamura S, Baratti D, Virzì S, Bonomi S, Iusco DR, Grassi A, et al. Learning curve for cytoreductive surgery and hyperthermic intraperitoneal chemotherapy in peritoneal surface malignancies: analysis of two centres. *J Surg Oncol.* (2013) 107:312–9. doi: 10.1002/jso.23231
30. Levine EA, Stewart IV JH, Shen P, Russell GB, Loggie BL, Votanopoulos KI. Intraperitoneal chemotherapy for peritoneal surface malignancy: Experience with 1,000 patients. *J Am Coll Surg.* (2014) 218:573–85. doi: 10.1016/j. jamcollsurg.2013.12.013
31. Passot G, Vaudoyer D, Villeneuve L, Kepenekian V, Beaujard AC, Bakrin N, et al. What made hyperthermic intraperitoneal chemotherapy an effective curative treatment for peritoneal surface malignancy: A 25-year experience with 1,125 procedures. *J Surg Oncol.* (2016) 113:796–803. doi: 10.1002/jso.24248
32. Rajeev R, Klooster B, Turaga KK. Impact of surgical volume of centers on post-operative outcomes from cytoreductive surgery and hyperthermic intra-peritoneal chemoperfusion. *J Gastrointest Oncol.* (2016) 7:122–8. doi: 10.3978/j.issn.2078-6891.2015.099

2

Neuraxial Anesthesia in the Geriatric Patient

Atanas G. Sivevski [1]****, Dafina Karadjova*** [1]***, Emilija Ivanov*** [1] ***and Andrijan Kartalov*** [2]

[1] Department of Anaesthesia, Clinical Center Mother Teresa, University Clinic for Gynecology and Obstetrics, Skopje, Macedonia, [2] Clinical Center Mother Teresa, University Clinic for TOARILUC, Skopje, Macedonia

***Correspondence:**
Atanas G. Sivevski
asivevski@yahoo.com

Neuraxial anesthesia is recommended as a well-accepted option to minimize the perioperative side effects in the geriatric patients. The available data from the current researches have shifted the focus from the conventional approach to spinal anesthesia to the concept of low dose local anesthetic combined with opioids. What remains clear from all these studies is that hemodynamic stability is much better in patients who received low-doses of intrathecal bupivacaine in combination with opioids, which is possibly result of a potent synergistic nociceptive analgesic effect and their minimal potential effects on sympathetic pathways thus minimizing spinal hypotension. Spinal anesthesia with 5–10 mg of 0.5% heavy bupivacaine, fentanyl 20 mcg and 100 mcg of long-acting morphine added to the perioperative plan decreased the incidence of spinal hypotension and improved perioperative outcomes in the geriatric patients undergoing (low segment) surgical procedures. These findings may be of interest in the gynecologic geriatric surgery also in which area there are very few studies concerning the use of low-dose concept.

Keywords: geriatric (aging), neuraxial anesthesia, low-dose, opoids, hypotension

INTRODUCTION

The European population is growing older. It is anticipated that in the next years more than 30% will be older than 65. Particularly fast growing sub-population is the one older than 85 (1). The anatomical and physiological changes of aging present challenge for the anesthetic and surgical management.

There is no ideal anesthetic for geriatric patients. More important than the choice of anesthetic technique is adequate pre-operative assessment and planning of appropriate monitoring. Together with tight control of the perioperative physiological parameters it will favor positive patient outcomes. The decrease of hospital stay in elderly patients undergoing surgery decreases the incidence of adverse events like reduction of both respiratory events and nosocomial infections, as well a less postoperative cognitive dysfunction (POCD) at 1 week in the postoperative period.

The physiological changes of aging have impact on neuraxial anesthesia techniques, both spinal and epidural. With advancing age, as a result of some anatomical irregularities (reduction in number of neurons, deterioration of myelin sheaths, sclerotic closure of the intervertebral foramens etc.) the level of analgesia increases after epidural administration of local anesthetics (LA) (2). With spinal anesthesia, the level of analgesia also increases after spinal administration of hyperbaric solutions (3).

CLINICAL RESEARCHES

There is no controlled trial that can demonstrate that either neuraxial or general anesthesia is clearly superior in terms of outcome in elderly patients. Cochrane systematic review of studies of hip surgeries in elderly, looked at 17 trials (2,567 patients) comparing general to neuraxial anesthesia. The review concluded that the long-term mortality was equal for both groups (4). However, neuraxial anesthesia remains a well-accepted option to: minimize the surgical stress (tachycardia and hypertension), reduce the pulmonary compromise (atelectasis, pneumonia, prolonged mechanical ventilation), thus showing superior postoperative pain control and reduction of perioperative opioids consumption, hence minimizing opioid side effects. Neuraxial anesthesia results in better peripheral vascular circulation and reduces total blood loss. Neuraxial anesthesia also reduces the incidence of POCD in the first postoperative week (4). In addition, neuraxial anesthesia favors early ambulation thus preventing deep venous thrombosis.

Results from the current research have shifted the focus from the conventional approach to spinal anesthesia (SA) to the concept of low dose LA combined with lipophilic opioids. The antinociceptive synergism between LA and intrathecal (IT) opioids is well known. This concept provides effective and superior analgesia and may prolong the duration and effectiveness of postoperative analgesia without associated motor blockade (5, 6). Most importantly, use of low dose of LA reduces the incidence of hemodynamic side effects in elderly (7). Carpenter at al. identified the high levels of sensory anesthesia and increasing age as two main risk factors for the development of spinal hypotension (8). In elderly, SA is associated with 25–69% incidence of hypotension (8). Decreased physiologic reserve and increased incidence of systemic disease, particularly cardiovascular disease, make the elderly population prone to long term complications even with brief episodes of uncorrected hypotension (9, 10).

Fentanyl is the most frequently used intrathecal lipophilic opioid and when administered in single dose of 10–30 mcg, it has a rapid onset (10–20 min) and short duration of action (4–6 h) with minimal cephalic spread. These properties minimize the risk of delayed respiratory depression and favor use of intrathecal fentanyl in ambulatory anesthesia where enhanced analgesia without prolonged hospital stay is important (11, 12).

Morphine is unsuitable for ambulatory surgery because of its slow onset time (30–60 min), dose-related duration of analgesia (13–33 h) and side-effect profile, particularly the delayed onset respiratory depression. Administration of up to 200 mcg of IT morphine with LA for peripheral vascular surgery in elderly patients (average age of 68) can be safely performed with minimal adverse respiratory risk (9). Two meta-analyses determined the incidence of respiratory depression in patients receiving low-dose (<0.2 and 0.2–0.3 mg) IT morphine to be 0–1.2% (13, 14). A retrospective audit of IT morphine in adult patients (409) where more than half the patients (57.2%) were aged 70 years or older and the doses of IT morphine used ranged from 0.1, 0.15, or 0.2 mg (22.9, 30.2, and 45.3%) only one patient, a 74 old-male with past history of cerebrovascular accident and epilepsy, developed respiratory depression (0.24%) (15).

Other researchers concluded that 100 mcg of morphine added to the spinal anesthetic (hip surgery) provided the most optimal balance between analgesia, pain relief and pruritus with acceptable risk of respiratory depression (16). There was no case of respiratory depression (Sat < 94%, RR < 8) or sedation score>2 in all of these studies. Therefore, we consider the risk of respiratory depression with 100 mcg of IT morphine added to low-dose mixture of LA plus fentanyl to be minimal and patients can leave the hospital the day after surgery. Also, the 100 mcg IT morphine could provide post-operative analgesia for the first 24 h, which is superior to the short-term fentanyl-analgesia in the immediate post-operative period.

Other studies with low dose bupivacaine and sufentanil showed similar results (17). Kumar et al reported hypotension in 44% in the conventional group (12.5 mg of 0.5% hyperbaric bupivacaine in a total 2.5 ml), and only 8% in the low-dose group, while Olofsson et al. treated 88% patients for hypotension in their conventional SA group (18, 19). The higher incidence of hypotension in these studies might be the different definition of hypotension. What remains clear from all these studies is that hemodynamic stability is much better in patients who received low-doses of intrathecal bupivacaine in combination with opioids, which is possibly result of a potent synergistic nociceptive analgesic effect and their minimal potential effects on sympathetic pathways thus minimizing spinal hypotension.

Besides lower incidence of hypotension, low-dose SA is characterized with less intense and shorter motor block, although the degree of motor block was not so important for this type of surgical procedure (17, 19). Nevertheless, the time in bed and ambulation was decreased, consequently reducing the incidence of potential postoperative complications. The post-operative pain was also at a satisfactory low level, while the percentage of side-effects minimal. Similar observations were found in other similar studies in the geriatric population (20, 21).

Elderly patients undergoing neuraxial anesthesia are at increased risk of hypothermia and shivering, which can lead to increased oxygen consumption, ventilation and cardiac output. There are studies showing that addition of fentanyl to low-dose bupivacaine decrease the incidence of shivering during spinal anesthesia in elderly patients (12, 18).

There are more options for adding adjuvants to LA in the SA. However, the opioids and α_2 adrenergic agonists are more commonly used as adjuvants in clinical practice. Dexmedetomidine, a selective α_2 adrenergic receptor agonist, has been shown to be a better adjuvant of LAs for neuraxial blocks although clonidine is the first clinically used intrathecal α_2-adrenoreceptor agonist.

Adding dexmedetomidine to LA in the SA is a relatively new area and there are almost no data on its use in an elderly population. In a systemic review and meta-analytic study dated from 2017, where researchers independently searched the PUBMED, EMBASE, Cochrane library and CBM for randomized controlled trials comparing the effects of dexmedetomidine and fentanyl as adjuvants to LAs for intrathecal injection (total of 639 patients from 9 studies), was reported that compared to fentanyl, dexmedetomidine as LA adjuvant in spinal anesthesia prolonged the duration of spinal anesthesia, improved postoperative analgesia, reduced the incidence of pruritus, and did not increase the incidence of hypotension and bradycardia (22).

There is no relevant evident data when comparing a dexmedetomidine with fentanyl-morphine combination as an adjuvant to LA in SA and especially applied in the elderly patients.

CONCLUSION

Current clinical evidence-based recommendations conclude that neuraxial opioid procedure must be one of the most important skills to master for the treatment of perioperative pain in the geriatric patients. This finding involves a broad type of surgical procedures that should benefit from the practice, ranging from minor (ambulatory) surgery to major procedures (23). Neuraxial anesthesia minimizes the risk of common postoperative side-effects seen with general anesthesia including POCD, fatigue, dizziness, pain, and gastrointestinal dysfunction while neuraxial opioids are safer and preferable to parenteral opioids.

A low-dose concept of SA, that consists of LA plus opioids, improved perioperative outcomes in the geriatric patients undergoing elective (low segment) surgery. A combination of intrathecal lipophilic and hydrophilic opioids, such as fentanyl and morphine added to a low dose LA, can improve and prolong perioperative analgesia in the first 24 h postoperatively. It is a simple and practical technique that decreases incidence of spinal hypotension, particularly undesirable in the elderly. The risk of respiratory depression is negligible when used in such a low dose settings. The SA with 5–10 mg 0.5% heavy bupivacaine mixed with fentanyl 20 mcg and morphine 100 mcg could be an acceptable choice in the growing segment of geriatric gynecological population also. There are very few studies concerning neuraxial low-dosage mixture in the geriatric gynecological surgery and more research must be done to confirm safety and efficacy of this concept.

AUTHOR CONTRIBUTIONS

AS, DK, EI, and AK declare that: (1) they made substantial contributions to the conception or design of the work; (2) they drafted the work and revised it; (3) they approve its publication; and (4) they agree to be held accountable for all aspects of the work in ensuring that questions related to the accuracy or integrity of any part of the work are appropriately investigated and resolved.

REFERENCES

1. Kalache A1, Keller I. The greying world: a challenge for the twenty-first century. *Sci Prog.* (2000) 83(Pt 1):33–54.
2. Simon MJ, Veering BT, Stienstra R, van Kleef JW, Burm AG. The effects of age on neural blockade and hemodynamic changes after epidural anesthesia with ropivacaine. *Anesth Analg.* (2002) 94:1325–30. doi: 10.1097/00000539-200205000-00052
3. Tsui BC, Wagner A, Finucane B. Regional anaesthesia in the elderly: a clinical guide. *Drugs Aging* (2004) 21:895–910. doi: 10.2165/00002512-200421140-00001
4. Rasmussen LS. Postoperative cognitive dysfunction: incidence and prevention. *Best Pract Res Clin Anaesthesiol.* (2006) 20:315–30. doi: 10.1016/j.bpa.2005.10.011
5. Guay J, Parker MJ, Gajendragadkar PR, Kopp S. Anaesthesia for hip fracture surgery in adults. *Cochrane Database Syst Rev.* (2016) 2:CD000521. doi: 10.1002/14651858.CD000521.pub3
6. Gwirtz KH, Young JV, Byers RS, Alley C, Levin K, Walker SG, et al. The safety and efficacy of intrathecal opioid analgesia for acute postoperative pain: seven years' experience with 5969 surgical patients at Indiana University Hospital. *Anesth Analg.* (1999) 88:599–604.
7. Gupta S, Sampley S, Kathuria S. Intrathecal sufentanil or fentanyl as adjuvants to low dose bupivacaine in endoscopic urological procedures. *J Anaesthesiol Clin Pharmacol.* (2013) 29:509–15. doi: 10.4103/0970-9185.119158
8. Carpenter RL, Caplan RA, Brown DL, Stephenson C, Wu R. Incidence and risk factors for side effects of spinal anesthesia. *Anesthesiology* (1992) 76:906–12. doi: 10.1097/00000542-199206000-00006
9. Critchley LAH. Hypotension, subarachnoid block and the elderly patient. *Anaesthesia* (1996) 5:1139–43. doi: 10.1111/j.1365-2044.1996.tb15051.x
10. Moore DC, Bridenbaugh LD. Spinal (subarachnoid) block. A review of 11 574 cases. *J Am Med Assoc.* (1995) 195:123–8.
11. DeSousa KA, Chandran R. Intrathecal morphine for postoperative analgesia: current trends. *World J Anesthesiol.* (2014) 3:191–202. doi: 10.5313/wja.v3.i3.191
12. Kararmaz A, Kaya S, Turhanoglu S, Ozyilmaz MA. Low-dose bupivacaine-fentanyl spinal anaesthesia for transurethral prostatectomy. *Anesthesia* (2003) 58:526–30. doi: 10.1046/j.1365-2044.2003.03153.x
13. Gehling M, Tryba M. Risks and side-effects of intrathecal morphine combined with spinal anaesthesia: a metaanalysis. *Anaesthesia* (2009) 64:643–51. doi: 10.1111/j.1365-2044.2008.05817.x
14. Meylan N, Elia N, Lysakowski C, Tramèr MR. Benefit and risk of intrathecal morphine without local anaesthetic in patients undergoing major surgery: meta-analysis of randomized trials. *Br J Anaesth.* (2009) 102: 156–67.
15. Lim PC, Macintype PE. An audit of intrathecal morphine analgesia for non-obstetrical patients in an adult tertiary hospital. *Anesth Intensive Care* (2006) 34:776–81.
16. Murphy PM, Stack D, Kinirons B, Laffey JG. Optimizing the dose of intrathecal morphine in older patients undergoing hip arthroplasty. *Anesth Analg.* (2003) 97:1709–15. doi: 10.1213/01.ANE.0000089965.75585.0D
17. Singh NP, Chhatrapati S. Efficacy of sufentanil with low dose bupivacaine on subarachnoid block for vaginal hysterectomy. *Anaesthesiology* (2007) 107:A884.
18. Kumar S, Bajwa SJ. Neuraxial opioids in geriatrics: a dose reduction study of local anesthetic with addition of sufentanil in lower limb surgery for elderly patients. *Saudi J Anaesth.* (2011) 5:142–9. doi: 10.4103/1658-354X.82781
19. Olofsson C, Nygards EB, Bjersten AB, Hessling A. Low dose bupivacaine with sufentanil prevents hypotention after spinal anaesthesia for hip repair in elderly patients. *Acta Anaesthesiol Scand.* (2004) 48:1240–4. doi: 10.1111/j.1399-6576.2004.00504.x
20. Asehnoune K, Larousse E, Tadie JM, Miniville V, Droupy S, Benhamou D. Small dose bupivacaine-sufentanil prevents cardiac output modifications after spinal anesthesia. *Anesth Analg.* (2005) 101:1512–5. doi: 10.1213/01.ANE.0000180996.91358.CC

21. Grewal P, Katyal S, Kaul TK, Narual N, Grewal A. A comparative study of effects of fentanyl with different doses of bupivacine in subarachnoid block. *J Anaesth Clin Pharmacol.* (2003) 19:193–7.
22. Sun SJ, Wang JM, Bao NR, Chen Y, Wang J. Comparison of dexmedetomidine and fentanyl as local anesthetic adjuvants in spinal anesthesia: a systematic review and meta-analysis of randomized controlled trials. *Drug Des Devel Ther.* (2017) 11:3413–24. doi: 10.2147/DDDT.S146092
23. Bujedo BM. Current evidence for spinal opioid selection in postoperative pain. *Korean J Pain* (2014) 27:200–9. doi: 10.3344/kjp.2014.27.3.200

3

Partial Nephrectomy Versus Radical Nephrectomy for Endophytic Renal Tumors: Comparison of Operative, Functional and Oncological Outcomes by Propensity Score Matching Analysis

Situ Xiong[1,2†], Ming Jiang[1,2†], Yi Jiang[2,3†], Bing Hu[1,2], Ru Chen[1,2], Zhijun Yao[1,2], Wen Deng[1,2†], Xianwen Wan[4], Xiaoqiang Liu[1*], Luyao Chen[1*] and Bin Fu[1,2*]*

[1] *Department of Urology, The First Affiliated Hospital of Nanchang University, Nanchang, China,* [2] *Jiangxi Institute of Urology, Nanchang, China,* [3] *Department of Urology, The Second Affiliated Hospital of Nanchang University, Nanchang, China,* [4] *Department of Anesthesiology, The First Affiliated Hospital of Nanchang University, Nanchang, China*

***Correspondence:**
Bin Fu
urofbin@163.com
Xiaoqiang Liu
shaw177@163.com
Luyao Chen
chenluyao301@163.com
Xianwen Wan
1017427059@qq.com

[†]These authors have contributed equally to this work

Purpose: The study aimed to compare operative, functional, and oncological outcomes between partial nephrectomy (PN) and radical nephrectomy (RN) for entophytic renal tumors (ERTs) by propensity score matching (PSM) analysis.

Methods: A total of 228 patients with ERTs who underwent PN or RN between August 2014 and December 2021 were assessed. A PSM in a 1:1 ratio was conducted to balance the differences between groups. Perioperative characteristics, renal functional, and oncological outcomes were compared between groups. Univariate and multivariate logistic and Cox proportional hazard regression analyses were used to determine the predictors of functional and survival outcomes.

Results: After PSM, 136 cases were matched to the PN group (n = 68) and the RN group (n = 68). Patients who underwent RN had shorter OT, less EBL, and lower high-grade complications (all p <0.05) relative to those who underwent PN. However, better perseveration of renal function was observed in the PN group, which was reflected in 48-h postoperative AKI (44.1% vs. 70.6%, p = 0.002), 1-year postoperative 90% eGFR preservation (45.6% vs. 22.1%, p = 0.004), and new-onset CKD Stage ≥III at last follow-up (2.9% vs. 29.4%, p <0.001). RN was the independent factor of short-term (OR, 2.812; 95% CI, 1.369–5.778; p = 0.005) and long-term renal function decline (OR, 10.242; 95% CI, 2.175–48.240; p = 0.003). Furthermore, PN resulted in a better OS and similar PFS and CSS as compared to RN (p = 0.042, 0.15, and 0.21, respectively). RN (OR, 7.361; 95% CI, 1.143–47.423; p = 0.036) and pT3 stage (OR, 4.241; 95% CI, 1.079–16.664; p = 0.039) were independent predictors of overall mortality.

Conclusion: Among patients with ERTs, although the PN group showed a higher incidence of high-grade complications than RN, when technically feasible and with experienced surgeons, PN is recommended for better preservation of renal function, longer OS, and similar oncological outcomes.

Keywords: endophytic renal tumor, partial nephrectomy, radical nephrectomy, propensity score matching, oncological outcomes, function outcomes, operative outcomes

INTRODUCTION

Endophytic renal tumors (ERTs) are tumors surrounded by normal renal parenchyma and attributed to three points of the E-element in the R.E.N.A.L. Nephrometry Score (RENAL-NS) system (1–3). Most ERTs are small spherical masses in deep locations and do not protrude from the renal surface of the tumor. Partial nephrectomy (PN) is the accepted standard treatment for normal small renal masses (4), with superior long-term benefit (5, 6).

Due to its highly complex anatomy, it is difficult to remove tumors and suture incised renal parenchyma, which requires considerable expertise and higher technical skills. Furthermore, these cases are related to higher intraoperative and perioperative complication rates, including positive resection margin caused by an unclear boundary, massive bleeding due to an accidental vascular injury, urine leakage caused by an accidental pelvicalyceal system injury, and renal vascular occlusion caused by inappropriate suture (7–9). Given the above risks and challenges, in the past, most urologists preferred RN for ERMs to avoid serious complications (10, 11). Owing to technological and conceptual advances, some authors have reported the successful application of PN for ERTs (9, 10, 12–14). These results demonstrate PN as a feasible technique for such anatomically complicated renal tumors. However, given technical difficulties due to this procedure, limited evidence of oncological and functional outcomes is available. Thus, it is unknown whether PN is more appropriate for ERTs than RN.

Thus far, no report of comparison between PN and RN for the treatment of ERTs has been published. We aimed to compare the operative, functional, and oncological outcomes for ERTs by PN or RN treatment by propensity score-matching (PSM) analysis; these findings may guide the treatment of ERTs.

MATERIALS AND METHODS

Patient Cohort

Patients with ERTs who underwent PN or RN between 1 August 2014 and 31 December 2021 at the First Affiliated Hospital of Nanchang University were assessed retrospectively. Of the 2,438 patients with a primary diagnosis of renal tumor or carcinoma, 228 patients with ERTs were identified and included in this study based on the following inclusion criteria: (1) imaging assessment of the location of the tumor was preserved in our radiographic database; (2) ERTs that were surrounded by normal renal parenchyma and attributed to three points for the E-element in the RENAL-NS system (3); (3) those who accepted surgical treatment by PN or RN, and (4) those without multiple lesions included endophytic masses (n >2), including multiple renal angiomyolipomas with endophytic lesion. The flowchart for the enrollment of patients with ERTs is shown in **Figure 1**. Patients who simultaneously met the above inclusion criteria (n = 228) were divided into the PN (n = 131) and RN (n = 97) groups according to the surgical method.

All operations were conducted by highly experienced urologists using laparoscopic or robot-assisted laparoscopic techniques; no open surgery was performed. After adequate exposure to the kidney and renal artery, intraoperative ultrasound was performed to locate the renal tumor during PN. The proximal renal artery away from the tumor was then clamped with bull's-head forceps to separate the tumor from the normal renal tissue with a pair of cold scissors, and two layers of suturing were performed to close the renal injury. Afterward, the bulldog forceps were removed for hemostatic evaluation, and the warm ischemia time was recorded. Apart from intraoperative ultrasound to locate tumors during PN, other detailed surgical procedures of PN and RN through laparoscopic or robot-assisted laparoscopic techniques for ERTs were the same as those for exophytic tumors described previously (14–16).

Research Materials

The demographic characteristics, including age, gender, body mass index (BMI), diabetes mellitus (DM), hypertension (HTN), chronic kidney disease (CKD) Stage ≥III, abdominal surgery history, age-adjusted Charlson's comorbidity index (ACCI), Eastern Cooperative Oncology Group Performance Status (ECOG PS), American Society of Anesthesiologists (ASA), preoperative serum creatinine (Scr), estimated glomerular filtration rates (eGFR), preoperative hemoglobin, and surgical technique were extracted from the prospectively managed clinical database. The Cockcroft-Gault (C–G) formula was used to calculate eGFR, and all values were standardized by body surface area of patients.

The oncology characteristics, including tumor size, location, laterality, clinical T stage (cTn), and RENAL-NS, were assessed by reviewing the computed tomography (CT) or magnetic resonance imaging (MRI) from our radiographic database. All the imaging information was blindly assessed and collected by urologists SX and Mj, and disputed cases were evaluated by a more senior urologist, LC.

Collected perioperative outcomes included operating time (OT), warm ischemia time (WIT), estimated blood loss (EBL), perioperative transfusion rate, surgery conversion rate, restoration time of bowel functions, drainage tube removal time, postoperative

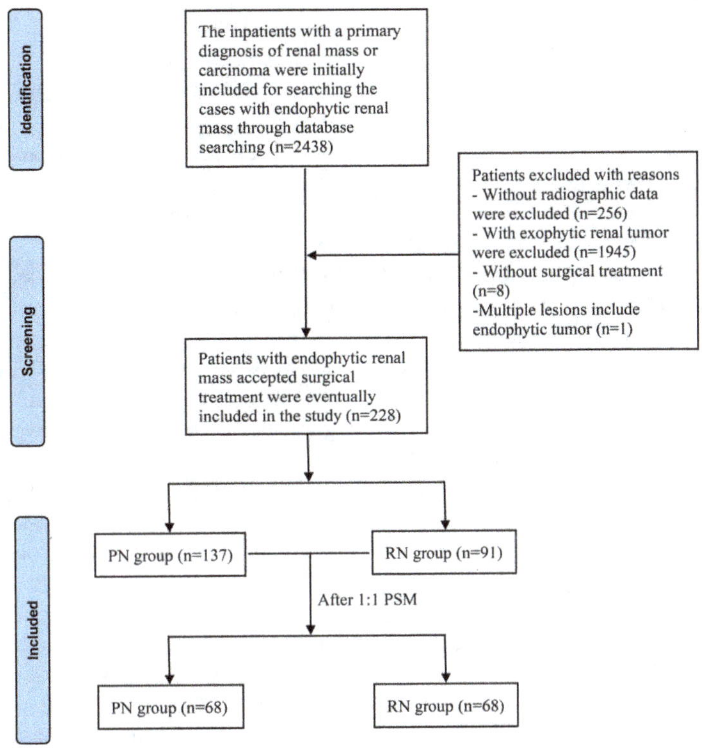

FIGURE 1 | Flow chart for inclusion of patients. PN, partial nephrectomy; RN, radical nephrectomy.

hospitalization time, postoperative complications, 48-h postoperative Scr, 48-h postoperative eGFR, 48-h postoperative eGFR descent, and 48-h postoperative acute kidney injury (AKI). Postoperative complications were determined by the Clavien–Dindo classification (17). AKI was defined as either a >50% increase in the postoperative serum creatinine relative to preoperative Scr or an absolute increase of >0.3 mg/dl according to the Acute Kidney Injury Network (AKIN) criteria (18).

All tumor specimens were reviewed for diagnosis by a single urological pathologist. The pathologic characteristics consisted of histological subtype, TNM stage, Fuhrman nuclear grade (I/II grade were classified into low grade and III/IV into high), parasitic (or tentacular) invasion, and distant extension according to the eighth edition of the American Joint Committee on Cancer (AJCC) cancer staging manual.

According to the standardized institutional postoperative protocol, the regular follow-up was conducted every 3 months after surgery for 6 months, every 6 months for the next 3 years, and annually after that. The essential oncology follow-up consisted of CT or MRI scans for the chest and entire abdomen. The changes in eGFR calculated using Scr followed up at postoperative 3-, 6-, and 12 months and 3- and 5 years reflected the renal function outcomes. Survival outcomes included cancer-specific survival (CSS), progression-free survival (PFS), and overall survival (OS), defined as the interval from the date of surgery to death related to the renal tumor; the first tumor recurrence, or metastasis, and death due to any cause, respectively.

Statistical Analysis

To eliminate differences between groups in preoperative demographic and tumor characteristics, PSM analysis was performed using variables of age, gender, BMI, DM, HTN, CKD, abdominal surgery history, ACCI, ECOG PG, ASA, preoperative Scr, preoperative eGFR, preoperative hemoglobin, tumor laterality, tumor size, clinical T stage, RENAL-NS, and surgical technique. The propensity score was evaluated by non-parsimonious multivariate logistic regression. Finally, 68 patients in the PN group were successfully matched with a nearest neighbor matching algorithm to the same number of patients in the RN group at a 1:1 ratio. The preoperative covariate differences between the two groups before and after PSM were compared.

All categorical variables compared using the Pearson χ^2 test were presented in the form of numbers and percentages. As for continuous variables, the normally distributed variables using the Student's t-test are presented as mean and standard deviation, and the non-normally distributed variables using the Wilcoxon rank sum test are presented as median and interquartile range. A Kaplan–Meier survival analysis was used to compare OS, PFS, and CSS outcomes between groups. Univariate and multivariate logistics and Cox proportional hazard regression were used to determine the predictors of functional and survival outcomes. The univariate results were used to determine the candidate variables for the final multivariate model. All statistical analyses were performed using SPSS 24.0 software (SPSS, Chicago, IL,

USA) and R software (version 4.1.0). The p <0.5 level was considered statistically significant.

RESULTS

During the study period, 228 patients with ERTs were included in the final analysis based on the inclusion and exclusion criteria. A total of 131 and 97 patients underwent PN and RN, respectively. According to the demographic and clinical characteristics shown in **Table 1**, statistically, significant differences are found for some variables before PSM. The patients in the RN group showed higher mean age (51.4 vs. 47.5 years, $p = 0.037$), lower mean BMI (22.9 vs. 23.7, $p = 0.039$), bigger tumor size (4.0 vs. 2.8 cm, $p < 0.001$), higher overall RENAL-NS (10.1 vs. 8.8, $p < 0.001$), higher R score (1.5 vs. 1.2, $p < 0.001$), higher N score (3.0 vs. 2.5, $p < 0.001$), and higher L score (2.6 vs. 2.2, $p < 0.001$) relative to the PN group. Furthermore, the RN group had a higher ratio of ECOG PS score of ≥2 (13.4% vs. 5.3, $p = 0.033$), clinical T stage ≥cT1b (49.5% vs. 15.3%, $p < 0.001$), hilar location (43.3% vs. 15.3%, $p < 0.001$), and a lower ratio of robot-assisted laparoscopic technique (18.6% vs. 37.4%, $p = 0.002$) compared to the PN group. No statistical difference was found in other variables between groups was observed. After performing 1:1 PSM, all statistically significant covariates achieved a good balance among the matched groups (with 68 patients in both PN and RN groups). The median follow-up duration in the PN and RN groups before the PSM was 41.2 and 45.3 months, respectively; after the PSM, the corresponding values were 44.8 and 45.2 months, respectively.

Operative, pathological, and renal functional outcomes for PN and RN groups after PSM are shown in **Table 2**. Patients in the PN group showed longer OT (194.4 vs. 171.3 mins, $p = 0.014$) and more EBL (198.5 vs. 140.7 ml, $p = 0.038$) than those in the RN group, whereas no statistical difference in required blood transfusion (2.9% vs. 5.9%, $p = 0.680$) was observed. Postoperative recovery indices, which included restoration time of bowel functions, drainage tube removal time, and postoperative hospitalization time, were similar between the groups. Two cases of surgical conversion (to RN) for intraoperative massive and repeated bleeding in the PN group, and no conversion in the RN group, or to open method were recorded. The mean warm ischemia time in the PN group was 27.6 min. No positive resection margins were observed in either group. Patients in the PN group had a similar ratio of overall and low-grade (Clavien–Dindo grades I–II) complications ($p = 0.060$ and $p = 0.341$, respectively) but showed a higher ratio of high-grade (Clavien–Dindo grades III–IV) complications (10.3% vs. 1.5%, $p = 0.029$) relative to the RN group. High-grade complications included ICU management (n = 1), urine leak

TABLE 1 | Preoperative basic characteristics of patients before and after propensity score matching.

Variables	Before propensity score matching			After propensity score matching		
	PN (n = 131)	RN (n = 97)	*p*-value	PN (n = 68)	RN (n = 68)	*p*-value
Age, years, mean (SD)	47.5 (12.7)	51.4 (15.3)	**0.037**	46.8 (13.7)	49.7 (14.8)	0.230
Gender (male), n (%)	75 (57.3%)	56 (57.7%)	0.942	35 (51.5%)	38 (55.9%)	0.606
BMI, mean (SD)	23.7 (2.8)	22.9 (2.9)	**0.039**	23.4 (2.8)	23.1 (2.9)	0.479
Diabetes mellitus, n (%)	12 (9.2%)	7 (7.2%)	0.529	7 (10.3%)	4 (5.9%)	0.345
Hypertension, n (%)	21 (16.0%)	17 (17.5%)	0.887	10 (14.7%)	9 (13.2%)	0.805
CKD Stage ≥III, n (%)	13 (9.9%)	12 (12.4%)	0.559	6 (8.8%)	7 (10.3%)	0.771
Abdominal surgery history, n (%)	23 (17.6%)	14 (14.4%)	0.527	10 (14.7%)	10 (14.7%)	NA
ACCI score, mean (SD)	4.1 (1.7)	4.3 (1.9)	0.265	4.0 (1.8)	4.2 (1.8)	0.534
ECOG PS score ≥2, n (%)	7 (5.3%)	13 (13.4%)	**0.033**	4 (5.8%)	6 (8.8%)	0.511
ASA score ≥2, n (%)	73 (55.7%)	53 (53.6%)	0.870	41 (60.3%)	37 (54.4%)	0.488
Scr, mg/dl, mean (SD)	0.88 (0.33)	0.86 (0.47)	0.726	0.83 (0.25)	0.82 (0.31)	0.791
eGFR, ml/min/1.73 m^2, mean **(SD)**	91.5 (26.4)	89.0 (26.7)	0.480	94.8 (26.9)	92.7 (26.8)	0.644
Hemoglobin, g/dl, mean (SD)	132.8 (15.6)	129.8 (16.4)	0.221	130.7 (16.6)	130.0 (14.8)	0.802
Laterality (left), n (%)	72 (55.0%)	48 (49.5%)	0.413	37 (54.4%)	36 (52.9%)	0.863
Tumor size, cm, mean (SD)	2.8 (1.0)	4.0 (1.5)	**<0.001**	3.3 (1.0)	3.6 (1.3)	0.077
Clinical T stage ≥cT1b, n (%)	20 (15.3%)	48 (49.5%)	**<0.001**	20 (29.2%)	28 (41.2%)	0.151
RENAL-NS, mean (SD)	8.8 (1.5)	10.1 (1.2)	**<0.001**	9.4 (1.3)	9.8 (1.2)	0.065
R score, mean (SD)	1.2 (0.4)	1.5 (0.6)	**<0.001**	1.3 (0.5)	1.4 (0.5)	0.149
N score, mean (SD)	2.5 (0.8)	3.0 (0.3)	**<0.001**	2.8 (0.6)	2.9 (0.4)	0.067
L score, mean (SD)	2.2 (0.9)	2.6 (0.7)	**<0.001**	2.4 (0.9)	2.5 (0.8)	0.309
Hilar location, n (%)	20 (15.3%)	42 (43.3%)	**<0.001**	17 (25.0%)	24 (35.3%)	0.191
Surgical Technique			**0.002**			0.252
Open	0	0		0	0	
Laparoscopic, n (%)	82 (62.6%)	79 (81.4%)		46 (67.6%)	52 (76.5%)	
Robot, n (%)	49 (37.4%)	18 (18.6%)		22 (32.4%)	16 (23.5%)	

RN, radical nephrectomy; PN, partial nephrectomy; SD, standard deviation; BMI, body mass index; CKD, chronic kidney disease, CKD Stage ≥III defined as eGFR<60 ml/min; Sc, serum creatinine; eGFR, estimated glomerular filtration rate; ACCI, age-adjusted Charlson's comorbidity index; ECOG PS, Eastern Cooperative Oncology Group Performance Status; ASA, American Society of Anesthesiologists; RENAL-NS, R.E.N.A.L. Nephrometry Score.
The bold numbers mean statistically difference.

TABLE 2 | Perioperative and oncological outcomes for PN and RN after propensity score matching.

Variables	PN (n = 68)	RN (n = 68)	*p*-value
OT, min, mean (SD)	194.4 (48.8)	171.3 (58.6)	**0.014**
WIT, min, median (IQR)	27.5 (26.3-29.0)	–	–
EBL, mL, median (IQR)	200 (100-200)	100 (100-150)	**<0.001**
Transfusion, n (%)	2 (2.9%)	4 (5.9%)	0.680
Surgery conversion, n (%)			
To RN	2 (2.9%)	–	–
Positive resection margin, n (%)	0	0	–
Restoration time of bowel functions, days, median (IQR)	2 (2-3)	2 (2-3)	0.305
Drainage tube removal time, days, median (IQR)	3 (3-5.75)	3 (3-4)	0.804
Postoperative hospitalization time, days, median (IQR)	7 (5-9)	6 (5-8)	0.061
Postoperative complications, n (%)	19 (27.9%)	10 (14.7%)	0.060
Clavien–Dindo grades I–II, n (%)	12 (17.6%)	9 (13.2%)	0.341
Clavien–Dindo grades III–IV, n (%)	7 (10.3%)	1 (1.5%)	**0.029**
ICU management	1 (1.5%)	0	–
Urine leak	3 (4.4%)	0	–
Hemorrhage treated by embolization	1 (1.5%)	0	–
Acute renal failure	1 (1.5%)	1 (1.5%)	–
Second operation	1 (1.5%)	0	–
Histologic subtype			0.062
Benign, n (%)	15 (22.1%)	7 (10.3%)	
Malignant, n (%)	53 (77.9%)	61 (89.7%)	
ccRCC, n (%)	46 (86.8%)	47 (77.1%)	–
pRCC, n (%)	2 (3.8%)	6 (9.8%)	–
chRCC, n (%)	1 (1.9%)	3 (4.9%)	–
Others, n (%)	4 (7.5%)	5 (8.2%)	–
Pathologic stage			0.115
pT1, n (%)	50 (94.3%)	52 (85.2%)	
pT3, n (%)	3 (5.7%)	9 (14.8%)	
Fuhrman grade			0.247
Low grade (I/II), n (%)	44 (91.7%)	42 (84.0%)	
High grade (III/IV), n (%)	4 (5.8%)	8 (16.0%)	
Lymph node metastasis, n (%)	0	2 (2.9%)	–

RN, radical nephrectomy; PN, partial nephrectomy; OT, operating time; WIT, warm ischemia time; EBL, estimated blood loss; SD, standard deviation; ICU, intensive care unit; ccRCC, clear cell renal cell carcinoma; pRCC, papillary renal cell carcinoma; chRCC, chromophobe renal cell carcinoma; eGFR, estimated glomerular filtration rate.
The bold numbers mean statistically difference.

(n = 3), hemorrhage treated by embolization (n = 1), acute renal failure (n = 1), and the second operation for suspected residual tumor (n = 1) in the PN group, and acute renal failure (n = 1) in the RN group.

Among pathologic characteristics, no statistically significant differences in histological subtype, pathological stage, or Fuhrman grade were observed between the two groups (all p >0.05).

Among postoperative renal functional outcomes (**Table 3**), the PN group showed a significant association with higher 48-h postoperative eGFR (70.5 vs. 57.4 ml/min/1.73m^2, p <0.001) than the RN group. Compared with preoperative eGFR, 48-h postoperative eGFR decreased in the PN and RN groups by 24.3 and 35.3 ml/min/1.73m^2, respectively (p = 0.002). Univariate and multivariate logistic analyses showed that RN

TABLE 3 | Preoperative functional outcomes for PN and RN after propensity score matching.

Variables	PN (n = 68)	RN (n = 68)	*p*-value
Preoperative Scr, mg/dl, mean (SD)	0.83 (0.25)	0.82 (0.31)	0.791
Preoperative eGFR, ml/min/1.73 m^2, mean (SD)	94.8 (26.9)	92.7 (26.8)	0.644
48-h postoperative Scr, mg/dl, mean (SD)	1.13 (0.42)	1.24 (0.47)	0.157
48-h postoperative eGFR, ml/min/1.73 m^2, mean (SD)	70.5 (22.8)	57.4 (17.5)	**<0.001**
48-h postoperative eGFR descend, ml/min/1.73 m^2, mean (SD)	23.9 (16.6)	35.3 (23.8)	**0.001**
48-h postoperative AKI, n (%)	30 (44.1%)	48 (70.6%)	**0.002**
1-year postoperative Scr, mg/dl, mean (SD)	0.98 (0.40)	1.19 (0.59)	**0.021**
1-year postoperative eGFR, ml/min/1.73 m^2, mean (SD)	84.4 (30.1)	66.7 (21.6)	**<0.001**
1-year postoperative 90% eGFR preservation, n (%)	31 (45.6%)	15 (22.1%)	**0.004**
Last follow-up Scr, mg/dl, mean (SD)	0.99 (0.43)	1.22 (0.74)	**0.028**
Last follow-up eGFR, ml/min/1.73 m^2, mean (SD)	82.1 (24.9)	66.1 (19.4)	**<0.001**
New-onset CKD Stage ≥III at last follow-up, n (%)	2 (2.9%)	20 (29.4%)	**<0.001**

RN, radical nephrectomy; PN, partial nephrectomy; SD, standard deviation; Scr, serum creatinine; eGFR, estimated glomerular filtration rate; AKI, acute kidney injury; CKD, chronic kidney disease.
The bold numbers mean statistically difference.

(OR, 2.812; 95% CI, 1.369–5.778; $p = 0.005$) was an independent risk factor for 48-h postoperative AKI (**Table 4**). Throughout the follow-up period, the renal function in the PN group was significantly better than that in the RN group (all $p < 0.001$) (**Figure 2**). One-year postoperative 90% eGFR preservation occurred in 45.6% of patients in the PN group and 22.1% in the RN group ($p = 0.004$). Furthermore, the patients in the PN group had a lower rate of new-onset CKD Stage ≥III at the last follow-up relative to the RN group (2.9% vs. 29.4%, $p < 0.001$). The results of univariate and multivariate logistic analyses suggested that hilar location (OR, 3.726; 95% CI, 1.283–10.823; $p = 0.016$) and RN (OR, 10.242; 95% CI, 2.175–48.240; $p = 0.003$) were independent risk factors for new-onset CKD Stage ≥III at the last follow-up (**Table 5**).

TABLE 4 | Univariate and multivariate Logistic analysis of independent risk factors for 48-h postoperative AKI.

Variables	Univariate Analysis		Multivariate Analysis	
	Crude OR (95% CI)	*p*-value	Adjusted OR (95% CI)	*p*-value
Age	1.01 (0.99–1.04)	0.260		
Gender				
Female (Re.) vs. male	0.90 (0.46–1.78)	0.763		
BMI	1.11 (0.98–1.26)	0.109		
Diabetes mellitus	0.59 (0.17–2.05)	0.409		
Hypertension	1.03 (0.38–2.74)	0.959		
Abdominal surgery history	0.71 (0.27–1.83)	0.473		
ACCI score	0.98 (0.81–1.19)	0.844		
ECOG PS score ≥2	0.73 (0.20–2.64)	0.626		
ASA score ≥2	0.81(0.41–1.61)	0.543		
Preoperative eGFR	1.01 (1.00–1.02)	0.201		
Preoperative hemoglobin	0.99 (0.96–1.01)	0.185		
Laterality				
Left (Re.) vs. Right	1.81 (0.91–3.62)	0.092		
Tumor size	0.98 (0.73–1.30)	0.865		
RENAL-NS	1.03 (0.80–1.34)	0.807		
R score	1.24 (0.60–2.57)	0.554		
N score	1.13 (0.58–2.17)	0.725		
L score	0.95 (0.63–1.42)	0.793		
Hilar location	0.81 (0.39–1.69)	0.567		
Technique				
Laparoscopic (Re.) vs. Robot	0.97 (0.45–2.07)	0.937		
Operating method				
PN (Re.) vs. RN	3.04 (1.50–6.17)	**0.002**	2.81 (1.37–5.78)	**0.005**
Operating time	1.00 (0.99–1.00)	0.154		
Estimated blood loss	1.00 (0.99–1.00)	0.199		
Transfusion	1.51 (0.27–8.56)	0.639		
Postoperative hospitalization time	0.85 (0.74–0.98)	**0.024**	0.87 (0.76–1.00)	0.055
Postoperative complications	1.96 (0.79–4.86)	0.144		
Histologic subtype				
Benign (Re.) vs. Malignant	1.77 (0.71–4.45)	0.221		
Pathologic stage				
pT1 (Re.) vs. pT3	0.88 (0.26–3.05)	0.844		
Fuhrman grade				
I/II (Re.) vs. III–IV	0.90 (0.26–3.06)	0.864		

BMI, body mass index; ACCI, age-adjusted Charlson's comorbidity index; ECOG PS, Eastern Cooperative Oncology Group Performance Status; ASA, American Society of Anesthesiologists; eGFR, estimated glomerular filtration rate; Re, reference; RENAL-NS, RENAL-Nephrometry Score; RN, radical nephrectomy; PN, partial nephrectomy.
The bold numbers mean statistically difference.

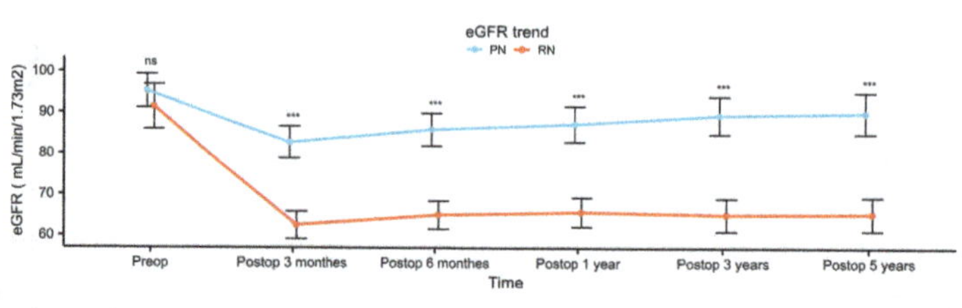

FIGURE 2 | Postoperative eGFR trend of patients in PN group and RN group after propensity score matching. eGFR, estimated glomerular filtration rate; PN, partial nephrectomy; RN, radical nephrectomy. "***" means p<0.001; "ns" means not statistically significant.

TABLE 5 | Univariate and multivariate Logistic analysis of independent risk factors for new onset CKD stage ≥ II at last follow-up.

Variables	Univariate Analysis		Multivariate Analysis	
	Crude OR (95% CI)	*p*-value	Adjusted OR (95% CI)	*p*-value
Age	1.04 (1.00–1.08)	**0.030**	1.04 (1.00–1.08)	0.060
Gender				
Female (Re.) vs. male	0.68 (0.27–1.69)	0.675		
BMI	0.88 (0.79–1.03)	0.110		
Diabetes mellitus	0.50 (0.06–4.08)	0.495		
Hypertension	1.47 (0.44–4.93)	0.536		
Abdominal surgery history	1.36 (0.41–4.54)	0.616		
ACCI score	1.14 (0.89–1.45)	0.305		
ECOG PS score ≥2	1.23 (0.67–2.27)	0.511		
ASA score ≥2	1.09 (0.43–2.75)	0.857		
Preoperative eGFR	0.99 (0.97–1.01)	0.361		
Preoperative hemoglobin	0.99 (0.97–1.02)	0.697		
Laterality				
Left (Re.) vs. Right	2.32 (0.90–5.97)	0.081		
Tumor size	0.99 (0.67–1.46)	0.961		
RENAL-NS	0.95 (0.67–1.34)	0.775		
R score	1.14 (0.44–2.96)	0.783		
N score	0.89 (0.39–2.06)	0.785		
L score	0.90 (0.53–1.53)	0.701		
Hilar location	3.52 (1.38–9.00)	**0.009**	3.73 (1.28–10.82)	**0.016**
Technique				
Laparoscopic (Re.) vs Robot	1.04 (0.37–2.90)	0.939		
Operating method				
PN (Re.) vs RN	13.8 (3.07–61.65)	**0.001**	10.24 (2.18–48.24)	**0.003**
Postoperative complications	1.35 (0.36–4.99)	0.655		
48-h postoperative AKI	2.95 (1.02–8.55)	**0.046**	1.79 (0.54–5.87)	0.339
Histologic subtype				
Benign (Re.) vs Malignant	1.27 (0.34–4.77)	0.724		
Pathologic stage				
pT1 (Re.) vs pT3	2.09 (0.51–8.60)	0.306		
Fuhrman grade				
I/II (Re.) vs III–IV	1.74 (0.42–7.24)	0.447		

BMI, body mass index; ACCI, age-adjusted Charlson's comorbidity index; ECOG PS, Eastern Cooperative Oncology Group Performance Status; ASA, American Society of Anesthesiologists; eGFR, estimated glomerular filtration rate; RENAL-NS, RENAL-Nephrometry Score; RN: radical nephrectomy; PN, partial nephrectomy.
The bold numbers mean statistically difference.

During the follow-up in the matched cohort, 8 and 16 patients developed local recurrence/distant metastasis in the PN and RN groups, respectively. The overall mortality was 4 patients in the PN group and 15 in the RN group. Cancer-related mortality occurred in 2 patients in the PN group and 8 in the RN group. Kaplan-Meier analyses suggested statistically significant differences in CSS, PFS, and OS in favor of PN (p = 0.006, 0.036, and 0.034, respectively) (**Figure 3**). Within the matched cohort, the patients in the PN group showed a longer OS compared with those in the RN group (p = 0.042). However, no statistically significant differences were observed in CSS and FPS between the two groups (p = 0.15 and 0.21, respectively). Univariate and multivariate Cox regression analyses showed that RN (OR, 7.36; 95% CI, 1.14–47.42; p = 0.036) and pathological T3 (pT3) stages were the predictors of overall mortality (OR, 4.241; 95% CI, 1.079–16.664; p = 0.039) (**Table 6**).

DISCUSSION

When technically feasible, the management of renal tumors has shifted from RN to PN to reduce the risk of CKD and cardiovascular diseases (6, 7). With the spread of this concept and improvements in surgical technology, the application of PN for renal tumors has been extended to more challenging cases, including ERTs (1). Although several authors have reported their successful experiences and beneficial results (19–21), the evidence in support of PN as a standard is weak. Due to the highly complex branching anatomical structure, it is challenging to remove deep endophytic tumors and suture incised renal parenchyma and hilar structures without increasing perioperative complications; this requires considerable anatomical knowledge and technical skill (2, 9). Park et al. showed that postoperative renal function and contralateral renal volume measured by 3D reconstructive technology according to the endophytic degree of tumors are similar between the OPN and ORN groups. Therefore, they recommended RN as a priority surgical option for ERTs (11). Superior surgical decisions regarding ERTs are of substantial importance; this debate is ongoing. The optimal management of ERTs should balance the potential benefits of intervention with competing risks of mortality in the best interests of these patients. Considering the various risks and benefits of different operating methods, we present here the first report on the perioperative, functional, and oncological outcomes of PN and RN for ERTs.

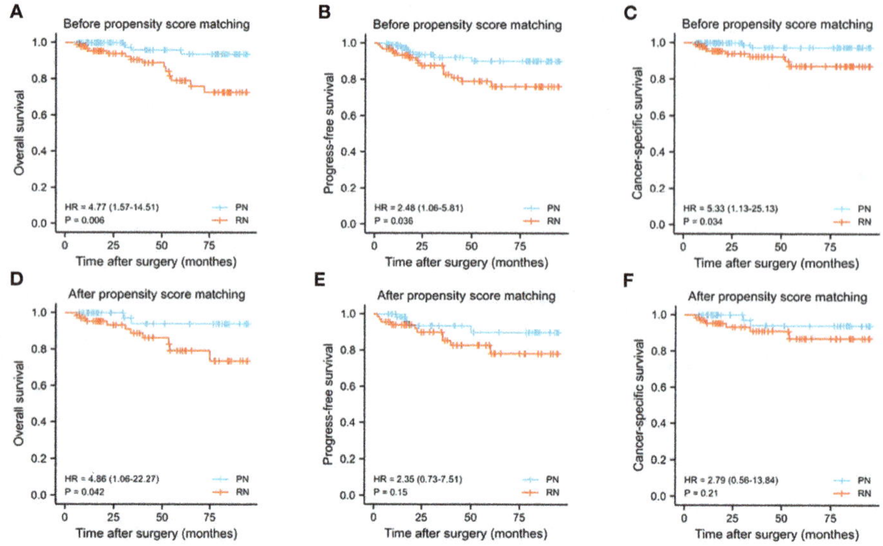

FIGURE 3 | Kaplan–Meier curves for overall survival **(A, D)**, progress-free survival **(B, E)**, cancer-specific survival **(C, F)** between the PN and RN groups before and after propensity score matching. PN, partial nephrectomy; RN, radical nephrectomy.

In this retrospective study, compared with patients who underwent PN, those who underwent RN were more likely to be the elderly with a poor general condition or larger tumor size, and highly complex tumors with high RENAL-NS. Such biases can be identified in other comparative studies between different surgical methods (partial and radical nephrectomy) (22–24). To eliminate selection bias and the influence of confounding factors, PSM analysis was conducted, as shown in **Table 1**. In the matched cohort, patients in the PN group showed a longer OT and more EBL relative to those in the RN group. A systematic review and meta-analysis by Yang et al. comprising 13 retrospective cohort studies with 13,269 patients showed that lower EBL was associated with PN and not RN for T1 renal tumor (25). Li et al. reported a similar result in another meta-analysis (26). Unlike PN, considering the omission in removing tumor and renorrhaphy during RN, the advantages of OT and EBL can be explained. Nevertheless, these advantages do not seem to be conducive to decreasing the length of postoperative hospital stays, which may be related to the similar transfusion rate, conversion rate, recovery time for postoperative bowel function, the duration of drainage, and incidence of overall complications between the two groups.

The occurrence of complications tended to be associated with the anatomical complexity of renal tumors and the basic characteristics of patients (27, 28). No statistically significant differences were observed in the incidence of overall complications between the two groups. However, after categorizing complications by Clavien–Dindo classification, in the intergroup comparison, the PN group was considerably higher than the RN group (10.3% vs. 1.5%, $p = 0.029$). Like in other retrospective studies on PN for the treatment of ERTs (29, 30), high-grade complications included urinary leakage, a requirement for ICU admission, excessive hemorrhage requiring embolization, acute renal failure, and a second operation for persistent drop in blood pressure and hemoglobin. In a meta-analysis involving 30,018 patients with RCC, Yang reported that PN is associated with an increased risk of postoperative hemorrhagic complications and urinary fistula as compared to RN (31). As a complex renal tumor, the risk of complications is higher for ERTs than for general renal tumors. The following surgical difficulties are the reasons for a higher incidence of high-grade complications in the PN group: first, ERTs are generally small in size, deep in location, and have invisible boundaries; thus, it takes a long time to locate and remove the tumor. Furthermore, the resection margin can be positive because of the indistinct tumor expansion during its removal (8), which has a major impact on the prognosis. Second, ERTs are prone to be close to the collecting system and renal sinus, wherein they are highly close to or even infiltrate into the secondary and tertiary renal arteries and veins. It is challenging to remove ERTs with a high risk of accidental vascular or pelvicalyceal system injury, which can lead to accidental rupture, massive bleeding, and urine leakage (7). Finally, even if the kidney tumor is successfully removed, the wound surface is so deep that sewing it up is challenging (9). Because the base of the wound is close to the collecting system or branch blood vessels, inappropriate suture may cause renal vascular occlusion or urine leak from the collecting system. Therefore, we recommend surgeons with rich experience and high technical skills perform PN for ERTs when a tumor-localizing device is available.

Removal of anatomically complicated tumors is inevitably associated with decreased preservation of normal parenchymal nephrons and prolonged WIT, both of which lead to increased renal impairment (32, 33). Despite these adverse factors, our findings showed that patients who underwent PN had less postoperative eGFR reduction (24.3 vs. 35.3 ml/min/1.73 m^2, $p = 0.002$) and a lower incidence of 48-h postoperative AKI

TABLE 6 | Univariate and multivariate Cox analysis of independent risk factors for overall mortality.

Variables	Univariate Analysis		Multivariate Analysis	
	Crude OR (95% CI)	*p*-value	Adjusted OR (95% CI)	-value
Age	1.11 (1.05–1.17)	**<0.001**	1.07 (0.95–1.20)	0.285
Gender				
Female (Re.) vs. male	1.89 (0.51–7.00)	0. 343		
BMI	1.04 (0.84–1.30)	0.725		
Diabetes mellitus	6.09 (1.63–22.70)	**0.007**	7.19 (0.98–36.45)	0.052
Hypertension	2.98 (0.79–11.30)	0.108		
Preoperative CKD	1.44 (0.19–11.29)	0.727		
Abdominal surgery history	2.36 (0.64–8.79)	0.200		
ACCI score	1.81 (1.36–2.41)	**<0.001**	1.34 (0.54–3.33)	0.533
ECOG PS ≥2	3.77 (2.41–6.93)	**<0.001**	0.40 (0.06–2.56)	0.332
ASA score ≥2	3.05 (0.82–11.32)	0.096		
Preoperative eGFR	0.98 (0.96–1.00)	0.086		
Preoperative hemoglobin	0.97 (0.94–1.00)	0.089		
Laterality				
Left (Re.) vs. Right	0.89 (0.28–2.81)	0.846		
Tumor size	1.29 (0.81–2.06)	0.279		
Clinical T stage ≥cT1b	3.42 (1.03–11.37)	**0.045**	1.42 (0.33–6.18)	0.642
RENAL-NS	1.79 (0.93–3.46)	0.084		
R score	2.75 (0.87–8.68)	0.084		
N score	5.77 (0.03–973.0)	0.503		
L score	1.70 (0.66–4.42)	0.275		
Hilar location	0.62 (0.17–2.29)	0.454		
Technique				
Laparoscopic (Re.) vs. Robot	0.77 (0.23–2.55)	0.665		
Operating method				
PN (Re.) vs. RN	7.36 (1.14–22.99)	**0.038**	7.36 (1.14–47.42)	**0.036**
Postoperative complications	1.02 (0.21–4.99)	0.981		
48-h postoperative AKI	2.72 (0.73–10.06)	0.135		
New onset CKD stage ≥III	1.37 (0.37–5.08)	0.637		
Histologic subtype				
Benign (Re.) vs. Malignant	2.65 (0.34–20.57)	0.351		
Pathologic stage				
pT1 (Re.) vs. pT3	4.24 (1.08–16.66)	**<0.001**	4.24 (1.30–33.21)	**0.039**
Fuhrman grade				
I/II (Re.) vs. III–IV	2.94 (0.58–14.78)	0.191		

BMI, body mass index; ACCI, age-adjusted Charlson's comorbidity index; ECOG PS, Eastern Cooperative Oncology Group Performance Status; ASA, American Society of Anesthesiologists; eGFR, estimated glomerular filtration rate; RENAL-NS, RENAL-Nephrometry Score; RN, radical nephrectomy; PN, partial nephrectomy.
The bold numbers mean statistically difference.

(44.1% vs. 70.6%, $p = 0.002$) relative to those who underwent RN. These results were similar to those of a recent study that investigated the impact factors of perioperative AKI (34). Multivariate analysis showed that the significant predictor of 48-h postoperative AKI was the surgical method, whereby the risk in the RN group was 2.812 times greater than the PN group ($p = 0.005$). In other comparative studies between PN and RN groups, significant differences in perioperative decreased renal function were observed not only for small tumors but also for anatomically complicated tumors (22, 35). The quality and quantity of preserved parenchyma are the main contributors to postoperative long-term renal function (36). The EORTC randomized trial 30904 compared the impact of NSS compared to RN on kidney function in patients with small (≤5 cm) renal tumors. The findings demonstrated that the incidence of at least moderate renal dysfunction was reduced substantially among patients who underwent NSS relative to RN (37). Our results showed similar functional outcomes. PN was more favorable for long-term renal function in patients with ERTs than RN, which was reflected in higher 48-h postoperative eGFR and a higher rate of 1-year postoperative 90% eGFR preservation. At the last follow-up, 20 of 22 cases showed new-onset CKD stage ≥III, wherein the kidney was removed completely. The significant predictors of new-onset CKD stage ≥III were hilar location and RN. It is well known that RN is the main cause of CKD stage ≥III after surgery. Additionally, by calculating the product of eGFR and relative change in renal function before and after surgery for patients with hilar renal tumors, Hinata et al. (38) reported a decrease in the 180-day postoperative renal function; resected weight was the independent predictor of the decrease in the function after PN. This was more likely correlated with preserved normal renal parenchyma and longer WIT due to the location of renal hilar tumors close to the main renal vessels (32, 33, 38).

The survival outcomes before PSM showed that the patients who underwent RN had worse OS relative to those who underwent PN. The loss of functional nephrons is related to a high likelihood of downstream metabolic disorders, including osteoporosis, anemia, and cardiovascular accidents (39, 40). Weight et al. (41) have shown that RN is associated with a 25% increased risk of cardiac death and a 17% increased risk of death due to any cause, ultimately leading to reduced OS (42). Additionally, age, BMI, and ACCI are influencing factors for OS (43–45). After eliminating these influencing factors by PSM, the RN group showed a worse OS status. Multivariate analysis confirmed that RN and pT3 stages were the predictors of overall mortality. The present results showed that non-metastatic pT3 RCC after laparoscopic management incurred metastatic progression of 26% and the three-year mortality rate was 33% (46). A study by Leibovich et al. (47) has shown that the risk ratio for death is 1.87 times higher in patients with peripheral perinephric or renal sinus fat invasion compared with those without fat invasion (p <0.001). Liu et al. (48) compared the survival benefit between PN and RN for renal tumors ≤7 cm with stage pT3a from the SEER database and found that PN yielded better OS for the ≤4 cm group than RN. Furthermore, the Cochrane meta-analysis by Chung et al. (49) compared the oncological outcomes between PN and RN among patients who were upstaged from cT1 renal tumor to pT3a renal cell carcinoma. Relative to RN, patients who underwent PN had better or at least similar oncological outcomes, with a significant improvement in OS, particularly. Therefore, if PN is feasible, RN should be avoided for better survival outcomes among patients with ERTs that can improve in stage.

Interestingly, significant differences between CCS and PFS disappeared after the selection bias and confounding factors of oncological characteristics, including tumor size and RENAL-NS, were balanced by PSM. The results of Palacios et al. (50) indicated that unfavorable oncological outcomes (i.e., CSS and RPS) for localized RCC were mostly associated with aggressive tumor characteristics, not renal function. Zhang et al. (51) reported that tumor size is significantly correlated with nuclear grade and pathological stage, and larger tumors are prone to higher grades and stages. Here, Fuhrman Grade III occurred in 6.9% of renal tumors, which were 2.1 to 4.0 cm in diameter, and 22.3% of tumors between 4.1 and 7 cm in diameter. A study comprising 886 cases of SRM confirmed that increased tumor anatomical complexity quantified by RENAL-NS was independently related to malignancy and high nuclear grade (52). Chen et al. (53) indicated that R- and N-scores were associated with higher postoperative pathological grades. In our study, before PSM, tumors in the RN groups showed larger size (4.1 vs. 2.8 cm, p <0.001), higher overall RENAL-NS (10.1 vs. 8.8, p <0.001), with higher R score (1.5 vs. 1.2, p <0.001), and higher N score (3.0 vs. 2.5, p <0.001) relative to the PN group. Thus, all the indicators favorable to tumor progression were skewed toward the RN group. When these significantly different indicators were balanced, the results of similar CSS and PFS in the matched cohort could be easily interpreted.

However, this study is not devoid of limitations. This study was retrospective and based on a single center database. Although PSM analysis was performed to account for the preoperative basic and oncological characteristics, the underlying selection biases or confounding factors may be uncontrollable to a certain extent. Anatomical features and oncological characteristics were assessed by two-dimensional cross-sectional imaging. Therefore, because of the experience and subjective factors of the observers, there might have been judgment biases in this study. Preoperative and postoperative renal functions were not estimated using radioisotope renography, the ideal tool but impractical for every patient. Thus, eGFR was calculated using the internationally recognized Cockgroft–Gault equation, and the results for all patients were standardized by body surface area to improve their reliability. Finally, considering the operating challenges, experienced urologists at a tertiary referral institution performed the procedures, and thus, these results cannot be generalized and should be interpreted with caution.

Despite these limitations, to our knowledge, this retrospective study is the first to evaluate the safety and efficacy of PN and RN for treating ERTs. Additionally, the results of this study are based on PSM analysis to balance influencing factors, which improved the reliability of these findings to a greater extent.

CONCLUSION

In conclusion, in the matched cohort of patients with ERTs, RN resulted in more favorable surgical outcomes, but these advantages did not translate into faster postoperative recovery. Additionally, RN was an independent risk factor for short-term and long-term renal function decline. The incidence of overall complications was comparable to that of RN, but PN was more prone to high-grade complications due to the complex anatomical structure of these tumors. Even so, patients who underwent PN showed better preservation of renal function, longer OS, and similar oncological outcomes compared to those who underwent RN. Therefore, we suggest that PN be preferentially considered for ERTs when technically feasible and the surgeon is experienced.

ETHICS STATEMENT

The studies involving human participants were reviewed and approved by Board and the ethical committee of the First Affiliated Hospital of Nanchang University. Written informed consent to participate in this study was provided by the participants' legal guardian/next of kin. Written informed consent was obtained from the individual(s), and minor(s)' legal guardian/next of kin, for the publication of any potentially identifiable images or data included in this article.

AUTHOR CONTRIBUTIONS

SX and MJ collected the data. SX and BF conceived the manuscript. SX wrote the manuscript. SX and YJ made tables and figures together. WD and BH provides guidance in statistical analysis. RC and ZY provides guidance on the making of figures. LC, XL and XW provided input into the revision of the manuscript. XW sent the manuscript to a native English speaker to correct spelling and grammatical errors. All authors listed have made a substantial, direct, and intellectual contribution to the work and approved it for publication.

ACKNOWLEDGMENTS

The authors thank all the people who support investigators to complete this article. We thank Bullet Edits Limited for the linguistic editing and proofreading of the manuscript.

REFERENCES

1. Perez-Ardavin J, Sanchez-Gonzalez JV, Martinez-Sarmiento M, Monserrat-Monfort García-Olaverri JJ, Boronat-Tormo J, F, et al. Surgical Treatment of Completely Endophytic Renal Tumor: A Systematic Review. *Curr Urol Rep* (2019) 20:3. doi: 10.1007/s11934-019-0864-x
2. Minoda R, Takagi T, Yoshida K, Kondo T, Tanabe K. Comparison of Surgical Outcomes Between Enucleation and Standard Resection in Robot-Assisted Partial Nephrectomy for Completely Endophytic Renal Tumors Through a 1:1 Propensity Score-Matched Analysis. *J Endourol* (2021) 35:1779–84. doi: 10.1089/end.2021.0213
3. Kutikov A, Uzzo RG. The R.E.N.A.L. Nephrometry Score: A Comprehensive Standardized System for Quantitating Renal Tumor Size, Location and Depth. *J Urol* (2009) 182:844–53. doi: 10.1016/j.juro.2009.05.035
4. Ljungberg B, Albiges L, Abu-Ghanem Y, Bensalah K, Dabestani S, Fernández-Pello S, et al. European Association of Urology Guidelines on Renal Cell Carcinoma: The 2019 Update. *Eur Urol* (2019) 75:799–810. doi: 10.1016/j.eururo.2019.02.011
5. Pierorazio PM, Johnson MH, Patel HD, Sozio SM, Sharma R, Iyoha E, et al. Management of Renal Masses and Localized Renal Cancer: Systematic Review and Meta-Analysis. *J Urol* (2016) 196:989–99. doi: 10.1016/j.juro.2016.04.081
6. Huang WC, Elkin EB, Levey AS, Jang TL, Russo P. Partial Nephrectomy Versus Radical Nephrectomy in Patients With Small Renal Tumors–is There a Difference in Mortality and Cardiovascular Outcomes? *J Urol* (2009) 181:55–61, 61-2. doi: 10.1016/j.juro.2008.09.017
7. Kim DK, Komninos C, Kim L, Rha KH. Robot-Assisted Partial Nephrectomy for Endophytic Tumors. *Curr urol Rep* (2015) 16:76. doi: 10.1007/s11934-015-0552-4
8. Dall'Oglio MF, Ballarotti L, Passerotti CC, Paluello DV, Colombo JJ, Crippa A, et al. Anatrophic Nephrotomy as Nephron-Sparing Approach for Complete Removal of Intraparenchymal Renal Tumors. *Int Braz J Urol* (2012) 38:356–61. doi: 10.1590/S1677-55382012000300008
9. Chung BI, Lee UJ, Kamoi K, Canes DA, Aron M, Gill IS. Laparoscopic Partial Nephrectomy for Completely Intraparenchymal Tumors. *J Urol* (2011) 186:2182–7. doi: 10.1016/j.juro.2011.07.106
10. Nadu A, Goldberg H, Lubin M, Baniel J. Laparoscopic Partial Nephrectomy (LPN) for Totally Intrarenal Tumours. *BJU Int* (2013) 112:E82–6. doi: 10.1111/bju.12168
11. Park DS, Hong YK, Lee SR, Hwang JH, Kang MH, Oh JJ. Three-Dimensional Reconstructive Kidney Volume Analyses According to the Endophytic Degree of Tumors During Open Partial or Radical Nephrectomy. *Int Braz J Urol* (2016) 42:37–46. doi: 10.1590/S1677-5538.IBJU.2014.0417
12. Fan G, Li J, Li M, Ye M, Pei X, Li F, et al. Three-Dimensional Physical Model-Assisted Planning and Navigation for Laparoscopic Partial Nephrectomy in Patients With Endophytic Renal Tumors. *Sci Rep* (2018) 8:582. doi: 10.1038/s41598-017-19056-5
13. Carbonara U, Simone G, Minervini A, Sundaram CP, Larcher A, Lee J, et al. Outcomes of Robot-Assisted Partial Nephrectomy for Completely Endophytic Renal Tumors: A Multicenter Analysis. *Eur J Surg Oncol* (2020) 47(5):1179–86. doi: 10.1016/S2666-1683(20)35531-2
14. Sun Y, Wang W, Zhang Q, Zhao X, Xu L, Guo H. Intraoperative Ultrasound: Technique and Clinical Experience in Robotic-Assisted Renal Partial Nephrectomy for Endophytic Renal Tumors. *Int Urol Nephrol* (2020) 53 (3):455–63. doi: 10.1007/s11255-020-02664-y
15. Qin B, Hu H, Lu Y, Wang Y, Yu Y, Zhang J, et al. Intraoperative Ultrasonography in Laparoscopic Partial Nephrectomy for Intrarenal Tumors. *PloS One* (2018) 13:e195911. doi: 10.1371/journal.pone.0195911
16. Mikhail D, Tabibzadeh A, Rai A, Richstone L. Laparoscopic Radical Nephrectomy. *J endourol* (2021) 35:S83–92. doi: 10.1089/end.2021.0626
17. Clavien PA, Barkun J, de Oliveira ML, Vauthey JN, Dindo D, Schulick RD, et al. The Clavien-Dindo Classification of Surgical Complications: Five-Year Experience. *Ann Surg* (2009) 250:187–96. doi: 10.1097/SLA.0b013e3181b13ca2
18. Mehta RL, Kellum JA, Shah SV, Molitoris BA, Ronco C, Warnock DG, et al. Acute Kidney Injury Network: Report of an Initiative to Improve Outcomes in Acute Kidney Injury. *Crit Care* (2007) 11:R31. doi: 10.1186/cc5713
19. Di Pierro GB, Tartaglia N, Aresu L, Polara A, Cielo A, Cristini C, et al. Laparoscopic Partial Nephrectomy for Endophytic Hilar Tumors: Feasibility and Outcomes. *Eur J Surg Oncol* (2014) 40:769–74. doi: 10.1016/j.ejso.2013.11.023
20. Harke NN, Mandel P, Witt JH, Wagner C, Panic A, Boy A, et al. Are There Limits of Robotic Partial Nephrectomy? TRIFECTA Outcomes of Open and Robotic Partial Nephrectomy for Completely Endophytic Renal Tumors. *J Surg Oncol* (2018) 118:206–11. doi: 10.1002/jso.25103
21. Pandolfo SD, Loizzo D, Autorino R. Editorial Comment to Expanding the Limits of Nephron-Sparing Surgery: Surgical Technique and Mid-Term Outcomes of Purely Off-Clamp Robotic Partial Nephrectomy for Totally Endophytic Renal Tumors. *Int J Urol* (2022) 29(4):288. doi: 10.1111/iju.14788
22. Kim H, Kim JK, Ye C, Choi JH, Lee H, Oh JJ, et al. Recurrence After Radical and Partial Nephrectomy in High Complex Renal Tumor Using Propensity Score Matched Analysis. *Sci rep-uk* (2021) 11:2919. doi: 10.1038/s41598-021-82700-8
23. Oh JJ, Byun S, Lee SE, Hong SK, Lee ES, Kim HH, et al. Partial Nephrectomy Versus Radical Nephrectomy for non-Metastatic Pathological T3a Renal Cell Carcinoma: A Multi-Institutional Comparative Analysis. *Int J Urol* (2014) 21:352–7. doi: 10.1111/iju.12283
24. Alvim R, Tin A, Nogueira L, Lebdai S, Wong N, Takeda T, et al. A Comparison of Oncologic and Functional Outcomes in Patients With Pt3a Renal Cell Carcinoma Treated With Partial and Radical Nephrectomy. *Int Braz J Urol* (2021) 47:777–83. doi: 10.1590/s1677-5538.ibju.2020.0149
25. Yang C, Liao Z. Comparison of Radical Nephrectomy and Partial Nephrectomy for T1 Renal Cell Carcinoma: A Meta-Analysis. *Urol Int* (2018) 101:175–83. doi: 10.1159/000490576
26. Li J, Zhang Y, Teng Z, Han Z. Partial Nephrectomy Versus Radical Nephrectomy for Ct2 or Greater Renal Tumors: A Systematic Review and Meta-Analysis. *Minerva Urol Nefrol* (2019) 71:435–44. doi: 10.23736/S0393-2249.19.03470-2
27. Ito T, Abbosh PH, Mehrazin R, Tomaszewski JJ, Li T, Ginzburg S, et al. Surgical Apgar Score Predicts an Increased Risk of Major Complications and Death After Renal Mass Excision. *J Urol* (2015) 193:1918–22. doi: 10.1016/j.juro.2014.11.085
28. Desantis D, Lavallée LT, Witiuk K, Mallick R, Kamal F, Fergusson D, et al. The Association Between Renal Tumour Scoring System Components and Complications of Partial Nephrectomy. *Can Urol Assoc J* (2015) 9:39–45. doi: 10.5489/cuaj.2303
29. Zapala P, Dybowski B, Miazek N, Radziszewski P. Open Partial Nephrectomy for Entirely Intraparenchymal Tumors: A Matched Case-Control Study of Oncologic Outcome and Complication Rate. *Int Braz J urol* (2017) 43:209–15. doi: 10.1590/s1677-5538.ibju.2016.0040
30. Kara O, Maurice MJ, Malkoc E, Ramirez D, Nelson R, Caputo P, et al. Comparison of Robot-Assisted and Open Partial Nephrectomy for Completely Endophytic Renal Tumours: A Single Centre Experience. *BJU Int* (2016) 118:946–51. doi: 10.1111/bju.13572
31. Yang Y. Partial Versus Radical Nephrectomy in Patients With Renal Cell Carcinoma: A Systematic Review and Meta-Analysis. *Urol J* (2020) 17:109–17. doi: 10.22037/uj.v0i0.5358
32. Mir MC, Pavan N, Capitanio U, Antonelli A, Derweesh I, Rodriguez-Faba O, et al. Partial Versus Radical Nephrectomy in Very Elderly Patients: A Propensity Score Analysis of Surgical, Functional and Oncologic Outcomes (RESURGE Project). *World J Urol* (2020) 38:151–8. doi: 10.1007/s00345-019-02665-2
33. Deng W, Liu X, Hu J, Chen L, Fu B. Off-Clamp Partial Nephrectomy has a Positive Impact on Short- and Long-Term Renal Function: A Systematic Review and Meta-Analysis. *BMC Nephrol* (2018) 19:188. doi: 10.1186/s12882-018-0993-3
34. Wenzel M, Kleimaker A, Uhlig A, Würnschimmel C, Becker A, Yu H, et al. Impact of Comorbidities on Acute Kidney Injury and Renal Function

Impairment After Partial and Radical Tumor Nephrectomy. *Scand J Urol* (2021) 55:377–82. doi: 10.1080/21681805.2021.1948916

35. Snow DC, Bhayani SB. Rapid Communication: Chronic Renal Insufficiency After Laparoscopic Partial Nephrectomy and Radical Nephrectomy for Pathologic T1a Lesions. *J Endourol* (2008) 22:337–41. doi: 10.1089/end.2007.0240
36. Rod X, Peyronnet B, Seisen T, Pradere B, Gomez FD, Verhoest G, et al. Impact of Ischaemia Time on Renal Function After Partial Nephrectomy: A Systematic Review. *BJU Int* (2016) 118:692–705. doi: 10.1111/bju.13580
37. Scosyrev E, Messing EM, Sylvester R, Campbell S, Van Poppel H. Renal Function After Nephron-Sparing Surgery Versus Radical Nephrectomy: Results From EORTC Randomized Trial 30904. *Eur Urol* (2014) 65:372–7. doi: 10.1016/j.eururo.2013.06.044
38. Hinata N, Shiroki R, Tanabe K, Eto M, Takenaka A, Kawakita M, et al. Robot-Assisted Partial Nephrectomy Versus Standard Laparoscopic Partial Nephrectomy for Renal Hilar Tumor: A Prospective Multi-Institutional Study. *Int J urol* (2021) 28:382–9. doi: 10.1111/iju.14469
39. Bagrodia A, Mehrazin R, Bazzi WM, Silberstein J, Malcolm JB, Stroup SP, et al. Comparison of Rates and Risk Factors for Development of Osteoporosis and Fractures After Radical or Partial Nephrectomy. *Urology* (2011) 78:614–9. doi: 10.1016/j.urology.2011.02.071
40. Woldrich J, Mehrazin R, Bazzi WM, Bagrodia A, Kopp RP, Malcolm JB, et al. Comparison of Rates and Risk Factors for Development of Anaemia and Erythropoiesis-Stimulating Agent Utilization After Radical or Partial Nephrectomy. *BJU Int* (2012) 109:1019–25. doi: 10.1111/j.1464-410X.2011.10432.x
41. Weight CJ, Larson BT, Fergany AF, Gao T, Lane BR, Campbell SC. Nephrectomy Induced Chronic Renal Insufficiency Is Associated With Increased Risk of Cardiovascular Death and Death From Any Cause in Patients With Localized Ct1b Renal Masses. *J Urol* (2010) 183:1317–23. doi: 10.1016/j.juro.2009.12.030
42. Thompson RH, Boorjian SA, Lohse CM, Leibovich BC, Kwon ED, Cheville JC, et al. Radical Nephrectomy for Pt1a Renal Masses may be Associated With Decreased Overall Survival Compared With Partial Nephrectomy. *J Urol* (2008) 179:468–71, 472-3. doi: 10.1016/j.juro.2007.09.077
43. Tang F, Lu Z, He C, Zhang H, Wu W, He Z. 53 Years Old is a Reasonable Cut-Off Value to Define Young and Old Patients in Clear Cell Renal Cell Carcinoma: A Study Based on TCGA and SEER Database. *BMC Cancer* (2021) 21:638. doi: 10.1186/s12885-021-08376-5
44. Farag KI, Makkouk A, Norian LA. Re-Evaluating the Effects of Obesity on Cancer Immunotherapy Outcomes in Renal Cancer: What Do We Really Know? *Front Immunol* (2021) 12:668494. doi: 10.3389/fimmu.2021.668494
45. Chang CM, Yin WY, Wei CK, Wu CC, Su YC, Yu CH, et al. Adjusted Age-Adjusted Charlson Comorbidity Index Score as a Risk Measure of Perioperative Mortality Before Cancer Surgery. *PloS One* (2016) 11:e148076. doi: 10.1371/journal.pone.0148076
46. Nayak JG, Patel P, Bjazevic J, Liu Z, Saarela O, Kapoor A, et al. Clinical Outcomes Following Laparoscopic Management of Pt3 Renal Masses: A Large, Multi-Institutional Cohort. *Can Urol Assoc J* (2015) 9:397–402. doi: 10.5489/cuaj.2848
47. Leibovich BC, Cheville JC, Lohse CM, Zincke H, Kwon ED, Frank I, et al. Cancer Specific Survival for Patients With Pt3 Renal Cell Carcinoma-can the 2002 Primary Tumor Classification be Improved? *J Urol* (2005) 173:716–9. doi: 10.1097/01.ju.0000151830.27750.d2
48. Liu S, Feng C, Liu C, Wang Z. Comparison of Prognosis Between Patients Undergoing Radical Nephrectomy Versus Partial Nephrectomy for Renal Cell Carcinoma ≤7 Cm T3aN0/xM0: Survival Benefit is Biased Toward Partial Nephrectomy. *Cancer Med-US* (2021) 10:8909–23. doi: 10.1002/cam4.4412
49. Chung DY, Kang DH, Kim JW, Kim DK, Lee JY, Cho KS. Comparison of Oncologic Outcomes Between Partial Nephrectomy and Radical Nephrectomy in Patients Who Were Upstaged From Ct1 Renal Tumor to Pt3a Renal Cell Carcinoma: An Updated Systematic Review and Meta-Analysis. *Ther Adv Urol* (2020) 12:2079203076. doi: 10.1177/1756287220981508
50. Palacios DA, Zabor EC, Munoz-Lopez C, Roversi G, Mahmood F, Abramczyk E, et al. Does Reduced Renal Function Predispose to Cancer-Specific Mortality From Renal Cell Carcinoma? *Eur urol* (2021) 79:774–80. doi: 10.1016/j.eururo.2021.02.035
51. Zhang C, Li X, Hao H, Yu W, He Z, Zhou L. The Correlation Between Size of Renal Cell Carcinoma and its Histopathological Characteristics: A Single Center Study of 1867 Renal Cell Carcinoma Cases. *BJU Int* (2012) 110:E481–5. doi: 10.1111/j.1464-410X.2012.11173.x
52. Mullins JK, Kaouk JH, Bhayani S, Rogers CG, Stifelman MD, Pierorazio PM, et al. Tumor Complexity Predicts Malignant Disease for Small Renal Masses. *J Urology* (2012) 188:2072–6. doi: 10.1016/j.juro.2012.08.027
53. Chen SH, Wu YP, Li XD, Lin T, Guo QY, Chen YH, et al. R.E.N.A.L. Nephrometry Score: A Preoperative Risk Factor Predicting the Fuhrman Grade of Clear-Cell Renal Carcinoma. *J Cancer* (2017) 8:3725–32. doi: 10.7150/jca.21189

4

A Survey of Enhanced Recovery After Surgery Protocols for Cesarean Delivery in Serbia

Borislava Pujic[1], Mirjana Kendrisic[2], Matthew Shotwell[3], Yaping Shi[3] and Curtis L. Baysinger[4]*

[1] Clinical Center Vojvodina, Obstetrics and Gynecology Hospital, Novi Sad, Serbia, [2] General Hospital, Sremska Mitrovica, Serbia, [3] Department of Biostatistics, School of Medicine, Vanderbilt University, Nashville, TN, United States, [4] Department of Anesthesiology, School of Medicine, Vanderbilt University, Nashville, TN, United States

***Correspondence:**
Borislava Pujic
borislava60@yahoo.com

Enhanced recovery after surgery (ERAS) protocols have been described for patients undergoing colon surgery. Similar protocols for cesarean delivery (CD) have been developed recently. CD is one of the most commonly performed surgical procedures, and adoption of ERAS protocols following CD might benefit patients and the health-care system. We aimed to determine which Serbian hospitals reported ERAS protocols, which elements of ERAS protocols were used in CD patients, and whether ERAS and non-ERAS hospitals differed. The survey was sent to all hospitals with obstetric services and 46 of 49 responded. The questionnaire asked whether ERAS protocols had been formally adopted for surgical patients and about their use in CD patients. Specific questions on elements described in other obstetric ERAS protocols for CD included preoperative patient preparation, type of anesthesia and temperature monitoring used for CD, maternal/neonatal contact, and time to discharge. ERAS protocols are used in 24% of surveyed hospitals, 84% admit the patient the day before elective CDs, 87% use a maternal bowel preparation morning on the day of CD, and 80% administer maternal deep venous thrombosis prophylaxis. Only 33% remove IV in the first postoperative day, and 89% of women do not eat solid food until the day following their CD. Neuraxial anesthesia is used in 46% of elective CDs in ERAS hospitals compared to 9% in non-ERAS hospitals ($P < 0.01$), and neuraxial narcotics for post CD analgesia are given more often in ERAS hospitals. Thirty-six percentage of ERAS patients are discharged within 3 days vs. none in the non-ERAS group. Few elements of ERAS protocols reported from other centers outside Serbia are employed in Serbian hospitals performing CD. Despite significant changes that have been made recently in CD care, enhanced recovery after CD could be significantly improved in Serbian hospitals.

Keywords: cesarean delivery, enhanced recovery, neuraxial anesthesia, length of stay, obstetric anesthesiology

INTRODUCTION

The significance of enhanced recovery after surgery (ERAS) protocols has been well established in non-obstetric surgery patients and was described by Wilmore and Kehlet, 15 years ago (1). Soon after ERAS protocol successes in speeding patient recovery, decreasing times to discharge form the hospital and improving patient outcomes were described in colorectal surgery patients (2), successful application was reported in urological, breast, pancreatectomy, liver resection, and gynecologic surgery (3–9). The ERAS approach emphasizes optimization of the processes of patient care, so that enhanced patient recovery can occur without decreasing the quality of care or patient satisfaction.

ERAS aims to return the patient to normal life quickly. The increased efficiencies have been demonstrated to reduce waste of scarce resources (10) and thus reduce the overall cost of care. While significant variations in ERAS protocols exist both within and between surgical specialties (11), common elements often include effective patient education and acceptance, good perioperative hydration and nutrition, use of surgical techniques associated with fastest patient recovery, maintenance of perioperative patient normothermia, early removal of urinary catheters, adequate pain relief that promotes early ambulation and minimal use of perioperative opioids (which helps the return of bowel function quickly). The multidisciplinary approach requires commitment from the patient, as well as all of the persons involved in their perioperative care: surgeons, anesthesiologists, pain specialists, nursing staff, physical and occupational therapists, social services, and hospital administration. Successful ERAS protocol implementation involves the creation of a core team of anesthesiologists, obstetricians, specialist nurses, and hospital managers (12). The large number of elements that are required for implementation of an ERAS protocol often requires significant culture change in the health organization (12).

Background and Rationale

Enhanced recovery after surgery protocols have been developed for patients undergoing cesarean delivery (CD) in recent years. CD is one of the most commonly performed operations worldwide, its incidence is increasing, and elective CD accounts for an increasing proportion of those operations (13). Therefore, CD represents an increasing burden on national health-care systems. Recent guidelines of the UK National Institute for Health and Care Excellence suggest that a majority of women undergoing elective CD could be discharged on the day after delivery (14). Such early discharges are not associated with either increased patient morbidity or higher readmission rates than in women discharged later (15). One recent report suggested that many women would prefer to be discharged a day earlier than occurred following their delivery (16). The widespread adoption of ERAS protocols for CD was recently advocated by Lucas and Gough as a means for achieving these positive outcomes (17).

Reports describing the implementation of ERAS protocols for CD have been recently published (13, 16, 18–21). In addition to the ERAS elements used in non-obstetric surgeries, these reports often describe early skin-to-skin contact in theater between mother and neonate, infant temperature monitoring to prevent neonatal hypothermia, delayed cord clamping, and early breastfeeding after maternal breast-feeding education. Most of these reports are from the UK, and two survey reports from there note a growing consensus of the elements that ERAS for CD should contain (21, 22).

No reports describing ERAS protocols for CD from Eastern European or middle-income countries have been published, and the number of institutions that use them are unknown. Accordingly, we aimed to determine the use of ERAS protocols for CD in Serbia and to determine the differences in use of common ERAS elements between those institutions that report the use of ERAS protocols and those that do not.

MATERIALS AND METHODS

A survey tool of 22 questions with multiple choice answers was sent by email to all hospitals in Serbia (4 university teaching hospitals and 45 general hospitals), which provide obstetric services (**Table 1**). This survey was approved by Ethical Committee at the Clinical Center of Vojvodina. The questionnaire was completed by either the Chief of Obstetrics or Chief of Anesthesiology who had knowledge of all aspects of perioperative care within the institution, and only one questionnaire per institution was

TABLE 1 | Questionnaire.

INSTITUTION ____________________
SPECIALTY (around)
- Obstetrics
- Anesthesiology

QUESTIONAIRE

In this research are included all hospitals in Serbia (4 university and 45 general Hospitals). Please answer the following questions by around the letter in front of the right answer or you write your answer. Filled questionnaire return by e-mail to following addresses:

borislava60@yahoo.com
mkendrisic@yahoo.co.uk

According to your answers, we shall try to understand which of the "Fast track" surgery criteria (ERAS: enhanced recovery after surgery) are implemented in our hospitals and to make some guidelines for cesarean delivery (CD).

1. Is the ERAS protocol for better and faster recovery after cesarean section introduced to the parturients in your institution?
   A. Yes
   B. No
   C. Sometimes
   D. ______________
2. Who inform the parturients preoperative?
   A. Obstetrician who takes care during the pregnancy
   B. Obstetrician who perform CS
   C. Anesthesiologist in anesthesia clinic
   D. Anesthesiologist who perform anesthesia for CS
   E. ______________________
3. In your hospital is usual patient's admission prior CS?
   A. Evening before schedule surgery
   B. 24 h before
   C. In the morning, on the surgery day
   D. ______________________
4. In your institution do you use bowel preparation before CS?
   A. Yes
   B. No
   C. Sometimes
   D. ______________
5. In your institution do you use antibiotics prophylaxis 30' before CS?
   A. Always
   B. Sometimes
   C. Never
   D. ______________
6. In your institution do you use DVT prophylaxis before or after CS?
   A. Always
   B. Sometimes
   C. Never
   D. ______________

(Continued)

TABLE 1 | Continued

7. What is the percentage of regional anesthesia (RA) for scheduled CS in your institution?
   A. <10%
   B. 10–29%
   C. 30–49%
   D. >50%

8. What is the percentage of RA for emergent CS in your institution?
   A. <10%
   B. 10–29%
   C. 30–49%
   D. >50%

9. Do you use opiates intrathecal for postoperative analgesia (morphine)?
   A. Always
   B. Sometimes
   C. Never
   D. _______________

10. Analgesia following CS is:
   A. IV
   B. IM
   C. combination (IV and IM)
   D. per oral
   E. _______________

11. How long parturients are on the IV infusion?
   A. < 24 h
   B. 24 h
   C. 48 h
   D. Depends of case
   E. _______________

12. When do you start with per oral liquids intake?
   A. Immediately postoperative
   B. Following 12 h
   C. Following 24 h
   D. Following 48 h

13. When do you start with per oral food intake?
   A. Following 12 h
   B. Following 24 h
   C. Following 48 h
   D. _______________

14. Do you use chewing gum following CS?
   A. Yes
   B. No
   C. Sometimes

15. When they start walking after CS?
   A. In the evening (On the day of CS)
   B. Tomorrow morning (following 24 h)
   C. Following 48 h
   D. _______________

16. When do you remove urinary catheter following CS?
   A. On the day of CS
   B. Tomorrow
   C. Following 48 h
   D. Depends of case

17. Do you use "skin to skin" contact on the operating table?
   A. Yes
   B. No

18. Do you use temperature checking intraoperative?
   A. Yes
   B. No

(Continued)

TABLE 1 | Continued

19. Do you use active warming during CS?
   A. Yes
   B. No
   C. Sometimes

20. Do you use medication to prevent chronic pain (gabapentin or pregabalin)?
   A. Yes
   B. No
   C. _______________

21. How many CS do you have at your hospital per year?
   A. <500
   B. 501–1,000
   C. >1,000

22. How long are parturients at the hospital following CS before discharge home?
   A. <3 days
   B. 4–6 days
   C. >6 days

returned. One of the authors (BP) followed up after distribution of the survey to answer all responder questions. The questionnaire asked for the presence of ERAS protocols for CD in the hospital, preoperative patient counseling of the elements within the protocol, time of admission to hospital and hospital stay, bowel preparation prior surgery, antibiotic prophylaxis prior to skin incision, prevention of deep venous thrombosis (DVT), percentage of neuraxial anesthesia (NA) for elective and emergency CD, use of intrathecal analgesia, medications for postoperative analgesia, oral intake after CD, use of chewing gum in the early postoperative period, duration of IV fluid therapy, urinary catheter removal, early mobilization of the parturient, skin-to-skin contact between mother and baby in the operating theater, monitoring of body temperature, and active maternal warming intraoperatively. Overall responses were recorded, and the responses between those hospitals with ERAS protocols in place were compared with those who did not report having them. Pearson' chi square test was used where appropriate for comparisons between groups in this prospective observational study (R version 3.3.3, R Core Team, R Foundation for Statistical Computing). Differences of $P \leq 0.05$ were considered significant.

RESULTS

Responses were obtained from 46 of 49 hospitals (3 university and 43 general hospitals; a 94% response rate). ERAS protocols were in use in 11 of 46 (24%) of surveyed hospitals and 63% of the time the responsibility for patients counseling was shared between the obstetrician and anesthesiologist (**Table 2**).

Survey Elements With Similar Responses Between ERAS and Non-ERAS Hospitals

Many surveyed items did not vary between institutions that reported ERAS use vs. those that did not. Surveyed hospitals reported admitting the patient the day before elective CD 84%

TABLE 2 | Survey items with similar responses from institutions with and without ERAS protocols.

Item	Overall	ERAS protocol	No ERAS protocol	*P* value
1. ERAS protocol is used	11 (24%)			
2. Who educates patient?				0.47
Obstetrician	9 (20%)	1 (9.1%)	8 (23%)	
Anesthesiologist	8 (17%)	3 (27%)	5 (14%)	
Either	29 (63%)	7 (64%)	22 (63%)	
3. When admitted for CD				0.17
Day before	37 (84%)	11 (100%)	26 (79%)	
Day of	7 (16%)	0	7 (21%)	
4. Bowel prep is used				0.35
Yes	39 (87%)	11 (100%)	28 (82%)	
No	4 (9%)	0	4 (9%)	
Sometimes	2 (4%)	0	2 (4%)	
5. Antibiotics 30 min before CD				0.08
Yes	21 (51%)	8 (73%)	13 (43%)	
No	5 (12%)	2 (18%)	3 (10%)	
Sometimes	15 (37%)	1 (9%)	14 (47%)	
6. DVT prophylaxis				0.29
Yes	37 (80%)	11 (100%)	26 (74%)	
No	1 (2%)	0	1 (3%)	
Sometimes	8 (17%)	0	8 (23%)	
7. Neuraxial narcotics for CD				0.09
Yes	4 (9%)	2 (18%)	2 (6%)	
No	25 (56%)	3 (27%)	22 (65%)	
Sometimes	16 (35%)	6 (55%)	10 (30%)	
8. Parenteral narcotics administration				0.56
IV	14 (36%)	2 (22%)	12 (40%)	
IM	1 (3%)	0	1 (3%)	
Both	24 (61%)	7 (78%)	17 (57%)	
9. When IV is removed				0.16
Immediately after CD	0	0	0	
<24 h after CD	13 (33%)	6 (55%)	7 (24%)	
24–48 h after CD	26 (65%)	5 (45%)	21 (72%)	
>48 h after CD	1 (2.5%)	0	1 (3%)	
10. When solid food is allowed				0.89
Immediately after CD	0	0	0	
12 h after CD	5 (11%)	1 (9%)	4 (12%)	
24 h after CD	20 (44%)	6 (55%)	14 (41%)	
48 h after CD	20 (44%)	4 (36%)	16 (47%)	
11. Chewing gum is used				0.15
Yes	0	0	0	
No	36 (86%)	10 (100%)	26 (74%)	
Sometimes	9 (20%)	0	9 (26%)	
12. Urinary catheter removed				0.44
Day of CD	2 (5%)	0	2 (6%)	
First post-operative day	26 (59%)	8 (73%)	18 (55%)	
Second post-operative day	11 (25%)	3 (27%)	8 (24%)	
Clinician judgment	5 (11%)	0	5 (15%)	
13. Skin to skin contact				0.09
Yes	22 (49%)	8 (73%)	14 (41%)	
No	23 (51%)	3 (27%)	20 (59%)	
14. Monitor maternal temp				0.32
Yes	5 (11%)	0	5 (14%)	
No	41 (89%)	11 (100%)	30 (86%)	
15. Active warming during CD				0.24
Yes	2 (4%)	0	2 (6%)	
No	34 (76%)	7 (64%)	27 (80%)	
Sometimes	9 (20%)	4 (36%)	5 (14%)	
16. Routinely give gabapentin				1.0
Yes	10 (22%)	2 (18%)	8 (23%)	
No	36 (78%)	9 (82%)	27 (77%)	

(*Continued*)

TABLE 2 | Continued

P values calculated using the Pearson Chi square test.

CD, cesarean delivery; NA, neuraxial anesthesia; h, hours; temp, temperature; admin, administration; DVT, deep venous thrombosis; min, minutes; ERAS, enhanced recovery after surgery.

of the time, use of maternal bowel preparation in the morning on the day of CD in 87% of patients, measures to prevent maternal DVT during the peri-partum period in 87% of mothers, administration of gabapentin approximately 22% of the time as an analgesic adjunct, with no differences between ERAS and non-ERAS groups.

Perioperative maternal temperature monitoring was reportedly used only 11% of the time and active warming of either IV fluids or other active measures was used less than 5% of the time; there were no differences between ERAS and non-ERAS groups. The maternal urinary catheter was nearly always retained until at least the first postoperative day and was removed in approximately a quarter of women on the second day, with removal in the rest after that. Only 5% of women had their IV removed within 24 h after delivery and 88% did not have solid food until the day following their CD. Among hospitals reporting ERAS use, 73% administered antibiotics within 30 min of a CD, compared to 43% in non-ERAS hospitals, and skin-to-skin contact during CD under NA occurred in 73% of ERAS institutions compared to less than 43% of non-ERAS hospitals, differences that nearly reach statistical significance. The use of neuraxial narcotics for postoperative analgesia is rare in Serbian hospitals, used 9% of the time overall, but 18% of ERAS protocol hospital reported using them vs. 6% of non-ERAS institutions, a difference that also nearly reached statistical significance.

Survey Elements With Differing Responses Between ERAS and Non-ERAS Hospitals

The use of NA for CD, time to ambulation, time to first PO fluids, and days to discharge varied between groups (**Table 3**). In the ERAS group, 46% of parturients received NA for elective CD and 36% were given NA for urgent CD over 50% of the time; only 9% of non-ERAS hospitals use NA for elective CD and 6% for urgent CD >50% of the time ($P < 0.01$ for both comparisons). PO fluid intake was allowed in 91% of patients in the ERAS group within 12 h of delivery, compared to 31% of the non-ERAS group ($P < 0.01$). Thirty-six percentage of ERAS group patients were discharged within 3 days of delivery, vs. none in the non-ERAS group, and no patient stayed after 6 days in the ERAS group compared to 20% in the non-ERAS group ($P < 0.01$). Hospitals in the ERAS group had significantly more deliveries and more patients walked on the day of their CD in the non-ERAS vs. the ERAS group.

TABLE 3 | Survey items with differing responses from institutions with and without ERAS protocols.

Item	Overall	ERAS protocol	No ERAS protocol	*P* value
1. NA for scheduled CD				<0.01
<10%	17 (39%)	1 (9%)	16 (49%)	
10–29%	13 (29%)	2 (18%)	11 (33%)	
30–49%	6 (14%)	3 (27%)	3 (9%)	
>50%	8 (18%)	5 (46%)	3 (9%)	
2. NA for urgent CD				<0.01
<10%	28 (62%)	2 (18%)	26 (77%)	
10–29%	8 (18%)	3 (27%)	5 (14%)	
30–49%	3 (7%)	2 (18%)	1 (3%)	
>50%	6 (13%)	4 (36%)	2 (6%)	
3. First ambulation				0.04
Day of CD	24 (53%)	3 (27%)	21 (62%)	
First post-operative day	20 (44%)	7 (64%)	13 (38%)	
Second post-operative day	1 (2%)	1 (9%)	0	
4. First PO fluids				<0.01
Immediately after CD	6 (13%)	2 (18%)	4 (11%)	
12 h after CD	15 (33%)	8 (73%)	7 (20%)	
24 h after CD	23 (50%)	1 (9%)	22 (63%)	
48 h after CD	2 (4%)	0	2 (6%)	
5. Number of deliveries				0.04
<500	28 (61%)	5 (46%)	23 (66%)	
501–1,000	12 (26%)	2 (18%)	10 (28%)	
>1,000	6 (13%)	4 (36%)	2 (6%)	
6. Days to discharge after CD				<0.01
<3 days	4 (9%)	4 (36%)	0	
3–6 days	35 (76%)	7 (64%)	28 (80%)	
>6 days	7 (15%)	0	7 (20%)	

P-values calculated using the Pearson Chi square test.
CD, cesarean delivery; NA, neuraxial anesthesia; h, hours; ERAS, enhanced recovery after surgery.

DISCUSSION

This is the first survey of ERAS use in obstetrics in a middle-income country. In Serbian hospitals, patients are not encouraged to eat solid food early after surgery, early mobilization is not encouraged, and a bowel preparation is mandatory in almost all hospitals. There is also a low percentage of NA for CD and a low rate of neuraxial narcotics use.

The low rate of skin-to-skin contact during CD may be due to a low rate of NA use and may interfere with successful breast feeding. Lack of successful breastfeeding is among those factors that have been associated with longer lengths of stay after CD in the UK (16).

A quarter of hospitals in Serbia reported having adopted ERAS protocols. A similar type survey conducted in the UK by Aluri and Wrench, showed that only 10 of 158 labor units in the UK were specifically following one (22). Despite this larger reported use, many elements in the ERAS protocols implemented elsewhere have not been routinely adopted by hospitals in Serbia. Most hospitals, both those with ERAS and those without ERAS, admit patients the night before elective CD, use a bowel preparation, do not allow oral intake up until a few hours before the procedure, do not routinely remove urinary catheters on the day of operation, do not monitor perioperative maternal temperature, and do not engage in active measures to avoid maternal hypothermia. These are practices that differ from hospitals outside Serbia that report using ERAS protocols. Although use of maternal temperature monitoring is routine in less than half of labor and delivery units in the UK, use of the other ERAS elements appears widespread among patients who undergo CD (21, 22).

In 2012, Abel et al. reported on a 2-month use of ERAS protocols for CD and compared two groups of 60 parturients who followed ERAS and non-ERAS pathways (19). Drinking in the recovery room was encouraged and patients were fed and mobilized early. The length of stay (LOS) decreased from 3.3 to 2.1 days, and the readmission rate was reduced from 8.3% to 3.3%. They showed that most of the patients in the ERAS group (97.8%) were satisfied and would recommend ERAS to others undergoing CD or would choose it for themselves in the future. We do not know if patient acceptance would be similar in Serbian mothers as we did not include measures of patient satisfaction in our survey.

Wrench et al. reported initiation of an ERAS for elective CD in 2012 and noted a decrease in LOS and patient satisfaction. Over 2 years, the maternal discharge rate on Day 1 increased from 1.6 to 25.2% (16). In Serbian hospitals, mothers are almost never discharged after CD on postoperative days 1 or 2, although many mothers express the desire to do so. Wrench et al. reported initiation of an ERAS for elective CD in 2012 and noted a decrease in LOS and patient satisfaction. Over 2 years, the maternal discharge rate on Day 1 increased from 1.6 to 25.2% (16). In Serbian hospitals, mothers are almost never discharged after CD on postoperative days 1 or 2, although many mothers express the desire to do so. One reason may be that the cost to the patient of in hospital care is low and patients may not feel an economic incentive to leave. Hospital administrators may also have little economic incentive to do so either. Finally, robust follow-up after patients are discharged may be necessary for patients discharged sooner after CD and the out of facility Serbian health-care system may not be able to assist parturients who are discharged home early.

We showed that Serbian hospitals that report ERAS use discharge patients home earlier than in non-ERAS groups. However, many ERAS hospitals reported a high number of discharges after 3 days compared to surveys of UK hospitals that show that a majority of women are eager go home and are discharged within 2 days of their CD. The elements of an ERAS program that are most associated with a greater chance for early discharge have not been determined. Although we showed that few elements of ERAS protocols reported elsewhere are routinely used in Serbian hospitals, adoption of an ERAS protocol lead to earlier patient discharges. We suggest that the adoption of an ERAS protocol leads to a greater effort on part of hospital staff and patients to achieve earlier maternal discharge, independent of the elements within the protocol. This change in organization and the re-setting of both staff and patient expectations may be the most important reason for reducing hospital stay, as has been suggested by others (12).

The lower rate of early ambulation in the ERAS group vs. the non-ERAS group may reflect the greater use of NA in the ERAS group. Practitioners in Serbia may discourage ambulation in patients for fear of post dural puncture headache (PDPH) after NA, despite substantial work that suggests that the rate of PDPH after NA is not influenced by patient activity.

The cost benefits of ERAS adoption for CD may be considerable. Pilkington et al. (16) reported a possible reduction of 200,000 euros in hospital expenses after implementation of ERAS protocol for CD in their hospital.

All patients may not be suitable candidates for ERAS. The factors suggesting which patients would benefit most from ERAS protocols have not been determined. However, Lucas and Gough suggested that a successful ERAS implementation for CD requires at a minimum good patient education, good in-hospital care, and good community out-of-hospital care for early discharged mothers and babies. Coates et al. showed how implementation of an ERAS program increased maternal satisfaction, primarily by increasing the number of earlier discharges (22). They also noted that a significant improvement in neonatal assessment and early determination of a neonate's status was essential for safe early discharge of both mother and child.

Our survey study has many limitations. As noted earlier, we did not survey for patient satisfaction, which would help in deciding if ERAS protocol introduction would be appropriate. We asked either the Chief of Obstetrics or Chief of Anesthesiology to complete the survey and there may be differences between groups of respondents, although follow-up to ensure understanding of the elements of the survey tool by author BP was rigorous and should have removed this bias. We did not ask the respondents about what barriers prevent the adoption of ERAS protocols, and thus using our data to affect change only identifies those elements for improvement, not how best to implement them. We asked many questions to help to describe perioperative CD care. This may have lead to our finding differences between ERAS and non-ERAS groups that may not be real. Finally, the elements of ERAS protocols which lead to improved maternal and neonatal outcomes have not been determined.

We found that hospitals that have adopted ERAS protocols discharge patients earlier than those that have not, although they do not use many of the elements reported from the UK. We simply do not know which elements are the most important. Patient education and institutional culture change may be the vital change needed. We suggest that setting the patient's expectation that they would be discharged home early and setting staff expectations for the same may be more important than other factors in determining time to discharge after CD; we cannot determine this from our study.

CONCLUSION

Enhanced recovery after surgery protocols are in use at some Serbian hospitals for surgical procedures (mostly colorectal procedures), and some report the use of some elements of ERAS protocols for have CD as well. The results showed uncommon use of antibiotic prophylaxis prior to skin incision but routine use of DVT prophylaxis, earlier oral intake, and earlier discharge from the hospital post CD compared to hospitals not reporting ERAS use. Successful ERAS protocol implementation for CD in Serbian hospitals will require the great efforts of a multidisciplinary medical staff team and the outside community.

AUTHOR CONTRIBUTIONS

BP, MK, MS, YS, and CB all made substantial contributions to the conceptual design of the work, in acquiring the data, and in its analysis. All helped draft the work and revised it critically. All the authors approved this copy for publication. All agreed to be accountable for all aspects of the work in ensuring its accuracy and integrity.

REFERENCES

1. Wilmore D, Kehlet H. Management of patients in fast track surgery. *BMJ* (2001) 322:473. doi:10.1136/bmj.322.7284.473
2. Fearona KC, Ljungqvist O, Von Meyenfeldt M, Revhaug A, Dejong CH, Lassen K, et al. Enhanced recovery after surgery: a consensus review of clinical care for patients undergoing colonic resection. *Clin Nutr* (2005) 24:466–447. doi:10.1016/j.clnu.2005.02.002
3. Kehlet H, Wilmore DW. Evidence-based surgical care and the evolution of fast-track surgery. *Ann Surg* (2008) 248(2):189. doi:10.1097/SLA.0b013e31817f2c1a
4. Ljungqvist O, Scott M, Fearon KC. Enhanced recovery after surgery: a review. *JAMA Surg* (2017) 152:292–8. doi:10.1001/jamasurg.2016.4952
5. Nygren J, Thacker J, Carli F, Fearon KC, Norderval S, Lobo DN, et al. Guidelines for perioperative care in elective rectal/pelvic surgery: enhanced recovery after surgery (ERAS) society recommendations. *World J Surg* (2013) 37:285–305. doi:10.1007/s00268-012-1787-6
6. Lassen K, Coolsen MM, Slim K, Carli F, de Aguilar-Nascimento JE, Schäfer M, et al. Guidelines for perioperative care for pancreaticoduodenectomy: enhanced recovery after surgery (ERAS®) society recommendations. *World J Surg* (2013) 37:240–58. doi:10.1007/s00268-012-1771-1
7. Cerantola Y, Valerio M, Persson B, Jichlinski P, Ljungqvist O, Hubner M, et al. Guidelines for perioperative care after radical cystectomy for bladder cancer: enhanced recovery after surgery (ERAS®) society recommendations. *Clin Nutr* (2013) 32:879–87. doi:10.1016/j.clnu.2013.09.014
8. Nelson G, Altman AD, Nick A, Meyer LA, Ramirez PT, Achtari C, et al. Guidelines for pre- and intra-operative care in gynecologic/oncology surgery: enhanced recovery after surgery (ERAS®) society recommendations – part I. *Gynecol Oncol* (2016) 140(2):313–22. doi:10.1016/j.ygyno.2015.11.015
9. Wang C, Zheng G, Zhang W, Zhang F, Lv S, Wang A, et al. Enhanced recovery after surgery programs for liver resection: a meta-analysis. *J Gastrointest Surg* (2017) 21(3):472–448. doi:10.1007/s11605-017-3360-y
10. Spanjersberg WR, Reurings J, Keus F, van Laarhoven CJ. Fast track surgery versus conventional recovery strategies for colorectal surgery. *Cochrane Database Syst Rev* (2011) 16(2):CD0077635. doi:10.1002/14651858.CD007635.pub2
11. Paton F, Chambers D, Wilson P, Eastwood A, Craig D, Fox D, et al. Initiatives to reduce the length of stay in acute hospital settings: a rapid synthesis of evidence relating to enhanced recovery programmes. *Health Serv Delivery Res* (2014) 2(21):434–75. doi:10.3310/hsdr02210
12. Maessen J, Dejong CH, Hausel J, Nygren J, Lassen K, Andersen J, et al. A protocol is not enough to implement an enhanced recovery program for colorectal resection. *Br J Surg* (2007) 94(2):224–31. doi:10.1002/bjs.5468
13. Corso E, Hind D, Beever D, Fuller G, Wilson M, Wrench IJ, et al. Enhanced recovery after elective caesarean: a rapid review of clinical protocols, and an umbrella review of systematic reviews. *BMC Pregnancy Childbirth* (2017) 17:91–100. doi:10.1186/s12884-017-1265-0

14. National Institute for Health and Care Excellence. *Clinical Guideline 132: Caesarean Section*. (2017). Available from: https://www.nice.org.uk/guidance/cg132/evidence (Accessed: April, 2018).
15. Chiong TP, Jin NM, Zawiah OS. Hospital discharge on the first compared with the second day after a planned cesarean delivery. *Obstet Gynecol* (2012) 120:1273–82. doi:10.1097/AOG.0b013e3182723a95
16. Wrench IJ, Allison A, Galimberti A, Radley S, Wilson MJ. Introduction of enhanced recovery for elective caesarean section enabling next day discharge: a tertiary centre experience. *Int J Obstet Anesth* (2015) 24(2):124–30. doi:10.1016/j.ijoa.2015.01.003
17. Lucas DN, Gough KL. Enhanced recovery in obstetrics – a new frontier? *Int J Obstet Anesth* (2013) 22:92–5. doi:10.1016/j.ijoa.2013.08.001
18. Vickers R, Das B. Enhanced recovery in obstetrics. *Int J Obstet Anesth* (2013) 22:349. doi:10.1016/j.ijoa.2013.05.011
19. Abell D, Long O, Skelton V, Penna L, Dasan J, Sharafudeen S. Enhanced recovery in obstetrics. *Int J Obstet Anesth* (2013) 22:349–50. doi:10.1016/j.ijoa.2013.05.001
20. Pilkington L, Curpad S, Parveen S. Enhanced recovery after surgery (ERAS) in obstetrics in Royal Gwent Hospital. *Eur J Obstet Gynecol Reprod Biol* (2016) 206:e92. doi:10.1016/j.ejogrb.2016.07.247
21. Coates E, Fuller G, Hind D, Wrench IJ, Wilson MJ, Stephens T. Enhanced recovery pathway for elective caesarean section. *Int J Obstet Anesth* (2016) 27:94–5. doi:10.1016/j.ijoa.2016.05.005
22. Aluri S, Wrench IJ. Enhanced recovery from obstetric surgery: a UK survey of practice. *Int J Obstet Anesth* (2014) 23(2):157–60. doi:10.1016/j.ijoa.2013.11.006

5

Endoscopic Endonasal Supraoptic and Infraoptic Approaches for Complex "Parasuprasellar" Lesions: Surgical Anatomy, Technique Nuances and Case Series

YouYuan Bao[†], YouQing Yang[†], Lin Zhou[†], ShenHao Xie, Xiao Wu, Han Ding, Jie Wu, Limin Xiao, Le Yang, Bin Tang and Tao Hong[*]

Department of Neurosurgery, The First Affiliated Hospital of Nanchang University, Nanchang, China

Correspondence:
Tao Hong
ht2000@vip.sina.com

[†]These authors have contributed equally to this work

Objective: The surgical management of lesions involving the lateral area of the suprasellar region, including the lateral aspect of the planum sphenoidale and the tight junction region of the optic canal (OC), anterior clinoid process (ACP), and internal carotid artery (ICA) and its dural rings, is extremely challenging. Here, these regions, namely, the "parasuprasellar" area, are described from the endonasal perspective. Moreover, the authors introduce two novels endoscopic endonasal supraoptic (EESO) and endoscopic endonasal infraoptic (EEIO) approaches to access the parasuprasellar area.

Methods: Surgical simulation of the EESO and EEIO approaches to the parasuprasellar area was conducted in 5 silicon-injected specimens. The same techniques were applied in 12 patients with lesions involving the parasuprasellar area.

Results: The EESO approach provided excellent surgical access to the lateral region of the planum sphenoidale, which corresponds to the orbital gyrus of the frontal lobe. With stepwise bone (OC, optic strut and ACP) removal, dissociation of the ophthalmic artery (OA) and optic nerve (ON), the EEIO approach enables access to the lateral region of the supraclinoidal ICA. These approaches can be used independently or in combination, but are more often employed as a complement to the endoscopic endonasal midline and transcavernous approaches. In clinical application, the EESO and EEIO approaches were successfully performed in 12 patients harboring tumors as well as multiple aneurysms involving the parasuprasellar area. Gross total and subtotal tumor resection were achieved in 9 patients and 1 patient, respectively. For two patients with multiple aneurysms, the lesions were clipped selectively according to location and size. Visual acuity improved in 7 patients, remained stable in 4, and deteriorated in only 1. No postoperative intracranial infection or ICA injury occurred in this series.

Conclusions: The EESO and EEIO approaches offer original treatment options for well-selected lesions involving the parasuprasellar area. They can be combined with the endoscopic endonasal midline and transcavernous approaches to remove extensive pathologies involving the intrasellar, suprasellar, sphenoid, and cavernous sinuses and even the bifurcation of the ICA. This work for the first time pushes the boundary of the endoscopic endonasal approach lateral to the supraclinoidal ICA and ON.

Keywords: endoscopic endonasal approach, parasuprasellar area, anterior clinoid process, optic canal, internal carotid artery, surgical technique

INTRODUCTION

With advances in surgical anatomy and endoscopic technology, the endoscopic endonasal approach (EEA) has been widely applied for ventral skull base lesions over the last several decades (1–3). Furthermore, this approach has been expanded to the lateral skull base, accompanied by the introduction of endoscopic transpterygoid route, such as the cavernous sinus (CS), pterygopalatine fossa and infratemporal fossa (4–9). The anatomy and related surgical nuances of these complex skull base areas have been well documented in a considerable amount of literature. Nevertheless, few reports exist on the detailed anatomy of the lateral area of the suprasellar region, including the lateral aspect of the planum sphenoidale and the tight junction region of the optic canal (OC), the anterior clinoid process (ACP), and the internal carotid artery (ICA) and its dural rings that fix its course (10, 11). There are essentially two reasons for such limited data: 1) limited access to these regions due to obstruction of vital neurovascular structures such as the optic nerve (ON) and ICA; 2) consideration of these regions as off-limits due to the lateral-seated location and intrinsic anatomical complexity. In fact, it is difficult to imagine the existence of such a high density of neurovascular and osseous as well as dural structures in such a narrow anatomical space.

Although not common, some different pathologies can afflict these regions, including primary lesions, such as ACP meningiomas and paraclinoid aneurysms, but more secondary tumors spread, such as tuberculum sellae meningiomas, invasive pituitary adenomas and craniopharyngiomas, from nearby regions. Pathologies encountered in these areas are typically intra- and extracranially. Moreover, these lesions tend to displace the ON from above and/or below, erode osseous and dural structures, and even encase the ICA and its bifurcation. Therefore, effective resection of these lesions poses a considerable challenge, even for skilled and experienced neurosurgeons.

Several traditional transcranial approaches (TCAs), including the standard or extended pterional approach (12, 13), orbital-zygomatic approach (14) and supraorbital approach (15), for accessing lesions in these areas have been described. Although TCAs can be good alternatives for subdural lesions, extradural lesions involving the intrasellar, sphenoid sinus and even CS are extremely difficult to manage because surgical corridors are inconsistent with the axis of tumor growth. In addition, inevitable brain retraction, extensive bone removal, and easy damage to important neurovascular elements make TCAs less favorable options.

In contrast, the EEA provides a direct corridor to access extradural lesions, with the advantage of easy removal of extensively involved osseous architectures and dural attachments. Additionally, a corridor to the subdural lesion is established when the lesion is removed. Most importantly, EEA allows for early identification and control of the paraclinoidal ICA, which is the main structure that must be crossed to expand laterally into these regions. These advantages are particularly promising for treating lesions involving these areas. Nevertheless, there are few reports regarding the endoscopic anatomy and how to effectively manage lesions involved these areas (10, 11).

For this reason, we sought to undertake a thorough anatomical description of the lateral aspect of the planum sphenoidale and the tight junction region of the OC, ACP, and ICA and its dural rings. These regions are located in the lateral area of the suprasellar region, the "parasuprasellar" area. Building on our detailed dissection, we introduce two novels endoscopic endonasal supraoptic (EESO) and endoscopic endonasal infraoptic (EEIO) approaches to access the parasuprasellar area. Indications and nuances of these approaches in treating 12 patients with tumors and aneurysms involving this area are also presented.

METHODS

Anatomical Dissection

Five embalmed and injected adult cadaveric heads were used for endoscopic and microsurgical dissection. The anatomy research was approved by our institutional ethics committee. Endoscopic endonasal anatomical dissections were performed using rod lens endoscopes (4-mm diameter, 18-cm length, 0° and 30°, Karl Storz). An extended EEA to the sella, parasellar and suprasellar areas, involving wide sphenoidotomy, posterior ethmoidectomy, and posterior septectomy, followed by a transpterygoid approach, was performed for all cadaveric heads in a stepwise manner, as previously described (2, 3, 16). All intrasphenoidal landmarks were exposed, including the sella, tuberculum sellae, optic protuberances, carotid protuberances, medial opticocarotid recesses (MOCRs) and lateral opticocarotid recesses (LOCRs). The posterior ethmoidal artery (PEA) was also skeletonized.

We defined the parasuprasellar area as a quadrangular space, and its main contents included the ON, the ICA and its proximal and distal dural rings, the ophthalmic artery (OA), and the ACP. The PEA is defined as the upper boundary of the parasuprasellar area. The inferior boundary is formed by the horizontal connection between the inferior edge of the LOCR and MOCR. The medial boundary is the vertical connection between the medial edge of the MOCR and the PEA, and the lateral boundary is the vertical connection between the lateral edge of the LOCR and the PEA. In addition, we divided the parasuprasellar area into 2 compartments based upon the ON: supraoptic and infraoptic compartments (**Figure 1A**). The EESO and EEIO approaches were performed to access the supraoptic and infraoptic regions, respectively.

Particular attention should be paid to the anatomy of the parasuprasellar area and its vicinity from an endoscopic perspective as well as to the stepwise surgical techniques related to the safe dissociation of the ON and OA. After completing the endonasal procedures, the extent of bone and dural removal from the parasuprasellar area was further evaluated from the intracranial superior view (**Figures 1E,F**). Several anatomical parameter measurements were also measured and recorded.

Patient Population

From January 2016 to March 2020, we retrospectively reviewed 12 patients with lesions invading the parasuprasellar area and for whom the EESO and EEIO approaches were performed either alone or in combination. T1/T2WI and Gd-enhanced T1WI were performed in 10 patients with tumors, and contrast-enhanced postoperative MRI was performed as follow-up on postoperative day 1 and at 3 months after surgery. The remaining two patients with multiple aneurysms underwent pre- and postoperative cerebrovascular examinations, including CT angiography and digital subtraction angiography (DSA). All patients also underwent preoperative thin-slice CT scans to evaluate the extent of OC and ACP involvement. Preoperative BOT was performed to evaluate whether collateral circulation could be compensated; if poor, an endovascular stent or bypass

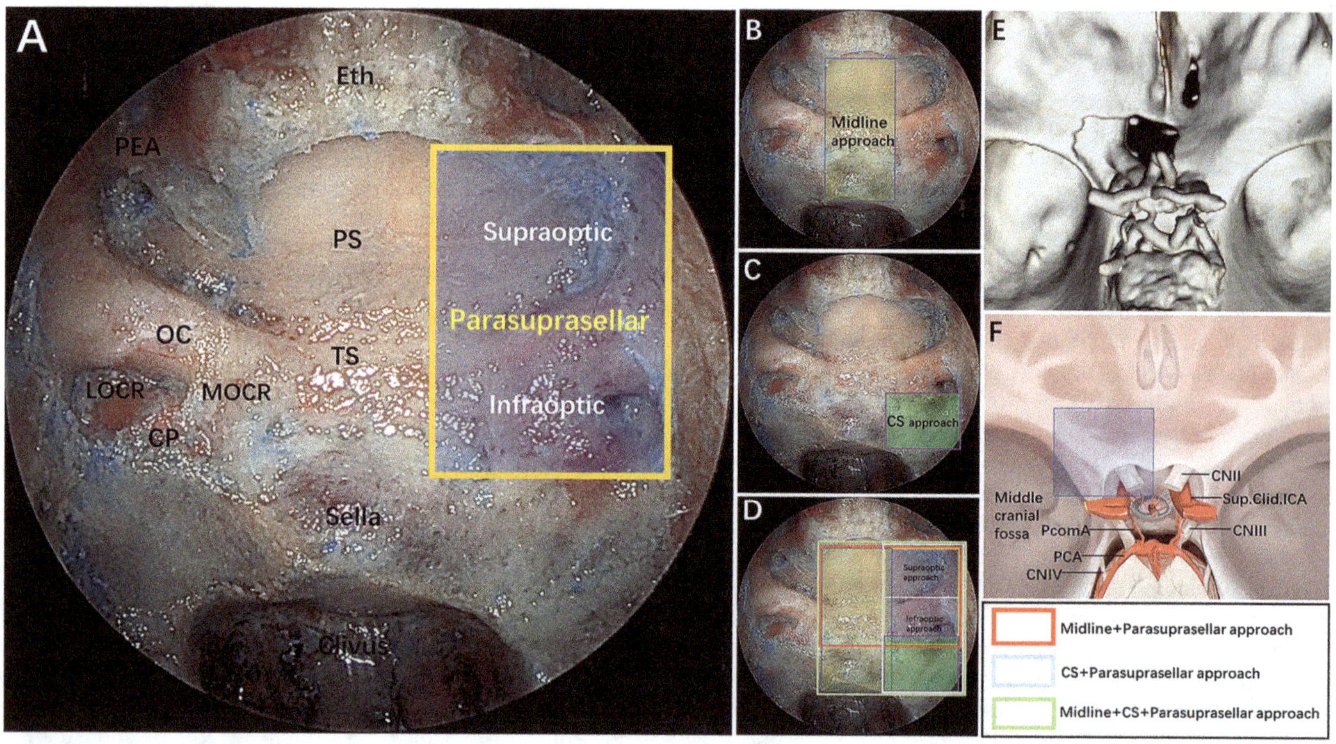

FIGURE 1 | **(A)** Endoscopic endonasal view of our proposed parasuprasellar area and its surrounding essential anatomical structures. The parasuprasellar area is delineated by the yellow quadrangular space, which is limited medially by the medial edge of the MOCR, laterally by the lateral edge of the LOCR, superiorly by the PEA, and inferiorly by the inferior edge of the MOCR and LOCR. In addition, as bounded by the optic nerve, it can be divided into supraoptic and infraoptic regions. **(B–D)** Illustration showing different combinations of surgical modules in both midline (transsellar/transtuberculum/transplanum approach) and/or lateral (transcavernous and parasuprasellar approach) planes. Note that the parasuprasellar approach includes supraoptic and infraoptic approaches. The various combinations of endoscopic corridors are indicated with different quadrangular colors (figure in the lower right corner). Red marks the combination of the endoscopic endonasal midline approach and parasuprasellar approach; blue represents the combination of the transcavernous approach and parasuprasellar approach; green shows the combination of the midline approach, transcavernous approach and parasuprasellar approach. **(E)** Three-dimensional (3D) reconstruction of a postoperative fine-slice CT scan showing the extent of bone removal through the supraoptic and infraoptic approaches. **(F)** Artistic illustration demonstrating maximum bone removal (blue square) in the parasuprasellar area *via* the supraoptic and infraoptic approach. Eth, cribriform plate of the ethmoid; PEA, posterior ethmoidal artery; PS, planum sphenoidale; OC, optic canal; TS, tuberculum sellae; MOCR, medial optocarotid recess; LOCR, lateral optocarotid recess; CP, carotid protuberance; CS, cavernous sinus; CN II, optic nerve; CN III, oculomotor nerve; CN IV, trochlear nerve; PcomA, posterior communication artery; Sup.Clid. ICA, supraclinoidal internal carotid artery; PCA, posterior cerebral artery. The figure is available in color only online.

would be prepared. Intraoperative electrophysiological monitoring, particularly visual evoked potentials (VEP), was used routinely throughout the procedure. Intraoperative neuronavigation and Doppler ultrasound were also applied to determine the exact course of the ICA. Additionally, the paraclival ICA was exposed in advance for proximal control. Special attention was given to the ophthalmological evaluation, including visual acuity and visual field, and limitations of ocular motility were observed by an ophthalmologist for all patients preoperatively and 3 to 6 months postoperatively. All medical records, including symptoms, neuroimaging, intraoperative videos, technical nuances, and surgical outcomes, were reviewed and analyzed retrospectively (**Table 1**).

RESULTS

EESO Approach to the Supraoptic Region

Stage 1: Recognition and Exposure of the Supraoptic Recess

After undergoing an initial extended EEA, the PEA located in its osseous canal is identified and serves as the upper boundary of the supraoptic region; the artery can be ligated and transected to facilitate lateral mobilization. The supraoptic recess is pyramid-shaped, with its base abutting the sphenoid sinus and apex corresponding intracranially to the body of the lesser sphenoid wing (**Figure 2A**) (11). The supraoptic recess needs to be identified and sufficiently delineated because its removal is one of the key steps to achieve further lateral extension over the planum sphenoidale.

Stage 2: Removal of the Medial Portion of the Lesser Sphenoid Wing and OC Unroofing

During this stage, the base of the supraoptic recess is drilled with a small diamond burr, proceeding deeply in a medial-to-lateral direction toward the body of the lesser sphenoid wing. As a consequence, the most medial portion of the lesser sphenoid wing overlying the orbit is exposed and progressively drilled out. However, removal of the lateral portion of the lesser sphenoid wing is limited inferiorly by the intracanalicular portion of the ON and the superior aspect of the medial orbital walls, which serves as the main anatomical landmark of the superolateral boundary of this exposure (**Figure 2B**). Afterward, the roof wall of the OC is drilled.

Stage 3: Resection of the Lateral Dura of the Planum Sphenoidale and Exposure of the Orbital Gyrus

The dura mater of the planum sphenoidale is opened in a posterior-to-anterior direction, after which the gyrus rectus of the frontal lobe and the olfactory nerve are visible at this level. The residual lateral part of the dura mater of the planum sphenoidale can be safely removed using an outward-facing Kerrison rongeur. This maneuver permits visualization of the medial orbital gyrus, anterior orbital gyrus and post orbital gyrus of the frontal lobe (**Figures 2C,D**). At this time, the distance from the lateral edge of the olfactory nerve to the outermost edge of the orbital gyrus is measured with a ruler (**Table 2**).

EEIO Approach to the Infraoptic Region

Stage 1: Removal of the Anterior Wall of the OC and Exposure of the Intracranial ON

After the bone of the anterior wall of the OC is removed in a medial-lateral direction up to the orbital apex, the dura overlying the intracranial ON is incised longitudinally to expose the origin of the OA (**Figures 3A–C**). Of note, the most common relationship of the origin of the OA to the intracranial ON is an inferomedial location; thus, opening the dura through a cut parallel to the ON in its upper half reduces the risk of damaging the artery (17, 18). To gain working space in the medial region of the paraclinoidal ICA, the diaphragm is incised toward the medial part of the distal dural ring (DDR). Following this, intradural exploration of the main neurovascular structures is performed. The pituitary stalk, superior hypophyseal artery (SHA) and its branches are exposed by gently lifting the ipsilateral ON (**Figure 3C**). Sliding deeper, the posterior communicating artery (PcomA) and the A1 segment of the anterior cerebral artery are identified using the space between the SHA and the ON (**Figure 3D**).

Stage 2: Drilling of the Optic Strut and Dissociation of the OA

Surgery in the lateral compartment of the paraclinoidal ICA requires removal of the optic strut, which corresponds to the LOCR from the endonasal perspective (19). Three vertices of this recess (resembling a triangle in shape) are identified: the superomedial, superolateral, and inferior vertices. The distance between each vertex of the LOCR is measured (**Table 2**). With regard to safe removal of the three vertices in turn to the base of the ACP, we have specifically discussed the relevant anatomical details and surgical nuances in a previous publication (20). Once drilling of the optic strut is concluded (**Figure 3E**), the DDR is opened to further safely dissociate the OA. Next, proper exposure of the ON and OA surrounded by the dural sheath is performed. At this stage, the courses of the precanalicular ON and OA are entirely exposed (**Figure 3F**). This maneuver aims to separate the ON from the OA, thus widening the surgical corridor of the infraoptic approach. The main structures are identified, including the PcomA, the anterior choroidal artery and its branches into the anterior perforating substance, the oculomotor nerve passing between the posterior cerebral artery and superior cerebellar artery into the CS, and the bifurcation of the ICA (**Figures 3G, H**).

Stage 3: Removal of the ACP and Severing of the OA

The ACP is now only connected to part of the lesser sphenoid wing. By using this ACP triangle space and following gentle medial mobilization of the paraclinoidal ICA, drilling and curettage of the base and tip of the ACP becomes feasible (**Figures 3I,J**). However, this step is performed with extreme care to avoid injury to the ICA, OA, ON and oculomotor nerve, and tailored bone drilling is strongly suggested according to disease-specific management. Once removal of the ACP tip is achieved, the dura of the inferior surface of the ACP is incised with angled scissors or coagulated. At this moment, the sylvian cistern is visible, and M1 is exposed between the frontal and temporal lobes; more laterally, the middle cerebral artery

TABLE 1 | Summary characteristics and outcomes of all 12 clinical cases.

Case No.	Age/Sex	Size(cm)	Diagnosis	Preop		Other Symptoms	ICA, ACA, MCA Involvement	Previous Treatment	Surgical Approach	Anterior Clinoidectomy	EOR	Postop		Complications	Follow-Up (months)
				Visual Acuity	Visual Field							Visual Acuity	Visual Field		
1	56/F	2.1×1.9×1.7	Lt ACP meningioma	Visual loss (lt)	Upper hemianopsia	Dizzy	No	None	TPA+SOA	No	GTR	Improvement	Normal	None	56
2	25/F	2.5×1.9×1.4	Rt ACP meningioma	Visual loss (rt)	Rt temporal hemianopsia	Headache	Yes, all attached	Pterional approach	TMA*+IOA	Yes	GTR	Worse (rt), unchanged (lt)	Rt temporal hemianopsia	None	50
3	56/F	2.1×1.8×1.7	Lt ACP meningioma	Normal	Normal	Dizzy	Yes, all attached	None	TMA+SOA +IOA	No	GTR	Stable	Normal	None	36
4	37/F	3.0×1.7×1.4	Lt ACP meningioma	Visual loss (lt)	Lt temporal hemianopsia	None	Yes, all encased	Pterional approach	TMA+TPA +TCA +SOA +IOA	Yes	STR	Stable	Lt temporal hemianopsia	CNIII pasly	45
5	12/M	2.8×3.1×3.9	Osteogenic meningioma	Visual loss	Lt amaurosis	None	No	None	TMA+TPA +SOA +IOA	Yes	GTR	Marked improvement	Lt temporal hemianopsia	Transient DI	18
6	45/F	3.7×4.0×3.9	Pituitary adenoma	Visual loss	Lt temporal hemianopsia	Headache	Yes, ICA and ACA encased	None	TMA+TPA +TCA +SOA +IOA	No	GTR	Stable	Lt temporal hemianopsia	CSF leak	30
7	52/F	3.5×2.7×2.9	Pituitary adenoma	Visual loss	Rt temporal hemianopsia	None	Yes, ICA encased, ACA and MCA attached	Endonasal endoscopic approach	TMA+TPA +TCA +SOA +IOA	Yes	GTR	Improvement	Normal	Panhypopituitarism Transient DI	22
8	56/M	4.5×2.7×3.0	Pituitary adenoma	Visual loss (rt)	Bitemporal hemianopsia	Headache, hypomnesis	Yes, ICA encased, ACA attached	Endonasal microscope approach	TMA+TPA +TCA +SOA +IOA	No	GTR	Marked Improvement	Normal	None	29
9	47/F	lt paraclinoid: 0.7×0.8 lt ophthalmic: 0.4×0.3 lt cav-ICA: 0.5×0.4	Multiple aneurysms: lt paraclinoid, lt ophthalmic, lt cav-ICA	Normal	Normal	Headache	NA	None	TMA+TPA +IOA	Yes	Clipping of lt paraclinoid, lt ophthalmic aneurysms	Stable	Normal	None	58
10	62/F	lt paraclinoid: 0.75×0.42 rt paraclinoid:2.26×2.17 Acom: 0.4×0.3	Multiple aneurysms: lt paraclinoid, rt paraclinoid, Acom	Visual loss	Normal	Dizzy	NA	None	TMA+IOA	No	Clipping of lt paraclinoid, Acom aneurysms	Marked improvement	Normal	None	44
11	30/M	2.3×2.2×1.9	Craniopharyngioma	Visual loss(rt)	Lower marginal field	None	Yes, all encased	Subfrontal approach, V-P shunting	TMA+SOA +IOA	No	GTR	Improvement	Rt hemianopsia	Hypothyroidism DI	26
12	37/F	1.8×1.4×1.0	Meningeal IgG4-related disease	Visual loss(rt)	Rt temporal hemianopsia	None	No	None	TMA+SOA +IOA	Yes	GTR	Improvement	Normal	CNIII pasly	52

*ICA, internal carotid artery; ACA, anterior cerebral artery; MCA, middle cerebral artery; EOR, extent of resection; ACP, anterior clinoid process; TPA, transpterygoid approach; TMA, transmidline approach;TCA, transcavernous approach; SOA, supraoptic approach; IOA, infraoptic approach; GTR, gross-total resection; STR, subtotal resection; DI, diabetes insipidus; NA, not applicable; Acom, anterior communicating;Cav-ICA=cavernous segment of ICA; * including endoscopic endonasal transsellar, transtuberculum, transplanumh and transclivus approaches.*

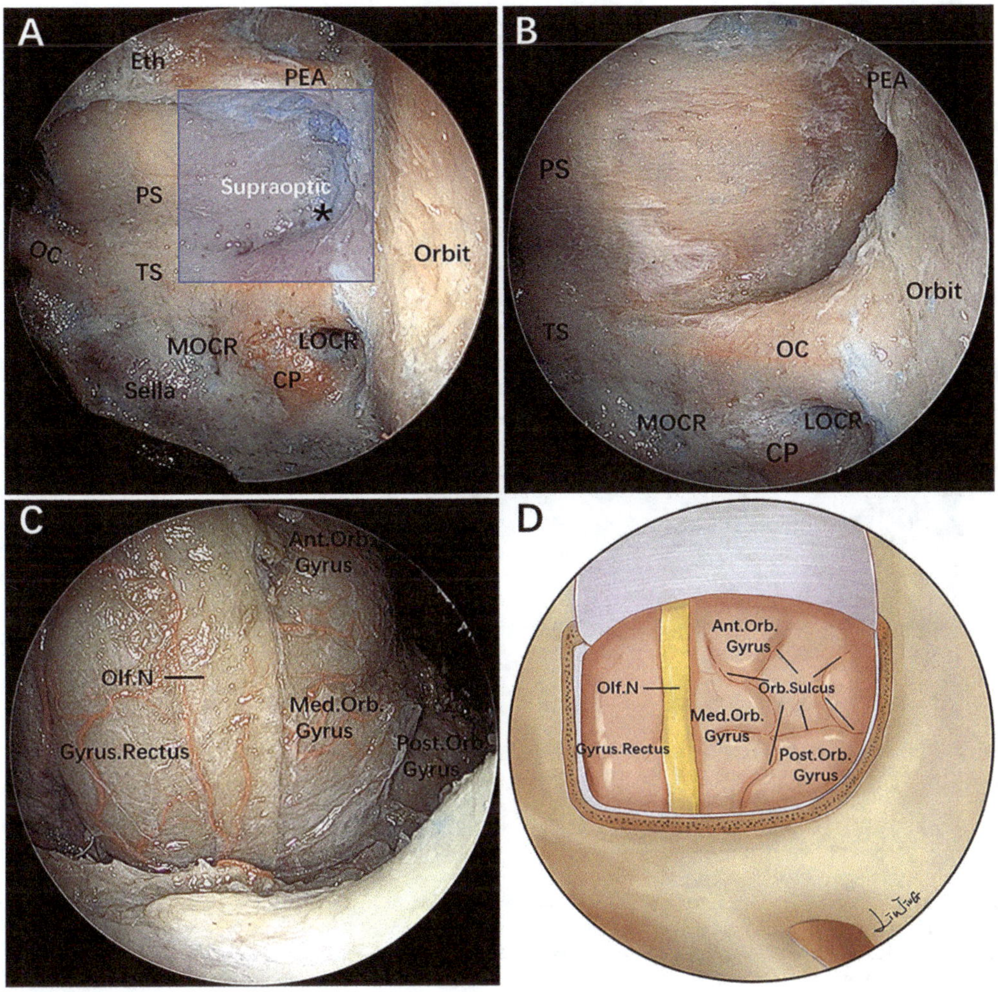

FIGURE 2 | Endoscopic endonasal supraoptic (EESO) approach: stepwise dissection to the supraoptic region in a colored silicone-injected cadaveric specimen. **(A)** Panoramic view of the sphenoid sinus floor with its anatomical landmarks. The blue quadrangular zone marks the supraoptic region, and the black asterisk represents the supraoptic recess. **(B)** A closer view of the supraoptic region after removal of the medial portion of the lesser sphenoid wing and OC unroofing. **(C)** After removing the bone and dura mater lateral to the planum sphenoidale, the gyrus rectus, olfactory nerve, medial orbital gyrus, anterior orbital gyrus and post orbital gyrus of the frontal lobes were exposed, viewed with a 0° endoscope. **(D)** Artistic illustration demonstrating the contents of the supraoptic region that can be reached *via* the EESO approach. Olf. N, olfactory nerve; Med.Orb. Gyrus, medial orbital gyrus; Ant.Orb. Gyrus, anterior orbital gyrus; Post.Orb. Gyrus, post orbital gyrus. The figure is available in color only online.

TABLE 2 | Relevant measurements.

Measurement	Mean ± SD, mm (right, n=5)	Mean ± SD, mm (left, n=5)	Mean ± SD, mm (total, n=10)
The length of the three sides of the ACP triangle:			
superomedial to superolateral vertices	4.30 ± 0.57	4.40 ± 0.65	4.35 ± 0.58
superomedial to inferior vertices	4.10 ± 0.55	4.20 ± 0.45	4.15 ± 0.47
superolateral to inferior vertices	3.80 ± 0.27	3.90 ± 0.42	3.85 ± 0.34
The lateral edge of the olfactory nerve to the outermost edge of the orbital gyrus	10.40 ± 0.65	10.30 ± 0.84	10.35 ± 0.71

bifurcation is observed at the level of its insular portion (**Figure 3K**). Some perforating vessels from M1 are also identified. Finally, the OA is transected, and the operating space of the infraoptic approach is further enlarged (**Figures 3L,M**).

Combined EESO and EEIO Approaches for the Parasuprasellar Area

After completing the above step-by-step dissection, combined EESO and EEIO approaches for accessing the parasuprasellar area were performed, as shown in **Figure 4**. It should be

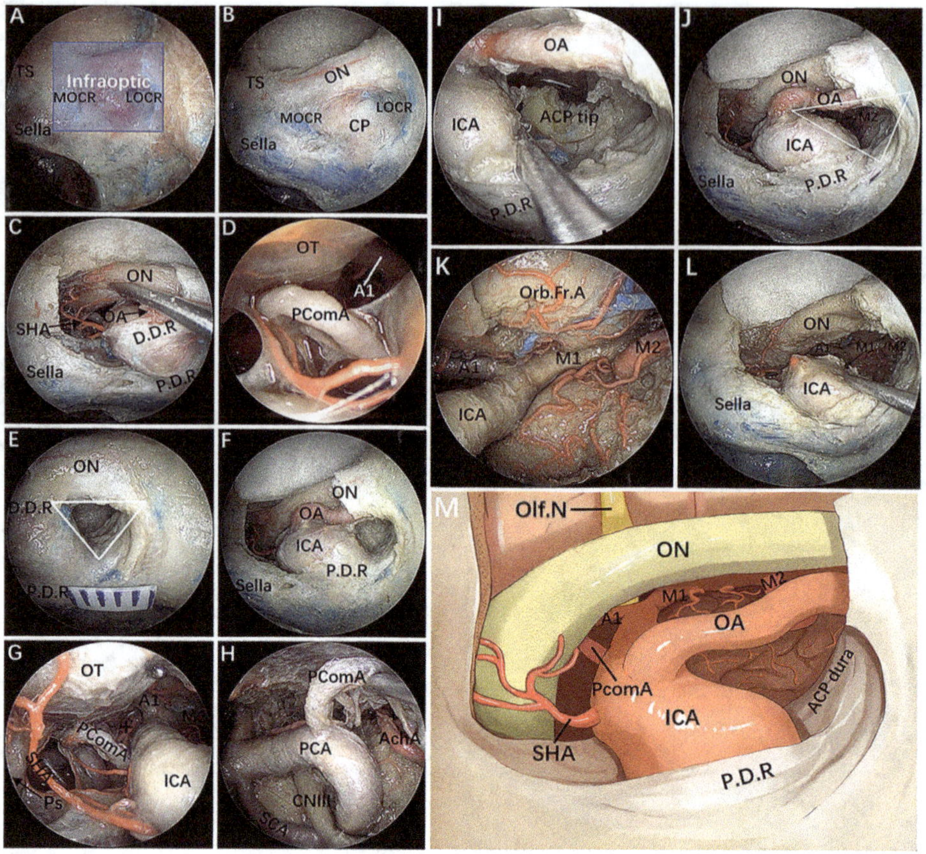

FIGURE 3 | Endoscopic endonasal infraraoptic (EEIO) approach: stepwise dissection to the infraoptic region in a colored silicone-injected cadaveric specimen. **(A)** The main anatomical landmarks in the infraoptic region (blue zone) are shown. **(B)** Removal of the anterior wall of the OC in a medial-lateral direction up the orbit apex. **(C)** The dura overlying the intracranial ON was incised longitudinally to expose the origin of the OA; the diaphragm was incised toward the medial part of the DDR, and SHA and its branches were exposed. **(D)** A closer view shows more subdural contents, including the PcomA, OT and A1 segments of the anterior cerebral artery. **(E)** Drilling of the optic strut and showing the ACP triangle. **(F)** The DDR and ON sheath are opened to further safely dissociate the OA and ON. **(G, H)** The subdural neurovascular structures were explored again by gently lifting of the ipsilateral ON. The main structures are identified, including the PcomA, pituitary stalk, AchA and its branches (black plus sign) into the anterior perforating substance in the crural cistern, the CNIII passing between the PCA and SCA into the cavernous sinus, and the bifurcation of the ICA. **(I)** The base and tip of the ACP can be further removed by gentle lifting of the OA or medial mobilization of the paraclinoidal ICA. **(J)** The ACP triangular is further enlarged. **(K)** The sylvian cistern was visible, and the ICA bifurcation was exposed between the frontal and temporal lobes; more laterally, the middle cerebral artery (MCA) bifurcation was observed at the level of its insular portion. **(L)** The OA was transected, and the operation space of the EEIO corridor was further enlarged. **(M)** Artistic illustration showing the main contents of the infraoptic region that can be reached *via* the EEIO approach. Note the ON has been slightly elevated. ON = optic nerve; OA = ophthalmic artery; SHA = superior hypophyseal artery; D.D.R, distal dural ring; P.D.R, proximal dural ring; ICA, internal carotid artery; OT, optic tract; AchA, anterior choroidal artery; SCA, superior cerebellar artery; Orb.Fr.A, orbital frontal artery; ACP, anterior clinoid process; M1, sphenoidal segment of the middle cerebral artery; M2, insular segment of the middle cerebral artery. The figure is available in color only online.

emphasized that the EESO and EEIO approaches can be used either alone or in combination; they can also be combined with the endoscopic endonasal midline approach (transsellar/transtuberculum/transplanum) and transcavernous approach according to the disease-specific location (**Figures 1B–D**).

EESO and EEIO Approaches: Case Series

The EESO and EEIO approaches were successfully performed either alone or in combination for 12 patients harboring tumors and aneurysms involving the parasuprasellar area (**Table 1**). The mean patient age was 42.9 years (range 12–62 years); there were 3 males and 9 females. The most common presenting symptom was visual deficit, including visual loss and visual field defects. Other symptoms were headache, dizziness, and hypomnesis. Three patients had previously undergone TCA, and 2 patients underwent an endonasal (microscope or endoscopic) approach at other institutions. The final diagnoses were meningiomas in 5 patients, pituitary adenoma in 3 patients, multiple aneurysms in 2 patients, and meningeal IgG4-related disease and craniopharyngioma in 1 patient each. Gross total tumor resection was achieved in 9 patients; subtotal resection was achieved in 1 patient. There were 2 patients with multiple aneurysms. One case of anterior communication and paraclinoid aneurysms were clipped *via* a pure EEIO approach; a contralateral giant paraclinoid aneurysm was secondarily

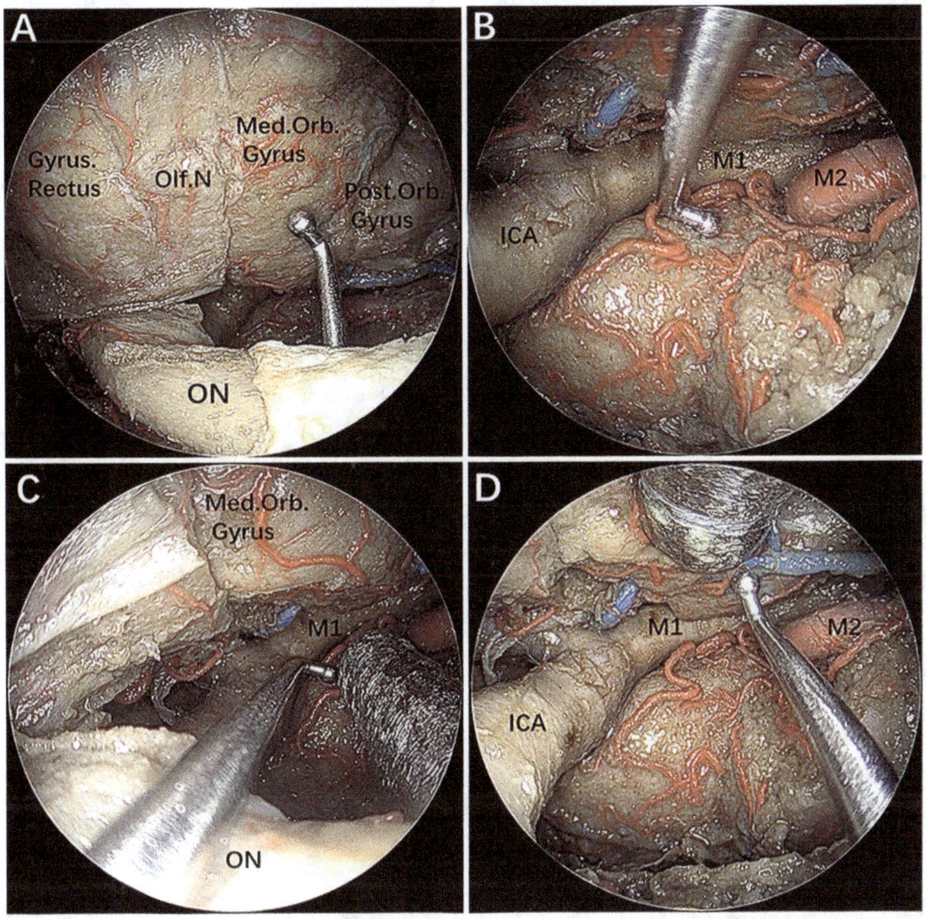

FIGURE 4 | (A–D) The instruments demonstrating a combined supraoptic and infraoptic approach to access the parasuprasellar area. The figure is available in color only online.

embolized at 2 months after the operation. The other patient harbored ophthalmic and paraclinoid aneurysms that were also clipped through the EEIO approach, although an intracavernous aneurysm was left untreated due to its location and size. Postoperative visual acuity improved in 7 patients, remained unchanged in 4 patients, and deteriorated in 1 patient in the right eye. The postoperative visual field was normal in 7 patients, whereas 5 still had unilateral temporal hemianopsia. Two patients experienced transient diabetes insipidus (DI), and 1 patient developed postoperative panhypopituitarism, which normalized by the 3-month follow-up. One patient experienced permanent DI and hypothyroidism, and postoperative hormone replacement therapy was required in the follow-up period. Postoperative cerebrospinal fluid (CSF) leakage occurred in 1 patient, and endoscopic endonasal repair was performed. Postoperative oculomotor nerve palsy developed in 2 patients; fortunately, it resolved completely in one patient by the 1-month follow-up, and significantly improved in the other patient by the 6-month follow-up. No postoperative intracranial infection or ICA injury occurred in this series.

DISCUSSION

Skull base pathologies encompassing the suprasellar lateral area, including the lateral aspect of the planum sphenoidale and the tight junction region of the OC, ACP, and ICA and its dural rings, still pose unique surgical challenges for neurosurgeons in terms of subsequent morbidity and gross total resection (10, 12, 20–22). These pathologies typically involve intra- and extracranially, tend to displace the ON from above and/or below, erode osseous and dural structures, and even involve the ICA bifurcation. Hence, TCAs for complete resection of these lesions have a high potential morbidity, even for skilled and experienced neurosurgeons. Today, endoscopy, which offers a wider, close-up view of the surgical field, is used broadly in skull base surgery. Although it has the disadvantage of increasing the rate of CSF leakage, the potential advantages of the EEA compared to conventional TCAs include avoiding brain retraction, improved visualization, better protection of surrounding neurovascular structures, and shorter hospital stay (1–3, 23–25). These advantages are similar when comparing the EEA and different TCAs for lesions involving the lateral area of the suprasellar region. The EEA not only provides the most straightforward surgical route parallel to the growth axis of the tumor but also, most importantly, allows for better control of the paraclinoidal ICA, which constitutes a lateral barrier to directly approaching these regions through the sphenoid sinus. However, the intricate anatomical complexity and lack of anatomical detail suitable for surgical exploration make these regions among the most challenging areas to approach.

In this paper, we describe the surgical anatomy of the lateral area of the suprasellar region, termed the "parasuprasellar" area, from the endoscopic perspective. Moreover, we introduce the EESO and EEIO approaches to access this complex area. The same techniques were applied in 12 consecutive patients harboring tumors and aneurysms involving the parasuprasellar area. To the best of our knowledge, this is the first report on the EESO and EEIO approaches.

Approach Selection and Technical Considerations

Our results validate the efficacy of the EESO and EEIO approaches in managing lesions involving the parasuprasellar area, as well demonstrated in our illustrations (**Figures 5–11**). In our experience, when tumors simultaneously invade the intrasellar, suprasellar and lateral to the parasuprasellar area, such as pituitary adenomas or craniopharyngiomas, the EEIO approach should be considered first. If the tumor is not safely exposed or still has an invisible portion, even after pulling it downward, the EESO approach should be selected to allow for additional exposure of the lateral tumor. When the lesion originates in the parasuprasellar area, such as ACP meningiomas or paraclinoid aneurysms, the EEIO approach can also be considered first to remove the lesion on the medial or lateral side of the paraclinoidal ICA. Similarly, if the lesion cannot be completely removed through the corridor below the ON, a combined EESO approach can be applied in most cases. It must be emphasized, however, that not all lesions involving this area are indications for EESO and EEIO approaches. Indeed, a primary TCA or staged operation may be indicated when the lesion involves the intracranial to the parasuprasellar area and is mainly located subdurally.

Of note, the use of the EESO or EEIO approach alone is rather rare and most often requires combination with the endoscopic endonasal midline approach and/or transcavernous approach. Different combinations of approaches can be selected according to the size and location of the lesion(s). For example, the transtuberculum/transplanum approach can be conveniently combined with the single EESO approach to provide better access to anterior cranial fossa meningiomas with lateral extension (case 1). Similarly, the combination of the transcavernous approach and EEIO approach has the potential for achieving complete resection of ACP meningiomas or pituitary adenomas involving the CS (cases 4, 6, 7 and 8). The EESO and EEIO approaches can be used as a complement to the midline approach and transcavernous approach and are

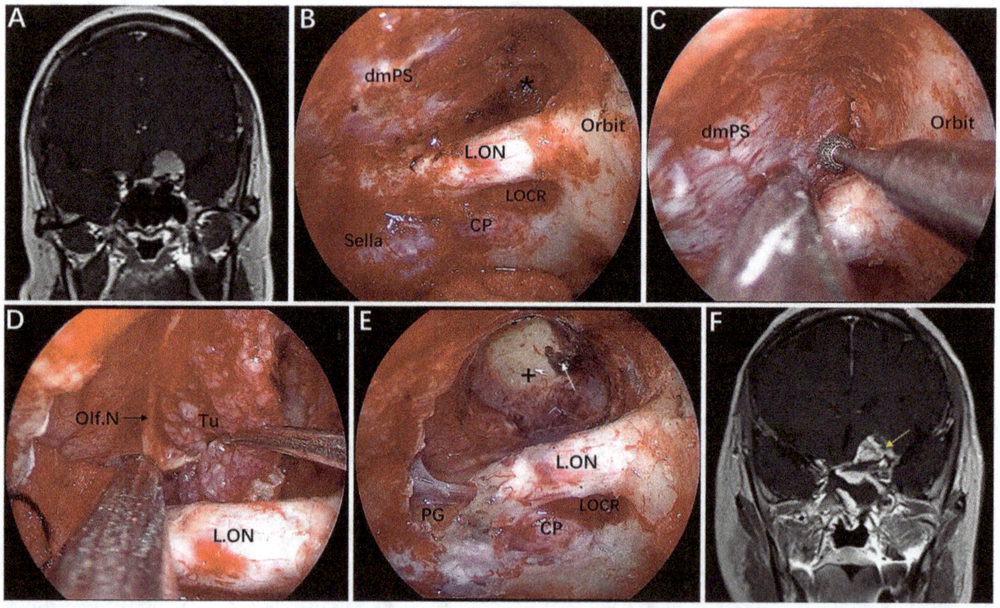

FIGURE 5 | Case 1, a 56-year-old woman, presented with a 1-year history of dizziness and progressive left visual loss for more than 1 month. **(A)** Preoperative coronal Gd-enhanced MRI showing a left ACP meningioma. **(B–E)** Intraoperative images. **(B)** Exposure of the lateral dura of the planum sphenoidale and supraoptic recess (black asterisk). **(C)** Drilling the roof wall of the optic canal and supraoptic recess in a medial-to-lateral direction toward the body of the lesser sphenoid wing. **(D)** Separation of the tumor from the olfactory nerve through the supraoptic approach. **(E)** Final endoscopic view after complete tumor removal. The white arrow represents the severed posterior ethmoidal artery. **(F)** Postoperative coronal MRI showing total tumor removal. The yellow arrow represents the autologous fat used during the operation. + = tumor cavity. The figure is available in color only online.

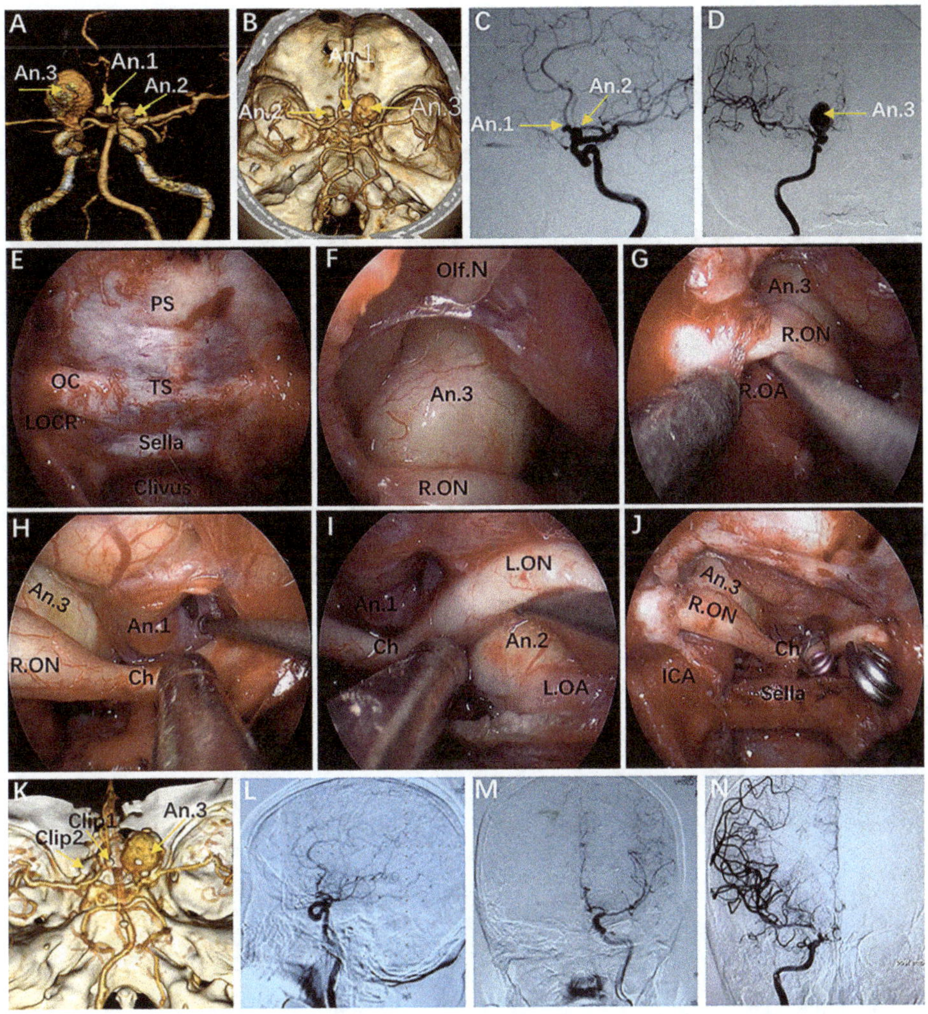

FIGURE 6 | Case 10, a 62-year-old woman, presented with visual loss for 2 months. **(A, B)** Preoperative CT angiography **(A)** and a 3-D reconstruction image **(B)** showing an Acom aneurysm (An1), a left praclinoid aneurysm (An2), and a large right paraclinoid aneurysm (An3). **(C, D)** Anteroposterior view **(C)** and lateral view **(D)** of bilateral internal carotid artery (ICA) injection of digital subtraction angiography (DSA) confirming an Acom aneurysm, a left praclinoid aneurysm, and a large right paraclinoid aneurysm. **(E–J)** Intraoperative images. **(E)** Endoscopic view of the skull base showing important bony landmarks. **(F, G)** Intraoperative image demonstrating an aneurysm body with a thrombus above the right optic nerve that cannot be clipped through an endonasal approach. **(H, I)** Exposure to the Acom aneurysm **(H)** and left paraclinoid aneurysm **(I)**. **(J)** Intraoperative picture showing that both aneurysms were clipped successfully after proximal control. **(K)** Postoperative CT angiography confirmed the patency of the bilateral A2 and distal ICA. **(L, M)** Postoperative lateral view **(L)** and anteroposterior view **(M)** of left ICA injection of DSA, revealing complete obliteration of An1 and An2. **(N)** Postoperative anteroposterior view of right ICA injection of DSA, showing complete obliteration of the An3 after second-stage coiling. An, aneurysm; R.OA, right ophthalmic artery; L.OA, left ophthalmic artery; Ch, optic chiasm. The figure is available in color only online.

extremely useful to access extensive pathologies for more complete resection while limiting morbidity.

Since the EESO and EEIO approaches require extensive removal of the skull base, strict cranial base reconstruction techniques for closure of the osteodural defect should be discussed. In our institution, we first use small pieces of autologous fat for intradural closure to eliminate the dead space. Then, we adopted the so-called sandwich technique, that is, two pieces of fascia lata or artificial dura were placed between the dura and bone as inlay substitutions and outside the bone as outlay substitutions, respectively. Finally, a vascularized pedicle nasoseptal flap harvested at the beginning of the procedure was positioned to cover the cranial defect, and each of the above layers was fixed with biological fibrin glue. However, it must be emphasized that, in the most lateral region of the cranial defect (where the ON stands), an inlay-overlay of dural substitutes will be difficult due to the irregularity of the osteodural defect. Therefore, autologous fat pieces should be placed across the intraextradural space.

Graduated, Stepwise EEIO Approach

In our practice, the EEIO is a graduated, stepwise approach based largely on the lesion location, size and extent. Our anatomical study and clinical cases demonstrate how to assemble multiple surgical

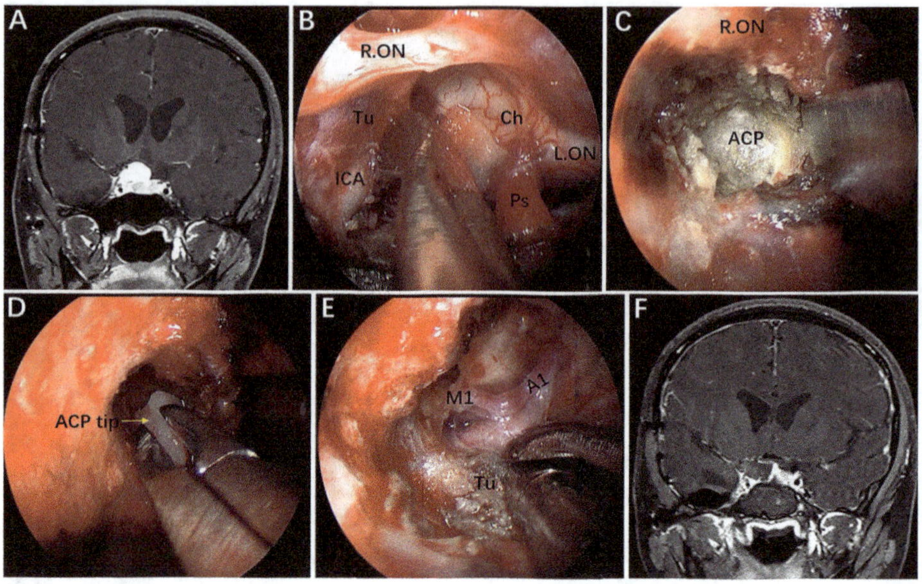

FIGURE 7 | Case 2, A 25-year-old woman presented with headache and decreased vision in her right eye for 6 months. **(A)** Preoperative coronal Gd-enhanced MRI demonstrating a right recurrent ACP meningioma. **(B)** Removal of the tumor on the medial and upper parts of the supraclinoidal ICA. **(C, D)** Removal of the ACP invaded by the tumor. **(E)** Separation of tumor adhering to the bifurcation of the ICA through the infraoptic corridor. **(F)** Postoperative MRI showing total tumor removal. Tu = tumor; Ps = pituitary stalk; ACP = anterior clinoid process. Some panels **(7A, D, F)** of the figure have been published in *Journal of Neurosurgery*. Published with permission. The figure is available in color only online.

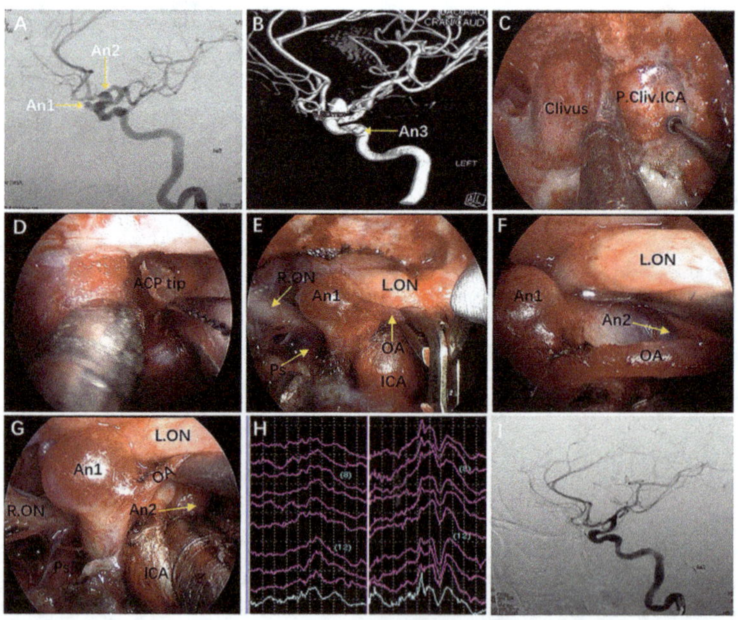

FIGURE 8 | Case 9, a 47-year-old woman, presented with headache for 3 months. **(A)** Preoperative lateral view of left internal carotid artery (ICA) injection for digital subtraction angiography (DSA) showing an ophthalmic aneurysm (An1) and a paraclinoid aneurysm (An2). **(B)** anteroposterior view of the 3D reconstruction images showing another aneurysm (An3) located in the cavernous segment of the ICA. C-G: Intraoperative images. **(C)** Exposure of the paraclival ICA for proximal control in advance. **(D)** Removal of the ACP tip. **(E)** Temporary occlusion of the OA. **(F)** Exposure of the An2 neck by lifting the ipsilateral optic nerve. **(G)** Clip application to the An2 neck after proximal control. **(H)** Intraoperative visual evoked potential monitoring changed after temporary occlusion of the OA. **(I)** Postoperative lateral view of DSA showing complete obliteration of An1 and An2. Some panels **(8A, B, G, I)** of the figure have been published in *Journal of Neurosurgery*.

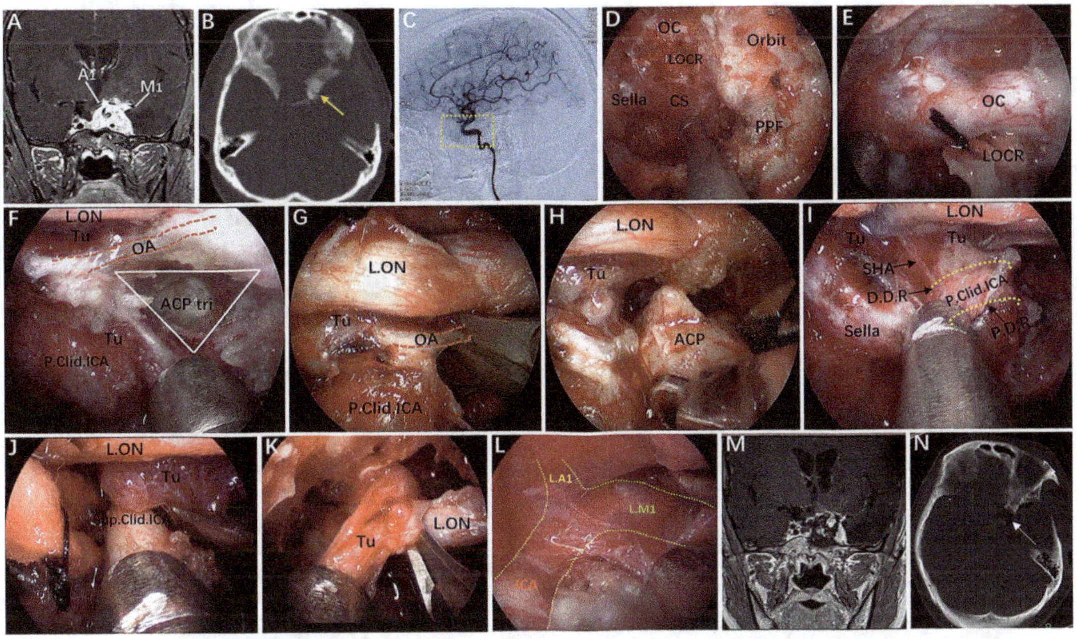

FIGURE 9 | Case 4, a 37-year-old woman, presented with progressive visual loss in the left eye for 2 years. **(A)** Preoperative coronal Gd-enhanced MRI showing a left recurrent ACP meningioma involving the right cavernous sinus and encasement of the ICA and its bifurcation. **(B)** Preoperative CT scans. The yellow arrow indicates the hyperplastic ACP. **(C)** Preoperative lateral view of left ICA injection of digital subtraction angiography (DSA) showing that the ophthalmic artery was not visible. **(D–L)** Intraoperative images. **(D)** Endoscopic view of important bony landmarks after the initial transpterygoid approach. **(E)** Exposure of the thickened OC and drilling of its roof and anterior walls. **(F)** Endoscopic exposure of the ACP triangle. The red dotted line indicates the course of the imaginary occluded OA. **(G)** Sacrifice of the OA surrounded by tumors and involving the dura. **(H)** Removal of the hyperplastic ACP. **(I–K)** Resection of the tumor on the medial and lateral sides of the supraclinoidal ICA through the combined supraoptic and infraoptic approaches. **(L)** Endoscopic exposure of the bifurcation of the ICA covered by arachnoid membrane. **(M)** Corresponding postoperative coronal MRI showing subtotal tumor resection, with part of the tumor remaining in the lateral wall of the left CS. **(N)** Postoperative CT scan showing ACP resection. The white arrow represents the removed ACP. Some panels **(9A, B, M, N)** of the figure have been published in *Journal of Neurosurgery*.

corridors to provide personalized access to complex parasuprasellar lesions. In Case 10, in which the left paraclinoid aneurysm was located just below the ON, successful clipping of the aneurysm was achieved using a pure EEIO approach (**Figure 6**).

Regarding Case 2, we found during the operation that a recurrent ACP meningioma was severely adhered to the ON and ICA and extended into the right OC. Thus, anterior clinoidectomy was applied, and the tumor, which was tightly attached to the ACP and the ICA bifurcation, was completely removed (**Figure 7**). It should be noted, however, that complete anterior clinoidectomy is not mandatory and that the extent of bony removal should be tailored to each case based on intraoperative need. If only the lateral region of the paraclinoidal ICA needs to be exposed or to obtain distal vascular control, partial anterior clinoidectomy should be considered; however, complete anterior clinoidectomy should be performed if the tumor involves the ACP and causes evident hyperplasia or the lesion has extended to involve the ICA bifurcation or even further. Such resection can reduce the risk of tumor recurrence. Most importantly, a corridor for accessing the lateral region of the supraclinoidal ICA is established while removing the involved ACP and the dura that envelops it. Nonetheless, this technique can only be implemented by experienced surgeons due to the complicated procedures and potential risks.

In Case 9, a lateral projecting paraclinoid aneurysm was encountered. In view of its position and orientation, we first performed anterior clinoidectomy to expose the lateral region of the paraclinoidal ICA. Then, the OA was dissociated and temporarily clipped, but the VEP changed, indicating that severing the OA would lead to serious visual impairment (**Figures 8E, H**). Finally, we attempted to expose the aneurysm neck between the OA and ON and successfully clipped the aneurysm through the ACP triangle (created by anterior clinoidectomy) (**Figures 8F, G**).

In Case 4, the tumor involved the intrasellar, suprasellar, CS, and encased the ICA and its bifurcation. The optic strut was drilled first, and the OA completely wrapped by the tumor was selectively dissected to further remove the hyperplastic ACP (**Figures 9F–H**). Thus, the tumor on the medial and lateral regions of the supraclinoidal ICA could be completely removed *via* an enlarged EEIO corridor (**Figures 9I, J**). This is the only case in our series, which preoperative DSA showed that the OA was not visible and the patient's intraoperative VEP stabilized,

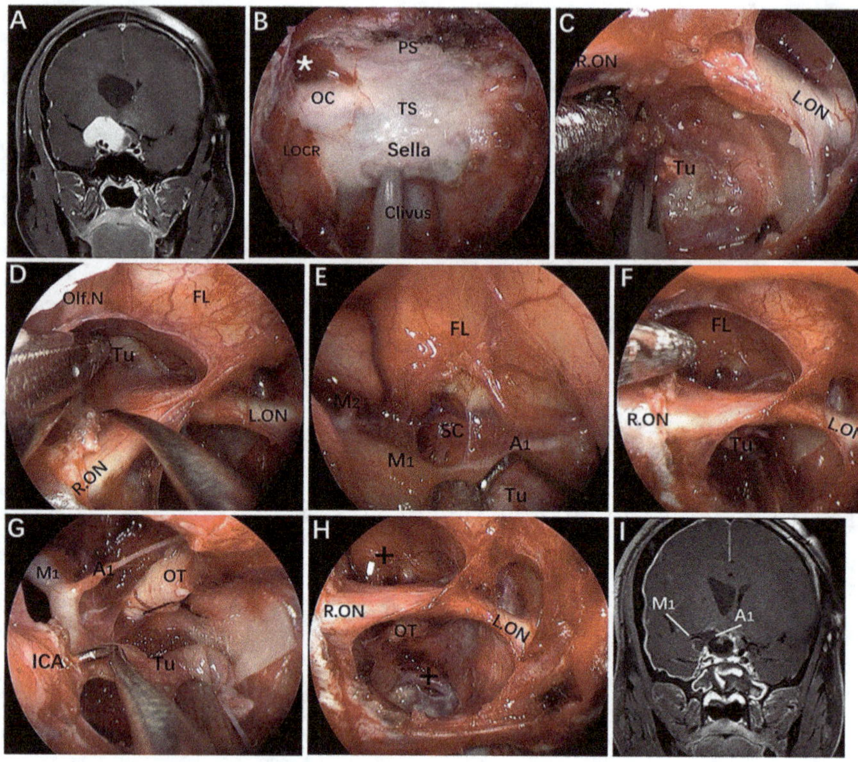

FIGURE 10 | Case 11, a 30-year-old man, presented with progressive loss of vision for 6 months. **(A)** Preoperative coronal Gd-enhanced MRI demonstrating a recurrent intra- and suprasellar craniopharyngioma with right sylvian fissure extension. **(B–H)** Intraoperative images. **(B)** Endoscopic view of the skull base showing important bony landmarks. The white asterisk marks the supraoptic recess. **(C)** Removal of intrasellar tumor. **(D)** Extracapsular separation of the tumor adhering to the frontal lobe through the supraoptic corridor. **(E)** Endoscopic view of the sylvian fissure during tumor removal. **(F, G)** Sharp dissection of the tumor away from the neurovascular structures by the infraoptic corridor. **(H)** Final endoscopic view after complete tumor removal. **(I)** Postoperative coronal MRI showing total tumor removal. The figure is available in color only online.

the OA was sacrificed. As expected, the patient's vision remained stable after surgery.

Visual Outcomes

The special location of such lesions is often responsible for vision loss related to intracranial and/or intracanalicular ON involvement. Ten patients in our series presented with varying degrees of vision loss; thus, improvement and preservation of visual function is a priority for this surgery. Remarkably, in our series, visual improvement occurred in 7 patients but was unchanged in 4 patients, and only 1 patient with recurrent ACP meningioma developed visual deterioration. This demonstrates that gentle pulling of the ON during resection will hardly affect visual function under VEP monitoring. Postoperative visual deterioration has been mainly related to injury of the subchiasmatic perforators, providing the main blood supply to the optic chiasma (26). Accordingly, the potential risk of injuring visual acuity may not be increased by extra manipulation in the supraoptic region. Furthermore, while applying the EEIO approach, endoscopy provides early and direct visualization of the subchiasmatic perforators, allowing for adequate dissection and protection. Last but most importantly, this approach allows for direct 270° decompression of the intracanalicular ON (10) and prompt removal of the involved dura and hyperostotic bone. Nevertheless, as mentioned above, these procedures must be carried out in an extremely delicate and careful manner. When removing bone, the egg-shelling technique with continuous saline irrigation must be followed to prevent thermal injury to the ON. We believe that if sufficient decompression is performed without the risk of further injury, vision problems may be reversed.

Limitations of the Study

The current study has several limitations that need to be considered. First, although no ICA or ON injury occurred in our series, these events are still our primary concern when managing parasuprasellar lesions. Second, cadaveric specimens are useful models to investigate surgical approaches, but they do not fully capture the clinical environment. Indeed, these corridors are relatively narrow in individuals who do not harbor such lesions. Finally, the learning curve is extremely steep and requires a high level of expertise in comprehensive skull base surgery, including both microsurgical cerebrovascular and endoscopic skills. Consequently, practice in the cadaver laboratory is mandatory to develop familiarity with these

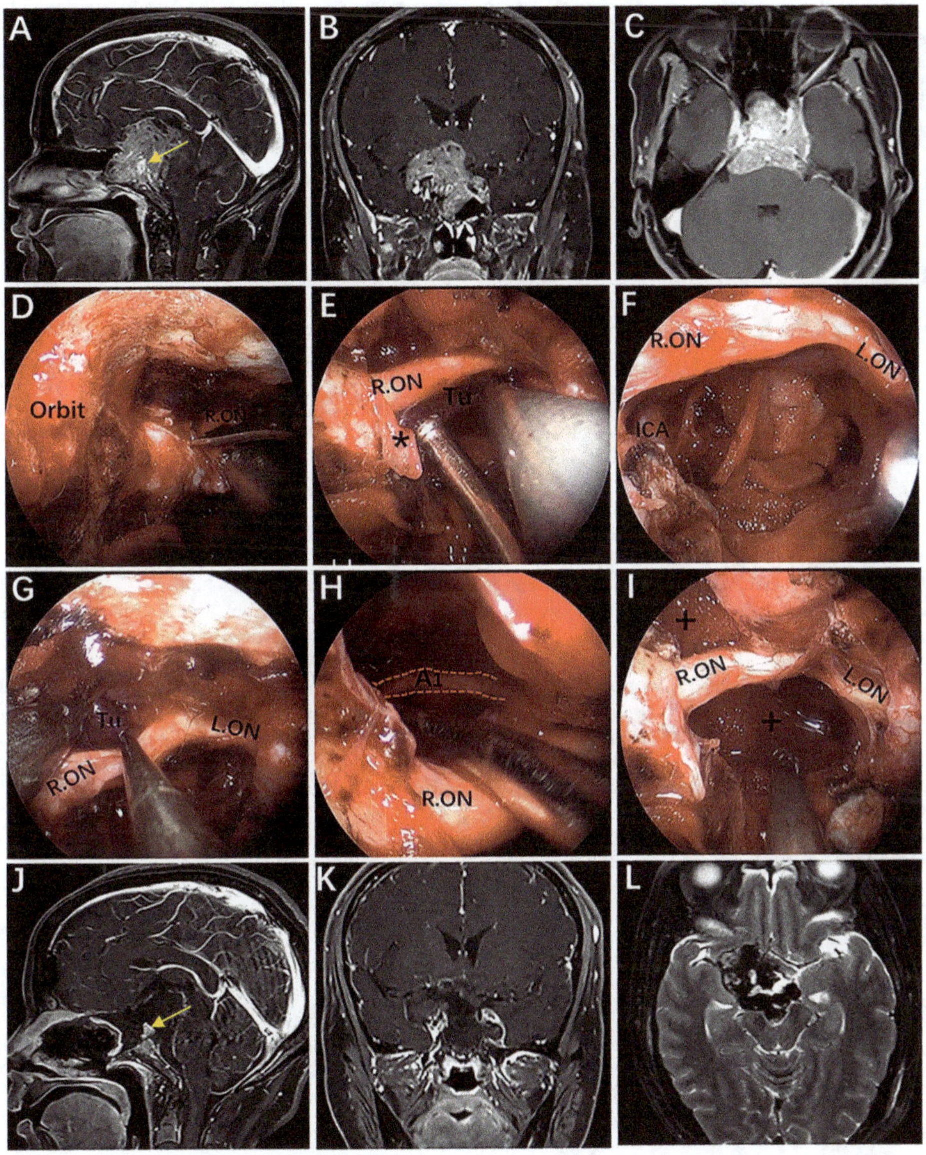

FIGURE 11 | Case 6, a 45-year-old woman presented with visual loss and headache for 2 years. **(A–C)** Preoperative Gd-enhanced MRI showing a multilobulated pituitary adenoma with bilateral cavernous sinus invasion, inferior extension into the clivus, superior compressed the third ventricle, and significantly encasement of the ICA and its bifurcation. **(D–I)** Intraoperative images. **(D)** Opening of the optic nerve sheath. **(E, F)** Removal of the tumor below the right optic nerve using a bimanual microsurgical technique and endoscopic view after resection. **(G)** Expose the tumor above the optic nerve. **(H)** Removal of the tumor using angled suction instruments through the supraoptic corridor. The red dotted line indicates the course of the A1 segments of the anterior cerebral artery. **(I)** Endoscopic view after tumor resection. **(J–L)** Postoperative MRI showing total tumor removal. The yellow arrow represents the normal pituitary gland. * = optic nerve sheath; + = tumor cavity. The figure is available in color only online.

precise and meticulous operations before they are applied clinically.

CONCLUSIONS

Based on our anatomical and surgical results, the EESO and EEIO approaches offer unique treatment options for well-selected lesions involving the parasuprasellar area. The approaches can be combined with the endoscopic endonasal midline approach and the transcavernous approach to remove extensive pathologies involving the intrasellar, suprasellar, sphenoid, and cavernous sinuses and even the bifurcation of the ICA. Our work for the first time pushes the boundary of the EEA lateral to the supraclinoidal ICA and ON.

ETHICS STATEMENT

The studies involving human participants were reviewed and approved by Institutional Ethics Committee of the First Affiliated Hospital of Nanchang University. The patients/participants provided their written informed consent to participate in this study.

AUTHOR CONTRIBUTIONS

TH contributed to the study conception and design. Material preparation and data collection were performed by YB, YY and LZ. Analysis of the data was performed by TH, YB, YY, LZ, SX, XW, HD, JW, LX, LY and BT. The first draft of the manuscript was written by YB. All authors commented on previous versions of the manuscript. All authors read and approved the final manuscript.

ACKNOWLEDGMENTS

We express our sincere appreciation to Miss Jing Liu for the illustration.

REFERENCES

1. Cavallo LM, Messina A, Cappabianca P, Esposito F, de Divitiis E, Gardner P, et al. Endoscopic Endonasal Surgery of the Midline Skull Base: Anatomical Study and Clinical Considerations. *Neurosurg Focus* (2005) 19(1):E2. doi: 10.3171/foc.2005.19.1.3
2. Kassam A, Snyderman CH, Mintz A, Gardner P, Carrau RL. Expanded Endonasal Approach: The Rostrocaudal Axis. Part I. Crista Galli to the Sella Turcica. *Neurosurg Focus* (2005) 19(1):E3. doi: 10.3171/foc.2005.19.1.4
3. Kassam A, Snyderman CH, Mintz A, Gardner P, Carrau RL. Expanded Endonasal Approach: The Rostrocaudal Axis. Part II. Posterior Clinoids to the Foramen Magnum. *Neurosurg Focus* (2005) 19(1):E4. doi: 10.3171/foc.2005.19.1.5
4. Alfieri A, Jho HD, Schettino R, Tschabitscher M. Endoscopic Endonasal Approach to the Pterygopalatine Fossa: Anatomic Study. *Neurosurgery* (2003) 52(2):374–78; discussion 8-80. doi: 10.1227/01.neu.0000044562.73763.00
5. Cavallo LM, Messina A, Gardner P, Esposito F, Kassam AB, Cappabianca P, et al. Extended Endoscopic Endonasal Approach to the Pterygopalatine Fossa: Anatomical Study and Clinical Considerations. *Neurosurg Focus* (2005) 19(1): E5. doi: 10.3171/foc.2005.19.1.6
6. Eloy JA, Murray KP, Friedel ME, Tessema B, Liu JK. Graduated Endoscopic Multiangle Approach for Access to the Infratemporal Fossa: A Cadaveric Study With Clinical Correlates. *Otolaryngology–Head Neck Surg Off J Am Acad Otolaryngology-Head Neck Surg* (2012) 147(2):369–78. doi: 10.1177/0194599812442612
7. Fernandez-Miranda JC, Zwagerman NT, Abhinav K, Lieber S, Wang EW, Snyderman CH, et al. Cavernous Sinus Compartments From the Endoscopic Endonasal Approach: Anatomical Considerations and Surgical Relevance to Adenoma Surgery. *J Neurosurg* (2018) 129(2):430–41. doi: 10.3171/2017.2.Jns162214
8. Hartnick CJ, Myseros JS, Myer CM3rd. Endoscopic Access to the Infratemporal Fossa and Skull Base: A Cadaveric Study. *Arch otolaryngology–head Neck Surg* (2001) 127(11):1325–7. doi: 10.1001/archotol.127.11.1325
9. Theodosopoulos PV, Guthikonda B, Brescia A, Keller JT, Zimmer LA. Endoscopic Approach to the Infratemporal Fossa: Anatomic Study. *Neurosurgery* (2010) 66(1):196–202; discussion -3. doi: 10.1227/01.Neu.0000359224.75185.43
10. Abhinav K, Acosta Y, Wang WH, Bonilla LR, Koutourousiou M, Wang E, et al. Endoscopic Endonasal Approach to the Optic Canal: Anatomic Considerations and Surgical Relevance. *Neurosurgery* (2015) 11 Suppl 3:431–45; discussion 45-6. doi: 10.1227/neu.0000000000000900
11. Di Somma A, Torales J, Cavallo LM, Pineda J, Solari D, Gerardi RM, et al. Defining the Lateral Limits of the Endoscopic Endonasal Transtuberculum Transplanum Approach: Anatomical Study With Pertinent Quantitative Analysis. *J Neurosurg* (2018) 130(3):848–60. doi: 10.3171/2017.9.Jns171406
12. Puzzilli F, Ruggeri A, Mastronardi L, Agrillo A, Ferrante L. Anterior Clinoidal Meningiomas: Report of a Series of 33 Patients Operated on Through the Pterional Approach. *Neuro-oncology* (1999) 1(3):188–95. doi: 10.1093/neuonc/1.3.188
13. Russell SM, Benjamin V. Medial Sphenoid Ridge Meningiomas: Classification, Microsurgical Anatomy, Operative Nuances, and Long-Term Surgical Outcome in 35 Consecutive Patients. *Neurosurgery* (2008) 62(3 Suppl 1):38–50. doi: 10.1227/01.neu.0000317372.92393.e8
14. Attia M, Umansky F, Paldor I, Dotan S, Shoshan Y, Spektor S. Giant Anterior Clinoidal Meningiomas: Surgical Technique and Outcomes. *J Neurosurg* (2012) 117(4):654–65. doi: 10.3171/2012.7.Jns111675
15. Romani R, Laakso A, Kangasniemi M, Lehecka M, Hernesniemi J. Lateral Supraorbital Approach Applied to Anterior Clinoidal Meningiomas: Experience With 73 Consecutive Patients. *Neurosurgery* (2011) 68(6):1632–47; discussion 47. doi: 10.1227/NEU.0b013e318214a840
16. Wu X, Xie SH, Tang B, Yang L, Xiao LM, Ding H, et al. Single-Stage Endoscopic Endonasal Approach for the Complete Removal of Trigeminal Schwannomas Occupying Both the Middle and Posterior Fossae. *Neurosurg Rev* (2021) 44(1):607–16. doi: 10.1007/s10143-020-01266-7
17. Naudy CA, Yanez-Siller JC, Mesquita Filho PM, Gomez GM, Otto BA, Carrau RL, et al. Anatomic Nuances of the Ophthalmic Artery Origin From a Ventral Viewpoint: Considerations and Implications for Endoscopic Endonasal Surgery. *Operative Neurosurgery (Hagerstown Md)* (2019) 16(4):478–85. doi: 10.1093/ons/opy188
18. Tayebi Meybodi A, Borba Moreira L, Lawton MT, Eschbacher JM, Belykh EG, Felicella MM, et al. Interdural Course of the Ophthalmic Artery in the Optic Canal. *J Neurosurg* (2019) 132(1):277–83. doi: 10.3171/2018.6.Jns18856
19. Peris-Celda M, Kucukyuruk B, Monroy-Sosa A, Funaki T, Valentine R, Rhoton ALJr. The Recesses of the Sellar Wall of the Sphenoid Sinus and Their Intracranial Relationships. *Neurosurgery* (2013) 73(2 Suppl Operative):ons117–31; discussion ons31. doi: 10.1227/neu.0000000000000184
20. Xiao L, Xie S, Tang B, Hu J, Hong T. Endoscopic Endonasal Anterior Clinoidectomy: Surgical Anatomy, Technique Nuance, and Case Series. *J Neurosurg* (2019) 133(2):451–61. doi: 10.3171/2019.4.Jns183213
21. Figueiredo EG, Tavares WM, Rhoton ALJr., De Oliveira E. Surgical Nuances of Giant Paraclinoid Aneurysms. *Neurosurg Rev* (2010) 33(1):27–36. doi: 10.1007/s10143-009-0224-2
22. Nozaki K, Kikuta K, Takagi Y, Mineharu Y, Takahashi JA, Hashimoto N. Effect of Early Optic Canal Unroofing on the Outcome of Visual Functions in Surgery for Meningiomas of the Tuberculum Sellae and Planum Sphenoidale. *Neurosurgery* (2008) 62(4):839–44; discussion 44-6. doi: 10.1227/01.neu.0000318169.75095.cb
23. de Divitiis E, Cavallo LM, Cappabianca P, Esposito F. Extended Endoscopic Endonasal Transsphenoidal Approach for the Removal of Suprasellar Tumors: Part 2. *Neurosurgery* (2007) 60(1):46–58; discussion -9. doi: 10.1227/01.Neu.0000249211.89096.25
24. Dehdashti AR, Ganna A, Witterick I, Gentili F. Expanded Endoscopic Endonasal Approach for Anterior Cranial Base and Suprasellar Lesions: Indications and Limitations. *Neurosurgery* (2009) 64(4):677–87; discussion 87-9. doi: 10.1227/01.Neu.0000339121.20101.85
25. Laufer I, Anand VK, Schwartz TH. Endoscopic, Endonasal Extended Transsphenoidal, Transplanum Transtuberculum Approach for Resection of Suprasellar Lesions. *J Neurosurg* (2007) 106(3):400–6. doi: 10.3171/jns.2007.106.3.400
26. Blunt MJ, Steele EJ. The Blood Supply of the Optic Nerve and Chiasma in Man. *J Anat* (1956) 90(4):486–93.

6

Enhanced Recovery in Surgical Intensive Care

Gordana Jovanović [1,2,3], Dea Karaba Jakovljević [3] and Mirka Lukić-Šarkanović [2]*

[1] University of Novi Sad, Faculty of Medicine, Department of Anesthesia and Perioperative Medicine, Novi Sad, Serbia, [2] Clinic for Anesthesia and Intensive Care Therapy, Clinical Center of Vojvodina, Novi Sad, Serbia, [3] University of Novi Sad, Faculty of Medicine, Department of Physiology and Sports Medicine, Novi Sad, Serbia

***Correspondence:**
Gordana Jovanović
gordana.jovanovic@mf.uns.ac.rs

Patients are admitted to the surgical intensive care (SICU) unit after emergency and elective surgery. After elective surgery, for further support, or to manage coexisting comorbidities. The implementation of the ERAS (Enhanced recovery after surgery) protocols in surgery should decrease the need for ICU beds, but there will always be unpredicted complications after surgery. These will require individual management. What we can do for our surgical patients in ICU to further enhance their recovery? To promote early enhanced recovery in surgical intensive care—SICU, three areas need to be addressed, sedation, analgesia, and delirium. Tools for measurement and protocols for management in these three areas should be developed to ensure best practice in each SICU. The fourth important area is Nutrition. Preoperative screening and post-operative measurement of the state of nutrition also need to be developed in the SICU. The fifth important area is early mobilization. ERAS protocols encourage early mobilization of the critically ill patients, even if on mechanical ventilation. Early mobilization is possible and should be implemented by special multidisciplinary ICU team. All team members must be familiar with protocols to be able to implement them in their field of expertise. Personal and professional attitudes are critical for implementation. In the core of all our efforts should be the patient and his well-being.

Keywords: ERAS protocol, surgical intensive care unit, recovery, perioperative care, early mobilization

INTRODUCTION

History of Enhanced Recovery Concept

Enhanced recovery concept was first introduced by Henrik Kehlet in 1990's. As a colorectal surgeon he developed the idea of "fast tracking" in major abdominal surgery, in order to promote faster recovery, and diminish complication after surgery.

Factors that limit early recovery include pain, post-operative paralytic ileus and different organ system dysfunctions. The traditional approach in use for decades, utilize only unimodal solutions for these problems (1–3).

For enhanced recovery, a multimodal, evidence - based approach is proposed.

Implementation of this innovative concept was facilitated by the simultaneous development of new regional anesthesia techniques for pain control, and minimally invasive laparoscopic techniques in abdominal surgery.

In 2010, ERAS (Enhanced recovery after surgery) Society was formed as a nonprofit, academic, international multidisciplinary society and has played an important role in helping to provide guidelines, educational meetings, and other support (www.erassociety.org) (2–4). The mission of the ERAS Society is to develop peri-operative care and improve recovery through research, education, audit and implementation of evidence-based practice.

To the present day 9 ERAS Society guidelines are available: for colonic surgery, pancreaticoduodenestomy, elective rectal/pelvic surgery, radical cystectomy, liver, bariatric, head and neck cancer surgery, gastrectomy and breast surgery (3). Modified ERAS guidelines exist for gynecology, thoracic, vascular, pediatric, urologic, orthopedic, esophagectomy, and colorectal liver metastasis surgery.

As authors, we are not aware of the existence of ERAS protocols specific for surgical intensive care, and although all existing ERAS protocols have an influence on patients being admitted in surgical intensive care unit, we think that more can be done, to further enhance recovery of these patients.

EARLY RECOVERY PROTOCOLS AS CONCEPT IN SURGICAL INTENSIVE CARE

Patients are admitted to the intensive care unit after emergency or elective surgery. In case of admission after elective surgery, for further support to manage coexisting comorbidities.

ERAS protocols in surgery starts in the preoperative period, and potential need for post-operative ICU admission should be discussed with the patient preoperatively.

Surgical Intensive Care Unit

As JL Vincent highlighted, a neglect of recovery is one of the ten big mistakes in intensive care medicine (5). Everyday battle for patient survival draws attention from recovery and period after leaving the intensive care unit.

In theory, the implementation of the ERAS protocols in surgery should decrease the need for ICU beds, but will always be unpredicted complications after surgery, which will be managed individually.

The next question is what can be done for our surgical patients in SICU to enhance their recovery?

The Role of Sedation and Analgesia in Enhanced Recovery After Surgery in the Intensive Care Unit

Sedation and analgesia are an integral part of care for critically ill, but sometimes with low priority, as care for other organ systems, as cardiac, pulmonary, or renal system are more acutely in focus. Only a small percentage of SICU patients need prolonged deep sedation. In the most cases the objective is for the patient to remain calm, cooperative and comfortable. The concept of "e CASH" (**e**arly **C**omfort using **A**nalgesia, minimal **S**edatives and maximal **H**uman care) is being introduced to guide clinicians (5–7).

Using this concept strategies for sedation and analgesia in SICU can be provided.

Analgesia

All critically ill adult patients in medical, surgical, and trauma ICUs typically experience pain. Providing analgesia should be a priority, on humanitarian grounds, and in keeping with the ERAS concept.

Essential for early mobilization, multimodal approach to pain should be implemented (8).

As stated in recent guidelines "Multimodal analgesia or balanced analgesia is approach that involves the use of more than one method or modality of controlling pain. These modalities may operate through different mechanisms or at different sites (i.e., peripheral vs. central actions). One example of multimodal analgesia is the use of various combinations of opioids and local anesthetics to manage post-operative pain" (9).

Pain management is the mainstay of treatment and precondition for other treatment options such as early mobilization where multimodal approach to pain should be implemented (8).

Pain should be measured in order to regularly reevaluate and optimize treatment.

There are many tools for measuring the pain in critically ill patient (Critical Care **Pain Observation Tool or BPS**—Behavioral Pain Scale) which can be used, or modified for local conditions (10).

Sedation and Delirium

Sedation is integral part of care in SICU to relieve discomfort and unnecessary suffering. Over sedation on the other hand is not beneficial and only a small percentage of patient need profound sedation and immobilization (5, 6). Benzodiazepines in the sedation of SICU patients should be avoided, and non-sedative drugs use such as propofol or dexmedetomidine should be encouraged (8).

Delirium is a common problem in some SICU patients affecting outcome in terms of prolonged ICU stay, persistent cognitive decline, reintubation, and worse overall outcome. Delirium is frequent in the medical and surgical Intensive Care Units (ICUs) with prevalence rates ranging from 32.3 to 77% and the incidence rates varying from 45 to 87% (11–14).

Currently there is a study recruiting patients "UNDERPIN-ICU" consisting of standardized protocols focusing on several modifiable risk factors for delirium, including cognitive impairment, sleep deprivation, immobility and visual and hearing impairment. The future results and maybe some implementation of the protocol remains to be seen (15).

In preventing delirium in ICU, there is a great potential in involving family members in activities that constantly serve as an orientation, cognitive or sensitive stimulus to the patients (16).

Abbreviations: RAS, Enhanced Recovery After surgery; ICU, intensive care unit; SICU, surgical intensive care unit; e CASH, early Comfort using Analgesia, minimal Sedatives and maximal Human care; ICU PAD, intensive care unit pain agitation delirium, ESPEN, European Society for Enteral and Parenteral Nutrition; A.S.P.E.N, American Society for Enteral and Parenteral Nutrition; ESICM, European Society of Intensive Care Medicine; BW, body weight ICUAW, intensive care unit-acquired weakness; ABCDEF bundle, Assess, Prevent, and Manage Pain, Both Spontaneous Awakening Trials and Spontaneous Breathing Trials, Choice of Sedation, Delirium: Assess, Prevent and Manage Early Mobility and Exercise, Family Engagement and Empowerment.

Patient-Centered Care

The patient should be in the center of all our efforts. Patient well-being and needs are our priority. Counseling, emotional support, and humanistic approach should be implemented in our everyday work. Many non-pharmacological modalities can be employed in sleep promotion and as alternative means of communication (5–7).

There are recent Clinical practice guidelines for the management of pain, agitation, and delirium in adult patients in the intensive care unit (8), that should be used according to local organization of the health care system.

The 2013 PAD guidelines (**P**ain **A**gitation **D**elirium) have been incorporated into the ICU PAD Care Bundle, with corresponding metrics developed to facilitate implementation. The bundle emphasizes an integrated approach to assessing, treating and preventing significant pain, over or under sedation, and delirium in critically ill patients (8, 12).

To promote early enhanced recovery in SICU, we should provide protocols for sedation and analgesia in the SICU (or develop local ones), implement tools for assessing the patient level of sedation and pain, develop and implement prevention and treatment strategies for post-operative delirium. The best practice will be to develop and implement care bundles for sedation, analgesia and post-operative delirium in each SICU.

THE ROLE OF NUTRITION IN ENHANCED RECOVERY AFTER SURGERY IN THE INTENSIVE CARE UNIT

Early Nutrition in SICU

Patients undergoing surgery are subjected to a catabolic state through activation of the inflammatory response and the release of stress hormones—cortisol, catecholamine, and glucagon. The stress hormones and inflammatory cytokines exert catabolic effects by depleting liver glycogen stores and causing lipolysis and proteolysis of fat and muscle protein stores. Additionally, surgery naturally induces a state of insulin resistance or decreased insulin sensitivity, with breakdown of lean body mass. This has been associated with increased morbidity, increased mortality, and increased length of hospital stay (17, 18).

Providing nutrition and correcting existing nutritional deficiencies is one of the mainstays in all surgical ERAS protocols. Nutrition support in SICU is also of high importance and interconnected with other elements of care. Nutritional support provides optimal wound healing and prevent loss of lean body mass. Prolonged period of fasting causes breakdown of the gastrointestinal tract barrier function, atrophy of endothelial *microvilli* and decrease of gut lymphoid tissue. This process increases infection and development of sepsis (17, 18).

At the present moment, there are two guidelines: one from ESPEN (European Society for Enteral and Parenteral Nutrition) and one from A.S.P.E.N (American Society for Enteral and Parenteral Nutrition). Both guidelines support the idea of early start with enteral nutrition in critically ill patients. The only contraindications for early enteral nutrition are the conditions of uncontrolled shock and high doses of vasoactive drugs, life threatening hypoxia, hypercapnia, acidosis, or bowel ischemia (19, 20).

The most recent guidelines developed by ESICM (European Society of Intensive Care Medicine) Working group on Gastrointestinal Function within the Metabolism, Endocrinology and Nutrition made 23 recommendations for early enteral nutrition in critically ill patient. Early enteral nutrition is recommended in cases of concomitant usage of neuromuscular blockade, therapeutic hypothermia, extracorporeal membrane oxygenation, prone positioning, for patients with traumatic brain injury, patients with stroke, spinal cord injury, severe acute pancreatitis, after gastrointestinal surgery, after abdominal aortic surgery, abdominal trauma after confirmed/restored gastrointestinal tract, diarrhea (21).

Apart from above mentioned contraindications, delayed enteral nutrition is considered in cases of high output intestinal fistulas, progressing intraabdominal hypertension, abdominal compartment syndrome, acute upper gastrointestinal bleeding, and life threatening metabolic derangements (20, 21).

The Amount of Protein in Critically Ill

The exact amount of protein required in critically ill patient is still a matter of the debate among nutritionists involved in ICU. For the first 12 days in the ICU, an average ICU patient worldwide receives 1,034 kcal/day and 0.6 g/kg/protein (22).

After the first phase of the critical illness ("ebb phase") the patient enters the recovery phase, total protein, and calorie delivery needs to increase significantly. The total recommended protein intake of 1,2 g/kg/BW /day should increase to 1.5–2 g/kg/BW/day (23, 24).

There is scientific evidence that adequate protein intake leads to better patient functional recovery and quality of life after ICU discharge (22–24).

To enhance further recovery of surgical critically ill patient, implementation of existing protocols should be a high priority. As for pain, agitation, and delirium, screening (measuring) for malnutrition is also very important, and should start preoperatively. Care bundles for early nutritional interventions and implementation of nutritional protocols should be developed by multidisciplinary ICU teams.

THE ROLE OF EARLY MOBILIZATION IN ENHANCED RECOVERY AFTER SURGERY IN THE INTENSIVE CARE UNIT

Bed rest was first introduced as a medical treatment in the Nineteenth-century to promote recovery, and remains unchanged even today in many hospitals. Critically ill patients are often seen as too sick to be involved in some form of rehabilitation treatment. The rehab programs are frequently perceived as potentially harmful and could cause injury (24).

Immobilization has many deleterious effects on a critically ill patient significantly on the musculoskeletal, cardiovascular, respiratory, and cognitive systems (25, 26).

TABLE 1 | Summary of recommendations for ERAS in SICU.

1.Pain agitation delirium	1.a Pain treatment is precondition for other treatment options 1.b Implement existing protocols for sedation and analgesia in the SICU (or develop local ones) 1.c Implement tools for assessing the patient level of sedation and pain. 1.d Implement prevention and treatment strategies for postoperative delirium. 1.e Development and implementation of CARE BUNDLES for sedation, analgesia and postoperative delirium in each SICU. **Guidelines:** Clinical practice guidelines for the management of pain, agitation, and delirium in adult patients in the intensive care unit. *Crit Care Med* (2013) 41:263–306.
2.Nutrition	2.a. Care bundles for early nutritional interventions and implementation of nutritional protocols should be developed by multidisciplinary ICU teams. **Guidelines:** 2016 Guidelines for the Provision and Assessment of Nutrition Support Therapy in the Adult Critically Ill Patient. *JPEN* (2016) 40(2): 159 –211.
3.Early mobilization	3.a ERAS protocols encourage early mobilization of the patients. 3.b Early mobilization is possible and should be implemented by special multidisciplinary ICU team. **Guidelines:** Physiotherapy for adult patients with critical illness: recommendations of the European Respiratory Society and European Society of Intensive Care Medicine Task Force on Physiotherapy for Critically Ill Patients. *Intensive Care Med* (2008) 34:1188–1199.
4.Logistic issues	4.a. All team members must be familiar with protocols in order to implement them in their field of expertise. 4.b Implementation will require an organizational modifications in the preoperative anesthesia visit, preoperative preparation, intraoperative pain management or fluid management, modifications in postoperative care **Guidelines**:www.erassociety.org

The development of intensive care unit-acquired weakness (ICUAW) is a longstanding problem in treatment of the critically ill patients and associated with a prolonged duration of mechanical ventilation, delayed rehabilitation, protracted ICU stay, and an increased risk for morbidity and mortality. The cause of ICUAW is multifactorial. There is no specific targeted treatment for prevention of ICUAW. Immobility and bed rest contribute to ICUAW and should be stopped as early as possible (27–29).

Mobilization and physiotherapy for mechanically ventilated patients is an even bigger challenge for health care workers in SICU. Only a small percentage of mechanically ventilated patients are regularly mobilized (<9%) (30, 31).

Prolonged (unnecessary) immobilization during hospitalization in SICU is still a frequent issue. There is mounting evidence that early physical activity and early mobilization are safe and effective. Despite this evidence implementation of this practice is still too low. All efforts aimed to promote this practice of early mobilization and rehabilitation will promote enhanced recovery in those patients (32–34).

ERAS protocols encourage early mobilization of the patients. Early mobilization is possible and should be implemented by special multidisciplinary ICU team.

CHALLENGES IN THE IMPLEMENTATION OF ENHANCED RECOVERY AFTER SURGERY IN THE INTENSIVE CARE UNIT

It has been more than 15 years from implementation of the first ERAS protocols and global and widespread implementation is yet to occur. It differs greatly among hospitals in different regions of the globe. There are many problems divided into two major categories: one category are caregivers and patients, and the other category are logistic issues (34).

Health Care Providers and Patients

The Health Care Providers

Implementing ERAS concept is more than making protocols. As mentioned above, there are vast scientific data from already existing ERAS protocols. Implementing them requires a multidisciplinary team of surgeons, anesthesiologists, nurses and other team members (nutritionist, physiotherapist, etc.). All team members must be familiar with protocols in order to implement them in their field of expertise. Personal and professional attitudes are critical for implementation. Sometimes enhanced recovery pathways may seem counterintuitive and contradict previous knowledge. For example, early nutrition and early mobilization, because bed rest and nil by mouth was the cornerstone of patient care for decades. All departments need some dedicated physician to promote the idea of enhanced recovery, but sometimes there is a "power play" among different professions over which profession should lead the program (35–37).

The Patient

As stated previously, in the core of our efforts should be the patient and his well-being.

Effective preoperative counseling is associated with improvements in post-operative recovery in terms of anxiety, faster return of bowel function and improved analgesia. Preoperative counseling is a very important component of the enhanced recovery protocol and should be done at all times. A realistic expectation and proper data are associated with more beneficial health outcomes. The informed patient is capable of making better decisions about their treatment (35, 37).

Logistic Issues

Organizational Issues

Analyzing enhanced recovery protocols, we come to the conclusion that some of them have more than 20 items.

Implementing all of them will require an organizational modifications in the preoperative anesthesia visit, preoperative preparation, intraoperative pain management or fluid management, modifications in post-operative care, which sometimes results in increased workload, it's time consuming or need additional training (37, 38).

Environmental Issues

Hospital environment has a positive impact on patient welfare. Specialized ICU, like geriatric ICU with a special features adjusted for geriatric patients, (e.g., single room), is the evidence that modern ICU gravitate to more "patient friendly" design. Enhanced recovery programs are sometimes perceived by health management as more expensive in terms of environmental and design alterations. Based on available data from the United States, ERAS programs lead to reductions in lengths of hospital stay that range from 0.7 to 2.7 days and substantial direct cost savings (39).

CONCLUSIONS AND FUTURE DIRECTIONS

The Society of Critical Care Medicine's ICU Liberation initiative aims to liberate patients from the harmful effects of pain, agitation, and delirium in the ICU. The Society of Critical Care Medicine introduced the concept of ABCDEF bundle for intensive care: **A**ssess, Prevent, and Manage Pain, **B**oth Spontaneous Awakening Trials and Spontaneous Breathing Trials, **C**hoice of Sedation, **D**elirium: Assess, Prevent and Manage **E**arly Mobility and Exercise, **F**amily Engagement and Empowerment. This concept and detailed care bundles can be found on the website www.iculiberation.org for details.

Future directions for the improvement and enhancement of the patient recovery in SICU is in development and implementation of specific care bundles (are being) carried out by SICU multidisciplinary teams. We can utilize existing ones or prepare and modify local ones.

Quality guidelines do already exist (8, 12, 19, 20, 33), therefore implementation in everyday practice is the key for impact and enhancement of the patients recovery in SICU. More emphasis on pain treatment, as well as treatment of delirium and agitation, early nutritional screening and interventions, early mobilization of critically ill patients, family member involvement and paradigm shift in our mentality as an ICU team members, is necessary for change to happen.

Summary recommendations for ERAS in SICU are in **Table 1**.

LIMITATATIONS OF THE REVIEW

One of the main limitations of this study is that these are recommendations for ERAS protocols in other settings, but there is not scientific data yet to show if they can be translated effectively into another (SICU) setting. This idea of incorporating ERAS protocols in SICU setting have great potential for future scientific research.

Second limitation pertains to the data we already have and that are proposed here to be used in SICU, such as existing protocols for assessment or management of sedation, analgesia, delirium, nutrition and early mobilization. Each and every item mentioned here is subject to some criticism in the present literature. For the present time, while waiting for further scientific refinement, those guidelines are the best scientific knowledge that we have. By using them we give structure and solid scientific background to our everyday work in SICU and their implementation can lead to optimization of various aspects of SICU practices.

AUTHOR CONTRIBUTIONS

GJ: conceptualization, investigation, literature review, visualization, and made a final version of manuscript, language supervision. DJ: conceptualization, literature review, writing the manuscript. ML-S: conceptualization, literature review, writing the manuscript, supervision.

REFERENCES

1. Kehlet H. Multimodal approach to control postoperative pathophysiology and rehabilitation. *Br J Anaesth.* (1997) 78:606–17.
2. Lassen K, Coolsen M, Slim K, Carli F, Aguilar-Nascimento E, Schäfer M, et al. Pancreaticoduodenectomy: ERAS recommendations. *Clin Nutr.* (2013) 32:870–1. doi: 10.1016/j.clnu.2012.08.011
3. Steenhagen E. Enhanced recovery after surgery: it's time to change practice! *Nutr Clin Pract.* (2016) 31:18–29. doi: 10.1177/0884533615622640
4. Cannesson M, Ani F, Mythen M, Kain Z. Anaesthesiology and perioperative medicine around the world: different names, same goals. *Br J Anaesth.* (2015) 114:8–9. doi: 10.1093/bja/aeu265
5. Vincent JL, Hall JB, Slutsky AS. Ten big mistakes in intensive care medicine. *Intensive Care Med.* (2014) 41:505–7. doi: 10.1007/s00134-014-3570-7
6. Vincent JL, Shehabi Y, Walsh TS, Pandharipande PP, Ball JA, Spronk P, et al. Comfort and patient-centered care without excessive sedation: the eCASH concept. *Intensive Care Med.* (2016) 42:962–71. doi: 10.1007/s00134-016-4297-4.7
7. Vincent JL. Optimizing sedation in the ICU: the eCASH concept. *Signa Vitae* (2017) 13:10–13. doi: 10.22514/SV133.062017.1
8. Barr J, Fraser GL, Puntillo K, Ely EW, Gélinas C, Dasta JF, et al. Clinical practice guidelines for the management of pain, agitation, and delirium in adult patients in the intensive care unit. *Crit Care Med.* (2013) 41:263–306. doi: 10.1097/CCM.0b013e3182783b72
9. Chou R, Gordon DB, de Leon-Casasola OA, Rosenberg JM, Bickler S5, Brennan T, et al. Management of Postoperative Pain: A Clinical Practice Guideline From the American Pain Society, the American Society of Regional Anesthesia and Pain Medicine, and the American Society of Anesthesiologists' Committee on Regional Anesthesia, Executive Committee, and Administrative Council. *J Pain* (2016) 17:131–57. doi: 10.1016/j.jpain.2015.12.008
10. Kotfis K, Zegan-Baranska M, Szydłowski L, Zukowski M, Ely E. Methods of pain assessment in adult intensive care unit patients — Polish version of the CPOT (Critical Care Pain Observation Tool) and BPS (Behavioral Pain Scale). *Anaesthesiol Intensive Ther.* (2017) 49:66–72. doi: 10.5603/AIT.2017.0010
11. Grover S, Sarkar S, Yaddanapudi LN, Ghosh A, Desouza A, Basu D. Intensive Care Unit delirium: A wide gap between actual prevalence and psychiatric referral. *J Anaesthesiol Clin Pharmacol.* (2017) 33:480–6. doi: 10.4103/0970-9185.222505
12. Baron R, Binder A, Biniek R, Braune S, Buerkle H, Dall P, et al. Evidence and consensus based guideline for the management of delirium, analgesia, and sedation in intensive care medicine. Revision 2015 (DAS-Guideline 2015) -short version. *Ger Med Sci.* (2015) 13:Doc19. doi: 10.3205/000223
13. Ely E, Gautam S, Margolin R, Francis J, May L, Speroff T, et al. The impact of delirium in the intensive care unit on hospital length of stay. *Intensive Care Med.* (2001) 27:1892–900. doi: 10.1007/s00134-001-1132-2
14. Mc Cusker J, Cole MG, Dendukuri N, Belzile E. Does delirium increase hospital stay? *J Am Geriatr Soc.* (2003) 51:539–46.
15. Wassenaar A, Rood P, Schoonhoven L, Teerenstra S, Zegers M, Pickkers P, et al. The impact of nUrsiNg DEliRium Preventive INnterventions in the Intensive Care Unit (UNDERPIN-ICU): a study protocol for a multi-centre, stepped wedge randomized controlled trial. *Int J Nurs Stud.* (2017) 68:1539–46. doi: 10.1016/j.ijnurstu.2016.11.018

16. Mitchell ML, Kean S, Rattray JE, Hull AM, Davis C, Murfield JE, et al.Family intervention to reduce delirium in hospitalized ICU patients: A feasibility randomized controlled trial. *Int Crit Care Nurs.* (2017) 40:77–84. doi: 10.1016/j.iccn.2017.01.001
17. Kehlet H. The stress response to surgery: release mechanisms and the modifying effect of pain relief. *Acta Chir Scand.* (1988) 550(Suppl):22–8.
18. Kehlet H. Surgical stress: the role of pain and analgesia. *Br J Anaesth.* (1989) 63:189–95.
19. McClave SA, Taylor BE, Martindale RG, Warren MM, Johnson DR, Braunschweig C, et al. 2016 Guidelines for the Provision and Assessment of Nutrition Support Therapy in the Adult Critically Ill Patient. *J Parenter Enteral Nutr.* (2016) 40: 159–211. doi: 10.1177/0148607115621863
20. Kreymann KG, Berger MM, Deutz NE, Hiesmayr M, Jolliet P, Kazandjiev G, Nitenberg G, et al. ESPEN Guidelines on enteral nutrition: intensive care. *Clin Nutr.* (2006) 25:210–23. doi: 10.1016/j.clnu.2006.01.021
21. Reintam BA, Starkopf J, Alhazzani W, Berger MM, Casaer MP, Deane AM, et al. Early enteral nutrition in critically ill patients: ESICM clinical practice guidelines. *Intensive Care Med.* (2017) 43:380–98. doi: 10.1007/s00134-016-4665-0
22. Wischmeyer PE. Tailoring nutrition therapy to illness and recovery. *Crit Care* (2017) 21(Suppl. 3):316. doi: 10.1186/s13054-017-1906-8
23. Hoffer LJ, Bistrian BR. What is the best nutritional support for critically ill patients? *Hepatobiliary Surg Nutr.* (2014) 3:172–4. doi: 10.3978/j.issn.2304-3881.2014.08.03
24. Hoffer LJ, Bistrian BR. Appropriate protein provision in critical illness: a systematic and narrative review. *Am J Clin Nutr.* (2012) 96:591–600. doi: 10.3945/ajcn.111.032078
25. Pavy-Le Traon A, Heer M, Narici MV, Rittweger J, Vernikos J. From space to Earth: advances in human physiology from 20 years of bed rest studies (1986–2006). *Eur J Appl Physiol.* (2007) 101:143–94. doi: 10.1007/s00421-007-0474-z
26. Dock W. The evil sequelae of complete bed rest. *JAMA* (1944) 125:1083–85. doi: 10.1001/jama.1944.02850340009004
27. Nordon-Craft A, Moss M, Quan D, Schenkman M. Intensive care unit-acquired weakness: implications for physical therapist management. *Phys Ther.* (2012) 92:1494–506. doi: 10.2522/ptj.201 10117
28. Stevens RD, Dowdy DW, Michaels RK, Mendez-Tellez PA, Pronovost PJ, Needham DM. Neuromuscular dysfunction acquired in critical illness: A systematic review. *Intensive Care Med.* (2007) 33:1876–91. doi: 10.1007/s00134-007-0772-2
29. Latronico N, Bolton CF. Critical illness polyneuropathy and myopathy: a major cause of muscle weakness and paralysis. *Lancet Neurol.* (2011) 10:931–41. doi: 10.1016/S1474-4422(11)70178-8
30. Hassan A, Rajamani A, Fitzsimons F. The 'MOVIN' project (Mobilization Of Ventilated Intensive care patients at Nepean): A quality improvement project based on the principles of knowledge translation to promote nurse-led mobilization of critically ill ventilated patients. *Int Critl Care Nurs.* (2017) 42:36–43. doi: 10.1016/j.iccn.2017.04.011
31. Li Z, Peng X, Zhu B, Zhang Y, Xi X. Active mobilization for mechanically ventilated patients: A systematic review. *Arch Phys Med Rehabil.* (2013) 94:551–61. doi: 10.1016/j.apmr.2012.10.023
32. Schweickert WD, Kress JP. Implementing early mobilization interventions in mechanically ventilated patients in the ICU. *Chest* (2011) 140:1612–7. doi: 10.1378/chest.10-2829
33. Gosselink R, Bott J, Johnson M, Dean E, Nava S, Norrenberg M, et al. Physiotherapy for adult patients with critical illness: recommendations of the European Respiratory Society and European Society of Intensive Care Medicine Task Force on Physiotherapy for Critically Ill Patients. *Intensive Care Med.* (2008) 34:1188–99. doi: 10.1007/s00134-008-1026-7
34. Adler J, Malone D. Early mobilization in the intensive care unit: A systematic review. *Cardiopulm Phys Ther J.* (2012) 23:5–13.
35. Kehlet H, Delaney CP, Hill AG. Perioperative medicine – the second round will need a change of tactics. *Br J Anaesth.* (2015) 115:13–4. doi: 10.1093/bja/aev098
36. Barber EA, Everard T, Holland AE, Tipping C, Bradley SJ, Hodgson CL. Barriers and facilitators to early mobilization in intensive care: A qualitative study. *Austr Crit Care* (2015) 28:177–82. doi: 10.1016/j.aucc.2014.11.001
37. Kehlet H. Fast-track surgery: A multidisciplinary collaboration. *ICU Manage Pract.* (2017) 17:138–9. doi: 10.1302/2058-5241.2.160060
38. Needham D, Feldman D, Kho M. The functional costs of ICU survivorship. Collaborating to improve post-ICU disability. *Am J Respir Crit Care Med.* (2011) 183:962–4. doi: 10.1164/rccm.201012-2042ED
39. Stone B, Grant C, Roda P, Hobson D, Pawlik T, Wu L, Wick E. Implementation costs of an enhanced recovery after surgery program in the United States: A financial model and sensitivity analysis based on experiences at a quaternary academic medical center. *J Am Coll Surg.* (2016) 222:219–25. doi: 10.1016/j.jamcollsurg.2015.11.021

7

Clinical Application of Indocyanine Green Fluorescence Technology in Laparoscopic Radical Gastrectomy

Meng Wei[1†]*, Yize Liang*[1†]*, Limei Wang*[2]*, Zhen Li*[2]*, Yuanyuan Chen*[3]*, Zhibo Yan*[1]*, Danping Sun*[1]*, Yadi Huang*[1]*, Xin Zhong*[1]*, Peng Liu*[1] *and Wenbin Yu*[1*]

[1] *Department of Gastrointestinal Surgery, General Surgery, Qilu Hospital, Cheeloo College of Medicine, Shandong University, Jinan, China,* [2] *Department of Gastroenterology, Qilu Hospital, Cheeloo College of Medicine, Shandong University, Jinan, China,* [3] *Nursing Department, Qilu Hospital, Cheeloo College of Medicine, Shandong University, Jinan, China*

Correspondence:
Wenbin Yu
wenbin_yu2003@163.com

[†]*These authors have contributed equally to this work and share first authorship*

Background: This study aimed to observe the application and evaluate the feasibility and safety of indocyanine green (ICG) fluorescence technology in laparoscopic radical gastrectomy (LRG).

Methods: Patients who underwent LRG & D2 lymphadenectomy at Qilu Hospital of Shandong University were included between January 2018 and August 2019. According to whether endoscopic injection of ICG was performed, patients were assigned to the ICG group (n=107) and the control group (n=88). The clinicopathologic features, retrieved lymph nodes, postoperative recovery, and follow-up data were compared between the two groups.

Results: Baseline characteristics are comparable. The ICG group had a significantly larger number of lymph nodes retrieved (49.55 ± 12.72 vs. 44.44 ± 10.20, P<0.05), shorter total operation time (min) (198.22 ± 13.14 vs. 202.50 ± 9.91, P<0.05), shorter dissection time (min) (90.90 ± 5.34 vs. 93.74 ± 5.35, P<0.05) and less blood loss (ml) (27.51 ± 12.83 vs. 32.02 ± 17.99, P<0.05). The median follow-up time was 29.0 months (range 1.5-43.8 months), and there was no significant difference between the ICG group and the control group in 2-year OS (87.8% vs. 82.9%, P>0.05) or DFS (86.0% vs. 80.7%, P>0.05).

Conclusions: ICG fluorescence technology in laparoscopic radical gastrectomy has advantages in LN dissection, operation time, and intraoperative blood loss. The 2-year OS and 2-year DFS rates between the two groups were comparable. In conclusion, ICG fluorescence technology is feasible and safe.

Keywords: indocyanine green (ICG), fluorescence, gastric cancer, laparoscopic gastrectomy (LG), lymph node

INTRODUCTION

Gastric cancer is the fifth most frequently diagnosed cancer and the fourth leading cause of death from cancer worldwide (1). Composing complete removal of the tumor and systemic lymph node (LN) dissection, radical surgery remains the mainstay frontline treatment for resectable gastric cancer (2–4). Adequate assessment of the lymph nodes is essential for its role in the disease stage and its prognostic value (5–10), and D2 lymphadenectomy is recommended for advanced gastric cancer (2–4, 11–13).

Laparoscopic gastrectomy (LG) was first reported by Kitano (14) in 1994 and applied in the treatment of advanced gastric cancer by Goh (15) in 1997. Possessing the advantages of minimal invasion and quick postoperative recovery, LG is gradually replacing open surgery as the first choice (16–19). However, because of the lack of tactile feedback and direct observation compared with open surgery, precise tumor positioning under laparoscopy is relatively difficult, especially for patients with early gastric cancer not invading the serosa and those who need additional surgery after noncurative ESD. In addition, the complexity and vastness of the layout of blood and lymphatic vessels contribute to the difficulty and risk of effective LN dissection. Decision and evaluation making done only by the means of surgeons' experience is extremely subjective and poses a danger of false negativity, which may cause insufficient LN dissection and poor prognosis of patients.

As a new surgery technology, dye-mediated surgical navigation (including carbon nanoparticles, indocyanine green, etc.) proved to supply surgeons with improved inspection of the complex perigastric anatomy during laparoscopic surgery. Studies have shown that carbon nanoparticle lymphatic mapping technology increases the number of LNs harvested and realizes tumor localization (20–22). Drawbacks exist, however, that once the carbon nanoparticles leaked into the abdominal cavity, the whole surgical field would be dyed black, thus interfering with the vision of the surgery field and increasing operation difficulty.

Approved by the US Food and Drug Administration (FDA) in the 1960s, ICG was applied to assess cardiac output and hepatic function in the early stage (23–26). Possessing the advantages of not interfering with the surgical field and high tissue penetration (27, 28), ICG fluorescence-guided laparoscopic surgery is therefore the subject of numerous studies (29–34). At present, the application of ICG in LRG has achieved certain success (35, 36) (37, 38). When injected into the gastric tissue around the tumor with endoscopy and exposed to a specific wavelength of near-infrared light, fluorescence emitted from ICG displays the tumor and perigastric LNs (39), making them visible and facilitating the surgery.

To further investigate the feasibility and safety of ICG fluorescence technology in LRG and provide valuable medicine evidence for clinical decision-making in radical gastric cancer resection, we conducted this retrospective study by evaluating the role of ICG fluorescence technology in surgical procedures, lymph node dissection, short-term survival, etc.

Abbreviations: ICG, indocyanine green; LRG, laparoscopic radical gastrectomy.

MATERIALS AND METHODS

Patients and Study Design

Patients who underwent LRG in the Department of Gastrointestinal Surgery, Qilu Hospital of Shandong University from January 2018 to August 2019 were considered for inclusion. According to whether endoscopic injection of ICG was performed, patients were assigned to the ICG group and the control group. Endoscopic ICG injection is an invasive procedure and can only be performed with the patient's consent. Some patients refused the endoscopic ICG injection.

The inclusion criteria were as follows: (1) Primary gastric adenocarcinoma in T1-T4a confirmed by postoperative pathology. (2) Underwent LRG + D2 lymphadenectomy.

The exclusion criteria were as follows: (1) History of previous gastrectomy, endoscopic mucosal resection, or endoscopic submucosal dissection. (2) History of other malignant diseases within the past five years. (3) History of previous neoadjuvant chemotherapy or radiotherapy. (4) Requirement of simultaneous surgery for other diseases. (5) Conversion to laparotomy.

The analyzed data were as follows: (1) Demographic data: age, sex, body mass index (BMI), American Society of Anesthesiology (ASA) physical status scores, and Eastern Cooperative Oncology ECOG performance status. (2) Perioperative outcomes: surgical procedure, operation time, blood loss, first flatus, first liquid diet, postoperative hospital stay, and postoperative complications. (3) Pathological outcomes: tumor diameter, histology, pT, and pN stage. (4) Assessment of D1 station LNs, D2 station LNS, and overall LNs. (5) Overall survival time (OS) and disease-free survival time (DFS).

The study protocol was approved by the Medical Ethics Committee of Qilu Hospital of Shandong University. All procedures were conducted under the ethical standards of the responsible committee on human experimentation (institutional and national) and with the Helsinki Declaration.

Preoperative ICG Injection

Endoscopy was performed 1 day (12-24 hours) before surgery for patients in the ICG group. Four points in the stomach (proximal, distal, and bilateral to the tumor region) were selected, and "sandwich injection methods" were used. In other words, 0.5 ml normal saline + 0.5 mL of ICG solution + 0.5 ml normal saline were injected sequentially into the submucosa layer of each point (**Figure 1**). ICG (25 mg/dose, produced by Dandong Yichuang Pharmaceutical Co., Dandong, China) was diluted with distilled water at a dose of 0.625 mg/ml. Well-trained endoscopists performed all the injections in this study to ensure accurate injection.

Surgery Procedure

In this study, a NOVADAQ fluorescence surgical system (Stryker Co., Kalamazoo, MI, USA) was applied. All patients underwent laparoscopic radical gastrectomy + D2 lymphadenectomy.

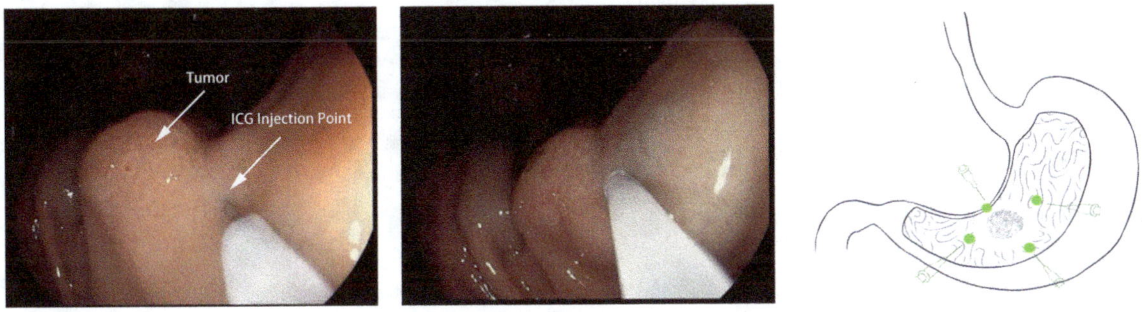

FIGURE 1 | Endoscopic peritumoral ICG injection one day before surgery. A site adjacent to the tumor is selected. Slight swelling of the mucosa without ICG leakage is a sign of successful injection.

During the procedure, the surgeon viewed the surgical field with frequent switching between white light view and near-infrared mode to enable accurate tumor localization (**Figures 2A, B**) and adequate lymphadenectomy at each LN station.

The gastric resection extent and lymphadenectomy were determined based on the tumor location, as stated in the Japanese guidelines (2). Total gastrectomy was performed with Roux-en-Y esophagojejunostomy, and distal gastrectomy was performed with Billroth II gastrojejunostomy + Braun anastomosis.

If fluorescent LNs were detected outside the planned dissection areas (stations 10 and 14v), excessive dissection beyond the scope of D2 lymphadenectomy was performed. (**Figures 2C, D**) In some areas with complex anatomy, such as the spleen vessels and No. 11P LNs, surgery was performed with the assistance of ICG fluorescence. (**Figures 2E–G**) After dissection of LNs in all stations, the near-infrared mode was used to assess the completeness of the lymphadenectomy and remove remnant fluorescent LNs.

Specimen Management

A surgeon from the surgical team performed specimen management immediately after the surgery. LNs of different stations were separated from the specimen according to "the Japanese Classification of Gastric Carcinoma: 3rd English edition" (40) and separately sent to the pathology department. In addition, LNs in the ICG group were examined according to different stations and whether they were fluorescent. (**Figures 2H, I**).

Follow Up

A minimum follow-up of 24 months was required and achieved for each patient after surgery. All enrolled patients underwent physical examination, blood testing, computed tomography, and upper gastrointestinal endoscopy regularly (41–43). Disease-free survival (DFS) time and overall survival time (DFS) were calculated.

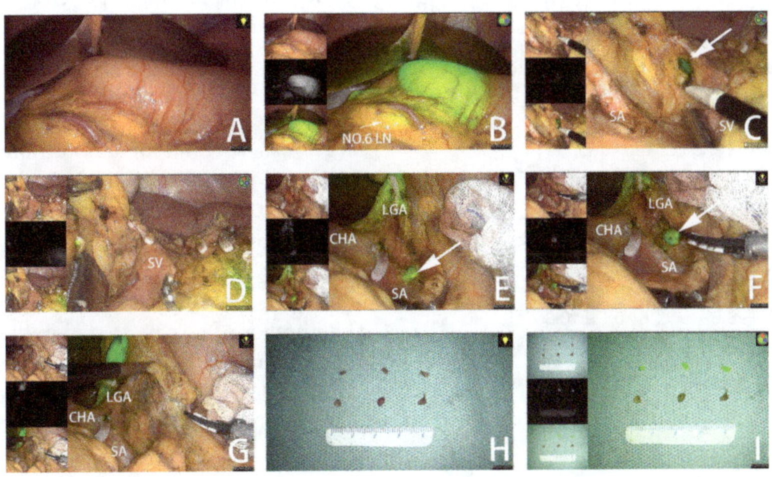

FIGURE 2 | **(A, B)** The tumor is observed under white light and fluorescent mode. **(C)** The fluorescent No.10 LNs are detected under fluorescent mode. **(D)** No remnant No.10 LNs are found after dissection. **(E)** Fluorescent No. 11P LNs are adjacent to splenic vessels. **(F)** No.11P LNs are separated from blood vessels. **(G)** No remnant No. 11P LNs are found after dissection. **(H)** LNs dissected from the specimen under white light. **(I)** LNs dissected from the specimen under fluorescent mode. The arrow points to the fluorescent LN. SA, spleen artery; SV, spleen vein; CHA, common hepatic artery; LGA, left gastric artery.

Statistical Analysis

The differences between the two groups were assessed using t tests, $\chi 2$ tests, or Fisher's exact tests as appropriate. The Kaplan–Meier method and the log-rank test were used for survival analysis. All tests were 2-sided with a significance level of $P < 0.05$. All data were analyzed using SPSS statistical software, version 24.0 (IBM Corp., Armonk, NY, USA). The data are presented as the mean ± standard deviation for continuous variables and as a number for categorical variables.

RESULTS

One hundred ninety-five patients (107 patients in the ICG group and 88 patients in the control group) were retrospectively analyzed. No significant differences were observed in sex, age, BMI, ASA score, or ECOG performance status between the two groups (P > 0.05), which indicates that the baseline characteristics of the two groups were comparable. (**Table 1**)

TABLE 1 | Baseline characteristics of ICG and control group.

	ICG n=107	Control n=88	P Value
Sex			0.859
Male	57 (53.3%)	48 (54.5%)	
Female	50 (46.7%)	40 (45.5%)	
Age (Years)	59.27 ± 8.99	61.53 ± 10.30	0.103
BMI (kg/m²)	24.60 ± 3.41	24.95 ± 2.65	0.424
ASA Score			0.490
I	16 (15.0%)	16 (18.2%)	
II	83 (77.5%)	62 (70.5%)	
III	8 (7.5%)	10 (11.4%)	
ECOG performance status			0.076
0	94 (87.9%)	69 (78.4%)	
1	13 (12.1%)	19 (21.6%)	

Data are shown as the mean ± standard deviation or number (%).
ICG, indocyanine green; BMI, body mass index; ASA, American Society of Anesthesiologists; ECOG, Eastern Cooperative Oncology Group.

Clinicopathologic Characteristics

Clinicopathologic characteristics are listed in **Table 2**. No significant differences between the two groups were observed in tumor diameter, histology, pathological stage, or surgical procedure (P>0.05). Compared to the control group, the ICG group had a significantly shorter total operation time (min) (198.22 ± 13.14 vs 202.50 ± 9.91, P<0.05), shorter dissection time (min) (90.90 ± 5.34 vs 93.74 ± 5.35, P<0.05), and less blood loss (ml) (27.51 ± 12.83 vs 32.02 ± 17.99, P<0.05). There were no significant differences between the two groups in anastomosis time (min) (65.04 ± 3.89 vs 65.82 ± 4.39, P>0.05). The data were compared between the two groups, and no significant differences were observed in terms of first flatus (hours) (63.50 ± 27.345 vs 68.26 ± 28.83, P>0.05), first water intake (hours) (85.51 ± 29.03 vs 92.43 ± 28.48, P>0.05), or postoperative hospital stay (days) (9.22 ± 2.48 vs 9.26 ± 3.04, P>0.05).

Postoperative complications occurred in 15 patients (14%) in the ICG group (anastomotic bleeding in one patient, delayed gastric emptying in one, inflammatory bowel obstruction in two, pneumonia in eight, cholecystitis in two, and lymphatic leakage in one) and 12 patients (13.6%) in the control group (anastomotic leakage in one patient, delayed gastric emptying in two, pneumonia in seven, and cholecystitis in two), and there were no significant differences in the overall postoperative complication rate. (P > 0.05). According to the Clavien–Dindo classification of surgical complications, in the ICG group, 11 patients were classified as grade II or lower, 3 patients as grade IIIa, 1 patient as grade IIIb, and no patient as grade V or higher; in the control group, 7 patients were classified as grade II or lower, 4 patients as grade III a, 1 patient as grade IIIb, and no patient as grade V or higher. The distribution of severity was similar between the 2 groups. Furthermore, 1 patient in the ICG group and 1 patient in the control group experienced a repeat of surgery as a result of anastomotic leakage and bleeding. All patients with complications in both groups were discharged successfully after conservative treatment or surgical interventions. (**Table 3**)

TABLE 2 | Perioperative outcomes of ICG and control group.

	ICG n=107	Control n=88	P Value
Tumor diameter (cm)	4.03 ± 2.48	4.09 ± 2.46	0.871
Histology			0.164
Poorly Differentiated	77 (72.0%)	52 (59.1%)	
Moderately Differentiated	21 (19.6%)	26 (29.5%)	
Well Differentiated	9 (8.4%)	10 (11.4%)	
pT stage			0.894
T1	35 (32.7%)	28 (31.8%)	
T2	18 (16.8%)	17 (19.3%)	
T3	37 (34.6%)	32 (36.4%)	
T4a	17 (15.9%)	11 (12.5%)	
pN stage			0.169
N0	50 (46.7%)	53 (60.2%)	
N1	13 (12.1%)	10 (11.4%)	
N2	11 (10.3%)	11 (12.5%)	
N3a	18 (16.8%)	7 (8.0%)	
N3b	15 (14.0%)	7 (8.0%)	
Surgical procedure			0.235
Distal gastrectomy	59 (55.1%)	41 (46.6%)	
Total gastrectomy	48 (44.9%)	47 (53.4%)	
Operation time (minute)	198.22 ± 13.14	202.50 ± 9.91	0.013
Dissection time	90.90 ± 5.34	93.74 ± 5.35	<0.001
Anastomosis time	65.04 ± 3.89	65.82 ± 4.39	0.190
Blood loss (ml)	27.51 ± 12.83	32.02 ± 17.99	0.043
First flatus (hour)	63.50 ± 27.35	68.26 ± 28.83	0.239
First water intake (hour)	85.51 ± 29.03	92.43 ± 28.48	0.096
Postoperative hospital stay (day)	9.22 ± 2.48	9.26 ± 3.04	0.931

Data are shown as the mean ± standard deviation or number (%).

Lymph Nodes Examination

The number of LNs harvested in the ICG group was significantly higher than that in the control group in terms of the overall LNs (49.55 ± 12.72 vs 44.44 ± 10.208, P<0.05) and the D1 station (28.54 ± 10.55 vs 24.13 ± 6.67, P<0.05), and no difference in the number of D2 station LNs was observed (21.05 ± 4.76 vs 20.38 ± 4.96, P>0.05).

The number of metastatic lymph nodes in the ICG group was significantly higher than that in the control group in terms of the overall LNs (6.45 ± 10.96 vs 3.33 ± 6.45, P<0.05) and the D1 station (5.06 ± 8.52 vs 2.40 ± 4.42, P<0.05), and no difference in

TABLE 3 | Postoperative complications of ICG and control group.

	ICG n=107	Control n=88	P Value
Postoperative complications	15 (14.0%)	12 (13.6%)	1.000
Anastomotic complication			
Bleeding	1 (0.9%)	0	1.000
Leakage	0	1 (1.1%)	1.000
Functional complication			
Delayed gastric emptying	1 (0.9%)	2 (2.3%)	1.000
Inflammatory bowel obstruction	2 (1.9%)	0	0.502
Others			
Respiratory infection	8 (7.5%)	7 (8.0%)	0.784
Cholecystitis	2 (1.9%)	2 (2.3%)	1.000
Lymphatic leakage	1 (0.9%)	0	1.000
In-hospital mortality	0	0	
Clavien–Dindo classification			0.678
I	2 (1.9%)	0	
II	9 (8.4%)	7 (8.0%)	
IIIa	3 (2.8%)	4 (4.5%)	
IIIb	1 (0.9%)	1 (1.1%)	
IV	0	0	
V	0	0	

Data are shown as number (%).

the number of metastatic D2 station LNs was observed (1.39 ± 2.93 vs 0.92 ± 2.32, P>0.05). No significant differences were found in the metastatic rate of LNs in any LN classification between the two groups.

In the ICG group, there was no significant difference in the positive rate of LNs between fluorescent and nonfluorescent LNs (**Table 4**).

Two Years Follow-Up

All patients were followed up, and data were collected: the median follow-up for all patients was 29.0 months (range 1.5-43.8 months). At the time of the last follow-up on August 31, 2021, 162 patients (83%) were alive without recurrence (90 in the ICG group and 72 in the control group), and 6 patients (3%) were alive with recurrence (4 in the ICG group and 2 in the control group). Twenty-seven of 195 patients (14%) had died; among them, 10 patients (5%) in the ICG group had recurrence at the time of death (2 patients with locoregional recurrence, 4 patients with local and distant recurrence, and 4 patients with distant recurrence) and 12 patients (6%) in the control group (2 patients with locoregional recurrence, 7 patients with local and distant recurrence, and 3 patients with distant recurrence), and 5 patients (3%) died due to other causes in the two groups (**Table 5**).

The long-term survival did not show differences between the ICG and control groups: the 2-year OS was 87.8% in the ICG group and 82.9% in the control group (log-rank p = 0.304). The 2-year DFS was 86.0% in the ICG group and 80.7% in the control group (log-rank p = 0.471). (**Figure 3**)

TABLE 4 | Number of retrieved lymph nodes in the ICG and control groups & Positive rate in the ICG group of fluorescent and nonfluorescent LNs.

	ICG n=107	Control n=88	P Value
Overall LNs			
Total LNs	49.55 ± 12.72	44.44 ± 10.20	0.002
Positive LNs	6.45 ± 10.96	3.33 ± 6.45	0.014
Positive rate	9.96 ± 17.83%	12.20 ± 22.38%	0.438
D1 Station LNs			
Total LNs	28.54 ± 10.55	24.13 ± 6.67	<0.001
Positive LNs	5.06 ± 8.52	2.40 ± 4.42	0.006
Positive rate	11.49 ± 18.84%	13.71 ± 21.74%	0.446
D2 Station LNs			
Total LNs	21.05 ± 4.76	20.38 ± 4.96	0.337
Positive LNs	1.39 ± 2.93	0.92 ± 2.32	0.221
Positive rate	5.07 ± 11.63%	5.55 ± 11.49%	0.774
	fluorescent LNs	**nonfluorescent LNs**	**P Value**
Positive rate	17.27 ± 27.58%	9.80 ± 21.39%	0.370

Data are shown as the mean ± standard deviation or number (%).

DISCUSSION

Recently, with the widespread application of laparoscopic surgery for patients with gastric cancer, ICG fluorescence-guided LRG has attracted much attention as a novel navigation technology. To evaluate the feasibility and safety of ICG in LRG, this study was conducted and indicated that compared with conventional LRG, ICG-guided LRG has the advantages of more lymph nodes dissected, less blood loss, and shorter operation time.

As a crucial step in gastric cancer surgery, adequate resection and assessment of LNs have been shown to be linked to disease staging, regional disease control, and long-term survival (6, 7, 44). Interestingly, fluorescence observation based on the absorption characteristics of ICG has been reported to make it possible to distinguish LNs containing ICG particles from surrounding tissue (45, 46), improving the chance of complete dissection. Kwon et al. (47) reported that ICG fluorescence-guided lymphography offered increased lymph node retrieval compared with conventional laparoscopic surgery. Chen et al.

TABLE 5 | Patients' status at last follow-up.

	ICG n=107	Control n=88	P Value
2-year OS	87.8%	82.9%	0.304
2-year DFS	86.0%	80.7%	0.471
2-year OS in T1	93.5%	92.0%	0.814
2-year DFS in T1	94.3%	92.9%	0.806
2-year OS in T2	94.4%	85.6%	0.472
2-year DFS in T2	94.4%	82.4%	0.275
2-year OS in T3	94.2%	85.0%	0.212
2-year DFS in T3	89.2%	87.5%	0.918
2-year OS in T4	52.9%	32.9%	0.191
2-year DFS in T4	52.9%	27.3%	0.175
Alive	94 (87.9%)	74 (84.1%)	
Alive without recurrence	90 (84.1%)	72 (81.8%)	
Alive with recurrence	4 (3.7%)	2 (2.3%)	
Death	13 (12.1%)	14 (15.9%)	
Death with other causes	3 (2.8%)	2 (2.3%)	
Death with recurrence	10 (9.3%)	12 (13.6%)	
Locoregional	2 (1.9%)	2 (2.3%)	
Local and distant	4 (3.7%)	7 (8.0%)	
Distant	4 (3.7%)	3 (3.4%)	

Data are shown as number (%).

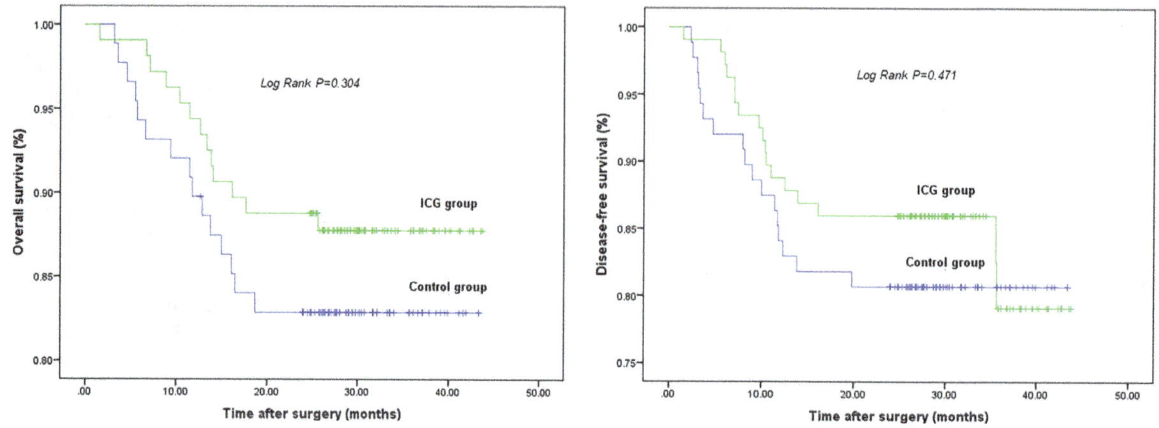

FIGURE 3 | 2-year overall survival (left) and 2-year disease-free survival (right). There is no difference in 2-year OS and 2-year DFS between two groups.

(48) suggested that more lymph nodes could be harvested during ICG-guided LRG with decreased lymph node noncompliance. Similar results are reported in this study; likewise, some new and interesting findings are yielded.

For example, the splenic artery may turn, twist, and become tortuous after originating from the celiac trunk, leading to the obscuration and difficulty of 11P LN dissection. However, possessing the property of strong tissue penetration, ICG fluorescence may highlight lymph nodes and enable the retrieval of a higher number of lymph nodes. In addition, because of the different diffusion and uptake rates of ICG in different tissues, perigastric blood vessels and associated lymphatic vessels can be accurately distinguished, making it possible to remove more lymph nodes adjacent to the blood vessel. Especially in the splenic hilum area, the relatively narrow operating space, the complexity of the vascular anatomy and the fragile texture of the spleen make ICG an indispensable tool to improve the safety and accuracy of surgery.

Since 1997, the Union for International Cancer Control (UICC) and American Joint Commission for Cancer (AJCC) have adopted the N stage of the tumor, node, metastasis (TNM) classification based on the number of metastatic lymph nodes (49). In our study, it seems that there were sufficient lymph nodes in the control group for positive lymph node status determination and more lymph nodes in the ICG group were unnecessary, but we should not ignore the fact that lymph node micrometastasis could not be exactly evaluated by routine H&E examination and is well associated with poor outcome in patients (50–54). Huang et al. (55) demonstrated that the number of dissected LNs is the only factor affecting negative lymph node counts. In other words, more lymph nodes dissected increases the number of positive lymph nodes and so-called negative nodes that may harbor micrometastases, thus leading to a better prognosis (56–58).

Although our study found that more overall LNs contributed to more positive LNs in the ICG group, we should take it into account that ICG is not a targeting marker for tumor cells (59) and is unable to trace positive LNs specifically. We also conducted a small sample (35 patients) study examining fluorescent and nonfluorescent LNs respectively in the ICG group, and no significant difference was found in the metastatic rate confirmed by pathology. Moreover, it is not uncommon to find discrepancies in which some obviously enlarged LNs are proven to be pathologically metastatic, but they are not fluorescent (60). This is considered to be partly because the lymphatic vessels were obstructed by a massive cancer embolus, the ICG cannot flow into these LNs (61). Therefore, ICG fluorescence technology can only be used to assist lymph node dissection, instead of being relied on to determine whether the lymph node is metastatic, which is consistent with the report of Cianchi et al. (62)

Another key step in curative gastric cancer surgery is the complete removal of the primary tumor with sufficient negative margins. Indeed, positive margins are associated with significantly worse survival (63–65). In fact, ICG fluorescence can improve the lack of visual inspection and palpation in traditional laparoscopic surgery and prove effective in the identification of tumors in our study. The surgeon can observe the tumor with frequent switching between white light view and near-infrared mode after endoscopic ICG injection around the tumor. As a consequence, it is possible to reduce the operation time and surgical invasion. In addition, the characteristics of ICG in distinguishing lymph nodes and surrounding tissues also enable prompt and accurate intraoperative decisions to speed up the surgical process and reduce the risk of blood vessel injury and bleeding.

It is reported that intraoperative blood loss and transfusion are associated with a higher risk of morbidity and mortality, although further investigation is needed (66–69). Yasuda et al. reported that not only the volume of blood loss, but the operation time is associated with morbidity after gastrectomy (70). In addition, cardiopulmonary adverse effects of general anesthesia and dioxide pneumoperitoneum are significant in laparoscopic surgery (71, 72). In this study, the ICG group was shown to provide the advantages of decreased intraoperative blood loss and shorter surgery time than the control group. The routine use of ICG fluorescence could potentially reduce the perioperative complications caused by blood loss and prolong dioxide pneumoperitoneum during LRG. In addition, the morbidity rates were 14.0% in the ICG group and 13.6% in the control group (P>0.05), which were similar to the rates reported in previous studies (73, 74). No intraoperative events or delayed complications during their hospital stay related to ICG were observed.

After a 2-year follow-up, there was no significant difference in long-term survival in each stage between the ICG group and the control group. This may be explained by the fact of the shorter follow up period of the present study. We also found that ICG-guided LRG obviously improved OS and DFS, because the number of harvested LNs in the ICG group was significantly larger and adequate numbers of LNs dissected in the standard lymphadenectomy region were necessary for accurate disease staging and avoiding LN micrometastasis, thus having a good impact on the prognosis of patients (75–77).

Currently, two ICG injection methods are used: preoperative endoscopic submucosal injection and intraoperative subserous injection. During the study, we found that the former is superior (61) since intraoperative injection may increase surgery risk caused by prolonged operation time and pneumoperitoneum time. In addition, the location of the tumor cannot be indicated accurately under laparoscopy if ICG was not injected around the tumor (78). There was also not sufficient time for ICG to diffuse from injection sites into the D2 station LNs. Of note, the concentration of ICG solution should not be too high; otherwise, the excessively strong fluorescence intensity may obstruct the observation of tissues. However, unlike carbon nanoparticles, low-dose of ICG is not visible in white light mode, so high concentrations or leakage of ICG do not interfere with the surgeon's vision.

There are some limitations to this study. First, compared with the control group, patients in ICG group had to bear more costs for indocyanine green and endoscopic injection. Second, there was no significant difference in long-term survival between the two groups due to the relatively short follow-up time, so a longer follow-up is necessary. Third, ICG is not a targeting tracer for tumor cells, so efforts to develop more targeted dyes are required. Fourth, this was not a strictly randomized controlled study, but patients almost randomly accept endoscopic ICG injections. The study was conducted at Qilu hospital of Shandong university that performs more than 1,000 gastrectomies for advanced gastric cancer each year. Considering the large number of patients, relatively few inpatient beds and the cost of hospitalization, the number of days in hospital before surgery was strictly controlled. In our hospital, gastroenterologists are also endoscopists, who are mainly responsible for the treatment of patients in addition to endoscopy. Inpatients waiting for surgery can receive endoscopic injection only after completing all preoperative examinations and making a successful appointment with an endoscopist. Those who do not meet these requirements cannot receive ICG injection.

In summary, a large randomized, multicenter trial is warranted to further evaluate the feasibility and safety of indocyanine green fluorescence technology in LRG for gastric cancer.

This study indicates that, with a shorter operation time, less blood loss, and no complications attributable to ICG, ICG fluorescence technology can guide surgeons to rapidly locate tumors and harvest more lymph nodes than conventional LRG. In addition, the two-year OS and DFS are comparable between two groups. In conclusion, ICG fluorescence technology in laparoscopic radical gastrectomy is safe and valuable.

AUTHORS CONTRIBUTIONS

WY is the corresponding author. MW and YZ are joint first authors. WY contributed to the study concept and design. WY, ZB and MW conducted the laparoscopic radical gastrectomy. LM and ZL conducted the endoscopy. MW and YZ wrote the manuscript. MW, YZ, LM, ZL, YY, ZB, DP, YD, XZ and PL conducted the data collection and analysis. WY revised and edited the manuscript. WY and YY are the guarantors of this study. All authors contributed to the article and approved the submitted version.

ETHICS STATEMENT

The studies involving human participants were reviewed and approved by the Medical Ethics Committee of Qilu Hospital of Shandong University. The patients/participants provided their written informed consent to participate in this study.

ACKNOWLEDGMENTS

We are grateful for all the patients who participated in this study.

REFERENCES

1. Sung H, Ferlay J, Siegel RL, Laversanne M, Soerjomataram I, Jemal A, et al. Global Cancer Statistics 2020: GLOBOCAN Estimates of Incidence and Mortality Worldwide for 36 Cancers in 185 Countries. *CA Cancer J Clin* (2021) 71(3):209–49. doi: 10.3322/caac.21660
2. Japanese Gastric Cancer A. Japanese Gastric Cancer Treatment Guidelines 2018 (5th Edition). *Gastric Cancer* (2021) 24(1):1–21. doi: 10.1007/s10120-020-01042-y
3. Smyth EC, Nilsson M, Grabsch HI, van Grieken NC, Lordick F. Gastric Cancer. *Lancet* (2020) 396(10251):635–48. doi: 10.1016/S0140-6736(20)31288-5
4. Guideline Committee of the Korean Gastric Cancer Association DWG, Review P. Korean Practice Guideline for Gastric Cancer 2018: An Evidence-Based, Multi-Disciplinary Approach. *J Gastric Cancer* (2019) 19 (1):1–48. doi: 10.5230/jgc.2019.19.e8
5. Wu CW, Hsiung CA, Lo SS, Hsieh MC, Chen JH, Li AF, et al. Nodal Dissection for Patients With Gastric Cancer: A Randomised Controlled Trial. *Lancet Oncol* (2006) 7(4):309–15. doi: 10.1016/S1470-2045(06)70623-4
6. Songun I, Putter H, Kranenbarg EM, Sasako M, van de Velde CJ. Surgical Treatment of Gastric Cancer: 15-Year Follow-Up Results of the Randomised Nationwide Dutch D1D2 Trial. *Lancet Oncol* (2010) 11(5):439–49. doi: 10.1016/S1470-2045(10)70070-X
7. Amin MB, Greene FL, Edge SB, Compton CC, Gershenwald JE, Brookland

RK, et al. The Eighth Edition AJCC Cancer Staging Manual: Continuing to Build a Bridge From a Population-Based to a More "Personalized" Approach to Cancer Staging. *CA Cancer J Clin* (2017) 67(2):93–9. doi: 10.3322/caac.21388

8. Wu CW, Hsieh MC, Lo SS, Tsay SH, Lui WY, P'Eng FK. Relation of Number of Positive Lymph Nodes to the Prognosis of Patients With Primary Gastric Adenocarcinoma. *Gut* (1996) 38(4):525–7. doi: 10.1136/gut.38.4.525
9. Siewert JR, Bottcher K, Stein HJ, Roder JD. Relevant Prognostic Factors in Gastric Cancer: Ten-Year Results of the German Gastric Cancer Study. *Ann Surg* (1998) 228(4):449–61. doi: 10.1097/00000658-199810000-00002
10. Smith DD, Schwarz RR, Schwarz RE. Impact of Total Lymph Node Count on Staging and Survival After Gastrectomy for Gastric Cancer: Data From a Large US-Population Database. *J Clin Oncol* (2005) 23(28):7114–24. doi: 10.1200/JCO.2005.14.621
11. Smyth EC, Verheij M, Allum W, Cunningham D, Cervantes A, Arnold D, et al. Gastric Cancer: ESMO Clinical Practice Guidelines for Diagnosis, Treatment and Follow-Up. *Ann Oncol* (2016) 27(suppl 5):v38–49. doi: 10.1093/annonc/mdw350
12. Hu Y, Huang C, Sun Y, Su X, Cao H, Hu J, et al. Morbidity and Mortality of Laparoscopic Versus Open D2 Distal Gastrectomy for Advanced Gastric Cancer: A Randomized Controlled Trial. *J Clin Oncol* (2016) 34(12):1350–7. doi: 10.1200/JCO.2015.63.7215
13. Degiuli M, Reddavid R, Tomatis M, Ponti A, Morino M, Sasako M, et al. D2 Dissection Improves Disease-Specific Survival in Advanced Gastric Cancer Patients: 15-Year Follow-Up Results of the Italian Gastric Cancer Study Group D1 Versus D2 Randomised Controlled Trial. *Eur J Cancer* (2021) 150:10–22. doi: 10.1016/j.ejca.2021.03.031
14. Kitano S, Iso Y, Moriyama M, Sugimachi K. Laparoscopy-Assisted Billroth I Gastrectomy. *Surg Laparosc Endosc* (1994) 4(2):146–8.
15. Goh PM, Khan AZ, So JB, Lomanto D, Cheah WK, Muthiah R, et al. Early Experience With Laparoscopic Radical Gastrectomy for Advanced Gastric Cancer. *Surg Laparosc Endosc Percutan Tech* (2001) 11(2):83–7. doi: 10.1097/00129689-200104000-00003
16. Lee HJ, Hyung WJ, Yang HK, Han SU, Park YK, An JY, et al. Short-Term Outcomes of a Multicenter Randomized Controlled Trial Comparing Laparoscopic Distal Gastrectomy With D2 Lymphadenectomy to Open Distal Gastrectomy for Locally Advanced Gastric Cancer (KLASS-02-RCT). *Ann Surg* (2019) 270(6):983–91. doi: 10.1097/SLA.0000000000003217
17. Katai H, Mizusawa J, Katayama H, Morita S, Yamada T, Bando E, et al. Survival Outcomes After Laparoscopy-Assisted Distal Gastrectomy Versus Open Distal Gastrectomy With Nodal Dissection for Clinical Stage IA or IB Gastric Cancer (JCOG0912): A Multicentre, Non-Inferiority, Phase 3 Randomised Controlled Trial. *Lancet Gastroenterol Hepatol* (2020) 5 (2):142–51. doi: 10.1016/S2468-1253(19)30332-2
18. Yu J, Huang C, Sun Y, Su X, Cao H, Hu J, et al. Effect of Laparoscopic vs Open Distal Gastrectomy on 3-Year Disease-Free Survival in Patients With Locally Advanced Gastric Cancer: The CLASS-01 Randomized Clinical Trial. *JAMA* (2019) 321(20):1983–92. doi: 10.1001/jama.2019.5359
19. Chen QY, Zhong Q, Liu ZY, Huang XB, Que SJ, Zheng WZ, et al. Advances in Laparoscopic Surgery for the Treatment of Advanced Gastric Cancer in China. *Eur J Surg Oncol* (2020) 46(10 Pt B):e7–e13. doi: 10.1016/j.ejso.2020.07.015
20. Yan J, Zheng XL, Liu ZYZ, Yu J, Deng ZW, Xue FQ, et al. A Multicenter Study of Using Carbon Nanoparticles to Show Sentinel Lymph Nodes in Early Gastric Cancer. *Surg Endosc* (2016) 30(4):1294–300. doi: 10.1007/s00464-015-4358-8
21. Feng Y, Yang K, Sun HH, Liu YP, Zhang D, Zhao Y, et al. Value of Preoperative Gastroscopic Carbon Nanoparticles Labeling in Patients Undergoing Laparoscopic Radical Gastric Cancer Surgery. *Surg Oncol* (2021) 38:101628. doi: 10.1016/j.suronc.2021.101628
22. Tian Y, Lin Y, Guo H, Hu Y, Li Y, Fan L, et al. Safety and Efficacy of Carbon Nanoparticle Suspension Injection and Indocyanine Green Tracer-Guided Lymph Node Dissection During Robotic Distal Gastrectomy in Patients With Gastric Cancer. *Surg Endosc* (2021). doi: 10.1007/s00464-021-08630-8
23. Alford R, Simpson HM, Duberman J, Hill GC, Ogawa M, Regino C, et al. Toxicity of Organic Fluorophores Used in Molecular Imaging: Literature Review. *Mol Imaging* (2009) 8(6):341–54. doi: 10.2310/7290.2009.00031
24. Cherrick GR, Stein SW, Leevy CM, Davidson CS. Indocyanine Green: Observations on its Physical Properties, Plasma Decay, and Hepatic Extraction. *J Clin Invest* (1960) 39:592–600. doi: 10.1172/JCI104072
25. Desmettre T, Devoisselle JM, Mordon S. Fluorescence Properties and Metabolic Features of Indocyanine Green (ICG) as Related to Angiography. *Surv Ophthalmol* (2000) 45(1):15–27. doi: 10.1016/S0039-6257(00)00123-5
26. Reinhart MB, Huntington CR, Blair LJ, Heniford BT, Augenstein VA. Indocyanine Green: Historical Context, Current Applications, and Future Considerations. *Surg Innov* (2016) 23(2):166–75. doi: 10.1177/1553350615604053
27. Schaafsma BE, Mieog JS, Hutteman M, van der Vorst JR, Kuppen PJ, Lowik CW, et al. The Clinical Use of Indocyanine Green as a Near-Infrared Fluorescent Contrast Agent for Image-Guided Oncologic Surgery. *J Surg Oncol* (2011) 104(3):323–32. doi: 10.1002/jso.21943
28. Vahrmeijer AL, Hutteman M, van der Vorst JR, van de Velde CJ, Frangioni JV. Image-Guided Cancer Surgery Using Near-Infrared Fluorescence. *Nat Rev Clin Oncol* (2013) 10(9):507–18. doi: 10.1038/nrclinonc.2013.123
29. Boni L, David G, Mangano A, Dionigi G, Rausei S, Spampatti S, et al. Clinical Applications of Indocyanine Green (ICG) Enhanced Fluorescence in Laparoscopic Surgery. *Surg Endosc* (2015) 29(7):2046–55. doi: 10.1007/s00464-014-3895-x
30. Boni L, David G, Dionigi G, Rausei S, Cassinotti E, Fingerhut A. Indocyanine Green-Enhanced Fluorescence to Assess Bowel Perfusion During Laparoscopic Colorectal Resection. *Surg Endosc* (2016) 30(7):2736–42. doi: 10.1007/s00464-015-4540-z
31. Wang X, Teh CSC, Ishizawa T, Aoki T, Cavallucci D, Lee SY, et al. Consensus Guidelines for the Use of Fluorescence Imaging in Hepatobiliary Surgery. *Ann Surg* (2021) 274(1):97–106. doi: 10.1097/SLA.0000000000004718
32. Aoki T, Koizumi T, Mansour DA, Fujimori A, Kusano T, Matsuda K, et al. Ultrasound-Guided Preoperative Positive Percutaneous Indocyanine Green Fluorescence Staining for Laparoscopic Anatomical Liver Resection. *J Am Coll Surg* (2020) 230(3):e7–12. doi: 10.1016/j.jamcollsurg.2019.11.004
33. Herrera-Almario G, Patane M, Sarkaria I, Strong VE. Initial Report of Near-Infrared Fluorescence Imaging as an Intraoperative Adjunct for Lymph Node Harvesting During Robot-Assisted Laparoscopic Gastrectomy. *J Surg Oncol* (2016) 113(7):768–70. doi: 10.1002/jso.24226
34. Yoshida M, Kubota K, Kuroda J, Ohta K, Nakamura T, Saito J, et al. Indocyanine Green Injection for Detecting Sentinel Nodes Using Color Fluorescence Camera in the Laparoscopy-Assisted Gastrectomy. *J Gastroenterol Hepatol* (2012) 27(Suppl 3):29–33. doi: 10.1111/j.1440-1746.2012.07067.x
35. Ushimaru Y, Omori T, Fujiwara Y, Yanagimoto Y, Sugimura K, Yamamoto K, et al. The Feasibility and Safety of Preoperative Fluorescence Marking With Indocyanine Green (ICG) in Laparoscopic Gastrectomy for Gastric Cancer. *J Gastrointest Surg* (2019) 23(3):468–76. doi: 10.1007/s11605-018-3900-0
36. Ikoma N, Badgwell BD, Mansfield P. Fluorescent-Image Guidance in Robotic Subtotal Gastrectomy. *Ann Surg Oncol* (2020) 27(13):5322. doi: 10.1245/s10434-020-08523-5
37. Shoji Y, Kumagai K, Kamiya S, Ida S, Nunobe S, Ohashi M, et al. Prospective Feasibility Study for Single-Tracer Sentinel Node Mapping by ICG (Indocyanine Green) Fluorescence and OSNA (One-Step Nucleic Acid Amplification) Assay in Laparoscopic Gastric Cancer Surgery. *Gastric Cancer* (2019) 22(4):873–80. doi: 10.1007/s10120-018-00919-3
38. Kim TH, Kong SH, Park JH, Son YG, Huh YJ, Suh YS, et al. Assessment of the Completeness of Lymph Node Dissection Using Near-Infrared Imaging With Indocyanine Green in Laparoscopic Gastrectomy for Gastric Cancer. *J Gastric Cancer* (2018) 18(2):161–71. doi: 10.5230/jgc.2018.18.e19
39. Luo S, Zhang E, Su Y, Cheng T, Shi C. A Review of NIR Dyes in Cancer Targeting and Imaging. *Biomaterials* (2011) 32(29):7127–38. doi: 10.1016/j.biomaterials.2011.06.024
40. Japanese Gastric Cancer A. Japanese Classification of Gastric Carcinoma: 3rd English Edition. *Gastric Cancer* (2011) 14(2):101–12. doi: 10.1007/s10120-011-0041-5
41. Hur H, Song KY, Park CH, Jeon HM. Follow-Up Strategy After Curative Resection of Gastric Cancer: A Nationwide Survey in Korea. *Ann Surg Oncol* (2010) 17(1):54–64. doi: 10.1245/s10434-009-0676-1
42. Whiting J, Sano T, Saka M, Fukagawa T, Katai H, Sasako M. Follow-Up of Gastric Cancer: A Review. *Gastric Cancer* (2006) 9(2):74–81. doi: 10.1007/s10120-006-0360-0

43. Zanotti D, Baiocchi GL, Coniglio A, Mohammadi B, Ministrini S, Mughal M, et al. Follow-Up After Surgery for Gastric Cancer: How to do it. *Updates Surg* (2018) 70(2):293–9. doi: 10.1007/s13304-018-0524-6
44. Maehara Y, Kakeji Y, Koga T, Emi Y, Baba H, Akazawa K, et al. Therapeutic Value of Lymph Node Dissection and the Clinical Outcome for Patients With Gastric Cancer. *Surgery* (2002) 131(1 Suppl):S85–91. doi: 10.1067/msy.2002.119309
45. Kim DW, Jeong B, Shin IH, Kang U, Lee Y, Park YS, et al. Sentinel Node Navigation Surgery Using Near-Infrared Indocyanine Green Fluorescence in Early Gastric Cancer. *Surg Endosc* (2019) 33(4):1235–43. doi: 10.1007/s00464-018-6401-z
46. Roh CK, Choi S, Seo WJ, Cho M, Son T, Kim HI, et al. Indocyanine Green Fluorescence Lymphography During Gastrectomy After Initial Endoscopic Submucosal Dissection for Early Gastric Cancer. *Br J Surg* (2020) 107(6):712–9. doi: 10.1002/bjs.11438
47. Kwon IG, Son T, Kim HI, Hyung WJ. Fluorescent Lymphography-Guided Lymphadenectomy During Robotic Radical Gastrectomy for Gastric Cancer. *JAMA Surg* (2019) 154(2):150–8. doi: 10.1001/jamasurg.2018.4267
48. Chen QY, Xie JW, Zhong Q, Wang JB, Lin JX, Lu J, et al. Safety and Efficacy of Indocyanine Green Tracer-Guided Lymph Node Dissection During Laparoscopic Radical Gastrectomy in Patients With Gastric Cancer: A Randomized Clinical Trial. *JAMA Surg* (2020) 155(4):300–11. doi: 10.1001/jamasurg.2019.6033
49. Sano T, Coit DG, Kim HH, Roviello F, Kassab P, Wittekind C, et al. Proposal of a New Stage Grouping of Gastric Cancer for TNM Classification: International Gastric Cancer Association Staging Project. *Gastric Cancer* (2017) 20(2):217–25. doi: 10.1007/s10120-016-0601-9
50. Kim JJ, Song KY, Hur H, Hur JI, Park SM, Park CH. Lymph Node Micrometastasis in Node Negative Early Gastric Cancer. *Eur J Surg Oncol* (2009) 35(4):409–14. doi: 10.1016/j.ejso.2008.05.004
51. Yasuda K, Adachi Y, Shiraishi N, Inomata M, Takeuchi H, Kitano S. Prognostic Effect of Lymph Node Micrometastasis in Patients With Histologically Node-Negative Gastric Cancer. *Ann Surg Oncol* (2002) 9 (8):771–4. doi: 10.1007/BF02574499
52. Lee E, Chae Y, Kim I, Choi J, Yeom B, Leong AS. Prognostic Relevance of Immunohistochemically Detected Lymph Node Micrometastasis in Patients With Gastric Carcinoma. *Cancer* (2002) 94(11):2867–73. doi: 10.1002/cncr.10562
53. Wu ZY, Li JH, Zhan WH, He YL, Wan J. Effect of Lymph Node Micrometastases on Prognosis of Gastric Carcinoma. *World J Gastroenterol* (2007) 13(30):4122–5. doi: 10.3748/wjg.v13.i30.4122
54. Zeng YJ, Zhang CD, Dai DQ. Impact of Lymph Node Micrometastasis on Gastric Carcinoma Prognosis: A Meta-Analysis. *World J Gastroenterol* (2015) 21(5):1628–35. doi: 10.3748/wjg.v21.i5.1628
55. Huang CM, Lin JX, Zheng CH, Li P, Xie JW, Lin BJ. Effect of Negative Lymph Node Count on Survival for Gastric Cancer After Curative Distal Gastrectomy. *Eur J Surg Oncol* (2011) 37(6):481–7. doi: 10.1016/j.ejso.2011.01.012
56. Harrison LE, Karpeh MS, Brennan MF. Extended Lymphadenectomy Is Associated With a Survival Benefit for Node-Negative Gastric Cancer. *J Gastrointest Surg* (1998) 2(2):126–31. doi: 10.1016/S1091-255X(98)80002-4
57. Saito H, Fukumoto Y, Osaki T, Fukuda K, Tatebe S, Tsujitani S, et al. Prognostic Significance of Level and Number of Lymph Node Metastases in Patients With Gastric Cancer. *Ann Surg Oncol* (2007) 14(5):1688–93. doi: 10.1245/s10434-006-9314-3
58. Deng JY, Liang H, Sun D, Pan Y, Zhang RP, Wang BG, et al. Outcome in Relation to Numbers of Nodes Harvested in Lymph Node-Positive Gastric Cancer. *Eur J Surg Oncol* (2009) 35(8):814–9. doi: 10.1016/j.ejso.2008.11.007
59. Egloff-Juras C, Bezdetnaya L, Dolivet G, Lassalle HP. NIR Fluorescence-Guided Tumor Surgery: New Strategies for the Use of Indocyanine Green. *Int J Nanomedicine* (2019) 14:7823–38. doi: 10.2147/IJN.S207486
60. Miyashiro I, Hiratsuka M, Kishi K, Takachi K, Yano M, Takenaka A, et al. Intraoperative Diagnosis Using Sentinel Node Biopsy With Indocyanine Green Dye in Gastric Cancer Surgery: An Institutional Trial by Experienced Surgeons. *Ann Surg Oncol* (2013) 20(2):542–6. doi: 10.1245/s10434-012-2608-8
61. Tajima Y, Yamazaki K, Masuda Y, Kato M, Yasuda D, Aoki T, et al. Sentinel Node Mapping Guided by Indocyanine Green Fluorescence Imaging in Gastric Cancer. *Ann Surg* (2009) 249(1):58–62. doi: 10.1097/SLA.0b013e3181927267
62. Cianchi F, Indennitate G, Paoli B, Ortolani M, Lami G, Manetti N, et al. The Clinical Value of Fluorescent Lymphography With Indocyanine Green During Robotic Surgery for Gastric Cancer: A Matched Cohort Study. *J Gastrointest Surg* (2020) 24(10):2197–203. doi: 10.1007/s11605-019-04382-y
63. Songun I, Bonenkamp JJ, Hermans J, van Krieken JH, van de Velde CJ. Prognostic Value of Resection-Line Involvement in Patients Undergoing Curative Resections for Gastric Cancer. *Eur J Cancer* (1996) 32A(3):433–7. doi: 10.1016/0959-8049(95)00591-9
64. Cho BC, Jeung HC, Choi HJ, Rha SY, Hyung WJ, Cheong JH, et al. Prognostic Impact of Resection Margin Involvement After Extended (D2/D3) Gastrectomy for Advanced Gastric Cancer: A 15-Year Experience at a Single Institute. *J Surg Oncol* (2007) 95(6):461–8. doi: 10.1002/jso.20731
65. Morgagni P, Garcea D, Marrelli D, de Manzoni G, Natalini G, Kurihara H, et al. Does Resection Line Involvement Affect Prognosis in Early Gastric Cancer Patients? An Italian Multicentric Study. *World J Surg* (2006) 30 (4):585–9. doi: 10.1007/s00268-005-7975-x
66. Glance LG, Dick AW, Mukamel DB, Fleming FJ, Zollo RA, Wissler R, et al. Association Between Intraoperative Blood Transfusion and Mortality and Morbidity in Patients Undergoing Noncardiac Surgery. *Anesthesiology* (2011) 114(2):283–92. doi: 10.1097/ALN.0b013e3182054d06
67. Al-Refaie WB, Parsons HM, Markin A, Abrams J, Habermann EB. Blood Transfusion and Cancer Surgery Outcomes: A Continued Reason for Concern. *Surgery* (2012) 152(3):344–54. doi: 10.1016/j.surg.2012.06.008
68. Spence RK, Carson JA, Poses R, McCoy S, Pello M, Alexander J, et al. Elective Surgery Without Transfusion: Influence of Preoperative Hemoglobin Level and Blood Loss on Mortality. *Am J Surg* (1990) 159(3):320–4. doi: 10.1016/S0002-9610(05)81227-9
69. Wu WC, Smith TS, Henderson WG, Eaton CB, Poses RM, Uttley G, et al. Operative Blood Loss, Blood Transfusion, and 30-Day Mortality in Older Patients After Major Noncardiac Surgery. *Ann Surg* (2010) 252(1):11–7. doi: 10.1097/SLA.0b013e3181e3e43f
70. Yasuda K, Shiraishi N, Adachi Y, Inomata M, Sato K, Kitano S. Risk Factors for Complications Following Resection of Large Gastric Cancer. *Br J Surg* (2001) 88(6):873–7. doi: 10.1046/j.0007-1323.2001.01782.x
71. Galizia G, Prizio G, Lieto E, Castellano P, Pelosio L, Imperatore V, et al. Hemodynamic and Pulmonary Changes During Open, Carbon Dioxide Pneumoperitoneum and Abdominal Wall-Lifting Cholecystectomy. A Prospective, Randomized Study. *Surg Endosc* (2001) 15(5):477–83. doi: 10.1007/s004640000343
72. Sharma KC, Brandstetter RD, Brensilver JM, Jung LD. Cardiopulmonary Physiology and Pathophysiology as a Consequence of Laparoscopic Surgery. *Chest* (1996) 110(3):810–5. doi: 10.1378/chest.110.3.810
73. Kim W, Song KY, Lee HJ, Han SU, Hyung WJ, Cho GS. The Impact of Comorbidity on Surgical Outcomes in Laparoscopy-Assisted Distal Gastrectomy: A Retrospective Analysis of Multicenter Results. *Ann Surg* (2008) 248(5):793–9. doi: 10.1097/SLA.0b013e3181887516
74. Kim HH, Han SU, Kim MC, Hyung WJ, Kim W, Lee HJ, et al. Long-Term Results of Laparoscopic Gastrectomy for Gastric Cancer: A Large-Scale Case-Control and Case-Matched Korean Multicenter Study. *J Clin Oncol* (2014) 32 (7):627–33. doi: 10.1200/JCO.2013.48.8551
75. Macalindong SS, Kim KH, Nam BH, Ryu KW, Kubo N, Kim JY, et al. Effect of Total Number of Harvested Lymph Nodes on Survival Outcomes After Curative Resection for Gastric Adenocarcinoma: Findings From an Eastern High-Volume Gastric Cancer Center. *BMC Cancer* (2018) 18(1):73. doi: 10.1186/s12885-017-3872-6
76. Pan S, Wang P, Xing Y, Li K, Wang Z, Xu H, et al. Retrieved Lymph Nodes From Different Anatomic Groups in Gastric Cancer: A Proposed Optimal Number, Comparison With Other Nodal Classification Strategies and its Impact on Prognosis. *Cancer Commun (Lond)* (2019) 39(1):49. doi: 10.1186/s40880-019-0394-4
77. Giuliani A, Caporale A, Corona M, Di Bari M, Demoro M, Ricciardulli T, et al. Lymphadenectomy in Gastric Cancer: Influence on Prognosis of Lymph Node Count. *J Exp Clin Cancer Res* (2004) 23(2):215–24.
78. Kitagawa Y, Fujii H, Kumai K, Kubota T, Otani Y, Saikawa Y, et al. Recent Advances in Sentinel Node Navigation for Gastric Cancer: A Paradigm Shift of Surgical Management. *J Surg Oncol* (2005) 90(3):147–51; discussion 51-2. doi: 10.1002/jso.20220

8

The Safety and Efficacy of the Continuous Peripheral Nerve Block in Postoperative Analgesia of Pediatric Patients

Dušica Simić[1,2], Marija Stević[1,2], Zorana Stanković[1], Irena Simić[1], Siniša Dučić[1,3], Ivana Petrov[1] and Miodrag Milenović[2,4]*

[1] Department of Anesthesiology and Intensive Care, University Children's Hospital, Belgrade, Belgrade, Serbia, [2] Medical Faculty University of Belgrade, Belgrade, Serbia, [3] Department of Orthopedic Surgery, University Children's Hospital, Belgrade, Belgrade, Serbia, [4] Department of Anesthesiology and Intensive Care, Clinical Center of Serbia, Belgrade, Serbia

***Correspondence:**
Dušica Simić
dusicasimic2@gmail.com

Postoperative analgesia is imperative in the youngest patients. Pain, especially if experienced during childhood, has numerous adverse effects—from psychological, through complications of the underlying disease (prolonged treatment, hospital stay, and increased costs of the treatment) to an increase in the incidence of death due to the onset of the systemic inflammatory response. Peripheral blocks provide analgesia for 12–16 h, and are safer due to rare side effects that are easier to treat. The continuous peripheral block (CPNB) has been increasingly used in recent years for complete and prolonged analgesia of pediatric patients, as well as a part of multidisciplinary treatment of complex regional pain syndrome. It has been shown that outpatient CPNB reduces the need for parenteral administration of opioid analgetics. It has also been proved that this technique can be used in pediatric patients in home conditions. Safety of CPNB is based on the increasing use of ultrasound as well as on the introduction of single enantiomers local anesthetics (ropivacaine and levobupivacaine) in lower concentrations. It is possible to discharge patient home with catheter, but it is necessary to provide adequate education for staff, patients, and parents, as well as to have dedicated anesthesiology team. Postoperative period without major pain raises the morale of the child, parents. and medical staff.

Keywords: pediatric anesthesia, continuous peripheral nerve block, postoperative analgesia, pain management, perineural catheters

MINI REVIEW

The pain, according to the new definition, is a disturbing experience associated with existing or potential tissue damage, with a sensory, emotional, cognitive, and social component (1). Postoperative analgesia is imperative in the youngest patients. Pain, especially experienced during childhood, has numerous adverse effects—from psychological, through complications of the underlying disease (prolonged treatment, hospital stay and increased costs of the treatment) to an increase in the incidence of death due to the onset of the systemic inflammatory response (2). It is clear that all those who deal with child health care have a moral obligation to prevent and adequately cure their pain.

Regardless of immaturity, the child can feel pain since birth (3). The pain sensitivity is greater in younger children and so analgesia should be provided to them during, before and after the surgery since birth. Repetition of painful procedures determines the threshold for pain for the whole life (4). Inadequate treatment of acute pain is one of the important prerequisites for the development of chronic pain.

The goal of analgesia in the postoperative period is to reduce or eliminate pain with minimal additional harmful effects and overall treatment costs. Adequate postoperative analgesia, especially during the first 48 h, reduces the stress response of the organism to the surgical procedure, thereby affecting endocrine, metabolic, and inflammatory changes. This reduces the incidence of postoperative complications and improves the outcome of surgical treatment (4–8).

Single shot peripheral regional blocks provide analgesia for 12–16 h, almost the same length as central blocks (9). Peripheral blocks are safer due to rare side effects that are easier to treat and their use has increased significantly over the last two decades (10). The continuous peripheral block (CPNB) has been increasingly used in recent years for complete and prolonged analgesia of pediatric patients, as well as a part of multidisciplinary treatment of complex regional pain syndrome (CRPS) or epidermolysis bullosa (11).

It has been proven that outpatient CPNB reduces the need for parenteral administration of opioid analgesics (12). It has also been proven that this technique can be used in pediatric patients in home conditions (13, 14). Patients can be released home even with a residual motor block, after prescribed additional oral analgesic therapy and after they received verbal and written instructions regarding the use of CPNB and the identification of possible complications (muscle weakness, less feeling for hot or sharp objects…) (13). There is currently no publication on the wound catheter technique in pediatric patients (11).

There are still not enough prospective studies to confirm the efficacy and safety of CPNB technique and the existing studies have numerous limitations. Comparison of studies is difficult due to differences in the definition of side effects.

Safety of CPNB is based on the increasing use of ultrasound (US) as well as on the introduction of single enantiomers local anesthetics (LA) (ropivacaine and levobupivacaine) in lower concentrations. Originally, bupivacaine had a primacy, while today ropivacaine (0.1–0.2% by infusion, average 0.25 mg/kg/h) is mainly used because of its lower toxicity (9, 15, 16). This LA also provides a better differential block (sensory block without motor nerve paresis) (17). It can also be used for a patient controlled administration (0.2% ropivacaine 0.02 ml/kg/h, bolus 0.1 ml/kg, lockout interval 30 min) (18). The risk of LA toxicity to muscle tissue is increased in infants, so it is advised to use the lowest possible doses and concentrations of LA (11, 19).

However, if catheter efficiency is suspected in the immediate postoperative period, it is recommended to perform a test bolus dose of 3 ml of lidocaine 1.5% with epinephrine 1:200,000 (15). If tachicardia appears, the catheter is placed intravascularly.

Peripheral regional block in children has faster onset but short duration. In children under 1 year of age, nerve fibers are thinner, myelination is scarce, and Ranvier's nodes are closer. The volume of distribution is higher (20, 21), clearance is smaller (22), and the free drug fraction (unbounded for proteins) is higher (20) so the doses are almost the same as in adults. Cytochrome CYP1A2 on which ropivacaine is metabolized matures around the age of 4–7 years old, and CYP3A4/7 on which levobupivacaine is metabolized matures at the end of the first year (23).

Catheters are placed in sterile conditions with the help of a nerve stimulator (4.6%), ultrasound (30.2%), or a combination of these two techniques (62.9%) (15). Placement of perineural catheters under the control of US is becoming more and more frequent and has an increasingly wider use nowadays. In the study of Walker et al. (9), the ultrasound has advantages (in up to 90% of the cases depending on the type of block). Advantages of using US are reflected in the fact that it is possible to monitor the path of anatomical structures to achieve a safe orientation. The latest US devices allow visualization of the needle itself and in that way they ensure the best position of the needle in relation to the anatomical structures, reduce the risk of nerve injury and surrounding structures. US enables monitoring of the distribution of LA, preventing intravascular injection and optimizes the amount of LA which reduces the risk of toxic reactions. The catheter was usually placed under general anesthesia [in 92.9% of patients by Visoiu et al. (15) and in 98.9% of cases by Gurnaney et al. (12)].

Patient satisfaction is a very important indicator of the quality of treatment and higher pain control satisfaction score (PCSS) is an indicator of better patient care. Pediatric patients have expressed satisfaction with the popliteal CPNB (24). For the first time, Visoiu et al. evaluated pediatric patient satisfaction with analgesic therapy using PCSS and 91.4% of patients were very satisfied (8–10 out of 10) (15). They reported home PCSS for parents (9–10 out of 10) and for medical staff (9–10 out of 10). In Visoiu et al. study, more patients reported pain at home than during the Postoperative Ambulatory Care Unit (PACU) stays. Pain scores were lower in the PACU and on postoperative day 0 than on postoperative day 1 and the following days (15).

In a study by Visoiu M et al., 31.4% of patients did not have pain and did not receive any additional analgesics during their stay in PACU. After the release from the hospital, 25% of the patients did not have any pain at home, although 97% of patients received at least 1 dose of opioids (15). According to Dadure et al. about 60% of patients received at least 1 additional dose of oral analgesics (25). Study of Ganesh et al. showed that about 56% of children received opioid during the first eight postoperative days (13). The average time for the first dose of opioids in Gurnaney's study was 16 h (12). 60% of their patients needed an opioid within the first 8 h 40% of which received the opioid already in the recovery room (12). The incidence of patients needing opioid analgesia increased to about 74% by 48 h with about 26% of the patients not requiring any opioid analgesics (11). The reason for the frequent use of opioids could have been due to the preference of lower concentration and infusion rate of LA to avoid motor block (recommended 0.4 mg/kg/h maximum infusion rate for ropivacaine). Another reason could be that multiple nerves need to be blocked, to provide complete sensory block after certain procedures.

Continuous peripheral block does not exclude the additional use of opioids (13). In the PACU surgical analgesia is usually achieved by CPNB but some other pains (tourniquet) or reasons to be restless remains (anxiety, due to the absence of the parents, emergence delirium associated with sevoflurane, etc.). Postoperative use of opioids in home conditions is likely to occur because parents are advised to give the prescribed medication (as needed) to the children with low intensity pain or before going to sleep (15).

Perineural catheter technique is used in chronic pain. The management of patient with CRPS is integrated in a multidisciplinar approach associating pain management with physiotherapy treatment and psychological management. The keys to success are active physiotherapy treatment and restoration of normal limb movement to which CPNB may contribute. Recurrent CRPS remains a therapeutic challenge in pediatric patients. Dadure et al (11), reported that a 4-day CPNB after an initial Bier block is effective against intractable and recurrent CRPS in 13 children, leading to pain reduction, physiotherapy facilitation, and functional rehabilitation. In this study, all children were able to move about easily after the initial 24-h period and continued the treatment at home using infusion pumps.

Complications are rare and minor, mainly mechanical (accidental catheter withdrawal, dislodgement, or occlusion), and nausea and vomiting (11). So far, the largest study on the safety of perineural catheters use in children on over 2,000 set up catheters in children demonstrated a low degree of complication, which is correlated with the percentage of complications in the adult population (15).

In the study by Visoiu et al., 14.4% of patients had subsequent catheter-related complications, mainly minimal catheter leakage that did not affect the analgesic effect (15). Dadure et al. reported 20.1% of mechanical problems associated with catheter (mainly leakage and dislodgement) (25). In a study by Ganesh et al. (13), the catheter was accidentally withdrawn in 40.5% of patients. Despite the use of good fixation, Walker et al. noticed the occurrence of subcutaneous catheter migration that may result in secondary block failure (9). Gurnaney et al. had 4.2% catheter complications, 1.9% catheter failure, and only 0.07% of local inflammation (12). There were no differences in the risks and complications in inpatients and outpatients. It is necessary to improve the technique of catheters positioning and fixing (12, 24). Some authors recommend the use of a small drop of Dermabond (Ethicon, Raleigh, NC, USA) at the insertion site (12, 15, 16) to prevent leaking.

Visoiu et al. reported that 28% of patients had postoperative nausea/vomiting and/or itching (15). The technique did not work in only 6.9% of cases, but even this small percentage is unacceptable for patients and medical staff. In the study by Dadure et al. 14.7% patients had nausea/vomiting and only 1.5% urinary retention and 0.9% pruritus (24). Gable et al. reported postoperative nausea and vomiting in 5.9% of patients (14).

In the study by Walkers et al. (9), there were no permanent neurological complications of deep infection or local anesthetic toxicity, but most patients were older than 10 years. There were no permanent neurological complications of deep infection or LA toxicity in other studies as well (10, 15). The most common local complications are rare: local inflammation at the site of catheter placement (redness, swelling, or pain) and abscess at the catheter insertion site. Ecoffey noticed only superficial infections or blood vessel puncture (10). Studies have shown that perineural catheters infections are a rare occurrence and that the incidence is in correlation with the time that has passed since the catheter is placed (9, 12, 13). It is considered that the perineural catheters should be removed 3 days after the placement which reduces complications to a minimum (15), except in cases where the benefits to the patient overcomes the clinical risk of infection.

Many complications (e.g., paresthesia) are difficult to diagnose in infants and nonverbal children who cannot describe their symptoms accurately. Nevertheless, in a study by Polaner et al. (26) the incidence of serious complications that was detected in prospectively acquired unselected population was extremely small, and no sequelae lasting >3 months were reported in close to 15,000 regional anesthetics. There were no serious complications such as persistent neurological deficit. In these instances, we must rely on confidence intervals to provide an upper limit of possible incidence rates (for example, although there was no mortality reported in 9,156 neuraxial blocks, a mortality of 0–3.3: 10,000 is still consistent) (26).

Krane and Polaner believe that it cannot be determined whether the rare symptoms of LA (e.g., tinnitus) are objective or only placebo responses in children who are told to pay attention to these symptoms of LA toxicity (27).

Absolute contraindications for placement of perineural catheters are: allergy to local anesthetic and infection at the site of planned puncture. Relative contraindications are sepsis, prolonged PT and PTT, heart failure, neurological diseases, and patient refusal. Due to the small number of contraindications and improvements in the clinical, economic, and humanistic approach, perineural catheters are used more often nowadays (15).

CONCLUSION

Regional anesthesia is commonly used in addition to general anesthesia to provide adequate postoperative analgesia and better comfort. It provides sufficient analgesia and better comfort and it is rarely performed in a wake state. Postoperative course without the significant pain raises the morale of the child, parents, and medical staff. The surgeon as well as the anesthesiologist is pleased to see a peaceful, alert and cooperative child in the immediate postoperative period. From an ethical point of view, it is not justifiable to allow the child to suffer pain, when simple and safe techniques of regional anesthesia are easily complementing or replacing conventional-general anesthesia. The goal of a physician should always be to minimize the psychological and physical trauma of the patient, regardless of how young and immature the child is. Hospital stay will be forever remembered as a traumatic experience if pain is not adequately treated. Therefore, proper care of pain is of great importance.

The use of any technique of regional anesthesia depends on the estimated risk/benefit ratio. No published study reported sustained neurological complications or serious side effects after use of CPNB. It is possible to discharge patient home with the catheter, but it is necessary to provide adequate education for staff, patients, and parents, as well as to have dedicated anesthesiology team. It is extremely important to organize adequate monitoring of these patients by phone calls and visits by trained medical workers. Regardless of the numerous ethical and security problems in the design of pediatric studies, more prospective studies are needed to provide adequate evidence.

AUTHOR CONTRIBUTIONS

DS: conceptualization, investigation, project administration, visualization, and wrote the manuscript. MS: investigation, visualization, literature review and wrote the manuscript. ZS: literature review, providing regional anesthesia, visualization and investigation. IS: placing perineural catheters, providing regional anesthesia, visualization, and investigation. SD: investigation and supervision. IP: providing regional anesthesia, language supervision and made a final version of manuscript. MM: visualization, analysis of literature, and investigation.

REFERENCES

1. Williams AC, Craig KD. Updating the definition of pain. *Pain* (2016) 157(11):2420–3. doi:10.1097/j.pain.0000000000000613
2. Kulshrestha A, Bajwa SJS. Management of acute postoperative pain in pediatric patients. *Anesth Pain Intens Care* (2014) 18(1):101–5.
3. Berry PH, Chapman CR, Covington EC, Dahl JL, Katz JA, Miaskowski C, et al. *Pain: Current Understanding of Assessment, Management and Treatments.* Pennsylvania Avenue: Joint Commission on Accreditation of Healthcare Organizations and the National Pharmaceutical Council, Inc. (2001).
4. Kehlet H, Holte K. Effect of postoperative analgesia on surgical outcome. *Br J Anaesth* (2001) 87:62–72. doi:10.1093/bja/87.1.62
5. Moraca RJ, Sheldon DG, Thirlby RC. The role of epidural anesthesia and analgesia in surgical practice. *Ann Surg* (2003) 238(5):663–73. doi:10.1097/01.sla.0000094300.36689.ad
6. Waurick R, Van Aken H. Update in thoracic epidural anaesthesia. *Best Pract Res Clin Anaesthesiol* (2005) 19(2):201–13. doi:10.1016/j.bpa.2004.12.001
7. Pasero C. Improving postoperative outcomes with epidural analgesia. *J Perianesth Nurs* (2005) 20(1):51–5. doi:10.1016/j.jopan.2004.11.007
8. Liu SS, Wu CL. Effect of postoperative analgesia on major postoperative complications: a systematic update of the evidence. *Anesth Analg* (2007) 104(3):689–702. doi:10.1213/01.ane.0000255040.71600.41
9. Walker BJ, Long JB, De Oliveira GS, Szmuk P, Setiawan C, Polaner DM, et al. Peripheral nerve catheters in children: an analysis of safety and practice patterns from the pediatric regional anesthesia network (PRAN). *Br J Anaesth* (2015) 115(3):457–62. doi:10.1093/bja/aev220
10. Ecoffey C, Lacroix F, Giaufré E, Orliaguet G, Courrèges P. Epidemiology and morbidity of regional anesthesia in children: a follow-up one-year prospective survey of the French-Language Society of Paediatric Anaesthesiologists (ADARPEF). *Paediatr Anaesth* (2010) 20:1061–9. doi:10.1111/j.1460-9592.2010.03448.x
11. Dadure C, Capdevila X. Peripheral catheter techniques. *Pediatr Anaesth* (2012) 22:93–101. doi:10.1111/j.1460-9592.2011.03730.x
12. Gurnaney H, Kraemer FW, Maxwell L, Muhly WT, Schleelein L, Ganesh A. Ambulatory continuous peripheral nerve blocks in children and adolescents: a longitudinal 8-year Single Center Study. *Anesth Analg* (2014) 118:621–7. doi:10.1213/ANE.0b013e3182a08fd4
13. Ganesh A, Rose JB, Wells L, Ganley T, Gurnaney H, Maxwell LG, et al. Continuous peripheral nerve blockade for inpatient and outpatient postoperative analgesia in children. *Anesth Analg* (2007) 105:1234–42. doi:10.1213/01.ane.0000284670.17412.b6
14. Gable A, Burrier C, Stevens J, Wrona S, Klingele K, Bhalla T, et al. Home peripheral nerve catheters: the first 24 months of experience at a children's hospital. *J Pain Res* (2016) 9:1067–72. doi:10.2147/JPR.S110947
15. Visoiu M, Joy LN, Grudziak JS, Chelly JE. The effectiveness of ambulatory continuous peripheral nerve blocks for postoperative pain management in children and adolescents. *Paediatr Anaesth* (2014) 24:1141–8. doi:10.1111/pan.12518
16. Aarons L, Sadler B, Pitsiu M, Sjovall J, Henriksson J, Molnar V. Population pharmacokinetic analysis of ropivacaine and its metabolite 2,6-pipecoloxylidide from pooled data in neonates, infants, and children. *Br J Anaesth* (2011) 107:409–24. doi:10.1093/bja/aer154
17. McClure JH. Ropivacaine. *Br J Anaesth* (1996) 76:300. doi:10.1093/bja/76.2.300
18. Dufflo F, Santouo-Miranda V, Pouyau A, Taylor P, Combet S, Chotel F, et al. Efficacy and plasma level of ropivacaine for children: controlled regional analgesia following lower limb surgery. *Br J Anaesth* (2006) 97:250–4. doi:10.1093/bja/ael145
19. Nouette G, Sirvent P, Canal Raffin M, Morau D, Malgat M, Molimard M, et al. Effects of intermittent femoral nerve injections of bupivacaine, levobupivacaine, and ropivacaine on mitochondrial energy metabolism and intracellular calcium homeostasis in rat psoas muscle. *Anesthesiology* (2007) 106:1026–34. doi:10.1097/01.anes.0000265164.29630.b4
20. Bosenberg B. Regional anesthesia: central neuraxial blocks. In: Bissonnette B, editor. *Pediatric Anesthesia.* USA: Peoples Medical Publishing House (2011). p. 806–7.
21. Palmon SC, Lloyd AT, Kirsch JR. The effect of needle gauge and lidocaine pH on pain during intradermal injection. *Anesth Analg* (1998) 86:379–81.
22. Suresh S, Polaner DM, Cote CJ. *Regional Anesthesia in: Cote and Lermans A Pediatrice of Anesthesia for Infants and Children.* Philadephia: Publishing Elsevier Saunders (2013). p. 835–79.
23. Johr M. Regional anaesthesia in neonates, infants and children. *Eur J Anaesthesiol* (2015) 32:289–97. doi:10.1097/EJA.0000000000000239
24. Ludot H, Berger J, Pichenot V, Belouadah M, Madi K, Malinovsky JM. Continuous peripheral nerve block for postoperative pain control at home: a prospective feasibility study in children. *Reg Anesth Pain Med* (2008) 33(1):52–6. doi:10.1016/j.rapm.2007.07.014
25. Dadure C, Bringuier S, Raux O, Rochette A, Troncin R, Canaud N, et al. Continuous peripheralnerve blocks for postoperative analgesia in children: feasibility and side effects in a cohort study of 339 catheters. *Can J Anaesth* (2009) 56:843–50. doi:10.1007/s12630-009-9169-8
26. Polaner DM, Taenzer AH, Walker BJ. Pediatric regional Anesthesia network (PRAN): a multi-instutional study of the use and incidence of comlications of pediatric regiona anesthesia. *Anesth Analg* (2012) 115(6):1353–64. doi:10.1213/ANE.0b013e31825d9f4b
27. Krane EJ, Polaner D. The safety and effectiveness of continuous peripheral nerve blockade in children. *Anesth Analg* (2014) 118:499–500. doi:10.1213/ANE.0000000000000110

9

Modified Leak-Proof Puncture Technique for the Aspiration of Giant Ovarian Cysts by Instantly Mounting a Plastic Wrap and Gauze with Cyanoacrylates

Hiroshi Ishikawa and Makio Shozu*

Department of Reproductive Medicine, Graduate School of Medicine, Chiba University, Chiba, Japan

**Correspondence:*
Hiroshi Ishikawa
ishikawa@chiba-u.jp

Objective: We developed a leak-proof puncture technique for giant ovarian cysts by instantly mounting a plastic wrap to the cysts using cyanoacrylates and aspirating cyst fluid over the wrap. Here, we modified it by inserting a gauze between the wrap and cyst to strengthen the mounting. This study aimed to clarify the feasibility of the modified procedure.

Method: A retrospective observational study was conducted in a single center. Surgical outcomes of 35 women who underwent the modified procedure from December 2013 to July 2020 were compared with those of 51 women who underwent the original procedure.

Results: Mean long-axis diameters of the cysts were 233.1 mm and 229.8 mm in the modified and original procedures, respectively. The median of surgical time, blood loss, and aspirated fluid volume were 109 min, 50 ml, and 3,050 ml, in the modified procedure, all of which were not significantly different from those of the original procedure. One case of mounting disruption and two (5.7%) cases of intraperitoneal spillage of the cyst fluid were observed in the modified procedure, whereas four (7.8%) cases of mounting disruption and five (9.8%) cases of intraperitoneal spillage occurred in the original procedure. These events were caused by aspiration difficulty of the high viscosity fluid and/or multilocular cysts. Laparotomy conversion was observed in five (14.3%) cases in the modified procedure.

Conclusion: Our modified procedure is feasible in select cases. The high viscosity of the cyst fluid and multilocular cyst may cause mounting disruption and intraperitoneal spillage of the cyst fluid.

Keywords: minimally invasive surgical procedures, ovarian cysts, cyanoacrylates, leak-proof puncture, minilaparotomy, plastic wrap

INTRODUCTION

The leak-proof puncture technique for the aspiration of cyst fluid in giant ovarian cysts is necessary for the removal of the cysts through small abdominal incisions and may prevent intraperitoneal spillage of cyst fluid during minimally invasive surgery. Several puncture techniques to aspirate the cyst contents without leakage during laparoscopic surgery have been reported (1–3). We had earlier reported a leak-proof puncture technique using cyanoacrylates and plastic wrap through mini laparotomy (4).

Our original technique consisted of instantly mounting a plastic wrap to the cyst using cyanoacrylates, followed by cyst fluid aspiration over this wrap. This technique is applicable to large and multiple cysts that exceed the umbilical height. However, the mounting between the wrap and the cyst was occasionally disrupted because of its fragility, resulting in the unexpected leakage of cyst fluid during aspiration. To reinforce the mounting between the wrap and the cyst, we modified the technique by inserting a gauze between the cyst and the wrap. Herein, we have reviewed a case series of the modified procedure and compared its surgical outcomes with those of the original procedure to clarify the feasibility and determine the appropriate recipients of the modified procedure.

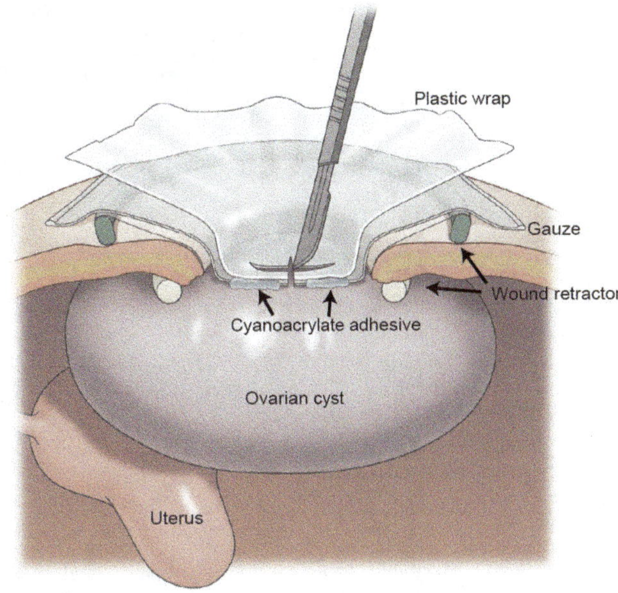

FIGURE 1 | Illustration of the modified leak-proof puncture technique for the aspiration of giant ovarian cysts. This illustration shows a cross-section of the modified leak-proof puncture technique for fluid aspiration of giant ovarian cysts. A wound retractor is attached to the abdominal small incision, and a plastic wrap and gauze are mounted to the cyst instantly using cyanoacrylate adhesive. After the mounting process, the cyst wall is cut and the cyst fluid is aspirated over the wrap.

MATERIALS AND METHODS

This is a retrospective observational study conducted in a single center. The study protocols for data analysis, including referring patient records, were approved by the Institutional Review Board at the Graduate School of Medicine, Chiba University (No. 2267). For this study, the opt-out method was applied to obtain consent for reviewing the patient records.

The study participants were women who underwent resection of giant ovarian cysts using the leak-proof puncture technique by instantly mounting a plastic wrap to the cysts using cyanoacrylates in the Chiba University Hospital. We have introduced the modified procedure in December 2013. Accordingly, we reviewed the medical records of 35 women who underwent the modified procedure in our facility from December 2013 to July 2020. To validate the modified procedure, we reviewed data of 51 women who underwent the original procedure for giant ovarian cyst fluid aspiration from January 2006 to September 2013.

The leak-proof puncture technique was applied to treat giant ovarian cysts that were determined to be benign tumors, including those which we cannot completely deny as borderline malignant tumors on preoperative imaging, mainly magnetic resonance imaging (MRI). Medical image interpretation specialists of our facility participated in a conference to determine the surgical indications relevant to the procedure.

An illustration of the modified procedure, consisting of the instant mounting of the plastic wrap and gauze to the cyst using cyanoacrylate adhesive and cyst fluid aspiration, is presented in **Figure 1**. First, we made a 3–5 cm transverse or vertical incision in the lower abdomen and attached a disposable retractor (Alexis® Wound Retractor; Applied Medical, Rancho Santa Margarita, CA, USA or other similar retractors) to visualize the cyst surface (**Figure 2A**). Then, we removed moisture from the cyst surface, placed a sterile gauze on the cyst, and applied cyanoacrylates (Aron Alpha®; Dai-ichi Sankyo, Tokyo, Japan) in a 2–4 cm diameter circle over the gauze (**Figure 2B**). Subsequently, we pressed a plastic wrap onto the gauze surface for 3 min (**Figure 2C**). The color of the adhesive changed from transparent to white following the completion of polymerization (**Figure 2D**). Subsequently, we punctured the cyst through the wrap with a sharp-pointed knife (**Figure 1**). The cyst fluid, with low viscosity, exuded from the cyst and was aspirated *via* the puncture hole (**Figure 3A**). Direct insertion of aspiration tubes into the puncture hole should be avoided to prevent the mounting from tearing. For multilocular cysts, initially, we aspirated the fluid in the largest cyst using the modified technique, punctured the adjacent cyst septum, and aspirated the cyst fluid. In cases where the adjacent cyst wall was not visible through the puncture hole, we pulled the cyst wall using forceps and extended the wall incision under direct vision. After the maximum possible aspiration of the cyst fluid, we lifted the cyst wall with the forceps (**Figure 3B**), placed it outside the body (**Figure 3C**), and performed cyst resection

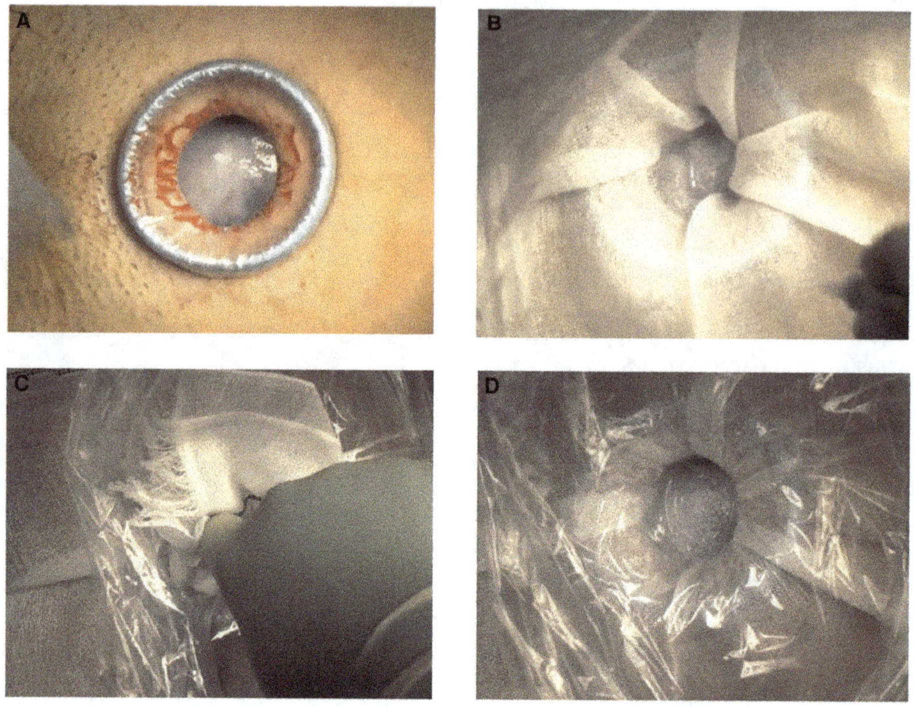

FIGURE 2 | Instant mounting of plastic wrap and gauze to the giant ovarian cyst. **(A)** Completion of the attachment of a wound retractor to the 3-cm lower abdominal transverse incision. **(B)** Condition immediately after applying cyanoacrylates on the cyst through the gauze. **(C)** Mounting the plastic wrap and gauze on the cyst. **(D)** Completion of the instant mounting to the cyst wall. The color of the adhesive has changed from transparent to white upon completion of cyanoacrylate polymerization.

(cystectomy) or oophorectomy (**Figure 3D**). We also presented a representative video (**Supplementary Material**).

We reviewed patients' age, body mass index (BMI), histories of laparotomy and/or laparoscopy as patients' characteristics and preoperative estimation of the long-axis diameter of the cysts that was measured by MRI. We also reviewed the surgical time, blood loss volume, and aspirated cyst fluid as surgical outcomes. Additionally, we analyzed the reasons for mounting disruption and/or intraperitoneal spillage of the cyst fluid. We also analyzed the reasons for conversion to laparotomy during the modified procedure. If the surgeon has little experience of the modified procedure, an experienced physician participated in the surgery as the first assistant.

JMP 14.0 (SAS Institute, Inc., Cary, NC) was used for statistical analyses. The comparison of continuous and categorical variables between women who underwent the modified procedure and those who underwent the original procedure was performed using the Student t-test and Pearson's chi-square test, respectively. Statistical significance was defined as $p < 0.05$.

RESULTS

Patient characteristics and surgical outcomes are presented in **Table 1**. Patients' age, BMI, and long-axis diameter of the cysts were not significantly different between women who underwent the modified and original procedures. The mean long-axis diameters of the cysts were 233.1 mm and 229.8 mm in the modified and original procedure, respectively. The median surgical time, blood loss volume, and aspirated cyst fluid in the modified procedure were 109 min, 50 ml, and 3,050 ml, respectively, whereas those in the original procedure were 118 min, 150 ml, and 2,800 ml, respectively. These parameters were not significantly different between the modified and original procedures except for blood loss volumea. Histopathology revealed that most of the ovarian cysts in the modified procedure were mucinous cyst adenomas.

Mounting disruption was observed in only one case in the modified procedure, whereas it was observed in four cases in the original procedure. Intraperitoneal spillage of the cyst fluid did not occur in the modified procedure because the fluid was highly viscous. Conversely, spillage was observed in all cases in the original procedure. The disruption and subsequent spillage occurred at the aspiration of multilocular cysts. Intraperitoneal spillage of the cyst fluid that was not accompanied by mounting disruption during surgery was observed in two cases in the modified procedure and two cases in the original procedure. The spillage occurred during the aspiration of multilocular cysts and/or the aspiration of the highly viscous fluid. Disruption of the cyst wall has occurred instead of the mounting disruption in these cases.

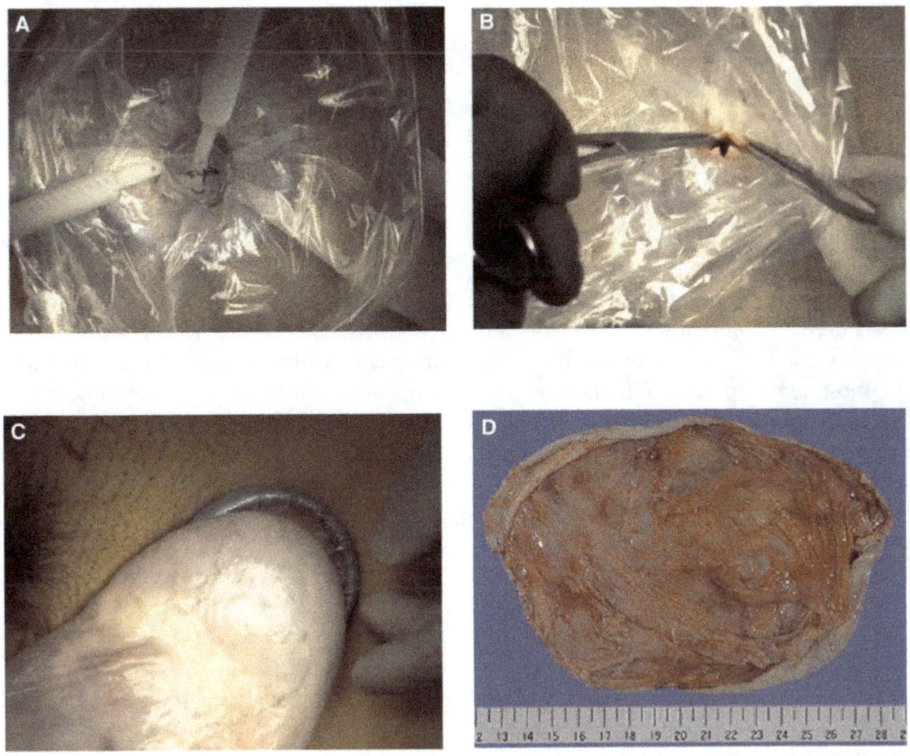

FIGURE 3 | Aspiration of the cyst fluid and cystectomy of the giant ovarian cyst. (**A**) Aspirating cyst fluid over the wrap. The cyst fluid of the serous cystadenoma flows from the puncture hole. (**B**) After cyst fluid aspiration, the mounting is pinched off with forceps to avoid intraperitoneal spillage of the cyst fluid. (**C**) The cyst is brought outside the body. (**D**) Resected giant ovarian cyst. The longitudinal diameter of the cyst is 205 mm. The pathological diagnosis was serous cystadenoma.

TABLE 1 | Patient characteristics and surgical outcomes.

	Modified procedure (n = 35)	Original procedure (n = 51)	p-value
Patient characteristics			
Age (year)[a]	50.3 ± 21.5	46.6 ± 23.0	0.4500
BMI (kg/m^2)[a]	22.6 ± 3.7	22.2 ± 4.0	0.6622
Long axis diameter of the cysts (mm)[a,c]	233.1 ± 61.9	229.8 ± 69.7	0.8246
Surgical outcomes			
Surgical time (min)[b]	109 (56–238)	118 (50–296)	0.1471
Volume of blood loss (ml)[b]	50 (5–590)	150 (10–5,335)	0.0387
Volume of aspirated cyst fluid (ml)[b]	3,050 (800–13,800)	2,800 (400–14,000)	0.6115

[a]*Data are presented as mean ± standard deviation.*
[b]*Data are presented as median (range).*
[c]*Diameter calculated by preoperative imaging evaluation.*

Conversion to laparotomy was observed in five cases in the modified procedure. Reasons for the conversion were as follows: difficulty of aspiration over the wrap because of the highly viscous cyst fluid (two cases), difficulty in picking up the entire cyst after cyst fluid aspiration due to broad and firm adhesions between the cyst and rectosigmoid colon caused by prior hysterectomy (two cases), and difficulty of mounting a plastic wrap and gauze due to the retroperitoneal location of the cyst (one case). No recurrent cases associated with intraperitoneal spillage of cyst fluid were observed.

DISCUSSION

Intraperitoneal spillage of the cyst fluid of ovarian cystic tumors should be avoided during resection, even if they are not suspected of malignancy, preoperatively. When intraperitoneal spillage of the cyst fluid occurs, peritoneal lavage is necessary. Before the introduction of the modified procedure, we had occasionally experienced intraperitoneal spillage of the cyst fluid because of the mounting disruption during the aspiration procedure. Mounting disruption may be due to the fragility of the adhesive surface. The gelatinous, highly viscous cyst fluid is challenging to aspirate over the wrap; hence, the fluid from inside the cyst is directly aspirated, leading to a strong tension over the mounting that causes its disruption. We had experienced four cases of mounting disruption out of 51 cases before the modification, and this disruption has shown an evident reduction with the modified technique (1 of 35 cases), though this difference was not significantly significant.

Although similar leak-proof puncture techniques using Dermabond and Dermabond plus (Johnson &Johnson Inc., NJ, USA) and BioGlue (CryoLife, GA, USA) for instant mounting of a plastic bag, vinyl membrane, and surgical glove to ovarian cysts have been reported (5–7), to the best of our knowledge, our modification to secure the mounting has not yet been reported. Similar to the original procedure, the modified procedure is safe, quick, and easy to perform, without requiring specialized training. In addition, it can be applied to giant ovarian cysts where the upper border is over the umbilicus. Laparoscopic surgery for the resection of huge ovarian cysts has also been reported; however, preventive methods for intraperitoneal spillage during the suction of the cyst fluid have not been mentioned in most of them. Our modification can also be applied during laparoscopic-assisted surgery.

Inadequate intraperitoneal observation throughout the small incision is a disadvantage of the modified technique at mini laparotomy, as with the original technique. Intraperitoneal adhesions between the tumor and other organs may be unidentifiable. Laparoscopy-assisted surgery could resolve this problem. Appropriate reduction of the cyst volume will enable the safe insertion of laparoscopic trocars into the abdominal wall, after pneumoperitoneum is achieved. The wound retractor, in our case series, was covered with a surgical glove and the cap closed to avoid air leakage during laparoscopy. Other authors have reported that a laparoscopic cap was put on to create and maintain pneumoperitoneum at the laparoscopy (8). The combination of laparoscopic observation and subsequent release of the adhesion may be useful in avoiding laparotomy conversion in cases of adhesion between the cyst and pelvic walls or other intraperitoneal organs.

A prior history of hysterectomy is associated with intraperitoneal adhesion between the ovarian tumor and intraperitoneal organs, including the pelvic peritoneum, gastrointestinal tract, and omentum (9). The remaining adnexa are occasionally fixed to the pelvic side wall during hysterectomy; in such cases, placing the entire ovarian cyst outside the body was observed to be difficult even after complete aspiration of the cyst contents. Therefore, careful attention must be paid to patients with prior history of hysterectomy before the application of the modified procedure.

Based on the instructions, the Aron alpha ethyl-2-cyanoacrylate used in this study, can be used below skin level and also for vessel adhesion. It has been used for soft tissue bonding in dermatologic surgeries (10) and surgical adhesion to blood vessels in vascular surgeries (11). No toxicity issues with the glue have been reported so far. Furthermore, we developed our modified procedure to reduce the risks of glue spillage inside the abdominal cavity. The gauze inserted between the plastic wrap and the cyst wall helps to trap all the glue. From this point of view, our modified procedure is much safer than the original procedure.

Cost-effectiveness including operative time in the modified procedure should be discussed. Compared with the original procedure, the modified procedure only adds a sterile gauze. It takes several seconds to insert the gauze between the plastic wrap and the cyst wall, and thus the operative time in the modified procedure may be delayed by several seconds. On the other hand, the enforcement of the bonding makes it easy to pick up the cyst outside the body. This may shorten the subsequent resection of the cyst. From this point of view, the modified procedure is also cost-effective.

This study has several limitations. First, the sample size is relatively small. Therefore, we could not detect any significance in the frequency of mounting disruption, intraperitoneal spillage of the cyst fluid, and conversion to laparotomy between the modified procedure and the original procedure. Second, we chose women who underwent the original procedure for the control. The surgeons who performed the two procedures were different, which might affect the surgical outcomes. Third, surgeons' experience in performing the procedure is a potential bias for the surgical outcomes. Finally, surgical outcomes included not only the leak-proof puncture procedures but also the subsequent cystectomy or resection of the cysts. Surgical time may extend, and blood loss volume may increase in cases of laparotomy conversion.

This procedure is important for decreasing the risk of ovarian cancer upstaging. Although we did not apply the modified procedure to apparent malignant ovarian cystic tumors in preoperative imaging diagnosis, we experienced several cases that showed malignancy in postoperative pathological diagnosis. Fortunately, intraperitoneal spillage of the cyst fluid did not occur in these cases; nevertheless, making an effort to avoid intraperitoneal spillage during the procedures was necessary.

In conclusion, we have modified our leak-proof puncture technique for fluid aspiration in giant ovarian cysts by inserting a gauze between the plastic wrap mounting and cyst. This modification reinforces the mounting and may prevent its disruption. This technique is safe, quick, and easy to perform without cyst fluid leakage. Additionally, it does not require pneumoperitoneum; therefore, it can be applied to patients in which long-term pneumoperitoneum may be avoided, for example, pregnant women. It can also be applied in laparoscopic-assisted surgery.

ETHICS STATEMENT

The studies involving human participants were reviewed and approved by The Institutional Review Board at Graduate School of Medicine, Chiba University. Written informed consent for participation was not required for this study in accordance with the national legislation and the institutional requirements.

AUTHOR CONTRIBUTIONS

HI and MS contributed to conception and design of the study. HI collected and analyzed data and wrote the first draft of manuscript. MS supervised the study and reviewed and edited the manuscript. All authors contributed to the article and approved the submitted version.

ACKNOWLEDGMENTS

We thank Medical Education Inc. for editing the illustration of the procedure and Dr. Yanruo Zhou for recording the narration of the video clip. We also thank Editage (www.editage.com) for English language editing.

REFERENCES

1. Alobaid A, Memon A, Alobaid S, Aldakhil L. Laparoscopic management of huge ovarian cysts. *Obstet Gynecol Int.* (2013) 2013:380854. doi: 10.1155/2013/380854.
2. Eltabbakh GH, Charboneau AM, Eltabbakh NG. Laparoscopic surgery for large benign ovarian cysts. *Gynecol Oncol.* (2008) 108:72–6. doi: 10.1016/j.ygyno.2007.08.085
3. Vlahos NF, Iavazzo C, Marcopoulos MC, Alamanou A, Kouiroukidou P, Chatzidakis V, et al. Laparoscopic management of large ovarian cysts. *Surg Innov.* (2012) 19:370–4. doi: 10.1177/1553350611432722
4. Shozu M, Segawa T, Sumitani H, Inoue M. Leak-proof puncture of ovarian cysts: instant mounting of plastic bag using cyanoacrylate adhesive. *Obstet Gynecol.* (2001) 97:1007–10. doi: 10.1016/s0029-7844(01)01364-3
5. Hicks-Courant K, Awtrey CS, Kim YB. Controlled decompression of large ovarian cystic tumors via mini-laparotomy using dermabond advanced™. *Gynecol Oncol Rep.* (2020) 32:100536. doi: 10.1016/j.gore.2020.100536.
6. Ehrlich PF, Teitelbaum DH, Hirschl RB, Rescorla F. Excision of large cystic ovarian tumors: combining minimal invasive surgery techniques and cancer surgery–the best of both worlds. *J Pediatr Surg.* (2007) 42:890–3. doi: 10.1016/j.jpedsurg.2006.12.069
7. Weng SS, Wang YL. Leak-proof extracorporeal drainage for management of large ovarian tumors. *Arch Gynecol Obstet.* (2012) 285:1079–82. doi: 10.1007/s00404-011-2115-3
8. Dubuisson J, Heersche S, Petignat P, Undurraga M. Laparoscopic management of giant ovarian cysts using the alexis laparoscopic system®: a case series. *Front Surg.* (2020) 7:24. doi: 10.3389/fsurg.2020.00024.
9. Al-Sunaidi M, Tulandi T. Adhesion-related bowel obstruction after hysterectomy for benign conditions. *Obstet Gynecol.* (2006) 108:1162–6. doi: 10.1097/01.AOG.0000239098.33320.c4
10. Tadokoro T, Kakinohana M, Navarro M, Goya M, Odo Y. The effectiveness of applying soft tissue bonding adhesive composed of 2-ethyl cyanoacrylate to epidural catheter fixations using film dressings: an open-label, randomized, parallel-group comparative study. *Anesth Analg.* (2019) 129:149–54. doi: 10.1213/ANE.0000000000003326
11. Kaplan M, Bozkurt S, Kut MS, Kullu S, Demirtas MM. Histopathological effects of ethyl 2-cyanoacrylate tissue adhesive following surgical application: an experimental study. *Eur J Cardiothorac Surg.* (2004) 25:167–72. doi: 10.1016/j.ejcts.2003.11.016

10

A Review of the Quadratus Lumborum Block and ERAS

Michael Akerman[1], Nada Pejčić[2] and Ivan Veličković[3]*

[1] Weill Cornell Medical College, Cornell University, New York City, NY, United States, [2] General Hospital Leskovac, Leskovac, Serbia, [3] SUNY Downstate Medical Center, Brooklyn, NY, United States

***Correspondence:**
Michael Akerman
michaelakerman10@gmail.com

The use of truncal nerve blocks has been described since 2001. Since then, there have been many studies trying to understand the ideal clinical scenarios for its use. Since 2001, the transversus abdominis plane block has evolved in many ways including from landmark based technique to ultrasound guided and more recently, into the quadratus lumborum (QL) block. Its anatomical placement, concentration of local anesthetic, volume of local anesthetic, and anatomic placement have all been raised as clinical questions. This article will discuss the literature of the QL block in an effort to understand how it is best used in a variety of clinical scenarios.

Keywords: quadratus lumborum, truncal block, quadratus lumborum block, transversus abdominis plane block, ultrasound

INTRODUCTION

The truncal nerve blocks, as a part of perioperative pain management, were introduced into clinical practice over 40 years ago. Primarily these were the ilioinguinal–iliohypogastric (II–IH) block (1–4) and the rectus sheath block (5), mostly used in the pediatric anesthesia population. In the early years of the 21st century, the transversus abdominis plane (TAP) block was introduced in everyday practice, providing a much wider field of analgesia (6, 7). At first, these blocks were performed without ultrasound guidance, using landmark techniques. However, the clinical use of truncal block techniques have developed over time and their expansion was driven by introducing ultrasound into anesthesiology practice. Although the anatomical markers are reliably detected by ultrasound, the blocks of the anterior abdominal wall vary in both the distribution of the local anesthetics and the field of coverage. In the search for the wider analgesia coverage and long-lasting postoperative analgesia, the transversalis fascia plane block and the quadratus lumborum block (QLB) have been developed.

Quadratus lumborum block is a block of the posterior abdominal wall, "interfascial plane block," which is performed exclusively under ultrasound guidance. It was described by anesthesiologist Dr. Rafael Blanco (8) as a variant of the TAP block in 2007. Much later, he gave a detailed description of the block technique using the name QLB (9). In the spring of 2013, Dr. Jens Børglum from the University Hospital in Copenhagen (Denmark) published a new ultrasound-guided transmuscular QL blockade, describing the so-called "Shamrock sign," the sign of a shamrock for the detection of a local anesthetic injection point (10). In autumn 2013, Dr. MihaelaVisoiu (11), a pediatric anesthesiologist from the University Children's Hospital in Pittsburgh (USA), published a case report with continuous QLB for postoperative analgesia. Subsequently, there has been an increasing interest of the anesthesia community in the use of truncal blocks, and the number of publications on the topic of QLB is progressively growing.

MECHANISM OF ACTION

The crucial ultrasound landmark for block performance is the quadratus lumborum muscle (QLM), and the key to the analgesia lies in the thoracolumbar fascia (TLF) (12–15). TLF is a complex, connective tissue tubular structure formed by binding aponeuroses and fascia layers, which, enveloping the back muscles, connects the anterolateral abdominal wall with the lumbar paravertebral region. The TLF is on its medial side attached to the thoracic and lumbar vertebrae, cranially continuing with endothoracic, and caudally with the fascia iliaca, potentially ensuring the spread of anesthetics in the craniocaudal direction (16). The true mechanism of analgesia provided by QLB has not yet been fully clarified. It is believed that the local anesthetics spread along the TLF and the endothoracic fascia into the paravertebral space, is responsible in part for the analgesia. In 2011, Carney et al. (17) showed that contrast spreads from the L1–T5 segment of the paravertebral space. However, a recent publication (18), shows that contrast injected into the area around QLM (QL plane) does not spread into the paravertebral space and contrast injected into the paravertebral space does not spread around QLM. Hence the assumption that visceral analgesia results from the spread of anesthetics to the celiac ganglion or sympathetic trunk *via* splanchnic nerves, as is the case with the paravertebral block. This remains to be confirmed or denied by future research. The most recent publication on this topic is the abstract presented at the American Society of Anesthesiologists meeting in October 2017, which shows local anesthetic spreading into the paravertebral space, cranially to the T10 segment (19).

An additional mechanism of action of local anesthetics can be explained by the anatomical-histological characteristics of the TLF. Namely, in the superficial layer of the TLF, there is a thick network of sympathetic neurons. In the fascia, there are the high-threshold and low-threshold mechanoreceptors and pain receptors sensitive to the effects of the local anesthetics. These receptors play a role in the development of both acute and chronic pain. The QLB analgesia could be, at least partially, explained by local anesthetic blockade of these receptors (15, 20).

Different approaches to block performance are applied in everyday clinical practice, and differences in the width of the anesthetized field and the duration of analgesia are significant. So far, studies done on cadavers (18, 21–24) show that the injected contrast can spread cranially to the thoracic paravertebral space and intercostal spaces covering somatic nerves and the thoracic sympathetic trunk up to the T4 level. Blockade of the subcostal, iliohypogastric, and ilioinguinal nerve is consistent. Sometimes, genitofemoral and lateral femoral cutaneous nerve could be blocked. Caudally, contrast can reach lumbar nerve roots, but the results vary and new studies are needed to clarify the link between the type of QLB and the achieved analgesic effect. All of these data indicate that the QLB provides somatic and visceral analgesia.

Obviously, there are variations in the width of achieved analgesia, and in the number of dermatomes covered by QLB. In most of the cases, analgesia is achieved in T7–L1 dermatomes (10–14, 24–28), although there are descriptions of cranial spread to T4–T5 (13), and caudal spread to L2–L3 (22) dermatomes. The height of the block can be influenced by the choice of the site for the application of local anesthetics, both in relation to QLM and in relation to the distance from the iliac crest and costal margin (12, 13). The rate of the drug application (29), and the individual anatomical variations can also influence the height of the block.

TYPES OF QLB

Since the initial description, the block has experienced several modifications and today four types of the block are performed, which differ by the site of drug application. These are QLB 1 or lateral QLB, QLB 2 or posterior QLB, QLB 3, or anterior/transmuscular QLB, and QLB 4 or intramuscular QLB.

Quadratus lumborum block 1 implies the application of local anesthetics on the lateral side of QLM in the area of its contact with the transversalis fascia, at the level where transversus abdominis muscle (TAM) tapers off into its aponeurosis (30). One group of authors (12) states that the target site is between the fascia and the muscle, which can be seen as expanding space upon local anesthetic injection. They emphasize that medication should not be given between the fascial layers as the nerve endings are between the fascia and the muscle. Another group of authors (13) states that drug is administered in the space between the common aponeurosis of internal oblique muscle (IOM) and TAM and the transversalis fascia.

Quadratus lumborum block 2 implies the application of medication on the posterior side of the QLM between the QLM and the medial lamina of TLF which separates QLM from the latissimus dorsi muscle and paraspinal muscles [erector spinae muscles (ESM)]. This is laterally from the attachment of IOM aponeurosis (30), in the to the so-called lumbar interfascial triangle (14).

Quadratus lumborum block 3 implies the application of medication at the front of the QLM, at the level of its attachment to the transverse process of L4 vertebra. This can be seen under ultrasound as spreading of the local anesthetic between the QLM and the psoas major muscle (PMM) (10, 31). This approach assumes during ultrasound one is viewing the "Shamrock sign"—the transverse process of L4 vertebra is seen as a stem with ESM as posterior leaf, PMM as anterior leaf, and QLM as lateral leaf.

Quadratus lumborum block 4 implies the application of medication in the muscle itself.

Murouchi states that for QLB 1 and 3 a local anesthetic needs to be applied between the anterior layers of TLF and that its intramuscular approach does not involve the spread of local anesthetics into the interfascial space (28).

BLOCK TECHNIQUE

We perform lateral QLB (QLB 1) and posterior QLB (QLB 2) in our practice. During the block performance, the patient is in the supine position. **Figure 1** shows the cross-section of the cadaver abdomen in supination and a schematic presentation of anatomical structures for better understanding and easier performance of the QLB. If QLB is performed on the operating table, the operating table can be gently tilted to the opposite side to achieve a better exposure. If QLB is performed on a regular bed, a pillow can be placed under the lumbar spine. Alternatively, the patient could be asked to turn to the opposite side. The procedure begins by placing a transversally oriented linear or convex ultrasound probe between two distinct markers—the iliac crest and the costal margin at the level of

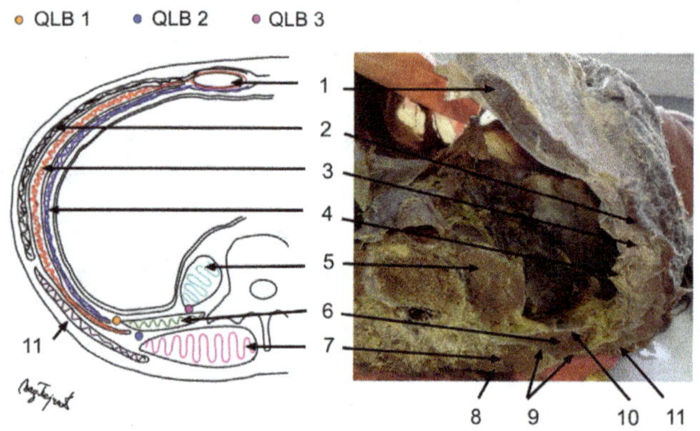

FIGURE 1 | Cross-section of the abdomen—a photo of cadaver and a scheme of anatomical structures. QLB 1—point of local anesthetic (LA) injection for QLB 1; QLB 2—point of LA injection for QLB 2; QLB 3—point of LA injection for QLB 3; 1—rectus abdominis muscle; 2—external oblique muscle; 3—internal oblique muscle; 4 -transversus abdominis muscle; 5—psoas major muscle; 6—quadratus lumborum muscle; 7—erectores spinae muscle; 8—lamina posterior of the thoracolumbar fascia; 9—lamina media of the thoracolumbar fascia; 10—lamina anterior of the thoracolumbar fascia; 11—latissimus dorsi muscle.

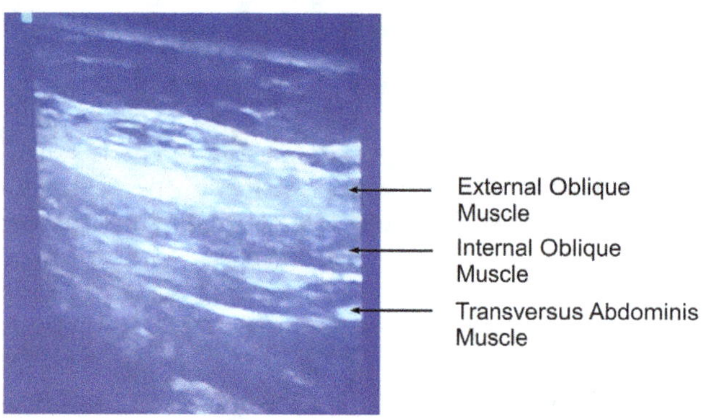

FIGURE 2 | Muscles of the anterolateral abdominal wall.

the anterior axillary line. The goal is to find three thin parallel muscles of the anterolateral abdominal wall, external oblique muscle, IOM, and TAM, from the outside to inside as in **Figure 2**. Moving the probe posteriorly, we follow narrowing of the muscles until the muscle fibers of TAM taper off into its aponeurosis at the level of the posterior axillary line. This is ultrasound-detected as a hyperechogenic sign (**Figure 3**), from which the QLM extends posteriorly and to the inside. Aponeuroses are seen as hyperechogenic structures, and muscles as hypoechogenic structures. If the image is lost during probe movement, we reposition probe to the starting point of scanning, looking for three parallel muscles, and then we continue scanning to the back, taking care that the probe is always perpendicularly placed on the skin surface and is following the body curvature. When we detect a remarkable hyperechogenic sign of the place where we want to inject a local anesthetic, we can improve the image by discrete tilting and rotation of

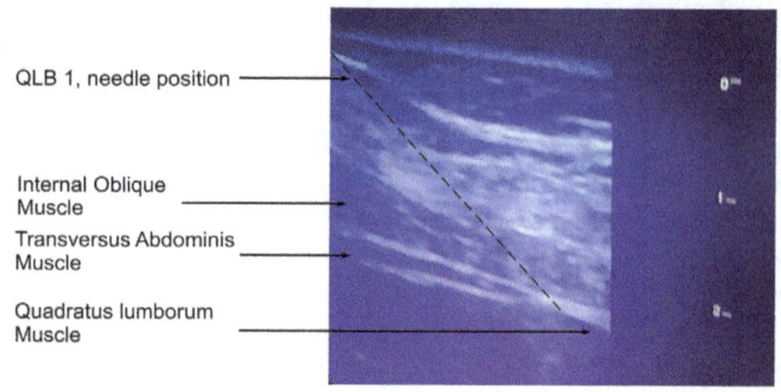

FIGURE 3 | Quadratus lumborum type 1 block—needle position.

the probe. If the hypoechogenic shadow blurs the image, it is necessary to add more gel that will improve the transmission of ultrasound waves from the probe to the skin.

The needle is introduced into the skin 1–2 cm above the probe (by "in plane" technique) and led through the muscles to the local anesthetic application site—posteriorly from the place where the TAM tapers off into its aponeurosis (we do not want the TAM perforation). The needle is advanced at 90° angle and only after the skin perforation we redirect needle in the desired direction. The TLF provides a characteristic elastic resistance to a blunt needle that is used for peripheral blocks, and TLF perforation is accompanied by double control—visual (ultrasound) and special tactile feeling due to loss of resistance. After a negative aspiration test, the injection of 1 ml of the solution provides visible hydrodisection—the accumulation of fluid in the form of a growing hypoechogenic shadow, which separates the muscle from the fascia, representing the third confirmation of the desired location. Then, the fractional administration of local anesthetics is performed. After every 5 ml of local anesthetic, it is necessary to do an aspiration test to confirm the extravascular location of the needle tip.

This technique is very easy to learn due to the fact that it is easy to find the key sonoanatomic markers for block performance. It can be learnt after only a few performance of the procedure (32).

When the catheter is placed for prolonged postoperative pain therapy, absolutely sterile working conditions are necessary (as for the epidural catheter placement or the central venous cannulation). This involves using caps, masks, sterile gloves, hand cleaning, sterile operating field, putting the probe into a sterile bag, and using sterile ultrasound gel. In the absence of sterile bags for the ultrasound probe and sterile gel, it is possible to improvise in the following way. An ultrasound probe with regular gel is placed in a sterile glove. The contact of the probe with skin can be improved by wetting skin with sterile saline.

For one-time administration of local anesthetic ("single shot" QLB), it is sufficient to apply clean technique according to many US regional anesthetic schools. This involves the use of regular gloves for single use without the preparation of a wide sterile field. It is necessary to use a cap and a mask. After identification of TAM and TLF, skin above the probe is cleaned with disinfectant. Insulated needle is held only at the "head," (without touching the metal part of the needle), and advanced through the cleaned skin. Only when we have an adequate ultrasound image and disinfected skin, we advance the needle through the skin and perform the block. A group of authors (33) recommends that a sterile transparent film (Tegaderm) should be placed over the probe and gel to additionally increase the safety and reduce the risk of infection.

For the performance of QLB, insulated block needles 50–150 mm in length are used, although for most patients the appropriate needle length is 100 mm.

There is still no consensus on the type, concentration, and volume of a local anesthetic used to perform QLB. QLB is performed by applying 15–30 mL (0.2–0.4 ml/kg) of a local anesthetic on the left and right side of the abdominal wall. 0.125–0.375% bupivacaine, levobupivacaine, or ropivacaine (12–14, 23, 25, 30, 34–37) can be used as local anesthetics. Many authors (26, 31, 35) recommend the addition of 2–4 mg dexamethasone to each side to extend the effect of the local anesthetic and, by some authors (38, 39), achieve the antiemetic effect. There is still no consensus on the effect of dexamethasone on the duration of peripheral nerve blocks either, but the most recent meta-analyses (39–41) indicate that perineurally administered dexamethasone prolongs the duration of the peripheral block and potentiates analgesia. We are currently complying with the recommended protocol from the Cornell Medical Center (Weill Cornell Medicine, New York, NY, USA), taking care that the patient does not receive a local anesthetic dose higher than the maximum allowed (2.5 mg/kg). We use 30 ml 0.25% bupivacaine/levobupivacaine with 2–4 mg dexamethasone per block. As a bilateral QLB is required for most procedures, the total dose is 60 ml of 0.25% (150 mg) bupivacaine/levobupivacaine with 4–8 mg of dexamethasone. For patients with a body weight of less than 60 kg, we use 20–30 ml of 0.20% bupivacaine/levobupivacaine with 2 mg dexamethasone per side.

The block can be performed postoperatively, on the operating table, immediately after waking up patient from general anesthesia, in the recovery room or in the intensive care unit. Patients who underwent neuraxial anesthesia are given QLB either before or after resolution of the block.

INDICATIONS

Quadratus lumborum block provides postoperative analgesia in a large number of surgical interventions and the list of indications is long.

The efficacy of QLB for postoperative analgesia following both cesarean section (8, 14, 30, 34, 35, 42–44) and gynecological laparoscopic procedures (25, 36) was shown. Additionally, the efficacy of QLB for postoperative analgesia was shown after abdominal surgery [small intestine (26) and colon (11, 27) resection, colostomy reconstruction (11), appendectomy (27), gastrectomy (45)], and for analgesia for anterior abdominal wall hernioplasty (46, 47) and orhcydopexy (47), both for open and laparoscopic procedures and for postoperative analgesia after open and laparoscopic nephrectomy (37, 48, 49).

As TAP block has its important place in postoperative analgesia after laparoscopic cholecystectomy, Elsharkawy (50) representing the American Society of Regional Anesthesia and Pain Medicine recommends the application of QLB for laparoscopic cholecystectomy (which we have confirmed in everyday practice on over 50 patients for the past 6 months).

There are more and more authors describing the application QLB for hip and femur surgery (31, 51–55) and lumbar vertebrae surgery (56, 57). A case study of the use of QLB for postoperative analgesia after femorofemoral bypass was published (58). A case of one-time administration of QLB in chronic pain treatment after the anterior abdominal wall hernia surgery with a multimonth effect after the block performance was also published (46).

QLB EFFICACY

All authors, which we have quoted so far, agree that QLB has an outstanding analgesic effect on pain reduction to 1–2/10 by Visual Analog Scale or Numeric Rating Scale pain scale, which usually last more than 24 h. Patients who receive QLB as part of a postoperative pain therapy, have lower pain levels both when resting and moving, which is important for early mobilization. The analgesic effect is as good as the one achieved by opioids, and there are no unwanted opioid effects such as nausea and vomiting (36). According to prospective studies published by Blanco et al.1 (4, 30) in 2015 and 2016, the need for morphine has been significantly reduced postoperatively in patients who received paracetamol, NSAID, and QLB as part of the multimodal postoperative analgesia compared to patients who received only paracetamol and NSAID, but did not receive QLB. Comparative studies have shown that the QLB covers a topographically broader field (Th7–Th12, compared to TAP Th10–Th12) (14, 25), and yields prolonged pain-free condition compared to the TAP block (24–48 h QLB versus 8–12 h TAP block) (14, 25, 47).

Quadratus lumborum block provides early and rapid pain relief in a high percentage of patients and allows early ambulation, which is one of the most important measures in the prevention of deep vein thrombosis and thromboembolic complications. So, this would be another important question that should be considered through future research—could QLB be used to reduce the incidence of postoperative thromboembolic complications?

QLB COMPLICATIONS

Complications associated with the performance of abdominal wall blocks are fortunately very rare and not described during QLB performance. Since QLB is a classical intramuscular medication injection, the possibility of infection is far lower than in performing the neuraxial blocks. So far, infections have not been described during the QLB performance. The advantage of QLB compared to other abdominal wall blocks is the fact that the passage of the needle and the site of the local anesthetic application are very distant from the peritoneal cavity, visceral abdominal organs, and large blood vessels. Therefore, needle trauma in terms of unintentional puncture of the peritoneum, intestine, liver, kidney, large blood vessels associated with blind methods (without ultrasound) of the TAP and II-IH block performance here is minimized. Performing a block under the control of ultrasound, with mandatory monitoring of the needle tip prior to injecting the drug, significantly increases the level of safety and efficiency of the technique. There are no data on neurological damage since the local anesthetic is not injected into the immediate proximity of the large nerve, but is injected into the space rich in small nerve endings. It is therefore generally accepted that QLB can be performed both under general and regional anesthesia (13).

An unwanted femoral nerve block is cited as a possible complication of QLB 3. A rational theoretical explanation lies in the immediate anatomical contact of the TLF and the iliac fascia and the possibility of spreading the anesthetic, down the iliac fascia causing weakness in the quadriceps (22, 52, 53, 59). Dam and associates (21) during the performance of QLB 3 do not puncture the PMM and do not get the contrast spreading caudally. This leaves us with a potential conclusion that if there are no punctures of the PMM, there is no unwanted quadriceps weakness.

Anterior abdominal wall blocks have the potential for local anesthetic systemic toxicity (LAST). For now, there is no LAST case with QLB. Namely, studies have shown that the concentration of local anesthetic (ropivacaine) in plasma is significantly lower after the performance of QLB comparing with than in the TAP block done by a lateral approach (13, 25). In any case, whenever regional blocks are performed, it is necessary to think of a potential LAST, take precautions to prevent LAST development and actively monitor the patient to timely spot the first signs and treat LAST.

As the QLB performance involves manipulation of the fascia where blood vessels exit from the paravertebral space, caution should be exercised in people receiving anticoagulant therapy due to the possible risk of hematoma (14).

As with any anesthetic procedure, it is necessary to take patient's written consent for the performance of the abdominal wall block, especially if the block is performed postoperatively in the intensive care unit or ward (13).

QLB AND ERAS PROTOCOL

Our review of literature did not result in any articles that would specifically discuss the role of QLB in ERAS protocols. Kim et al. recently published review on the role of TAP block as a part of ERAS protocol (60). They found that the use of TAP block resulted in significantly less opioid use, less postoperative pain and non inferiority was shown in comparison with thoracic epidural. Since QLB is similar to TAP block all of these findings should be subjects of new research. Other studies have shown less post-operative nausea and vomiting (36, 61), decreased post-operative sedation (62, 63), decreased length of hospital stay (64), earlier urinary catheter removal (65) when abdominal trunk blocks are used. This is another area where extensive research is needed. Improved early oral intake and early mobilization can be more easily achieved with good pain control and QLB has a great potential in this area of ERAS.

CONCLUSION

Quadratus lumborum block is a new form of the abdominal wall block which is relatively easily performed thanks to clear ultrasound anatomic markers. The block effect lasts 24–48 h and until now no complications have been described during the block performance. QLB is safe and has found its place in multimodal postoperative pain therapy in patients undergoing abdominal surgery, gynecological and obstetric procedures, and orthopedic interventions on hips, whether interventions are performed in general or spinal anesthesia, both in adults and in children. It follows from the above that QLB has the potential to significantly facilitate and improve postoperative pain therapy.

AUTHOR CONTRIBUTIONS

MA performed the proofreading of the translation of the article. NP and IV did the writing in Serbian and the literature search for the article.

REFERENCES

1. Bowen JR, Thompson WR, Dorman BA, Soderberg CH Jr, Shahinian TK. Change in the management of adult groin hernia. *Am J Surg* (1978) 135:564–9. doi:10.1016/0002-9610(78)90038-7
2. Bainton A. Ilioinguinal/ iliohypogastric nerve block. *Anaesthesia* (1982) 37:696–7.
3. Hannallah RS, Broadman LM, Belman AB, Abramowitz MD, Epstein BS. Comparison of caudal and ilioinguinal/iliohypogastric nerve blocks for control of post-orchiopexy pain in pediatric ambulatory surgery. *Anesthesiology* (1987) 66:832–4. doi:10.1097/00000542-198706000-00023
4. Markham SJ, Tomlinson J, Hain WR. Ilioinguinal nerve block in children. A comparison with caudal block for intra and postoperative analgesia. *Anaesthesia* (1986) 41:1098–103. doi:10.1111/j.1365-2044.1986.tb12956.x
5. Smith BE, Suchak M, Siggins D, Challands J. Rectus sheath block for diagnostic laparoscopy. *Anaesthesia* (1988) 43:947–8. doi:10.1111/j.1365-2044.1988.tb05658.x
6. O'Donnell BD, McDonnell JG, McShane AJ. The transversus abdominis plane (TAP) block in open retropubicprostatectomy. *Reg Anesth Pain Med* (2006) 31:91. doi:10.1016/j.rapm.2005.10.006
7. McDonnell JG, O'Donnell B, Curley G, Heffernan A, Power C, Laffey JG. The analgesic efficacy of transversus abdominis plane block after abdominal surgery: a prospective randomized controlled trial. *Anesth Analg* (2007) 104:193–7. doi:10.1213/01.ane.0000250223.49963.0f
8. Blanco R. TAP block under ultrasound guidance: the description of a 'non pops technique'. *Reg Anesth Pain Med* (2007) 32:130. doi:10.1016/j.rapm.2007.06.268
9. Blanco R. Optimal point of injection: the quadratus lumborum type I and II blocks. *Anesthesia* (2013) 68:4.
10. Børglum J, Moriggl B, Jensen K, Lönnqvist PA, Christensen AF, Sauter A, et al. Ultrasound-guided transmuscular quadratus lumborum blockade. *Br J Anaesth* (2013) 110:3. Available at http://bja.oxfordjournals.org/forum/topic/brjana_el%3b9919
11. Visoiu M, Yakovleva N. Continuous postoperative analgesia via quadratus lumborum block – an alternative to transversus abdominis plane block. *Paediatr Anaesth* (2013) 23:959–61. doi:10.1111/pan.12240
12. Ueshima H, Otake H, Lin JA. Ultrasound-guided quadratus lumborum block: an updated review of anatomy and techniques. *Biomed Res Int* (2017) 2017:2752876. doi:10.1155/2017/2752876
13. Chin KJ, McDonnell JG, Carvalho B, Sharkey A, Pawa A, Gadsden J. Essentials of our current understanding: abdominal wall blocks. *Reg Anesth Pain Med* (2017) 42:133–83. doi:10.1097/AAP.0000000000000545
14. Blanco R, Ansari T, Riad W, Shetty N. Quadratus lumborum blockversus transversus abdominis plane block for postoperative pain after cesarean

delivery: a randomized controlled trial. *Reg Anesth Pain Med* (2016) 41:757–62. doi:10.1097/AAP.0000000000000495
15. Benetazzo L, Bizzego A, De Caro R, Frigo G, Guidolin D, Stecco C. 3D reconstruction of the crural and thoracolumbar fasciae. *Surg Radiol Anat* (2011) 33:855–62. doi:10.1007/s00276-010-0757-7
16. El-Boghdadly K, Elsharkawy H, Short A, Chin KJ. Quadratus lumborum block nomenclature and anatomical considerations. *Reg Anesth Pain Med* (2016) 41:548–9. doi:10.1097/AAP.0000000000000411
17. Carney J, Finnerty O, Rauf J, Bergin D, Laffey JG, Mc Donnell JG. Studies on the spread of local anaesthetic solution in transversus abdominis plane blocks. *Anaesthesia* (2011) 66:1023–30. doi:10.1111/j.1365-2044.2011.06855.x
18. Kumar A, Sadeghi N, Wahal C, Gadsden J, Grant SA. Quadratus lumborum spares paravertebral space in fresh cadaver injection. *Anesth Analg* (2017) 125:708–9. doi:10.1213/ANE.0000000000002245
19. Tamura T, Shuichi Y, Ito S, Shibata Y, Nishiwaki K. *A Crossover Healthy Volunteers Study of Quadratus Lumborum Block to Detect the Paravertebral Space Dissemination*. Boston: ASA Annual Meeting (2017).
20. Tesarz J, Hoheisel U, Wiedenhöfer B, Mense S. Sensory innervation of the thoracolumbar fascia in rats and humans. *Neuroscience* (2011) 194:302–8. doi:10.1016/j.neuroscience.2011.07.066
21. Dam M, Moriggl B, Hansen CK, Hoermann R, Bendtsen TF, Børglum J. The pathway of injectate spread with the transmuscular quadratus lumborum block: a cadaver study. *Anesth Analg* (2017) 125:303–12. doi:10.1213/ANE.0000000000001922
22. Carline L, McLeod GA, Lamb C. A cadaver study comparing spread of dye and nerve involvement after three different quadratus lumborum blocks. *Br J Anaesth* (2016) 117:387–94. doi:10.1093/bja/aew224
23. Adhikary SD, El-Boghdadly K, Nasralah Z, Sarwani N, Nixon AM, Chin KJ. A radiologic and anatomic assessment of injectate spread following transmuscularquadratus lumborum block in cadavers. *Anaesthesia* (2017) 72:73–9. doi:10.1111/anae.13647
24. Elsharkawy H, El-Boghdadly K, Kolli S, Esa WAS, DeGrande S, Soliman LM, et al. Injectate spread following anterior subcostal and posterior approaches to the quadratus lumborum block: a comparative cadaveric study. *Eur J Anaesthesiol* (2017) 34:587–95. doi:10.1097/EJA.0000000000000680
25. Murouchi T, Iwasaki S, Yamakage M. Quadratus lumborum block: analgesic effects and chronological ropivacaine concentrations after laparoscopic surgery. *Reg Anesth Pain Med* (2016) 41:146–50. doi:10.1097/AAP.0000000000000349
26. Kadam VR. Ultrasound-guided quadratus lumborum block as a postoperative analgesic technique for laparotomy. *J Anaesthesiol Clin Pharmacol* (2013) 29:550–2. doi:10.4103/0970-9185.119148
27. Ueshima H, Hiroshi O. Intermittent bilateral anterior subcostal quadratus lumborum block for effective analgesia in lower abdominal surgery. *J Clin Anesth* (2017) 43:65. doi:10.1016/j.jclinane.2017.09.018
28. Murouchi T. Reply to Dr El-Boghdadly et al. *Reg Anesth Pain Med* (2016) 41:549. doi:10.1097/AAP.0000000000000431
29. El-Boghdadly K, Elsharkawy H, Short A, Chin KJ. Reply to Drs La Colla and Ben-David. *Reg Anesth Pain Med* (2017) 42:128. doi:10.1097/AAP.0000000000000535
30. Blanco R, Ansari T, Girgis E. Quadratus lumborum block for postoperative pain after caesarean section: a randomised controlled trial. *Eur J Anaesthesiol* (2015) 32:812–8. doi:10.1097/EJA.0000000000000299
31. La Colla L, Uskova A, Ben-David B. Single-shot quadratus lumborum block for postoperative analgesia after minimally invasive hip arthroplasty: a new alternative to continuous lumbar plexus block? *Reg Anesth Pain Med* (2017) 42:125–6. doi:10.1097/AAP.0000000000000523
32. Pejčić N, Mitić R, Veličković I. Quadratus lumborum blok – metodpostoperativneanalgezijestiže u Srbijukrozvrata OB Leskovac. *Apollinem Med Aesculapium* (2017) 15:16–20.
33. Alakkad H, Naeeni A, Chan VW, Abbas S, Oh J, Ami N, et al. Infection related to ultrasound-guided single-injection peripheral nerve blockade: a decade of experience at Toronto Western Hospital. *Reg Anesth Pain Med* (2015) 40:82–4. doi:10.1097/AAP.0000000000000181
34. Sebbag I, Qasem F, Dhir S. Ultrasound guided quadratus lumborum block for analgesia after cesarean delivery: case series. *Rev Bras Anestesiol* (2017) 67:418–21. doi:10.1016/j.bjan.2017.03.002
35. Maenchen N, Hansen CK, Dam M, Børglum J. Ultrasound-guided transmuscular quadratus lumborum (TQL) block for pain management after caesarean section. *Int J Anesth Anesthesiol* (2016) 3:048. doi:10.23937/2377-4630/3/2/1048
36. Ishio J, Komasawa N, Kido H, Minami T. Evaluation of ultrasound-guided posterior quadratus lumborum block for postoperative analgesia after laparoscopic gynecologic surgery. *J Clin Anesth* (2017) 41:1–4. doi:10.1016/j.jclinane.2017.05.015
37. Chakraborty A, Goswami J, Patro V. Ultrasound-guided continuous quadrates lumborum block for postoperative analgesia in a pediatric patient. *A A Case Rep* (2015) 4:34–6. doi:10.1213/XAA.0000000000000090
38. Børglum J, Gögenür I, Bendtsen TF. Abdominal wall blocks in adults. *Curr Opin Anaesthesiol* (2016) 29:638–43. doi:10.1097/ACO.0000000000000378
39. Zorrilla-Vaca A, Li J. Dexamethasone injected perineurally is more effective than administered intravenously for peripheral nerve blocks: a meta-analysis of randomized controlled trials. *Clin J Pain* (2018) 34(3):276–84. doi:10.1097/AJP.0000000000000519
40. Baeriswyl M, Kirkham KR, Jacot-Guillarmod A, Albrecht E. Efficacy of perineural vs systemic dexamethasone to prolong analgesia after peripheral nerve block: a systematic review and meta-analysis. *Br J Anaesth* (2017) 119:183–91. doi:10.1093/bja/aex191
41. Chong MA, Berbenetz NM, Lin C, Singh S. Perineural versus intravenous dexamethasone as an adjuvant for peripheral nerve blocks: a systematic review and meta-analysis. *Reg Anesth Pain Med* (2017) 42:319–26. doi:10.1097/AAP.0000000000000571
42. Kerai S, Saxena KN. Quadratus lumborum block for post-caesarean analgesia. *Indian J Anaesth* (2017) 61:364. doi:10.4103/ija.IJA_220_17
43. Nair A. Bilateral quadratus lumborum block for post-caesarean analgesia. *Indian J Anaesth* (2017) 61:362–3. doi:10.4103/ija.IJA_204_17
44. Krohg A, Ullensvang K, Rosseland LA, Langesaeter E, Sauter A. The analgesic effect of ultrasound-guided quadratus lumborum block after cesarean delivery: a randomized clinical trial. *Anesth Analg* (2018) 126(2):559–65. doi:10.1213/ANE.0000000000002648
45. Cardoso JM, Sá M, Reis H, Almeida L, Sampaio JC, Pinheiro C, et al. Type II quadratus lumborum block for a subtotal gastrectomy in a septic patient. *Rev Bras Anestesiol* (2016). doi:10.1016/j.bjan.2016.09.009
46. Carvalho R, Segura E, Loureiro MD, Assunção JP. Quadratus lumborum block in chronic pain after abdominal hernia repair: case report. *Braz J Anesthesiol* (2017) 67:107–9. doi:10.1016/j.bjane.2014.08.010
47. Öksüz G, Bilal B, Gürkan Y, Urfalioğlu A, Arslan M, Gişi G, et al. Quadratus lumborum block versus transversus abdominis plane block in children undergoing low abdominal surgery: a randomized controlled trial. *Reg Anesth Pain Med* (2017) 42:674–9. doi:10.1097/AAP.0000000000000645
48. Chakraborty A, Khemka R, Datta T. Ultrasound-guided truncal blocks: a new frontier in regional anaesthesia. *Indian J Anaesth* (2016) 60:703–11. doi:10.4103/0019-5049.191665
49. Sindwani G, Sahu S, Suri A, Saeed Z. Bilateral quadratus lumborum block for postoperative analgesia in a Von Hippel-Lindau syndrome patient undergoing laparoscopic radical nephrectomy. *Saudi J Anaesth* (2017) 11:513–4. doi:10.4103/sja.SJA_263_17
50. Elsharkawy H. Quadratus lumborum blocks. *Adv Anesth* (2017) 35:145–57. doi:10.1016/j.aan.2017.07.007
51. Sato M, Hara M, Uchida O. An antero-lateral approach to ultrasound-guided lumbar plexus block in supine position combined with quadratus lumborum block using single-needle insertion for pediatric hip surgery. *Paediatr Anaesth* (2017) 27:1064–5. doi:10.1111/pan.13208
52. Ueshima H, Yoshiyama S, Otake H. The ultrasound-guided continuous transmuscular quadratus lumborum block is an effective analgesia for total hip arthroplasty. *J Clin Anesth* (2016) 31:35. doi:10.1016/j.jclinane.2015.12.033
53. Parras T, Blanco R. Randomised trial comparing the transversus abdominis plane block posterior approach or quadratus lumborum block type I with femoral block for postoperative analgesia in femoral neck fracture, both ultrasound-guided. *Rev Esp Anestesiol Reanim* (2016) 63:141–8. doi:10.1016/j.redar.2015.06.012
54. Hockett MM, Hembrador S, Lee A. Continuous quadratus lumborum block for postoperative pain in total hip arthroplasty: a case report. *A A Case Rep* (2016) 7:129–31. doi:10.1213/XAA.0000000000000363
55. Ben-David B, La Colla L. Extravasated fluid in hip arthroscopy and pain: is quadratus lumborum block the answer? *Anesth Analg* (2017) 125:364. doi:10.1213/ANE.0000000000002198

56. Ueshima H, Hiroshi O. Lumbar vertebra surgery performed with a bilateral posterior quadratus lumborum block. *J Clin Anesth* (2017) 41:61. doi:10.1016/j.jclinane.2017.06.012
57. Iwamitsu R, Ueshima H, Otake H. Intermittent bilateral posterior quadratus lumborum block was effective for pain management in lumbar spinal fusion. *J Clin Anesth* (2017) 42:16. doi:10.1016/j.jclinane.2017.08.012
58. Watanabe K, Mitsuda S, Tokumine J, Lefor AK, Moriyama K, Yorozu T. Quadratus lumborum block for femoral-femoral bypass graft placement: a case report. *Medicine (Baltimore)* (2016) 95:e4437. doi:10.1097/MD.0000000000004437
59. Wikner M. Unexpected motor weakness following quadratus lumborum block for gynaecologicall aparascopy. *Anaesthesia* (2017) 72:230–2. doi:10.1111/anae.13754
60. Kim AJ, Yong RJ, Urman RD. The role of transversus abdominis plane blocks in enhanced recovery after surgery pathways for open and laparoscopic colorectal surgery. *J Laparoendosc Adv Surg Tech A* (2017) 27(9):909–14. doi:10.1089/lap.2017.0337
61. Johns N, O'Neill S, Ventham NT, Barron F, Brady RR, Daniel T. Clinical effectiveness of transversus abdominis plane (TAP) block in abdominal surgery: a systematic review and meta-analysis. *Colorectal Dis* (2012) 14:e635–42. doi:10.1111/j.1463-1318.2012.03104.x
62. Bharti N, Kumar P, Bala I, Gupta V. The efficacy of a novel approach to transversus abdominis plane block for postoperative analgesia after colorectal surgery. *Anesth Analg* (2011) 112:1504–8. doi:10.1213/ANE.0b013e3182159bf8
63. Brady RR, Ventham NT, Roberts DM, Graham C, Daniel T. Open transversus abdominis plane block and analgesic requirements in patients following right hemicolectomy. *Ann R Coll Surg Engl* (2012) 94:327–30. doi:10.1308/003588412X13171221589856
64. Walter CJ, Maxwell-Armstrong C, Pinkney TD, Conaghan PJ, Bedforth N, Gornall CB, et al. A randomised controlled trial of the efficacy of ultrasound-guided transversus abdominis plane (TAP) block in laparoscopic colorectal surgery. *Surg Endosc* (2013) 27:2366–72. doi:10.1007/s00464-013-2791-0
65. Niraj G, Kelkar A, Hart E, Horst C, Malik D, Yeow C, et al. Comparison of analgesic efficacy of four-quadrant transversus abdominis plane (TAP) block and continuous posterior TAP analgesia with epidural analgesia in patients undergoing laparoscopic colorectal surgery: an open-label, randomised, noninferiority trial. *Anaesthesia* (2014) 69:348–55. doi:10.1111/anae.12546

11

The Transumbilical Laparoendoscopic Single-Site Extraperitoneal Approach for Pelvic and Para-Aortic Lymphadenectomy: A Technique Note and Feasibility Study

Shiyi Peng[1,2]*, Ying Zheng*[1,2*]*, Fan Yang*[1,2]*, Kana Wang*[1,2]*, Sijing Chen*[1,2] *and Yawen Wang*[3]

[1] *Department of Gynecology, West China Second Hospital, Sichuan University, Chengdu, China,* [2] *Key Laboratory of Obstetrics, Gynecologic and Pediatric Diseases and Birth Defects of Ministry of Education, West China Second Hospital, Sichuan University, Chengdu, China,* [3] *Department of Obstetrics and Gynecology, Shanxi Bethune Hospital, Taiyuan, China*

Correspondence:
Ying Zheng
zhy_chd@126.com

Background: Nowadays, lymphadenectomy could be performed by the transperitoneal or extraperitoneal approach. Nevertheless, each approach has its own advantages and disadvantages. Under these circumstances, we developed a transumbilical laparoendoscopic single-site (TU-LESS) extraperitoneal approach for lymphadenectomy. In this research, the primary goal is to demonstrate the feasibility of the novel approach in systematic lymphadenectomy and present the surgical process step-by-step.

Methods: Between May 2020 and June 2021, patients who had the indications of systematic lymphadenectomy underwent lymphadenectomy via the TU-LESS extraperitoneal approach. This new approach was described in detail, and the clinical characteristics and surgical outcomes were collected and analyzed.

Results: Eight patients with gynecological carcinoma were included in the research, including four with high-risk endometrial cancer and four with early-stage ovarian cancer. The TU-LESS extraperitoneal approach for pelvic and para-aortic lymphadenectomy was successfully performed in all patients without conversion. In all, a median of 26.5 pelvic lymph nodes (range 18–35) and 18.0 para-aortic lymph nodes (range 7–43) were retrieved. There was a median of 166.5 min of surgical time (range 123–205). Patients had speedy recoveries without complications. All patients had positive pain responses after surgery, as well as satisfactory cosmetic and body image outcomes.

Conclusion: Our initial experience showed that it is feasible to perform systematic lymphadenectomy with the TU-LESS extraperitoneal approach. And this new approach may provide a new measure or a beneficial supplement for lymphadenectomy in gynecologic cancer.

Keywords: extraperitoneal approach, pelvic lymphadenectomy, para-aortic lymphadenectomy, laparoendoscopic single-site (LESS) surgery, ovarian cancer, endometrial cancer

INTRODUCTION

Lymphadenectomy is paramount for precise staging and tailoring treatment of gynecological malignancies. Compared to laparotomy, laparoscopic surgery caused less surgical trauma and fewer wound complications. The feasibility and safety of minimally invasive surgery for lymphadenectomy has been well-investigated and proved (1, 2). Currently, laparoscopic lymphadenectomy is performed either trans- or extraperitoneally. Dissection of the pelvic lymph nodes (LNs) is easier with the transperitoneal approach; however, the intestinal disruption is a major barrier for para-aortic lymphadenectomy (PALN) (**Figure 1**). The extraperitoneal approach has been described as a solution to resolve this problem. Without the interference of bowels, the extraperitoneal approach provides an easier access to the infrarenal para-aortic LNs with lower risk of intestinal and urinary injuries (3). The full exposure of surgical field achieved a higher para-aortic LN yield compared to the transperitoneal route (4, 5).

Laparoendoscopic single-site (LESS) surgery has emerged as a minimal invasive surgical approach, which could further minimize the surgical trauma compared to multi-port laparoscopy surgery (6). LESS is as safe and effective as the traditional laparoscopy in the gynecologic surgery (7). Compared to patients in the multi-port laparoscopy group, patients in the single-port laparoscopy group attained mild pain with less analgesic consumption and shorter hospital stay (8–11). The single-port left iliac extraperitoneal PALN was first described by Guoy et al. (12). Subsequently, Lambaudie et al. (13) and Beytout et al. (14) introduced similar single-port lateral approaches. These results indicated that the number of para-aortic LNs retrieved by the single-port lateral extraperitoneal approach was compatible with that of the multi-port extraperitoneal route (3, 10, 13). In spite of this, the most common lateral extraperitoneal technique restraints access to the obturator fossa which impedes pelvic lymphadenectomy (PLN) (15) (**Figure 2**). Under these circumstances, PLN and other staging procedures sometimes need extra incisions, which increases the amount of trauma experienced throughout the operation. Thus, the TU-LESS extraperitoneal approach, which combines the strengths of LESS with that of extraperitoneal approach was developed to achieve PLN and PALN in a minimal invasive way. This study aims to describe the details of surgical procedures and present our preliminary experience with the TU-LESS extraperitoneal approach for PLN and PALN in order to further evaluate its feasibility.

METHODS

Patients

This study included eight patients from May 2020 to June 2021. Patients who had indications of systematic lymphadenectomy and were candidates for LESS surgery were eligible for inclusion. Clinical data were collected, including demographics, pathological features, and perioperative outcomes of patients who had the surgery. The study was approved by the institutional review board of the West China Second Hospital, Sichuan University, and all participants provided their written informed consent to participate in this study. The duration of lymphadenectomy time was defined as the interval from the first incision of skin to completion of lymphadenectomy, excluding subsequent procedures such as hysterectomy. The failure of the TU-LESS extraperitoneal approach was defined as the conversion to a transperitoneal approach *via* laparoscopy or open surgery; and intraoperative complications included peritoneal rupture and damage to intestines, bladder, ureters, nerves, or blood vessels. Postoperative complications included any adverse event that occurred within 30 days after surgery, including lymphocysts, thrombosis, infection, and chyle leakage. Visual analog scoring was used to assess the degree of postoperative pain of umbilical incision 24 h after surgery in the range of 0–10, 0 for no pain, 1–3 for mild pain, 4–6 for moderate pain, and 7–10 for severe pain (16). The body image questionnaire (BIQ) was administered 7 and 30 days after the surgery to assess patient satisfaction with the surgical intervention (17). The BIQ consists of two subscales: body image scale and cosmetic scale (**Supplementary Data Sheet 1**). With a score from 5 to 20, the body image scale measures perception of patients and their attitude to physical condition. The cosmetic scale evaluates the satisfaction of patients to their umbilical scars with a score from 3 to 24. The higher the score, the more satisfied the patient was with body image and cosmetic effect.

Lymphadenectomy Indications

Dissection of LNs should be recommended for endometrial cancer (EC) patients who are at high risk of recurrence, including those with deep myometrial invasion, high-grade histology, lymphatic vascular invasion, or type II tumors (2). For early-stage EC, the biopsy of sentinel lymph node (SLN) has been proved to be an accurate and effective alternative to lymphadenectomy. However, the use of SLN in high-risk group is controversial, lacking adequate high-level evidences to prove its safety. As a result, systematic lymphadenectomy was nevertheless conducted in this trial on individuals who were considered to be at high risk. In addition, systematic lymphadenectomy was indicated in patients with stage IA-IIA epithelial ovarian carcinoma (OC), except for the mucinous type without suspicious LNs), including those who wished to preserve fertility. Laparoscopy could be employed for patients with early-stage OC by an experienced surgeon (1).

Surgical Technique

All surgical procedures were performed by an experienced gynecologic oncologist. The patient was placed in trendelenburg position with the primary surgeon on the left and the assistant on the opposite sides. First, the primary surgeon made a 2 cm umbilical incision and a multichannel single port (Kangji, Hangzhou, China) was inserted into the intraperitoneal space (**Figure 3**). Careful transperitoneal exploration was conducted to exclude intra-abdominal carcinomatosis and collect peritoneal washing for cytologic evaluation.

Second, we had to identify the posterior peritoneum above the aortic bifurcation at first and execute a figure-of-eight suture subsequently. The surgeon pulled the thread and the sutured

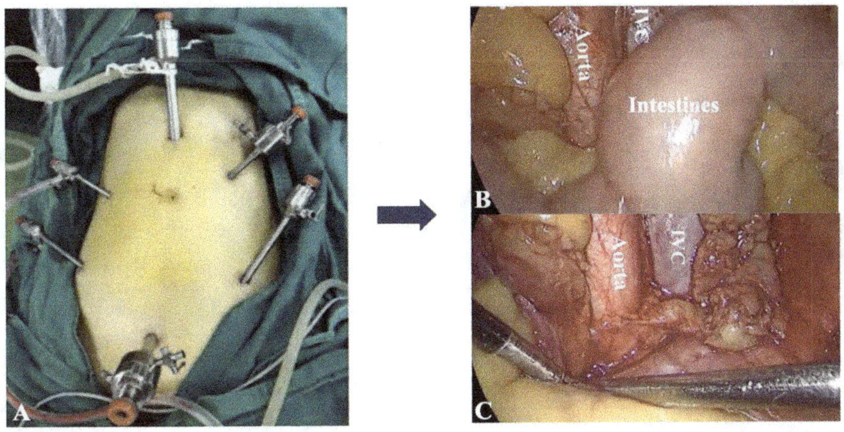

FIGURE 1 | The transperitoneal approach for PALN. **(A)** The placement of trocars. It was difficult to achieve adequate exposure of para-aortic regions for PALN because of the interference of intestines **(B,C)**. IVC: Inferior vena cava.

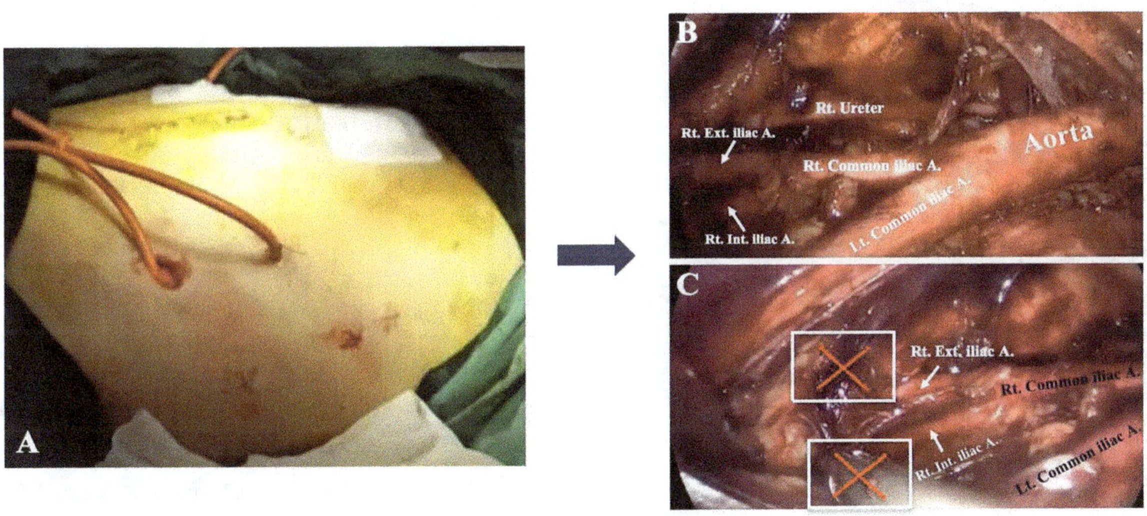

FIGURE 2 | The lateral extraperitoneal approach for lymphadenectomy. **(A)** The lateral incisions. **(B)** Para-aortic LN dissection. Bilateral obturator fossae were challenging to reach when performing pelvic lymphadenectomy **(C)**.

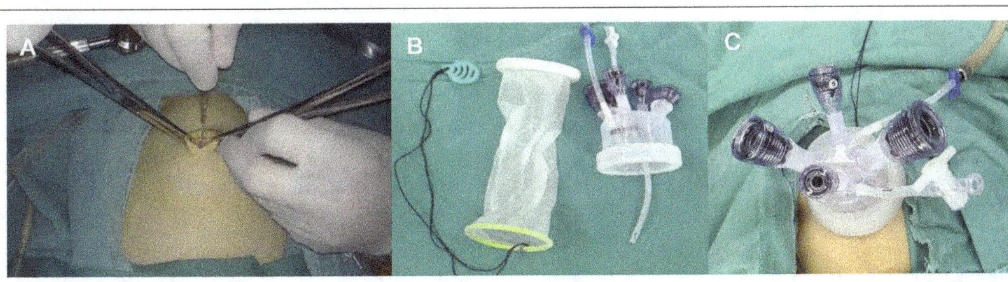

FIGURE 3 | (A) Make a 2-cm umbilical incision. **(B)** The multichannel single port (Kangji). **(C)** Set up the port into the intraperitoneal space.

posterior peritoneum was gently raised toward the umbilical incision. Using a purse-string suture, the suspended posterior peritoneum was held in place and marked. Afterwards, the center portion of the suspended posterior peritoneum was gently sliced open (**Figure 4**, **Supplementary Video 1**). The third step was to separate the extraperitoneal soft tissues that attached to the

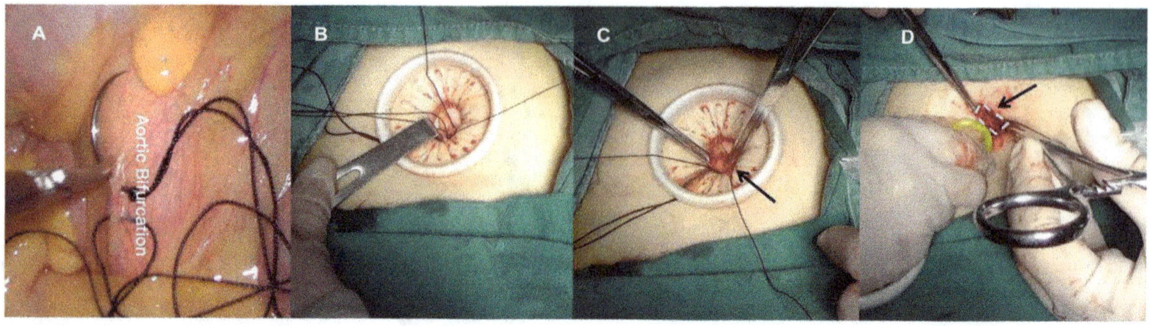

FIGURE 4 | (A) Make a figure-of-eight on the posterior peritoneum above the aortic bifurcation. **(B)** Raise the sutured posterior peritoneum to the umbilical incision. **(C)** Cut open the suspended posterior peritoneum. **(D)** Reset the port into the retroperitoneal space.

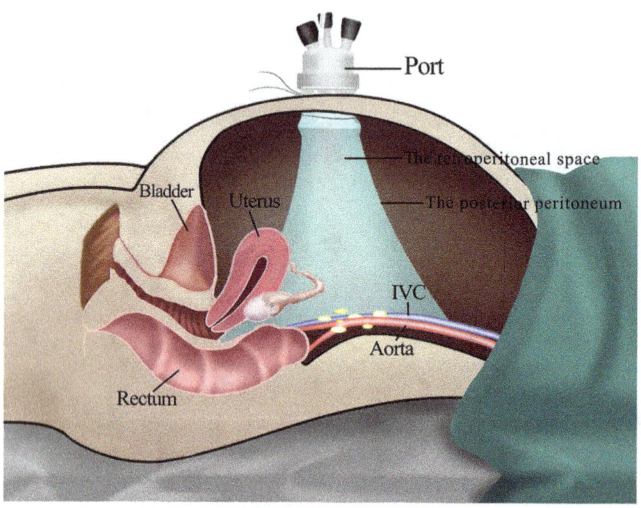

FIGURE 5 | The establishment of the retroperitoneal space. IVC, inferior vena cava.

anterior peritoneum with blunt-finger dissection in order to expand the extraperitoneal space. Subsequently, the port was repositioned into the retroperitoneal space with the purse-string suture tightened and secured. The microvessels were coagulated by a harmonic scalpel (HARMONIC, Ethicon, America), and carbon dioxide was insufflated at the maximum pressure of 14–20 mmHg to establish the retropneumoperitoneum (**Figure 5, Supplementary Video 1**).

Procedures were carried out for systematic PLN that included removal of the common iliac, external iliac, internal iliac, obturator, and deep inguinal nodes (**Figure 6, Supplementary Video 1**). During PALN operations, the surgeon stood between the legs of the patient and the assistant on the right. Para-aortic LNs were dissected from the aortic bifurcation to the left renal vein (RV) (**Figure 7, Supplementary Video 1**). All surgical specimens were taken out in bags in time to prevent the spillage of tumor cells. And the surgeon sprayed the porcine fibrin sealant kit (Bioseal, Guangzhou, China) onto the surgical field to prevent lymphatic leakage and lymphocyst (18).

After the extraperitoneal surgery, the port was reset into the intraperitoneal space for other transperitoneal procedures (i.e., hysterectomy, omentectomy, or salpinx oophorectomy) according to the different types of tumor.

RESULTS

Patient Information

A total of eight patients underwent lymphadenectomy via the TU-LESS extraperitoneal approach. Half of patients were suffering from high-risk EC (one dedifferentiated carcinoma, two grade 3 serous carcinoma with deep myometrial infiltration, and one clear cell carcinoma). The other four patients were diagnosed with early-stage epithelial OC (two serous carcinoma, one clear cell carcinoma, and one endometrioid carcinoma), and three of them opted for fertility-sparing surgery (i.e., preservation of the uterus and contralateral adnexa). The median age was 44 years (range 22–64), and the median BMI was 23.1 kg/m^2 (range 20.7–28.4). According to the Chinese criteria, two patients were classified as obese (BMI = 28.2 and 28.4 kg/m^2) (19). In this group, half had a history of abdominal surgery, and one even had undergone four surgeries. The clinical characteristics of patients are summarized in **Table 1**.

Surgical Outcomes

Table 2 displays the operative outcomes. The upper limit of PALN for all patients was at the renal vascular level. The median time of LN dissection was 166.5 min (range 123–205). During the procedure, no intraoperative complications were observed and no conversion to transperitoneal approach or multiport laparoscopic surgery occurred. The median blood loss was 100 ml (range 100–300) and no patient required blood transfusion. Concerning the LN yields, the median count of para-aortic LNs was 18 (range of 7–30), and the retrieved pelvic LNs was 26.5 (range 18–35). Three EC patients had positive LNs, two with pelvic nodal metastasis and one with para-aortic nodal involvement. Furthermore, there was no evidence of LN metastasis in OC patients. The median flatus time was 23.0 h (range 16.0–38.0) and the median hospital duration was 3 days (range of 2–4). All patients felt mild pain for 24 h after surgery with a median score of 2

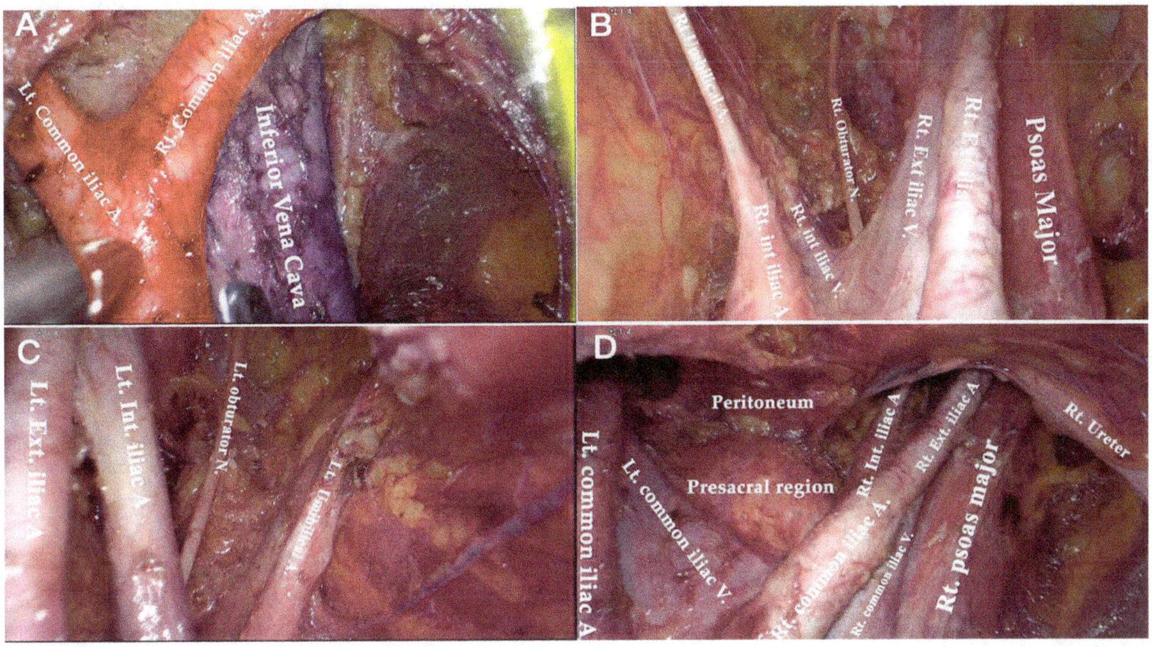

FIGURE 6 | Anatomical overview of pelvic area after PLN. **(A)** The aortic bifurcation and inferior vena cava. **(B)** The right obturator fossa. **(C)** The left obturator fossa. **(D)** The view of presacral area.

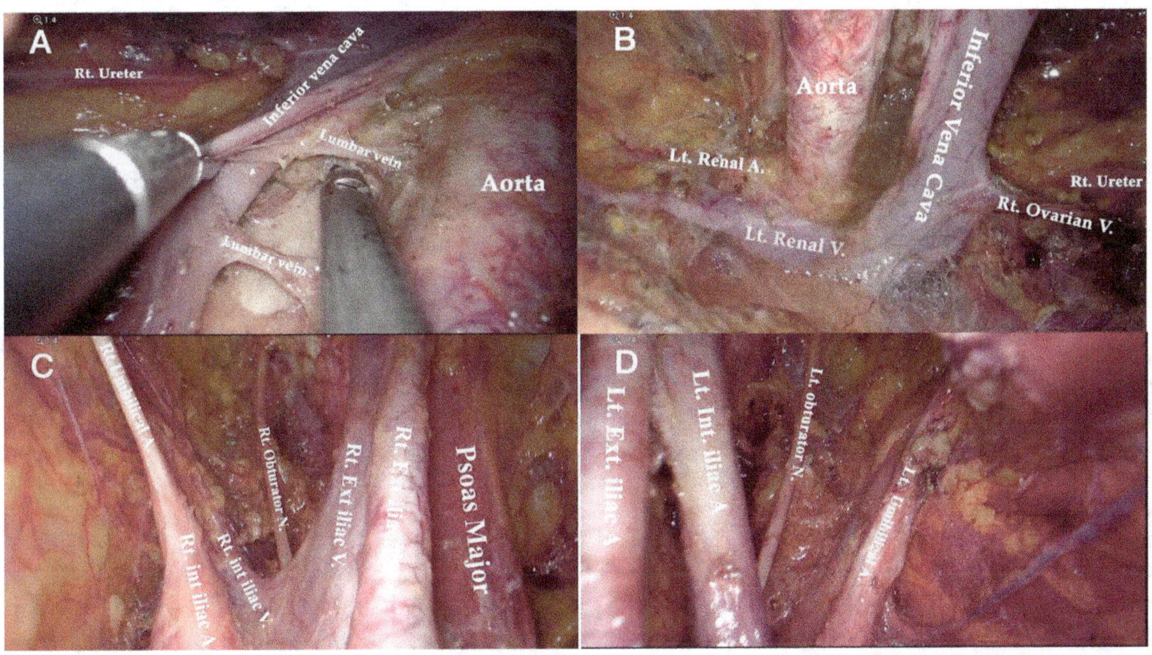

FIGURE 7 | Anatomical overview of para-aortic area. **(A)** Lymphadenectomy up to the left renal vein. **(B)** The right para-aortic region. **(C)** Dissection of the interaortocaval and retrocaval lymph nodes. **(D)** The infrarenal region after PALN.

(range 1–3). The median satisfaction value for body image was 17 (range 16–19) 7 days after surgery and increased to 19.5 (range 18–20) a month after surgery; while the median score of cosmetic effects was 18 (range 15–19) 1 week after surgery and improved to 22.5 (range 21–23) after 30 days (**Figure 8**).

TABLE 1 | Patient characteristics.

Case	Age, y	BMI, kg/m^2	Histologic type	FIGO staging	Number of previous abdominal surgeries	Conversion
1	48	21.0	Dedifferentiated EC	IIIC	0	N
2	54	23.0	Serous EC	IB	0	N
3	29	28.2	Serous OC	IC	1	N
4	50	26.0	Serous EC	IB	1	N
5	22	22.5	Endometrioid OC	IA	1	N
6	64	28.4	Clear cell EC	IIIC	0	N
7	40	20.7	Serous OC	IA	4	N
8	28	23.1	Clear cell OC	IC	0	N

TABLE 2 | Surgical and postoperative information.

Case	Operative time, min	Aortic dissection level	Para-aortic LNs, *n*	Pelvic LNs, *n*	Blood loss, ml	Complications	Flatus time, h	Postoperative pain score, 24 h	Body image scale (range 5–20) 7/30 days	Cosmetic scale (range 3–24), 7/30 days	Hospital duration, days
1	205	Infrarenal	14	33	100	N	38	2	16/18	18/22	4
2	173	Infrarenal	43	18	100	N	21	2	17/20	17/23	2
3	163	Infrarenal	12	35	200	N	22	2	18/20	19/23	3
4	165	Infrarenal	19	27	100	N	18	1	19/20	17/23	4
5	175	Infrarenal	30	20	300	N	16	3	16/19	15/22	4
6	168	Infrarenal	17	23	100	N	27	1	16/20	18/22	3
7	158	Infrarenal	21	28	200	N	24	2	17/19	19/21	2
8	123	Infrarenal	7	26	100	N	26	2	18/19	18/23	3
Median	166.5	/	18.0	26.5	100	/	23	2	17/19.5	18/22.5	3

DISCUSSION

Lymph node status evaluation is a critical component of thorough surgical staging for ovarian and EC (20–22). Laparoscopic lymphadenectomy has been proven safe for surgical staging in EC and early-stage OC patients with less complications and faster recovery (1, 2, 23). Previous studies have shown that extraperitoneal lymphadenectomy is superior to the transperitoneal approach for PALN, because it could avoid intestinal interference and allow an easier access to supramesenteric LNs (5, 24, 25). We initially attempted to employ the TU-LESS extraperitoneal approach in the surgical staging procedures for a patient with advanced cervical cancer in order to accurately delineate the radiographic field. The PALN and right enlarged obturator LN biopsy were performed easily via this novel technique (26). Further exploration and practice of this technique were conducted, and the primary findings of our study confirmed that the TU-LESS extraperitoneal approach is feasible for systematic PLN and PALN.

Compared to the node counts of laparoscopic transperitoneal procedure (range 14–22) (11, 13, 27–29), our method yielded a comparable number of pelvic LNs. The median count of para-aortic LNs (18, range 7–30) in our investigation was equivalent to that of the largest case series of single-port lateral extraperitoneal approach reported by Guoy (median 18, range 2–47) (3), but was higher than that of left-sided extraperitoneal approach using multiport laparoscopy (range 9.5–15) (3, 5, 14, 30). Despite the left extraperitoneal approach being viable for completing the aortic nodal dissection, Dargent asserted that the number of right-sided aortic sampling had reduced compared to bilateral extraperitoneal approach ($p < 0.01$) (31). Furthermore, being limited in access to the deep obturator fossae was one of major technical difficulties of the left-sided approach, which was mainly due to the poor angle of view (13, 15, 32) (as **Figure 2C** shows). Some technique modifications were made to overcome this difficulty, such as addition of different incisions. Querleu added two incisions on the basis of the left-sided extraperitoneal approach in order to achieve obturator node sampling for patients with locally advanced cervical cancer (32). However, whether this technique could be applied in systematic PLN remains to be verified, and the authors further noted that right obturator fossa was obviously difficult to reach with this technique. Other methods for pelvic LN dissection were also reported, such as combining a right extraperitoneal approach (33). Nonetheless, these modifications would increase surgical trauma, and there were few studies that investigated the feasibility for systematic PLN. One of the greatest merits of the TU-LESS extraperitoneal approach is that it allows equal access to the bilateral pelvic and para-aortic areas through the same extraperitoneal approach because the umbilical

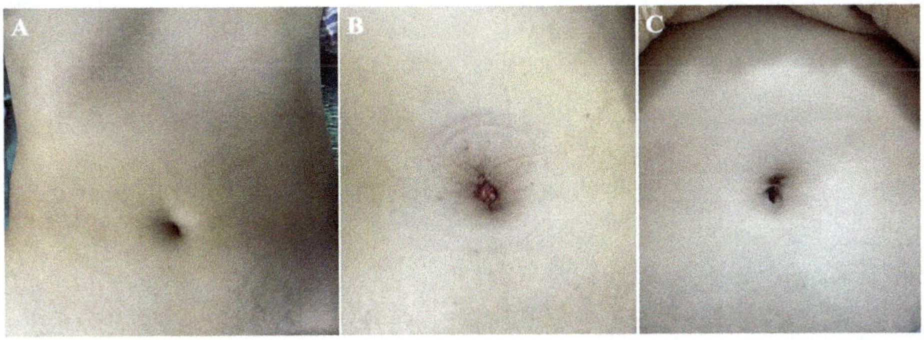

FIGURE 8 | The umbilical incisions of the TU-LESS extraperitoneal approach. **(A)** The preoperative appearance. **(B)** The postoperative appearance. **(C)** The appearance 3 months after surgery.

incision is centrally located, which facilitates the obturator and infrarenal LN dissection (**Figures 6, 7**). Additionally, careful contrast of **Figures 2C, 6, 7** showed that the anatomic angles during the lateral extraperitoneal procedures were altered, adding to identification complexity for surgeons. However, surgeons did not need to readapt to the changing anatomic angles with the TU-LESS extraperitoneal approach, since the angle of view was the same as the transperitoneal approach or laparotomy which many surgeons have been accustomed to.

Reducing intraperitoneal adhesion is another significant advantage of the extraperitoneal approach. Occelli et al. compared the adhesion rate of laparoscopic transperitoneal vs. extraperitoneal PALN on pigs. The results showed that the extraperitoneal group had a lower adhesion formation rate than the transperitoneal group ($p = 0.04$) (15). Abdominal adhesion is likely to increase the morbidity associated with radiotherapy and may result in adnexal adhesion or even infertility (34, 35). The TU-LESS extraperitoneal approach also theoretically has this advantage, because it could minimize peritoneal injury and leave the peritoneal cavity intact after surgery. For these reasons, in our research, the TU-LESS extraperitoneal approach was considered to be an optimal treatment for young patients who wish to preserve their fertility. Three patients with epithelial OC received the fertility preservation surgery. All of them completed the comprehensive assessment of LNs and dissected lesions with little peritoneal damage. While peritoneal cavity could remain intact with our technique, however, the fertility outcomes ought to be followed. Additionally, patients who underwent abdominal surgeries might potentially benefit from the TU-LESS extraperitoneal approach since it avoids adhesiolysis, and thus it could reduce the risk of intra-abdominal organ injury. In our analysis, half of the patients had surgical history, and none of them had intraperitoneal complications. To sum up, different approaches for lymphadenectomy have their own strengths and limitations; and the concerned summarization from our current exploration and prior studies are presented in **Table 3**.

In previous studies, the lymphadenectomy time of the lateral extraperitoneal approach was varied (range 125–339.5 min) (3, 25, 30, 36). The time required for lymphadenectomy

TABLE 3 | Advantages and limitations of three approaches for lymphadenectomy.

	Transperitoneal approach	Lateral extraperitoneal approach	TU-LESS extraperitoneal approach (current work)
PLN	Easy	Difficult	Easy
PALN(RV level)	Difficult	Easy	Easy
Risk of abdominal adhesion	Increase	Decrease	Decrease
Changes in anatomic recognition	No change	Change	No change
Surgical trauma	Small	Small	Minimal

RV, renal vein.

in this study was in concordance with the prior findings, but it was less than the time of early practice of the single-port extraperitoneal approach for PALN (average 240 min, range 180–270 min) described by Guoy et al. (37). However, our lymphadenectomy time was somewhat longer than the single-port transperitoneal approach for PLN and PALN (range 60–185 min) (13), which might be explained by the extra time needed to establish the retropneumoperitoneum. The operation time may decrease when the learning curve climbs.

In our research, there were no complications during or after surgery, nor was there a conversion to the transperitoneal route. The procedural failure of the extraperitoneal approach was attributed to the peritoneal rupture (38). Peritoneal rupture occurred in seven patients (16%) during the lateral single-port extraperitoneal lymphadenectomy according to Beytout (14). Neither a peritoneal rupture nor any other technical problems have ever caused abortion of extraperitoneal operation in our series.

Additionally, some studies indicated that the extraperitoneal approach may be an optimal option for patients with a high

BMI. Dowdy et al. (39) and Pakish et al. (25) confirmed that patients with BMI >35 kg/m^2, who had extraperitoneal PALN, harvested more para-aortic nodes than those who underwent abdominal or transperitoneal PALN. BMI had no effect on the duration of surgery, and the area of visceral adipose tissues did not affect the extraperitoneal approach of PALN (40). According to earlier studies, the maximum BMI of patients who underwent the extraperitoneal lymphadenectomy was ranging from 31 to 40 kg/m^2 (1, 3, 9, 11, 20). Nonetheless, we successfully performed the TU-LESS extraperitoneal technique on two obese patients who satisfied Chinese diagnostic criteria (BMI ≥28 kg/m^2). However, since this was a primary exploration with a limited number of patients, we did not try to use this measure for systematic lymphadenectomy in patients with BMI more than 30 kg/m^2. We were exploring an easier method for establishing extraperitoneal space in obese patients. The feasibility and safety of robotic technology for lymphadenectomy in gynecologic cancer have been validated, with the benefits of a three-dimensional vision, scaled movement, and short learning curves (41). Gallotta demonstrated that the robotic technology is conducive for PALN. The results showed that aortic LN yields were comparable when patients with BMI >30 kg/m^2 were compared with those with BMI <30 kg/m^2 (42).The robotic surgery was likely to be a preferable approach for obese patients, and the node counts were not affected by increasing BMI (43). Combining robotic technology and the TU-LESS extraperitoneal approach for lymphadenectomy may provide a potential and feasible option for obese patients. Robotic technology may facilitate in shortening the learning curve of the TU- LESS extraperitoneal approach and implementing it.

CONCLUSION

In conclusion, the TU-LESS extraperitoneal approach for pelvic and PALN is feasible with a practical application. It significantly improves the exposure and visualization for PLN and PALN, while causing minimal surgical trauma. Depending on the results of our study, this innovative approach may become an effictive alternative measure to the transperitoneal and lateral extraperitoneal approach. However, further studies are required to compare the surgical outcomes like LN yields, surgical trauma, cosmesis, and other index among three approaches. Additionally, based on the current research, a long-term clinical application on a larger sample would be required to evaluate the effects in a more objective manner.

ETHICS STATEMENT

The studies involving human participants were reviewed and approved by the Medical Institutional Review Board of West China Second Hospital of Sichuan University. The patients/participants provided their written informed consent to participate in this study. Written informed consent was obtained from the individual(s) for the publication of any potentially identifiable images or data included in this article.

AUTHOR CONTRIBUTIONS

SP contributed to writing the manuscript and drawing pictures. YZ designed the study and revised the manuscript. FY and KW analyzed and interpreted the data. SC and YW made the video and collected the data. All authors contributed to the manuscript and approved the final manuscript.

SUPPLEMENTARY MATERIAL

Supplementary Video 1 | The TU-LESS extraperitoneal approach for systematic lymphadenectomy.

Supplementary Data Sheet 1 | The Body Image Questionnaire (BIQ).

REFERENCES

1. Armstrong DK, Alvarez RD, Bakkum-Gamez JN, Barroilhet L, Behbakht K, Berchuck A, et al. Ovarian cancer, version 2.2020, Nccn clinical practice guidelines in oncology. *J Natl Compr Canc Netw.* (2021) 19:191–226. doi: 10.6004/jnccn.2021.0007
2. Abu-Rustum NR, Yashar CM, Bradley K, Campos SM, Chino J, Chon HS, et al. Nccn guidelines® insights: uterine neoplasms, version 3.2021. *J Natl Compr Canc Netw.* (2021) 19:888–95. doi: 10.6004/jnccn.2021.0038
3. Gouy S, Uzan C, Scherier S, Gauthier T, Bentivegna E, Kane A, et al. Single-port laparoscopy and extraperitoneal para-aortic lymphadenectomy for locally advanced cervical cancer: assessment after 52 consecutive patients. *Surg Endosc.* (2014) 28:249–56. doi: 10.1007/s00464-013-3180-4
4. Díaz-Feijoo B, Bebia V, Hernández A, Gilabert-Estalles J, Franco-Camps S, de la Torre J, et al. Surgical complications comparing extraperitoneal vs transperitoneal laparoscopic aortic staging in early stage ovarian and endometrial cancer. *Gynecol Oncol.* (2021) 160:83–90. doi: 10.1016/j.ygyno.2020.10.038
5. Zhang W, Xia L, Han X, Ju X, Wu X, Chen X. Extraperitoneal laparoscopy for para-aortic lymphadenectomy in endometrial carcinoma staging: an approach with higher efficiency. *World J Surg Oncol.* (2021) 19:323. doi: 10.1186/s12957-021-02416-x
6. Spana G, Rane A, Kaouk JH. Is robotics the future of laparoendoscopic single-site surgery (less)? *BJU Int.* (2011) 108:1018–23. doi: 10.1111/j.1464-410X.2011.10513.x
7. Song T, Kim ML, Jung YW, Yoon BS, Joo WD, Seong SJ. Laparoendoscopic single-site versus conventional laparoscopic gynecologic surgery: a metaanalysis of randomized controlled trials. *Am J Obstet Gynecol.* (2013) 209:317.e1–9. doi: 10.1016/j.ajog.2013.07.004
8. Michener CM, Lampert E, Yao M, Harnegie MP, Chalif J, Chambers LM. Meta-analysis of laparoendoscopic single-site and vaginal natural orifice transluminal endoscopic hysterectomy compared with multiport hysterectomy: real benefits or diminishing returns? *J Minim Invasive Gynecol.* (2021) 28:698–709.e1. doi: 10.1016/j.jmig.2020.11.029
9. Yuan JB, Chen MF, Qi L, Li Y, Li YL, Chen C, et al. Preservation of the saphenous vein during laparoendoscopic single-site inguinal lymphadenectomy: comparison with the conventional laparoscopic technique. *BJU Int.* (2015) 115:613–8. doi: 10.1111/bju.12838
10. Hudry D, Cannone F, Houvenaeghel G, Buttarelli M, Jauffret C, Chéreau E, et al. Comparison of single-port laparoscopy and conventional laparoscopy for extraperitoneal para-aortic lymphadenectomy. *Surg Endosc.* (2013) 27:4319–24. doi: 10.1007/s00464-013-3051-z
11. Fagotti A, Boruta DM, 2nd, Scambia G, Fanfani F, Paglia A, Escobar PF. First 100 early endometrial cancer cases treated with laparoendoscopic single-

site surgery: a multicentric retrospective study. *Am J Obstet Gynecol.* (2012) 206:353.e1–6. doi: 10.1016/j.ajog.2012.01.031

12. Gouy S, Uzan C, Kane A, Gauthier T, Morice P. Single-port laparoscopy and extraperitoneal para-aortic lymphadenectomy: 3 consecutive cases. *Int J Gynecol Cancer.* (2011) 21:1695–7. doi: 10.1097/IGC.0b013e31822a0175
13. Lambaudie E, Cannone F, Bannier M, Buttarelli M, Houvenaeghel G. Laparoscopic extraperitoneal aortic dissection: does single-port surgery offer the same possibilities as conventional laparoscopy? *Surg Endosc.* (2012) 26:1920–3. doi: 10.1007/s00464-011-2126-y
14. Beytout C, Laas E, Naoura I, Bendifallah S, Canlorbe G, Ballester M, et al. Single-port extra- and transperitoneal approach for paraaortic lymphadenectomy in gynecologic cancers: a propensity-adjusted analysis. *Ann Surg Oncol.* (2016) 23:952–8. doi: 10.1245/s10434-015-4874-8
15. Occelli B, Narducci F, Lanvin D, Querleu D, Coste E, Castelain B, et al. De novo adhesions with extraperitoneal endosurgical para-aortic lymphadenectomy versus transperitoneal laparoscopic para-aortic lymphadenectomy: a randomized experimental study. *Am J Obstet Gynecol.* (2000) 183:529–33. doi: 10.1067/mob.2000.105736
16. Fagotti A, Bottoni C, Vizzielli G, Gueli Alletti S, Scambia G, Marana E, et al. Postoperative pain after conventional laparoscopy and laparoendoscopic single site surgery (less) for benign adnexal disease: a randomized trial. *Fertil Steril.* (2011) 96:255–9.e2. doi: 10.1016/j.fertnstert.2011.04.006
17. Dunker MS, Stiggelbout AM, van Hogezand RA, Ringers J, Griffioen G, Bemelman WA. Cosmesis and body image after laparoscopic-assisted and open ileocolic resection for crohn's disease. *Surg Endosc.* (1998) 12:1334–40. doi: 10.1007/s004649900851
18. Gasparri ML, Ruscito I, Bolla D, Benedetti Panici P, Mueller MD, Papadia A. The efficacy of fibrin sealant patches in reducing the incidence of lymphatic morbidity after radical lymphadenectomy: a meta-analysis. *Int J Gynecol Cancer.* (2017) 27:1283–92. doi: 10.1097/IGC.0000000000001051
19. Coorperative Meta analysis Group of China Obesity Task Force. Predictive values of body mass index and waist circumference to risk factors of related disease in Chinese adult population. *Chin J Epidemiol.* (2002) 1:10–5.
20. O'Hanlan KA, Sten MS, O'Holleran MS, Ford NN, Struck DM, McCutcheon SP. Infrarenal lymphadenectomy for gynecological malignancies: two laparoscopic approaches. *Gynecol Oncol.* (2015) 139:330–7. doi: 10.1016/j.ygyno.2015.09.019
21. Koo YJ, Kim JE, Kim YH, Hahn HS, Lee IH, Kim TJ, et al. Comparison of laparoscopy and laparotomy for the management of early-stage ovarian cancer: surgical and oncological outcomes. *J Gynecol Oncol.* (2014) 25:111–7. doi: 10.3802/jgo.2014.25.2.111
22. Kong Q, Wei H, Zhang J, Li Y, Wang Y. Comparison of the survival outcomes of laparoscopy versus laparotomy in treatment of early-stage ovarian cancer: a systematic review and meta-analysis. *J Ovarian Res.* (2021) 14:45. doi: 10.1186/s13048-021-00793-1
23. Gallotta V, Petrillo M, Conte C, Vizzielli G, Fagotti A, Ferrandina G, et al. laparoscopic versus laparotomic surgical staging for early-stage ovarian cancer: a case-control study. *J Minim Invasive Gynecol.* (2016) 23:769–74. doi: 10.1016/j.jmig.2016.03.006
24. Prodromidou A, Machairas N, Spartalis E, Kostakis ID, Iavazzo C, Moris D, et al. Transperitoneal versus extraperitoneal laparoscopic lymphadenectomy for gynecological malignancies: a systematic review and meta-analysis. *Anticancer Res.* (2018) 38:4677–81. doi: 10.21873/anticanres.12773
25. Pakish J, Soliman PT, Frumovitz M, Westin SN, Schmeler KM, Reis RD, et al. A Comparison of extraperitoneal versus transperitoneal laparoscopic or robotic para-aortic lymphadenectomy for staging of endometrial carcinoma. *Gynecol Oncol.* (2014) 132:366–71. doi: 10.1016/j.ygyno.2013.12.019
26. Chen S, Zhou J, Zheng Y, Wang K, Yang X. Para-aortic and right obturator lymphadenectomy for surgical staging of advanced cervical cancer through the tu-less extraperitoneal approach. *J Minim Invasive Gynecol* . 2021) 28:1140. doi: 10.1016/j.jmig.2020.12.014
27. Boruta DM, Fagotti A, Bradford LS, Escobar PF, Scambia G, Kushnir CL, et al. Laparoendoscopic single-site radical hysterectomy with pelvic lymphadenectomy: initial multi-institutional experience for treatment of invasive cervical cancer. *J Minim Invasive Gynecol.* (2014) 21:394–8. doi: 10.1016/j.jmig.2013.10.005
28. Paik ES, Baek SH, Kang JH, Jeong SY, Kim MS, Kim WY, et al. Comparison of laparoscopy and laparotomy for para-aortic lymphadenectomy in women with presumed stage i-ii high-risk endometrial cancer. *Front Oncol.* (2020) 10:451. doi: 10.3389/fonc.2020.00451
29. Larciprete G, Casalino B, Segatore MF, Jarvis S, Catarinella V, Cirese E. Pelvic lymphadenectomy for cervical cancer: extraperitoneal versus laparoscopic approach. *Eur J Obstet Gynecol Reprod Biol.* (2006) 126:259–63. doi: 10.1016/j.ejogrb.2005.09.019
30. Iacoponi S, De Santiago J, Diestro MD, Hernandez A, Zapardiel I. Single-port laparoscopic extraperitoneal para-aortic lymphadenectomy. *Int J Gynecol Cancer.* (2013) 23:1712–6. doi: 10.1097/IGC.0000000000000006
31. Dargent D, Ansquer Y, Mathevet P. Technical development and results of left extraperitoneal laparoscopic paraaortic lymphadenectomy for cervical cancer. *Gynecol Oncol.* (2000) 77:87–92. doi: 10.1006/gyno.1999.5585
32. Querleu D, Ferron G, Rafii A, Bouissou E, Delannes M, Mery E, et al. Pelvic lymph node dissection via a lateral extraperitoneal approach: description of a technique. *Gynecol Oncol.* (2008) 109:81–5. doi: 10.1016/j.ygyno.2007.12.031
33. Pan XY, Lin H, Wang YN, Zhao YW, Cheng JY, Sun AP. Feasibility of laparoscopic extraperitoneal pelvic lymphadenectomy in gynecologic malignancies. *Gynecol Oncol.* (2011) 122:281–4. doi: 10.1016/j.ygyno.2011.04.048
34. Vergote I, Pouseele B, Van Gorp T, Vanacker B, Leunen K, Cadron I, et al. Robotic retroperitoneal lower para-aortic lymphadenectomy in cervical carcinoma: first report on the technique used in 5 patients. *Acta Obstet Gynecol Scand.* (2008) 87:783–7. doi: 10.1080/00016340802146946
35. Mabuchi S, Kimura T. Extraperitoneal radical trachelectomy with pelvic lymphadenectomy: a novel fertility-preserving option for early stage cervical cancer patients. *Int J Gynecol Cancer.* (2017) 27:537–42. doi: 10.1097/IGC.0000000000000918
36. Schuman S, Lucci JA 3rd, Twiggs LB. Laparoendoscopic single-site extraperitoneal aortic lymphadenectomy: first experience. *J Laparoendosc Adv Surg Tech A.* (2011) 21:251–4. doi: 10.1089/lap.2010.0362
37. Gouy S, Uzan C, Kane A, Scherier S, Gauthier T, Bentivegna E, et al. A new single-port approach to perform a transperitoneal step and an extraperitoneal para-aortic lymphadenectomy with a single incision. *J Am Coll Surg.* (2012) 214:e25–30. doi: 10.1016/j.jamcollsurg.2012.02.012
38. Morales S, Zapardiel I, Grabowski JP, Hernandez A, Diestro MD, Gonzalez-Benitez C, et al. Surgical outcome of extraperitoneal paraaortic lymph node dissections compared with transperitoneal approach in gynecologic cancer patients. *J Minim Invasive Gynecol.* (2013) 20:611–5. doi: 10.1016/j.jmig.2013.03.009
39. Dowdy SC, Aletti G, Cliby WA, Podratz KC, Mariani A. Extra-peritoneal laparoscopic para-aortic lymphadenectomy–a prospective cohort study of 293 patients with endometrial cancer. *Gynecol Oncol.* (2008) 111:418–24. doi: 10.1016/j.ygyno.2008.08.021
40. Nakao K, Sasaki H, Nishimura T, Banno H, Otsuka K, Hirabuki S, et al. Periaortic abdominal fat area as a predictor of surgical difficulties during extraperitoneal laparoscopic para-aortic lymphadenectomy. *J Minim Invasive Gynecol.* (2020) 27:1377–82. doi: 10.1016/j.jmig.2019.10.016
41. Gallotta V, Giudice MT, Conte C, Sarandeses AV, D'Indinosante M, Federico A, et al. Minimally invasive salvage lymphadenectomy in gynecological cancer patients: a single institution series. *Eur J Surg Oncol.* (2018) 44:1568–72. doi: 10.1016/j.ejso.2018.08.006
42. Gallotta V, Federico A, Gaballa K, D'Indinosante M, Conte C, Giudice MT, et al. The role of robotic aortic lymphadenectomy in gynecological cancer: surgical and oncological outcome in a single institution experience. *J Surg Oncol.* (2019) 119:355–60. doi: 10.1002/jso.25335
43. Cunningham MJ, Dorzin E, Nguyen L, Anderson E, Bunn WD Jr. Body mass index, conversion rate and complications among patients undergoing robotic surgery for endometrial carcinoma. *J Robot Surg.* (2015) 9:339–45. doi: 10.1007/s11701-015-0538-8

12

A Scientometric Analysis and Visualization Discovery of Enhanced Recovery After Surgery

*Mingjie Zhang[1], Xiaoxue Wang[2], Xueting Chen[2], Zixuan Song[3], Yuting Wang[3], Yangzi Zhou[3] and Dandan Zhang[3]**

[1]Department of Surgery, Shengjing Hospital of China Medical University, Shenyang, China, [2]Department of Health Management, Shengjing Hospital of China Medical University, Shenyang, China, [3]Department of Obstetrics and Gynecology, Shengjing Hospital of China Medical University, Shenyang, China

**Correspondence:*
Dandan Zhang
zhangdd@sj-hospital.org

Background: Enhanced recovery after surgery (ERAS), a new clinical surgical concept, has been applied in many surgical disciplines with good clinical results for the past 20 years. Bibliometric analysis is an effective method to quantitatively evaluate the academic productivity. This report aimed to perform a scientometric analysis of the ERAS research status and research hotspots.

Methods: Comprehensive scientific mapping analysis of a wide range of literature metadata using the scientometric tools, including the Bibliometrix R Package, Biblioshiny, and CiteSpace. Data were retrieved from the Web of Science Core Collection database of original articles from 2001 to 2020. Specific indicators and maps were analyzed to show the co-authorship, co-institute, co-country, co-citation, and international cooperation. Automatic literature screening, unsupervised cluster filtering, and topic cluster identification methods were used to display the conceptual framework and thematic evolution.

Results: A total of 1,403 research projects drafted by 6,966 authors and published in 413 sources were found. There was an exponential growth in the number of publications on ERAS. There were 709 collaborations between authors from different countries, and the US, China, and the UK had the greatest number of publications. The WORLD JOURNAL OF SURGERY, located in Bradford's Law 1, had the highest number of published articles ($n = 1{,}276$; total citations $= 3{,}193$). CiteSpace network analysis revealed 15 highly correlated cluster ERAS studies, and the earliest study was on colonic surgery, and ERAS was recently applied in cardiac surgery. The etiology of ERAS is constantly evolving, with surgery and length of hospital as the main topics. Meta-analyses and perioperative care have tended to decline.

Conclusion: This is the first scientometric analysis of ERAS to provide descriptive quantitative indicators. This can provide a better understanding of how the field has evolved over the past 20 years, help identify research trends, and provide insights and

---

Abbreviations: ERAS, Enhanced recovery after surgery; TC, total citations; NP, Net output; FTS, Fast-track surgery.

research directions for academic researchers, policymakers, and medical practitioners who want to collaborate in these areas in the future.

Keywords: enhanced recovery after surgery, fast-track surgery , bibliometrics, bibliometrix, citespace

INTRODUCTION

Enhanced recovery after surgery (ERAS) was first proposed by Kehlet et al. at the University of Copenhagen in Denmark in the late 1990s and has been applied clinically (1, 2). ERAS was initially used primarily in Europe and North America to study the effects of surgical stress response on open colorectal surgery in terms of rapid recovery. ERAS represents the idea of synergy through a combination of effective measures, with the central aim of reducing trauma and stress. ERAS is the best result of multidisciplinary collaboration that perfectly blends the latest research findings from surgery, anesthesia, and nursing into an integrated innovative concept that represents an optimized clinical pathway. This optimized clinical pathway involves the whole process of patient diagnosis and treatment, emphasis on the patient-centered concept. The implementation of the ERAS pathway can improve perioperative safety and the satisfaction in surgical patients, shorten the postoperative hospital stay, and help reduce the incidence of postoperative complications (3). Using the ERAS, patients can be identified, compartmentalized, and accommodated at every step throughout the perioperative period to facilitate an effective and safe process from preoperative evaluation through discharge to recovery. The advantages of ERAS have been recognized by operators and specialists worldwide, and its application in the medical field has been actively promoted. The ERAS Society has developed numerous perioperative guidelines for ERAS for various specialties and disciplines since 2005 (4–11).

The postoperative rehabilitation of patients undergoing surgery is affected by various factors, such as stress response, pain, and postoperative intestinal paralysis (12). stress response after surgery is a physiological and pathological process in the body, including changes in the nerve, endocrine, metabolic, and immune functions. Similarly, pain can adversely affect patient recovery. Postoperative intestinal paralysis aggravates postoperative discomfort, especially in patients undergoing abdominal surgery, affecting oral feeding and delaying the recovery of patients. Therefore, the combination of new techniques in anesthesiology, pain control, and surgical methods with the improvement of the traditional postoperative nursing methods can reduce the postoperative stress reaction, incidence of postoperative complications and mortality, postoperative hospital stay, and hospitalization cost. This finding is consistent with the concept of minimally invasive surgery. ERAS generally includes the following: (1) Preoperative patient education. (2) better anesthesia, analgesia, and surgical techniques can reduce surgical stress, pain, and discomfort. (3) enhanced postoperative rehabilitation including early ambulation and enteral nutrition. Several surgical studies have shown that ERAS can significantly shorten the postoperative hospitalization time, reduce hospitalization costs, and maximize the use of limited hospital resources without increasing the incidence of complications and mortality, which will become the trend of surgery (13, 14).

ERAS has been applied and supplemented for 20 years since it was first proposed in 2001, and is now being developed in a more refined direction. Its research direction is not limited to the surgical field, and future research directions and current research hotspots need to be clarified. Bibliometric analysis is the application of statistical and mathematical tools to books and media communications (15). Bibliometric analysis is a transparent, systematic, and repeatable review process that significantly improves the quality of literature review. This provides a means of mapping research fields and influential work without subjective bias.

This study aimed to identify research flows and topics by analyzing the citation dynamics in ERAS studies from to 2001–2020 to measure their impact on the scientific community (qualitative indicators). These topics and streams of research can guide scholars to find directions for future research and to find answers to current questions.

MATERIALS & METHOD

Study Design/Ethics Statement

This was a bibliometric network study using metadata from the Web of Science Core Collection on July 12, 2021. This is described in accordance with the STROBE guidelines (16). This was not a human-focused study and, as such, neither the institutional review board approval nor informed consent was required. This study was divided into five steps, known as the document metering workflow proposed by Zupic and Ater (17). **Figure 1** represents the five steps used to complete the bibliometric analysis of ERAS.

Data Sources

The original data for this article were obtained from the Web of Science core collection database, including SCI-EXPAND and SSCI. This following titles were used for the selection: "enhanced recovery after surgery" or "enhanced postsurgical recovery" or "enhanced recovery program" or "enhanced recovery pathways" or "accelerated rehabilitation" or "fast track surgery." The publication date was restricted from January 1, 2001 to December 31, 2020. The manuscript type was "article" and the target results were filtered. The file format recorded content was set to "plain text" and was exported as "full record".

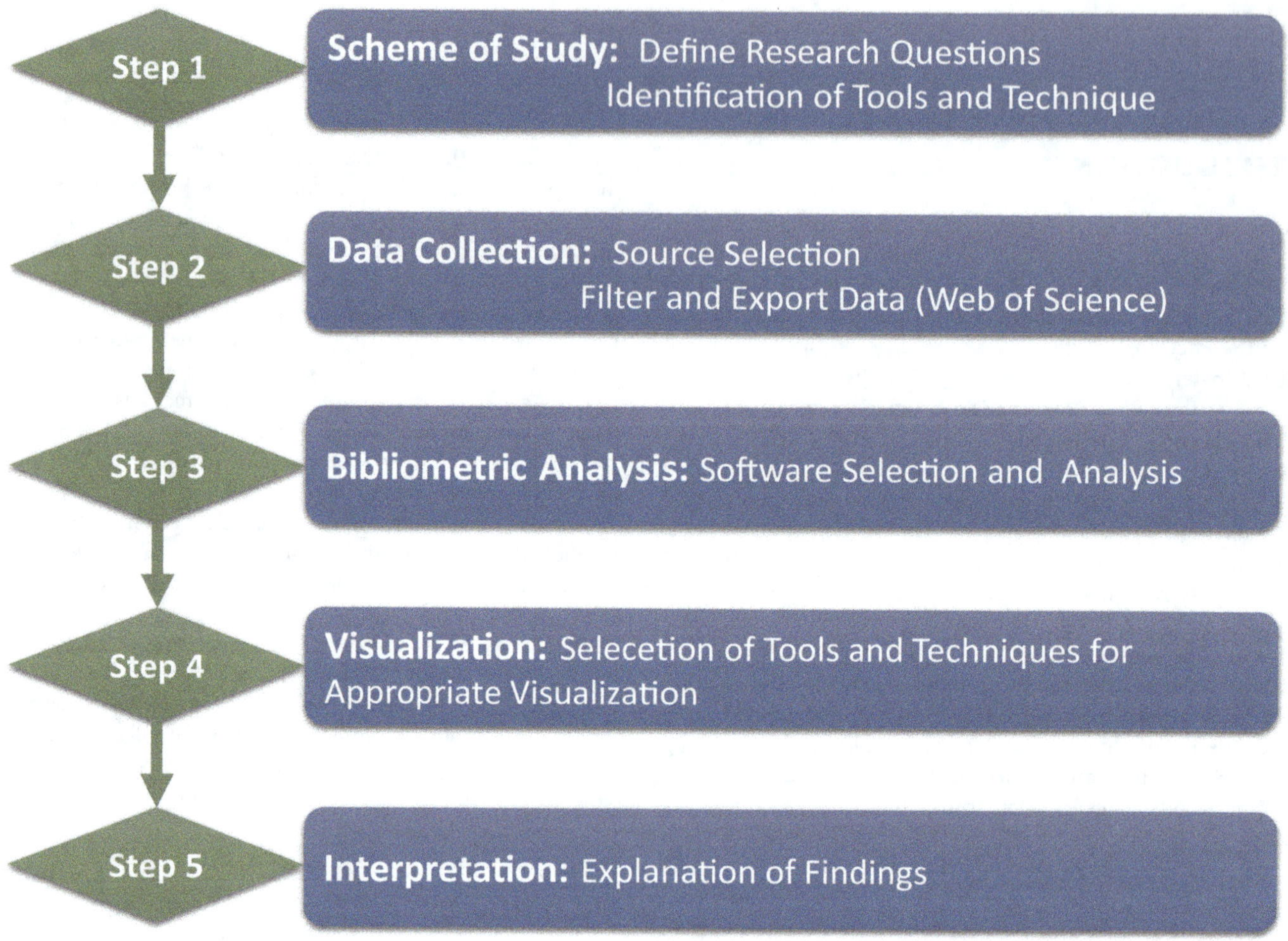

FIGURE 1 | The Procedure of Bibliometric Analysis.

Analysis Tool

Bibliometrix is an R language based bibliometric software with multiple toolkits for full-process bibliometrics and visual presentation of scientific documents, which was developed by Aria (18). Based on the data exported from the WOS database and then completed by the team researchers (XX Wang and ZX Song), the bibliometric analysis was conducted using the R software version 3.6.2 (R Foundation for Statistical Computing, Vienna, Austria; http://www.r-project.org) through the Bibliometrix R package.

CiteSpace is a visual tool for bibliometric analysis developed by Chaomei Chen, based on the Java platform (19). As an interactive analysis tool, it combines bibliometrics and data-mining algorithms to complete scientific mapping through the visualization of results. CiteSpace can be used to analyze cooperative networks and co-citations (20). Version 5.8.3 was used in this study for the analysis of the co-authorship, co-institute, co-country, and document co-citation of the articles published from 2001 to 2020. The time slice was two years, and the selection criterion was the first 50% of each time period. In collaborative networks, the size of the circles represents the number of studies published; the shorter the distance between the circles, the greater the collaboration between the two authors/institutions/countries. The blue-purple nodes represented earlier studies, whereas the yellow-red nodes represented more recent studies. In the co-citation analysis, the size of the nodes represented the frequency of citations, nodes with different colors represented different years, the line between the nodes represented the relationship between the co-citations, and the thickness of the line represented the strength of the relationship. The color corresponds to the time of the node's first co-citation, and the color from cold to warm represented early to recent co-citation. The thickness of the tree-ring was proportional to the number of citations in a given time zone. Modularity (Q) and weighted mean silhouette (S) were the two indicators used to evaluate clustering in the co-citation analysis. A Q value >0.3 meant very important network and an S value >0.5 meant reasonable clustering results.

Measurement

Descriptive analysis was used to explain the core sources, authors, countries, publications, and affiliations of publications. Price's law was used to assess whether the growing trend in the ERAS was scientific. Simultaneously, we identified the core sources using the Bradford's law (21). According to the Bradford's law, the data was divided into three regions. Zone 1 was highly productive and was considered a nuclear zone.

The author/publication-level metrics, such as the h-, m-, and g indices were determined (22, 23). In addition, we used keyword plus for the analysis, which was provided by the database to describe the knowledge structure of the study more concisely and standardized. The core research areas and key themes were essential for determining the direction of future research, therefore, thematic maps and thematic evolution were used.

In the thematic maps, each quadrant could be separated by centrality and density to form a two-dimensional graph. Centrality was the importance of a topic in the research field, and the density was used to measure the development of the topic. Quadrant I, located in the upper-right quadrant, named motor themes, suggested that the themes of the region have developed and formed important pillars that shape the field of research. Quadrant II, located in the upper left quadrant, named niche themes, reflected highly developed but isolated themes. Quadrant III, located in the lower-left quadrant and named emerging or declining themes, suggested weak development and marginalization of the research field. Quadrant IV, located in the lower-right quadrant, was named as basic themes. Although these topics are less developed, they are important to the field of study.

RESULTS

Overall Publication Performance and Growth Rate

Table 1 presents the descriptive features of the ERAS literature. A total of 1,403 studies were selected according to the search strategy. We identified 1,320 articles and 81 articles and proceedings papers. A total of 2,098 keywords plus 1,991 author keywords were used. Furthermore, 6,966 authors wrote the documents; among them, only 26 articles were written by one author. The collaboration index was 5.07, which showed the highly collaborative nature of ERAS publications. The document-per-author ratio was 0.201, implying that, on average, approximately five authors wrote a document.

By summarizing the number of papers published over the years, **Figure 2A** shows the overall trend of ERAS studies published worldwide from 2001 to 2020. ERAS research has an overall upward trend, and according to the curves analyzed from the data, it was found to be more suitable for exponential adjustment than linear adjustment, thus satisfying the Price's law. The correlation coefficient (r) after mathematical adjustment of the exponential curve was 0.9804, while the linear adjustment of the measured values, R, was 0.8051. Therefore, the percentage of unexplained variation was 19.49%.

Figure 2B shows three sets of data: simple-country authors, multicountry authors, and the citation rate of each country. The USA was at the top with several publications, China was ranked second, and the UK was ranked third, but concerning citations, China's total citations were worse than those of the UK. In contrast, although Sweden has a relatively small number of publications, it was at the top four the most cited countries, after the USA, the UK, and Canada. The country with the highest international cooperation was the USA, followed by Canada and the France. The most relevant affiliations are reported in **Figure 2C**. The McGill University was the first, and provided a strong basis for ERAS. The University of Texas MD Anderson Cancer Center and Maastricht University were the second and third affiliations of most publications, respectively.

In addition to the annual production, major topics, locations, and affiliations of ERAS-related publications were viewed. **Figure 2D** shows a threefold analysis of the ERAS publications, with keywords plus on the left, affiliations on the right, and relevant countries in the middle. The chart shows that the USA was working with most of the top agencies to focus on ERAS-related topics. In addition, China, Canada, and

TABLE 1 | Descriptive characteristics of ERAS literature.

Description	Results
Main information about data	
Timespan	2001:2021
Sources (Journals, Books, etc)	413
Documents	1,403
Average years from publication	5.27
Average citations per documents	26.72
Average citations per year per doc	3.939
References	21,902
Document types	
article	1,320
article; proceedings paper	81
Document contents	
Keywords Plus (ID)	2,098
Author's Keywords (DE)	1,991
Authors	
Authors	6,966
Author Appearances	9,558
Authors of single-authored documents	26
Authors of multi-authored documents	6,940
Authors collaboration	
Single-authored documents	33
Documents per Author	0.201
Authors per Document	4.97
Co-Authors per Documents	6.82
Collaboration Index	5.07

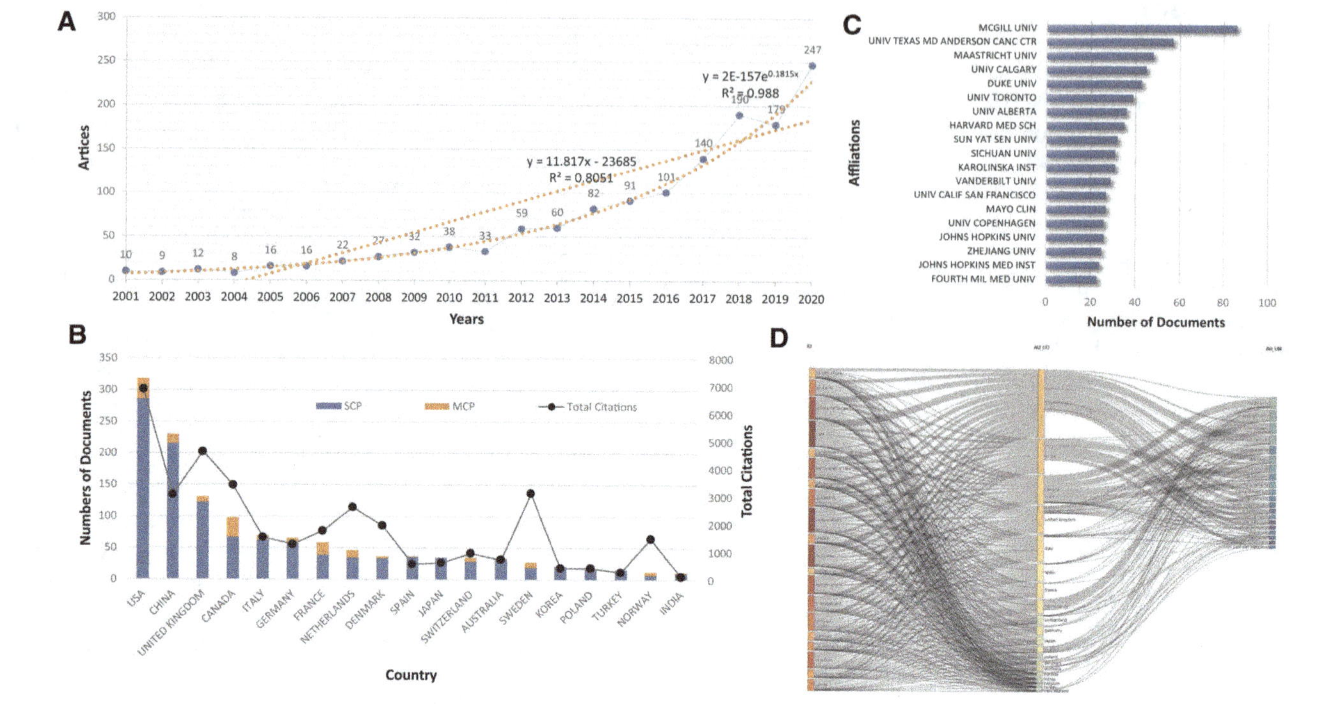

FIGURE 2 | **(A)** Growth of scientific production on ERAS from 2001 to 2020. A linear adjustment of the data and an adjustment to the exponential curve were made, in order to assess whether the production fulfilled the Price's Law. Linear adjustment: $y = 11.8176x - 23685$, $R^2 = 0.8051$; Exponential adjustment: $y = 2E\text{-}157e0.1815x$, $R^2 = 0.9804$. **(B)** The countries of the top 20 most relevant corresponding authors of the articles on ERAS. MCP, Multi-country publications; SCP, simple-country publications. **(C)** Top 20 of the Most Relevant Affiliations. **(D)** R Studio - Three-fields plot: left – keywords plus from the data records, middle – countries, right – authors affiliations.

the UK have made significant contributions to ERAS science topics. Issues related to outcomes and care are the most widely studied in most countries.

Core Journals, Core Journal Articles and Core Words of ERAS

We used source impact and Bradford's Law to find publications on ERAS in the core journals in the scientific literature. **Table 2** ranks the articles by h, M, G-index, total citations (TC), net output (NP), and pub year of publication (PYstart), and represents the Bradford's Law (**Figure 3A**), which divides journals into three regions. We found that 24 of the 413 journals were in core zone 1, and the top 24 journals were the core publishing sources for corona literature in the social sciences.

Table 3 lists the top 20 most-cited articles in the database along with their global citations. **Figure 3B** shows the local and global citations for highly cited papers. **Table 4** provides the most frequent words used in the ERAS literature, which is divided into four parts: keywords plus, authors' keywords, abstracts, and titles. **Figure 3C** shows the word cloud created using keyword plus. Words with a high frequency in the literature were larger in size.

Co-authorship, Co-institute, Co-country and Document Co-citation Analysis

The results of the generating collaborator mappings using CiteSpace were 676 nodes and 1,440 links (**Figure 4A**), which means that 1,401 articles were published by 676 authors. As shown in **Figure 4A**, many authors preferred to combine with relatively stable collaborators, resulting in a relatively large cluster of authors. In earlier studies, only a few core authors cooperated less with the central clusters. The most representative author was LJUNGQVIST O, who published 33 studies, followed by DEMARTINES N and KEHLET H. The top-ranked item by centrality was O LJUNGQVIST (2005) with a centrality of 30, and the second one was OLLE LJUNGQVIST (2010) with a centrality of 28. The third was H KEHLET (2002) and GREGG NELSON (2016), with centralities of 25.

The institute of the two authors appeared in the same article as a cooperative organization, namely, the co-institute. The Citesapce software was used to calculate the co-occurrence frequency matrix to determine the degree of cooperation. **Figure 4B** shows the collaborative institutes in the era domain, with an institution map of 367 nodes and 848 links. Generally, the institutions were concentrated in universities and a few in hospitals.

TABLE 2 | Zone 1 journals according Bradford's law and the source impact.

Element	Source impact							Bradford's law			
	Articles	h_index	g_index	m_index	TC	NP	PY_start	Rank	Freq	cumFreq	Zone
World journal of surgery	1,276	26	44	1.857143	3,193	44	2008	1	44	44	Zone 1
Surgical endoscopy and other interventional techniques	714	15	24	1.363636	666	37	2011	2	38	82	Zone 1
Colorectal disease	792	18	31	1.125	990	33	2006	3	34	116	Zone 1
International journal of colorectal disease	480	16	26	1.066667	693	31	2007	4	32	148	Zone 1
Journal of cardiothoracic and vascular anesthesia	260	16	22	0.761905	513	23	2001	5	24	172	Zone 1
Obesity surgery	398	13	22	0.8125	517	22	2006	6	23	195	Zone 1
Journal of laparoendoscopic & advanced surgical techniques	73	9	15	0.692308	255	17	2009	7	20	215	Zone 1
Journal of gastrointestinal surgery	530	14	18	0.933333	706	18	2007	8	19	234	Zone 1
Surgical clinics of North America	68	9	13	1	192	19	2013	9	19	253	Zone 1
British journal of surgery	2,355	17	18	0.809524	1,912	18	2001	10	18	271	Zone 1
Diseases of the colon & rectum	951	13	17	0.722222	1,171	17	2004	11	17	288	Zone 1
International journal of clinical and experimental medicine	20	1	2	0.142857	11	6	2015	12	16	304	Zone 1
International journal of surgery	253	11	16	1.375	383	16	2014	13	16	320	Zone 1
American surgeon	91	6	11	0.3	127	13	2002	14	15	335	Zone 1
Anesthesia and analgesia	1,102	11	15	0.52381	680	15	2001	15	15	350	Zone 1
Journal of the american college of surgeons	694	12	15	1.333333	645	15	2013	16	15	365	Zone 1
BMJ open	94	10	14	1	311	14	2012	17	14	379	Zone 1
American journal of surgery	474	7	13	0.538462	202	13	2009	18	13	392	Zone 1
Gynecologic oncology	385	9	13	1.5	601	13	2016	19	13	405	Zone 1
Annals of surgery	2,424	10	12	0.5	1,291	12	2002	20	12	417	Zone 1
Journal of surgical research	150	7	11	0.538462	172	11	2009	21	12	429	Zone 1
Medicine	98	7	11	1.166667	133	11	2016	22	12	441	Zone 1
American journal of obstetrics and gynecology	173	9	11	2.25	395	11	2018	23	11	452	Zone 1
Clinical nutrition	1,031	10	11	0.588235	3,219	11	2005	24	11	463	Zone 1

Authors from two different countries appear in the same article; that is, a co-country. **Figure 4C** shows the results for co-countries in the era domain. As shown in **Figure 4C**, although the United States was ranks first worldwide in terms of publication volume, European countries had a relatively close cooperative relationship.

After analysis using CiteSpace, **Figure 4D** shows a document co-citation network diagram containing 832 nodes, 3,503 links, and 15 main clusters. The modularity Q value was 0.7918, and the weighted mean silhouette S was 0.9004.

A literature co-citation analysis of ERAS studies yielded 15 co-citation categories, marked by their citation index terms. To obtain the key cluster of the cited references, log-likelihood tests (LLR) were used to select the noun phrase from the title of the article in Citespace. The contour value of each cluster was >0.9, indicating reliable and meaningful results. **Figure 4E** summarizes the details of the 15 clusters using a timeline view to reflect the research patterns and emerging trends in the network map. Articles with the strongest citation bursts showed a significant increase in interest in ERAS. **Figure 4F** shows the 25 strongest references from 2008 to 2020.

Collaborative World Map as a Measure of the Social Structure: There were 709 collaborations between authors from different countries. The world map (**Figure 4G** and **Supplementary material**) shows that the most frequent cooperation was between the United States and Canada (24), followed by the United Kingdom and Canada (25), Canada and Sweden, and the United Kingdom and Sweden (23).

Conceptual Framework and Thematic Evolution

Based on the relationship between the keywords plus, the research content was roughly divided into several topics. The identified topics were categorized into a strategic map to analyze the importance and development of the research topic. The strategy map was based on the full-time span from

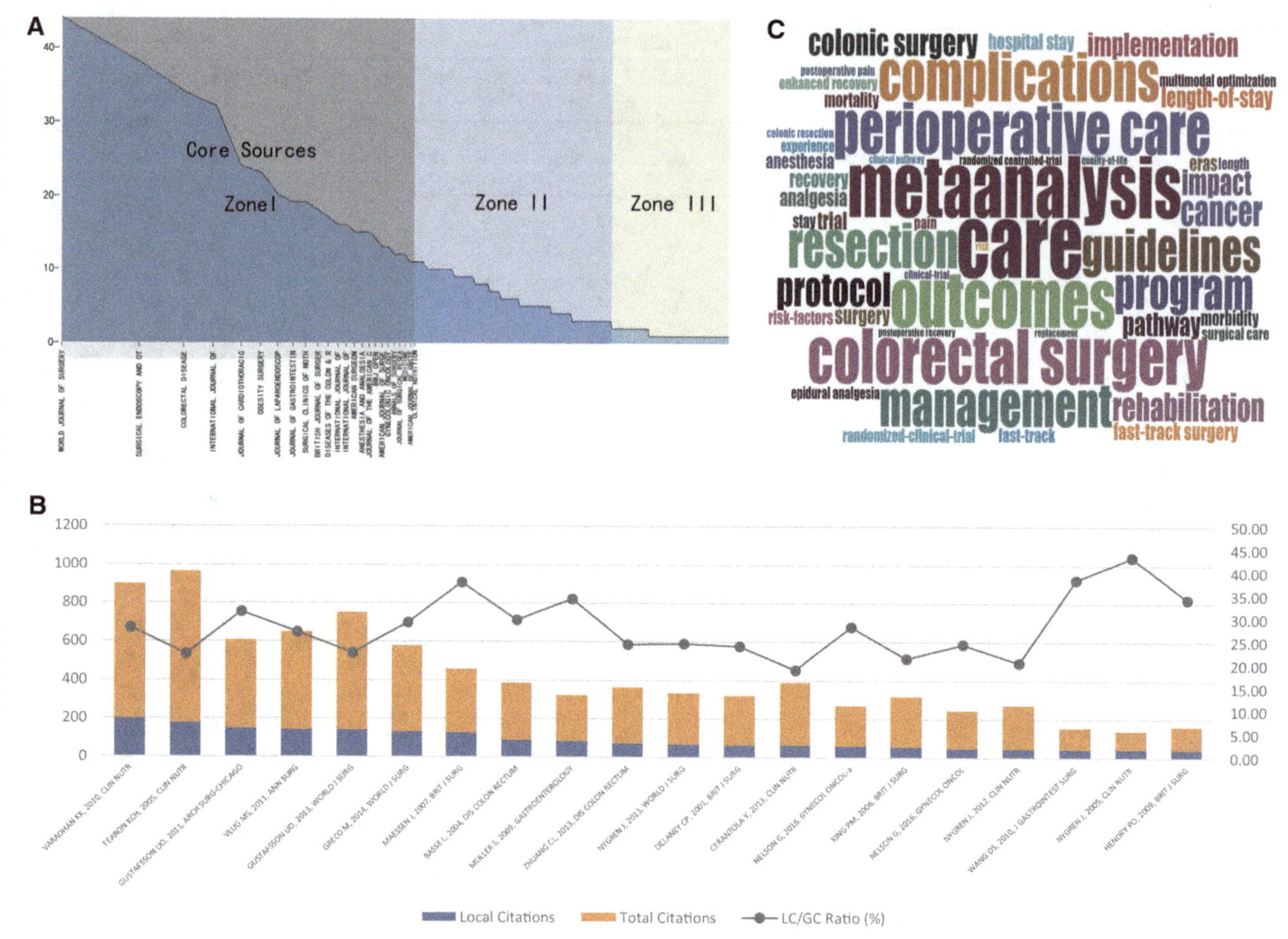

FIGURE 3 | **(A)** Journal Rankings According to the Bradford Law. **(B)** Top 20 of the Most Globally Cited Article and their located cited. **(C)** Word cloud based on the most frequent words (Keywords Plus) used in the articles on ERAS.

2001 to 2020. We used the first 400 keywords, but the items displayed in the cluster were set to a minimum frequency of 40. The number of representative labels in each theme was set to three so that the thematic map based on density (Y-axis) and centrality (X-axis) could be obtained, as shown in **Figure 5**. The centrality measured the importance of a topic, and density measured the development of the topic. The topics appearing in the lower left were the emerging or declining topics, which are new topics that can emerge better or decline from the research field. The upper right panel represented high density and high centrality. The developed theme of this section was the motor theme, and was necessary.

Thematic evolution showed the historical development of the ERAS literature. The use of keywords and topic evolution described the history and evolution of the topics. This time division was based on the author's subjective judgment while allowing for a better representation of the evolution of the subject. The first part was from 2001 to 2006, the second from 2007 to 2011, the third from 2012 to 2016, and the last from 2017 to 2021. **Figure 6** shows the topic evolution of the keyword plus (**Supplementary material**).

DISCUSSION

Fast-track surgery (FTS) or ERAS is the inevitable result of the development of medical theory and technology, "Pain and Risk "Free" was the goal of surgery (26). The connotation of ERAS was to reduce the body's stress response to trauma, promote rapid functional recovery, reduce the incidence of clinical complications, and shorten the length of hospital stay. A large number of clinical studies have proven that perioperative process optimization and multidisciplinary collaboration of minimally invasive techniques can improve the treatment effects, reduce medical interventions (over-treatment), and promote patient recovery (27). For ERAS to be practiced clinically, its philosophy and associated pathways must be based on evidence-based medicine and multidisciplinary

TABLE 3 | Top 20 most cited articles.

Paper	Most local cited				Most global cited			
	Local citations	Normalized local citations	Normalized global citations	Total citations	TC per year	Normalized TC	LC/GC ratio (%)	Year
The enhanced recovery after surgery (ERAS) pathway for patients undergoing major elective open colorectal surgery: a meta-analysis of randomized controlled trials	196	16.44	12.87	701	58.4167	12.8686	27.96	2010
Enhanced recovery after surgery: a consensus review of clinical care for patients undergoing colonic resection	175	11.72	10.48	787	46.2941	10.4846	22.24	2005
Adherence to the enhanced recovery after surgery protocol and outcomes after colorectal cancer surgery	145	10.22	7.83	462	42	7.8345	31.39	2011
Laparoscopy in combination with fast track multimodal management is the best perioperative strategy in patients undergoing colonic surgery: a randomized clinical trial (LAFA-study)	138	9.73	8.67	511	46.4545	8.6655	27.01	2011
Guidelines for perioperative care in elective colonic surgery: Enhanced Recovery After Surgery (ERAS(®)) Society recommendations	138	12.12	10.15	611	67.8889	10.1523	22.59	2013
Enhanced recovery program in colorectal surgery: a meta-analysis of randomized controlled trials	130	15.23	11.71	447	55.875	11.7105	29.08	2014
A protocol is not enough to implement an enhanced recovery programme for colorectal resection	125	10.11	5.33	331	22.0667	5.327	37.76	2007
Colonic surgery with accelerated rehabilitation or conventional care	88	5.46	3.56	297	16.5	3.5569	29.63	2004
A fast-track program reduces complications and length of hospital stay after open colonic surgery	82	7.09	5.13	240	18.4615	5.1268	34.17	2009
Enhanced recovery after surgery programs versus traditional care for colorectal surgery: a meta-analysis of randomized controlled trials	71	6.24	4.84	291	32.3333	4.8352	24.40	2013
Guidelines for perioperative care in elective rectal/pelvic surgery: Enhanced Recovery After Surgery (ERAS(®)) Society recommendations	66	5.80	4.45	268	29.7778	4.4531	24.63	2013
'Fast track' postoperative management protocol for patients with high co-morbidity undergoing complex abdominal and pelvic colorectal surgery	62	6.89	4.34	258	12.2857	4.3361	24.03	2001
Guidelines for perioperative care after radical cystectomy for bladder cancer: Enhanced Recovery After Surgery (ERAS(®)) society recommendations	62	5.45	5.45	328	36.4444	5.45	18.90	2013
Guidelines for pre- and intra-operative care in gynecologic/oncology surgery: Enhanced Recovery After Surgery (ERAS®) Society recommendations–Part I	59	10.44	8.00	209	34.8333	8.0019	28.23	2016
Randomized clinical trial comparing laparoscopic and open surgery for colorectal cancer within an enhanced recovery programme	56	5.37	5.95	261	16.3125	5.9487	21.46	2006
Guidelines for postoperative care in gynecologic/oncology surgery: Enhanced Recovery After Surgery (ERAS®) Society recommendations–Part II	48	8.49	7.50	196	32.6667	7.5042	24.49	2016
Guidelines for perioperative care in elective rectal/pelvic surgery: Enhanced Recovery After Surgery (ERAS®) Society recommendations	46	4.61	3.55	224	22.4	3.5527	20.54	2012

(continued)

TABLE 3 | Continued

Paper	Most local cited				Most global cited			
	Local citations	Normalized local citations	Normalized global citations	Total citations	TC per year	Normalized TC	LC/GC ratio (%)	Year
Fast-track surgery improves postoperative recovery in patients with gastric cancer: a randomized comparison with conventional postoperative care	43	3.61	2.06	112	9.3333	2.056	38.39	2010
A comparison in five European Centres of case mix, clinical management and outcomes following either conventional or fast-track perioperative care in colorectal surgery	42	2.81	1.29	97	5.7059	1.2923	43.30	2005
Determinants of outcome after colorectal resection within an enhanced recovery programme	41	3.55	2.56	120	9.2308	2.5634	34.17	2009

collaboration. It should not only reflect the core concept of accelerating recovery, but should consider the patient's underlying diseases, types of surgery, perioperative complications, and other specific conditions. Moreover, in-depth clinical studies are required to demonstrate the safety, feasibility, and necessity of ERAS-related pathways.

According to a bibliometric analysis, the United States has the largest number of ERAS-related articles published followed by China. Despite the large number of published reports in China, there were fewer citations. Most of the top 20 most-cited articles were published in the early period of ERAS in Europe and the United States because ERAS originated in Europe and the United States, and were the first to carry out relevant research on ERAS (28, 29). In contrast, as a North American country, Canada was ranks fourth in the total number of articles published; however, the proportion of multi-country publications was high, and most of the articles were from the McGill University, which reflects the high concentration of research. The university with the second highest research focus was the MD Anderson Cancer Center in the United States, which may be due to the fact that the previous studies on ERAS were on radical surgery for patients with tumor.

Earlier researches on ERAS were mainly related to surgery, therefore, the most cited journals in zone 1 of the Bradford's Law were journals of the surgery discipline, such as the WORLD JOURNAL OF SURGERY, SURGICAL ENDOSCOPY AND OTHER INTERVENTIONAL TECHNIQUES, and COLORECTAL DISEASE. According to the Word Cloud, "colorectal surgery" and "resection" played important roles in surgery and colorectal surgery was the most mature surgical method that used ERAS. With ERAS, the hospital stay and complications in patients who underwent colorectal surgery effectively reduced without an increase in the readmission rates (30).

The ERAS Society was founded in 2001, and in 2005, the first worldwide expert consensus on accelerated recovery for colon resection was developed (29). In addition, relevant studies on ERAS mainly focused on research directions, such as meta-analysis and perioperative care. Randomized controlled trials and meta-analyses have been used in ERAS studies, and a large number of high-quality clinical studies are important for further evidence-based practice and guidelines development. Meta-analysis and clinical research have mainly focused on perioperative nursing, postoperative complications, length of hospital stay, final results, and process management (25, 31). In addition to the ERAS, perioperative care was very important in the implementation to surgical management. Currently, the relevant care specifications are clearly specified in the guidelines for various specialties (7–9). Clinical evidence has shown that perioperative FTS care can promote postoperative rehabilitation and shorten the hospitalization time of patients with gynecological diseases (32). Magheli provided FTS care to 50 patients undergoing laparoscopic radical prostatectomy, which significantly improved the recovery time of the bowel function and defecation time, shortened the postoperative hospital stay, and improved the overall satisfaction rate of patients (33).

Among the 15 clusters obtained through CiteSpace cluster analysis, most studies on ERAS were still related to surgery, but were developed from colorectal surgery in the early stages of cardiac surgery, neurosurgery, and other surgical disciplines. Guidelines are emerging for other general surgery procedures (pancreaticoduodenectomy, elective colon surgery, and elective rectal and pelvic surgery) (10, 11, 24). ERAS has gained acceptance worldwide over time and is widely used in a range of surgical specialties, such as urology, orthopaedics, and obstetrics and gynecology. Although a study on FTS was published in cardiac surgery as early as 1994 (34), it was not until 2015 that Zaouter from France first reported the systematic application of ERAS in cardiac surgery (35). In 2018, Noss systematically reviewed the relevant issues of ERAS in cardiac surgery and provided an in-depth consideration of the existing problems (36). Many urological studies have

TABLE 4 | Most frequent words.

Keywords plus		Author keywords	
Words	**Occurrences**	**Words**	**Occurrences**
care	285	enhanced recovery after surgery	301
metaanalysis	254	eras	159
outcomes	231	enhanced recovery	149
colorectal surgery	222	colorectal surgery	117
perioperative care	209	fast-track surgery	85
complications	200	length of stay	84
resection	183	fast track	71
management	180	perioperative care	70
guidelines	174	laparoscopy	60
program	168	fast-track	52
protocol	141	surgery	49
cancer	122	enhanced recovery after surgery (eras)	46
rehabilitation	115	rehabilitation	38
colonic surgery	111	colorectal cancer	36
impact	104	complications	34
implementation	98	fast track surgery	33
pathway	96	outcomes	31
randomized clinical-trial	96	postoperative complications	31
length-of-stay	83	bariatric surgery	30
surgery	73	colorectal	29
Titles		**Abstracts**	
Words	**Occurrences**	**Words**	**Occurrences**
surgery	1,363	patients	5,596
recovery	1,092	surgery	3,898
enhanced	981	eras	3,540
patients	316	recovery	2,527
fast_track	241	postoperative	2,454
colorectal	237	stay	1,859
program	226	hospital	1,726
Eras	185	study	1,515
protocol	178	enhanced	1,507
Study	167	days	1,467
pathway	163	care	1,291
cancer	156	protocol	1,254
laparoscopic	153	complications	1,226
undergoing	140	length	1,221
postoperative	124	results	1,169
randomized	122	compared	1,028
implementation	120	outcomes	999
Trial	120	time	969
Care	119	undergoing	950
perioperative	109	significantly	932

reported the use of ERAS in the perioperative period of laparoscopic nephrectomy (37), open partial nephrectomy (38), laparoscopic radical prostatectomy (39), and TVT or TVT-O (40). Compared to the control group, the duration of hospital-stay in the patients who underwent ERAS was significantly shorter, with better pain control and patient satisfaction. Similarly, to promote and regulate the use of ERAS in gynecology, the International ERAS Society in 2016 proposed guidelines for the use of ERAS in gynecology/gynecological oncology (41, 42).

After more than 20 years of research, evidence-based medicine demonstrated the effectiveness of ERAS in a rational manner, and ERAS models have demonstrated unprecedented advantages in the recovery of patients undergoing surgery (28). From the thematic maps, studies on complications, impact, length of hospital stay, resection, and cancer were mature, and several of the research directions were supported by evidence-based evidence in the guide. However, research topics such as meta-analyses, colorectal surgery, and perioperative care are declining despite the current large number of studies. Similarly, the thematic evolution of ERAS research in the past 20 years showed that ERAS application and anesthesiology research in tumor surgery were prominent in 2006–2010, while in the next five years, more attention will be paid to the comprehensive management of the perioperative period and the emergence of large randomized controlled clinical trials. Simultaneously, ERAS-related meta-analyses began to appear (43). After 2015, patient-reported outcomes were the purpose of ERAS. More attention has been paid to the comfort and safety of patients in hospitals, as well as the reduction of surgical complications, rather than the reduction of hospital days and cost alone (44–47).

ERAS is not a new technology but an integrated and innovative management mode. Its theoretical system has been relatively well-developed after more than 20 years of development. ERAS concepts and models in different disciplines need to consider the characteristics of their respective disciplines; therefore, there are some differences. Despite the success of the ERAS concept, it still has several challenges. The implementation of the ERAS protocol requires good patient and doctor compliance. A multicenter study found that a reduction in the complications was positively correlated with ERAS compliance ($OR = 0.69$, $P < 0.001$) (48, 49). At the same time, team cooperation and continuous quality improvement plans are required. The team will formulate the ERAS plan and target management, such as the length of stay, and continue to adhere to and learn the summarized strategies (50). For example, many hospitals in Canada have continuously improved and perfected the clinical practice guideline (CPG) with the application of the "Knowledge-to-Action Cycle" (51), thus slimming the ERAS protocol and increasing the clinical application compliance. Preoperative assessment, preparation, and treatment of patients with high-risk factors and reduction in the failure rate of the ERAS protocols are the major measures to increase

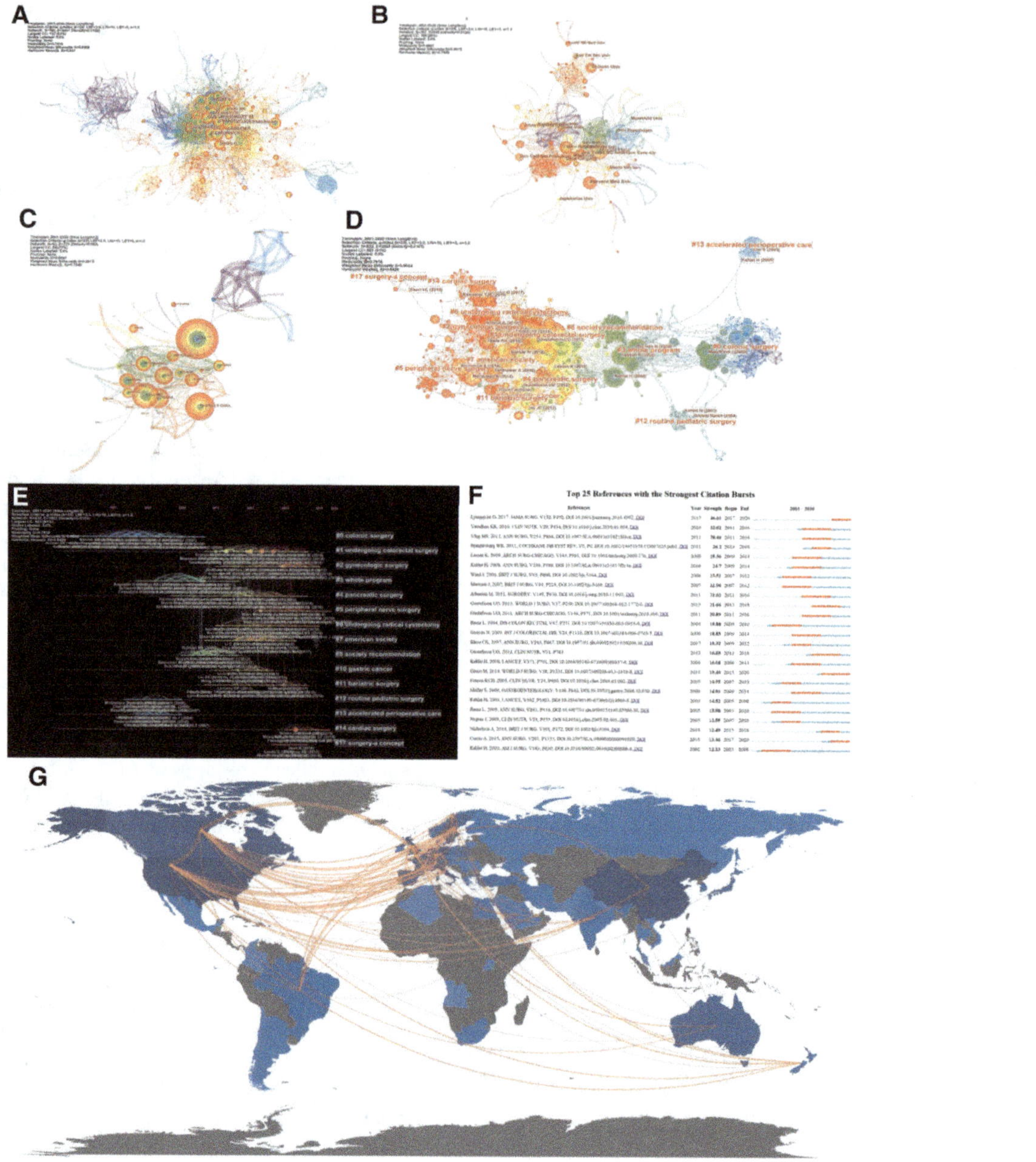

FIGURE 4 | **(A)** An author cooperation map related to ERAS research from 2001 to 2020. **(B)** An institution cooperation map related to ERAS research from 2001 to 2020. **(C)** A country cooperation map related to ERAS research from 2001 to 2020. **(D)** Reference co-citation map related to ERAS research from 2001 to 2020. **(E)** The timeline view of cited reference related to ERAS. **(F)** Top 25 references with the strongest citation bursts. **(G)** The country collaboration map of the global authors of the ERAS research.

patient compliance (52–54). Based on multimodal or multidisciplinary collaboration, the preoperative emphasis on patient education, communication, and collaboration underpins the success of ERAS (55, 56).

Although ERAS has many advantages and is accepted by doctors, there may be limitations to its future use. ① Firstly, the doctors and patients rely on "traditional practices" and "safety considerations." ② Secondly, from the different systemic conditions, diseases, surgical procedures and hospitals, it was concluded that the ERAS protocols must be "diversified and individualized," which makes them less evidence-based. ③ Thirdly, the combination of different disciplines may make ERAS processes too convoluted, impeding accelerated recovery. The payment system of medical insurance and cultural background influence the promotion of ERAS programs.

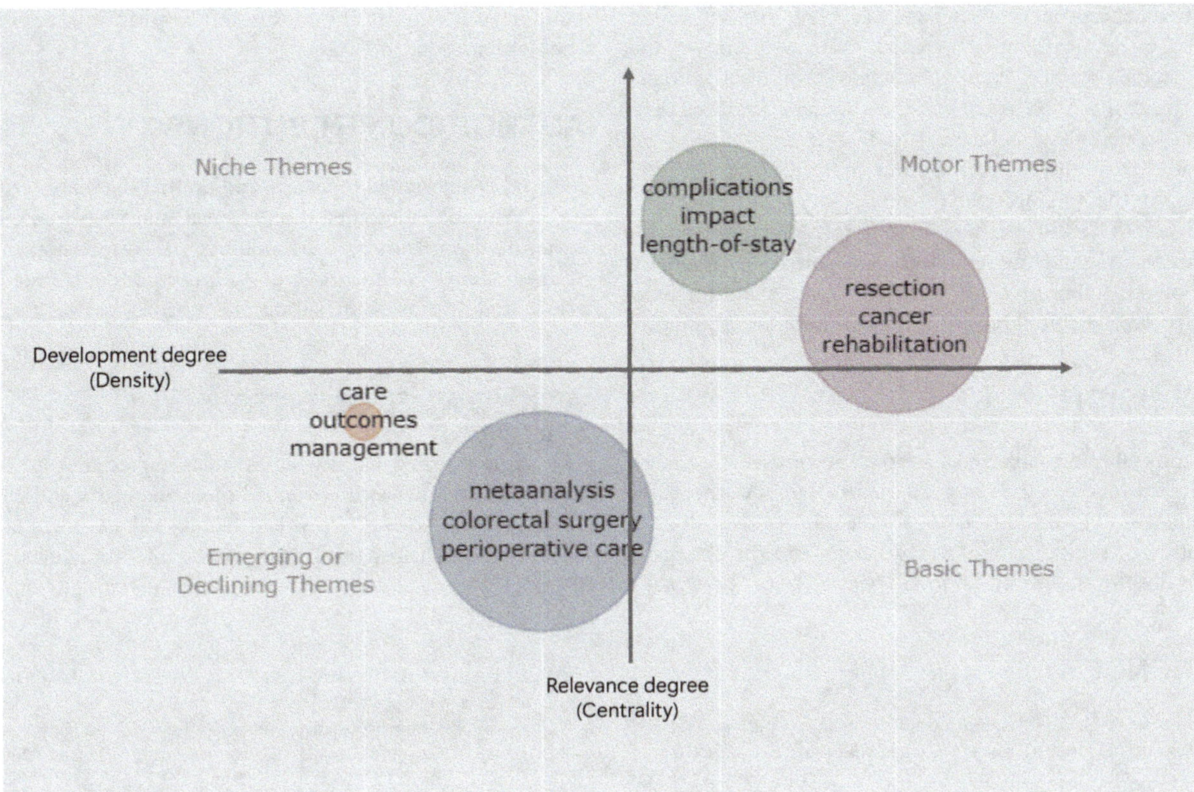

FIGURE 5 | The strategy map of identified topics clustered by keywords plus.

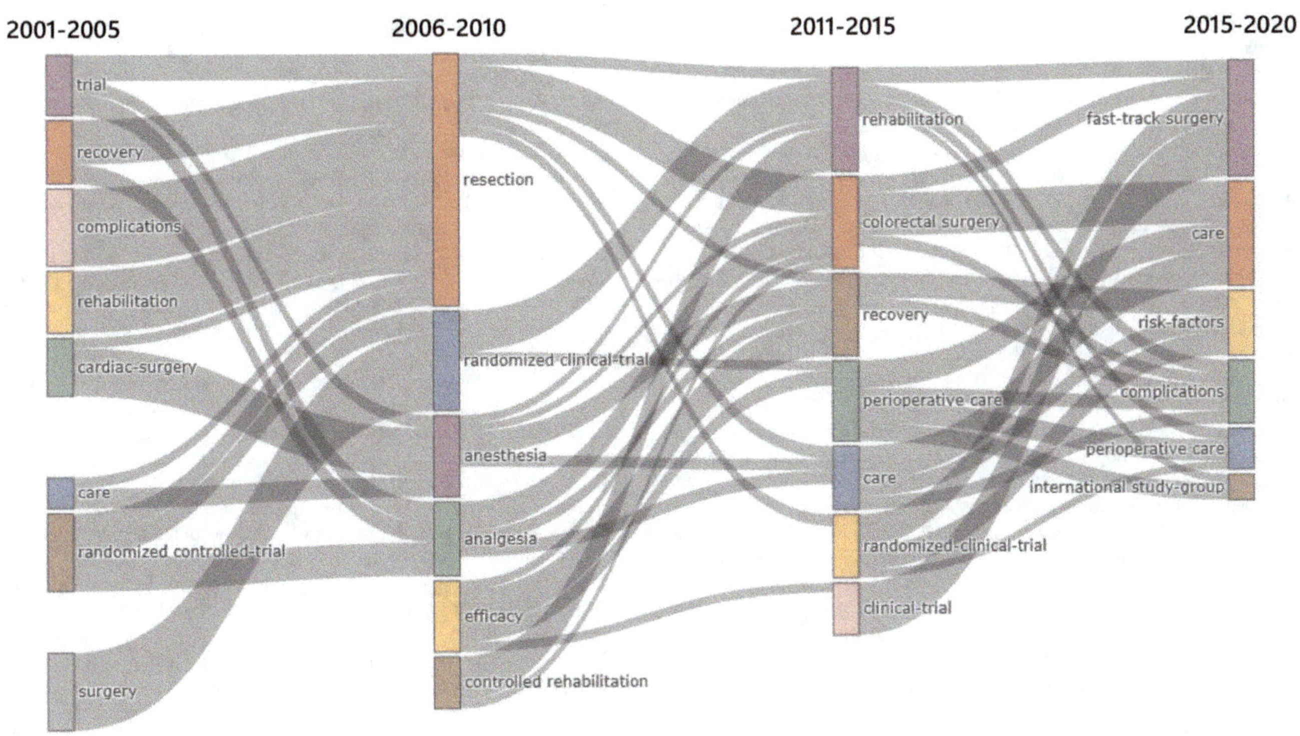

FIGURE 6 | Thematic Evolution of ERAS research from 2001 to 2020.

The literature included in this study is from the core collection database of WOS, which has high quality studies, but selection bias cannot be avoided. It is well known that various databases have their advantages and disadvantages, but we chose the WoS over PubMed because PubMed does not store reference metadata, and references were an important part of the research output indicators. In addition, according to the bibliometric research principles, there is a potential length time-lapse bias that puts newer articles at a disadvantage in receiving citations. Of course, bibliometric analyses of the same topic will be used by other authors, and our results may be compared with those of others in the future.

CONCLUSION

In this study, Bibliometrix and Citespace were used to analyze ERAS literature over the past 20 years. Despite the rapid development of ERAS in various disciplines, the effective coordination of multidisciplinary physicians and the change in patients' deeply rooted traditional views were the major obstacles to its further development. The bibliometric analysis conducted in this study is expected to provide a reference for the development of ERAS.

AUTHOR CONTRIBUTIONS

MZ and DZ designed the study and drafted the manuscript. XW, XC, YW and YZ designed the statistical analysis plan. ZS and DZ reviewed the manuscript. All authors take responsibility for the appropriateness of the content. All authors contributed to the article and approved the submitted version.

ACKNOWLEDGMENTS

The authors would like to express their appreciation to Massimo Aria and CM Chen, who invented the bibliometrix and CiteSpace, which are free to use. We would like to express our gratitude to all those who helped us in the writing of this manuscript. We thank all peer reviewers for their opinions and suggestions.

REFERENCES

1. Wilmore DW, Kehlet H. Management of patients in fast track surgery. *BMJ (Clin Res Ed).* (2001) 322(7284):473–6. doi: 10.1136/bmj.322.7284.473
2. Kehlet H, Wilmore DW. Multimodal strategies to improve surgical outcome. *Am J Surg.* (2002) 183(6):630–41. doi: 10.1016/s0002-9610(02)00866-8
3. Sun YM, Wang Y, Mao YX, Wang W. The safety and feasibility of enhanced recovery after surgery in patients undergoing pancreaticoduodenectomy: an updated meta-analysis. *BioMed Res Int.* (2020) 2020:7401276. doi: 10.1155/2020/7401276
4. Batchelor TJP, Rasburn NJ, Abdelnour-Berchtold E, Brunelli A, Cerfolio RJ, Gonzalez M, et al. Guidelines for enhanced recovery after lung surgery: recommendations of the Enhanced Recovery After Surgery (ERAS®) Society and the European Society of Thoracic Surgeons (ESTS). *Eur J Cardiothorac Surg.* (2019) 55(1):91–115. doi: 10.1093/ejcts/ezy301
5. Beverly A, Kaye AD, Ljungqvist O, Urman RD. Essential elements of multimodal analgesia in enhanced recovery after surgery (ERAS) guidelines. *Anesthesiology Clin.* (2017) 35(2):e115–43. doi: 10.1016/j.anclin.2017.01.018
6. Brindle M, Nelson G, Lobo DN, Ljungqvist O, Gustafsson UO. Recommendations from the ERAS® Society for standards for the development of enhanced recovery after surgery guidelines. *BJS Open.* (2020) 4(1):157–63. doi: 10.1002/bjs5.50238
7. Brindle ME, McDiarmid C, Short K, Miller K, MacRobie A, Lam JYK, et al. Consensus guidelines for perioperative care in neonatal intestinal surgery: enhanced recovery after surgery (ERAS(®)) society recommendations. *World J Surg.* (2020) 44(8):2482–92. doi: 10.1007/s00268-020-05530-1
8. Brustia R, Monsel A, Skurzak S, Schiffer E, Carrier FM, Patrono D, et al. Guidelines for perioperative care for liver transplantation: enhanced recovery after surgery (ERAS) recommendations. *Transplantation.* (2022) 106(3):552–61. doi: 10.1097/tp.0000000000003808
9. Cerantola Y, Valerio M, Persson B, Jichlinski P, Ljungqvist O, Hubner M, et al. Guidelines for perioperative care after radical cystectomy for bladder cancer: enhanced recovery after surgery (ERAS(®)) society recommendations. *Clin Nutr.* (2013) 32(6):879–87. doi: 10.1016/j.clnu.2013.09.014
10. Gustafsson UO, Scott MJ, Hubner M, Nygren J, Demartines N, Francis N, et al. Guidelines for perioperative care in elective colorectal surgery: enhanced recovery after surgery (ERAS(®)) society recommendations: 2018. *World J Surg.* (2019) 43(3):659–95. doi: 10.1007/s00268-018-4844-y
11. Melloul E, Lassen K, Roulin D, Grass F, Perinel J, Adham M, et al. Guidelines for perioperative care for pancreatoduodenectomy: enhanced recovery after surgery (ERAS) recommendations 2019. *World J Surg.* (2020) 44 (7):2056–84. doi: 10.1007/s00268-020-05462-w
12. Basse L, Raskov HH, Hjort Jakobsen D, Sonne E, Billesbølle P, Hendel HW, et al. Accelerated postoperative recovery programme after colonic resection improves physical performance, pulmonary function and body composition. *Br J Surg.* (2002) 89(4):446–53. doi: 10.1046/j.0007-1323.2001.02044.x
13. de Groot JJ, van Es LE, Maessen JM, Dejong CH, Kruitwagen RF, Slangen BF. Diffusion of enhanced recovery principles in gynecologic oncology surgery: is active implementation still necessary? *Gynecol Oncol.* (2014) 134(3):570–5. doi: 10.1016/j.ygyno.2014.06.019
14. Pędziwiatr M, Kisialeuski M, Wierdak M, Stanek M, Natkaniec M, Matłok M, et al. Early implementation of enhanced recovery after surgery (ERAS®) protocol - compliance improves outcomes: a prospective cohort study. *Int J Surg.* (2015) 21:75–81. doi: 10.1016/j.ijsu.2015.06.087
15. Andrés A. *Measuring academic research: How to undertake a bibliometric study.* Witney: Oxford: Chandos Publishing (2009). ISBN: 978 1 84334-528-2.
16. Vandenbroucke JP, von Elm E, Altman DG, Gøtzsche PC, Mulrow CD, Pocock SJ, et al. Strengthening the reporting of observational studies in epidemiology (STROBE): explanation and elaboration. *Int J Surg.* (2014) 12 (12):1500–24. doi: 10.1016/j.ijsu.2014.07.014
17. Zupic I, Čater T. Bibliometric methods in management and organization. *Organ Res Methods.* (2015) 18(3):429–72. doi: 10.1177/1094428114562629
18. Aria M, Cuccurullo C. Bibliometrix: an R-tool for comprehensive science mapping analysis. *J Informetrics.* (2017) 11(4):959–75. doi: 10.1016/j.joi.2017.08.007
19. Chen C. Searching for intellectual turning points: progressive knowledge domain visualization. *Proc Natl Acad Sci U S A.* (2004) 101(Suppl 1):5303–10. doi: 10.1073/pnas.0307513100
20. Chen C. Science mapping: a systematic review of the literature. *J Data Inf Sci.* (2017) 02/20(2):1–40. doi: 10.1515/jdis-2017-0006
21. Joshi SB, Mamdapur G, Rajgoli IU. *Application of bradford's law of sattering to the literature of stellar.* Physics. Pearl: A Journal of Library and Information Science (2015) p. 133–40. doi: 10.5958/0975-6922.2015.00018.2
22. Koo M. Systemic lupus erythematosus research: a bibliometric analysis over a 50-year period. *Int J Environ Res Public Health.* (2021) 18(13). doi: 10.3390/ijerph18137095
23. Martynov I, Klima-Frysch J, Schoenberger J. A scientometric analysis of neuroblastoma research. *BMC Cancer.* (2020) 20(1):486. doi: 10.1186/s12885-020-06974-3
24. Nygren J, Thacker J, Carli F, Fearon KC, Norderval S, Lobo DN, et al. Guidelines for perioperative care in elective rectal/pelvic surgery: enhanced recovery after surgery (ERAS(®)) society recommendations. *World J Surg.* (2013) 37(2):285–305. doi: 10.1007/s00268-012-1787-6

25. Hajibandeh S, Hajibandeh S, Bill V, Satyadas T. Meta-analysis of enhanced recovery after surgery (ERAS) protocols in emergency abdominal surgery. *World J Surg.* (2020) 44(5):1336–48. doi: 10.1007/s00268-019-05357-5
26. Steenhagen E. Enhanced recovery after surgery: it's time to change practice!. *Nutr Clin Pract.* (2016) 31(1):18–29. doi: 10.1177/0884533615622640
27. Hoffmann H, Kettelhack C. Fast-track surgery–conditions and challenges in postsurgical treatment: a review of elements of translational research in enhanced recovery after surgery. *European Surg Res.* (2012) 49(1):24–34. doi: 10.1159/000339859
28. Ljungqvist O, Scott M, Fearon KC. Enhanced recovery after surgery: a review. *JAMA Surg.* (2017) 152(3):292–8. doi: 10.1001/jamasurg.2016.4952
29. Fearon KC, Ljungqvist O, Von Meyenfeldt M, Revhaug A, Dejong CH, Lassen K, et al. Enhanced recovery after surgery: a consensus review of clinical care for patients undergoing colonic resection. *Clin Nutr.* (2005) 24 (3):466–77. doi: 10.1016/j.clnu.2005.02.002
30. Ban KA, Berian JR, Ko CY. Does implementation of enhanced recovery after surgery (ERAS) protocols in colorectal surgery improve patient outcomes? *Clin Colon Rectal Surg.* (2019) 32(2):109–13. doi: 10.1055/s-0038-1676475
31. Noba L, Rodgers S, Chandler C, Balfour A, Hariharan D, Yip VS. Enhanced recovery after surgery (ERAS) reduces hospital costs and improve clinical outcomes in liver surgery: a systematic review and meta-analysis. *J Gastrointestinal Surg.* (2020) 24(4):918–32. doi: 10.1007/s11605-019-04499-0
32. Ottesen M, Sørensen M, Rasmussen Y, Smidt-Jensen S, Kehlet H, Ottesen B. Fast track vaginal surgery. *Acta Obstet Gynecol Scand.* (2002) 81(2):138–46. doi: 10.1034/j.1600-0412.2002.810209.x
33. Magheli A, Knoll N, Lein M, Hinz S, Kempkensteffen C, Gralla O. Impact of fast-track postoperative care on intestinal function, pain, and length of hospital stay after laparoscopic radical prostatectomy. *J Endourol.* (2011) 25 (7):1143–7. doi: 10.1089/end.2011.0020
34. Engelman RM, Rousou JA, Flack 3rd JE, Deaton DW, Humphrey CB, Ellison LH, et al. Fast-track recovery of the coronary bypass patient. *Ann Thorac Surg.* (1994) 58(6):1742–6. doi: 10.1016/0003-4975(94)91674-8
35. Zaouter C, Imbault J, Labrousse L, Abdelmoumen Y, Coiffic A, Colonna G, et al. Association of robotic totally endoscopic coronary artery bypass graft surgery associated with a preliminary cardiac enhanced recovery after surgery program: a retrospective analysis. *J Cardiothorac Vasc Anesth.* (2015) 29(6):1489–97. doi: 10.1053/j.jvca.2015.03.003
36. Noss C, Prusinkiewicz C, Nelson G, Patel PA, Augoustides JG, Gregory AJ. Enhanced recovery for cardiac surgery. *J Cardiothorac Vasc Anesth.* (2018) 32(6):2760–70. doi: 10.1053/j.jvca.2018.01.045
37. Recart A, Duchene D, White PF, Thomas T, Johnson DB, Cadeddu JA. Efficacy and safety of fast-track recovery strategy for patients undergoing laparoscopic nephrectomy. *J Endourol.* (2005) 19(10):1165–9. doi: 10.1089/end.2005.19.1165
38. Chughtai B, Abraham C, Finn D, Rosenberg S, Yarlagadda B, Perrotti M. Fast track open partial nephrectomy: reduced postoperative length of stay with a goal-directed pathway does not compromise outcome. *Adv Urol.* (2008) 2008:507543. doi: 10.1155/2008/507543
39. Gralla O, Haas F, Knoll N, Hadzidiakos D, Tullmann M, Romer A, et al. Fast-track surgery in laparoscopic radical prostatectomy: basic principles. *World J Urol.* (2007) 25(2):185–91. doi: 10.1007/s00345-006-0139-2
40. McAchran SE, Goldman HB. Contemporary length of stay and resource utilization when using a fast-track regimen for mid-urethral sling surgery. *Urology.* (2009) 74(3):531–4. doi: 10.1016/j.urology.2009.04.039
41. Nelson G, Altman AD, Nick A, Meyer LA, Ramirez PT, Achtari C, et al. Guidelines for pre- and intra-operative care in gynecologic/oncology surgery: enhanced recovery after surgery (ERAS®) society recommendations–Part I. *Gynecol Oncol.* (2016) 140(2):313–22. doi: 10.1016/j.ygyno.2015.11.015
42. Bisch SP, Jago CA, Kalogera E, Ganshorn H, Meyer LA, Ramirez PT, et al. Outcomes of enhanced recovery after surgery (ERAS) in gynecologic oncology - a systematic review and meta-analysis. *Gynecol Oncol.* (2021) 161(1):46–55. doi: 10.1016/j.ygyno.2020.12.035
43. Varadhan KK, Neal KR, Dejong CH, Fearon KC, Ljungqvist O, Lobo DN. The enhanced recovery after surgery (ERAS) pathway for patients undergoing major elective open colorectal surgery: a meta-analysis of randomized controlled trials. *Clin Nutr.* (2010) 29(4):434–40. doi: 10.1016/j.clnu.2010.01.004
44. Taniguchi H, Sasaki T, Fujita H, Kobayashi H, Kawasaki R, Goloubev M, et al. Modified ERAS protocol using preoperative oral rehydration therapy: outcomes and issues. *J Anesth.* (2014) 28(1):143–7. doi: 10.1007/s00540-013-1769-3
45. Zhou B, Ji H, Liu Y, Chen Z, Zhang N, Cao X, et al. ERAS reduces postoperative hospital stay and complications after bariatric surgery: a retrospective cohort study. *Medicine.* (2021) 100(47):e27831. doi: 10.1097/md.0000000000027831
46. Tweed TTT, Woortman C, Tummers S, Bakens M, van Bastelaar J, Stoot J. Reducing hospital stay for colorectal surgery in ERAS setting by means of perioperative patient education of expected day of discharge. *Int J Colorectal Dis.* (2021) 36(7):1535–42. doi: 10.1007/s00384-021-03948-0
47. Tamang T, Wangchuk T, Zangmo C, Wangmo T, Tshomo K. The successful implementation of the Enhanced Recovery After Surgery (ERAS) program among caesarean deliveries in Bhutan to reduce the postoperative length of hospital stay. *BMC Pregnancy Childbirth.* (2021) 21(1):637. doi: 10.1186/s12884-021-04105-9
48. Currie A, Burch J, Jennie JT, Faiz O, Kennedy RH, Ljungqvist O, et al. The impact of enhanced recovery protocol compliance on elective colorectal cancer resection: results from an international registry. *Ann Surg.* (2015) 261(6):1153–9. doi: 10.1097/sla.0000000000001029
49. Geltzeiler CB, Rotramel A, Wilson C, Deng L, Whiteford MH, Frankhouse J. Prospective study of colorectal enhanced recovery after surgery in a community hospital. *JAMA Surg.* (2014) 149(9):955–61. doi: 10.1001/jamasurg.2014.675
50. Ament SM, Gillissen F, Moser A, Maessen JM, Dirksen CD, von Meyenfeldt MF, et al. Identification of promising strategies to sustain improvements in hospital practice: a qualitative case study. *BMC Health Serv Res.* (2014) 14:641. doi: 10.1186/s12913-014-0641-y
51. McLeod RS, Aarts MA, Chung F, Eskicioglu C, Forbes SS, Conn LG, et al. Development of an enhanced recovery after surgery guideline and implementation strategy based on the knowledge-to-action cycle. *Ann Surg.* (2015) 262(6):1016–25. doi: 10.1097/sla.0000000000001067
52. Renz BW, Kasparek MS, Seeliger H, Worthley DL, Jauch KW, Kreis ME, et al. The CR-POSSUM risk calculator predicts failure of enhanced recovery after colorectal surgery. *Acta Chir Belg.* (2015) 115(1):20–6. doi: 10.1080/00015458.2015.11681062
53. Chaudhary A, Barreto SG, Talole SD, Singh A, Perwaiz A, Singh T. Early discharge after pancreatoduodenectomy: what helps and what prevents? *Pancreas.* (2015) 44(2):273–8. doi: 10.1097/mpa.0000000000000254
54. Carli F, Scheede-Bergdahl C. Prehabilitation to enhance perioperative care. *Anesthesiol Clin.* (2015) 33(1):17–33. doi: 10.1016/j.anclin.2014.11.002
55. Lyon A, Solomon MJ, Harrison JD. A qualitative study assessing the barriers to implementation of enhanced recovery after surgery. *World J Surg.* (2014) 38(6):1374–80. doi: 10.1007/s00268-013-2441-7
56. Pearsall EA, Meghji Z, Pitzul KB, Aarts MA, McKenzie M, McLeod RS, et al. A qualitative study to understand the barriers and enablers in implementing an enhanced recovery after surgery program. *Ann Surg.* (2015) 261(1):92–6. doi: 10.1097/sla.0000000000000604

13

Epidural Analgesia with Surgical Stabilization of Flail Chest Following Blunt Thoracic Trauma in Patients with Multiple Trauma

Darko Aleksa Golic*, Dragan Svraka, Nataša Keleman and Snjezana Petrovic

Medical Faculty of Banja Luka, University Clinical Center of Republic of Srpska, University Banja Luka, Banjaluka, Bosnia and Herzegovina

***Correspondence:**
Darko Aleksa Golic
darko.golic@kc-bl.com

Flail chest, often defined as the fracture of three or more ribs in two or more places, represents the most severe form of rib fractures. Conservative treatment, consisting of respiratory assistance with endotracheal intubation and mechanical ventilation (internal pneumatic stabilization) and pain control, are the current treatments of choice in the majority of patients with multiple rib fractures. However, the use of mechanical ventilation may create complications. In selected patients, operative fixation of fractured ribs within 72 h post injury may lead to better outcomes. We conducted a retrospective analysis of a series of nine cases of patients who developed flail chest after blunt trauma, and were treated with surgical osteofixation of the chest wall and postoperative epidural analgesia at the University Clinical Center of the Republic of Srpska during the period from January 2015. to December 2016. Two patients had trauma to the chest only, and the other patients had associated injuries to the head, abdomen, spine, and fractures of the pelvis and long bones. In the majority of patients (77.7%), surgical stabilization of the chest was performed on the second day following the injury, (mean, 2.33 days) and no later than 5 days after the injury. All patients received epidural analgesia with 0, 25% bupivacaine and 0, 01% morphine and intravenous multimodal analgesia, beginning 6 h after thoracotomy. The average length of ICU stay was 14.7 days (range 2–36), while the average number of days of mechanical ventilation was 8.1. The average duration of hospitalization was 25.4 days. Tracheotomy was performed in 33.3% of study patients. Mortality in the observed group was 44.4%. This study shows that surgical stabilization and epidural analgesia reduced ventilator support, shortened trauma intensive care unit stay, and reduced medical costs vs internal pneumatic stabilization.

Keywords: thoracic epidural analgesia, blunt thoracic trauma, multimodal analgesia, operative fixation of ribs, retrospective analysis

INTRODUCTION

Traumatic flail chest is a potentially life threatening injury, often associated with prolonged mechanical ventilation and intensive care unit stay. Unfortunately, there is little literature describing the incidence of admission to the ICU following blunt trauma. In one small series of patients, Veysi et al. found that 37.5% of their blunt trauma population were admitted to the ICU and reported a mortality rate of 18.7%. Their mortality rate is similar to that in other published series (1). These patients often have multiple other injuries that complicate thoracic wall treatment options. Rib fractures occur in 10% of all trauma patients, and in approximately 30% of all patients with significant chest trauma, and are cause of significant morbidity (2, 3). Flail chest, generally defined as the fracture of three or more ribs in two or more places, represents the most severe form of rib fractures. Conservative therapies, consisting of respiratory assistance and pain control, are the current treatments for the majority of patients with multiple rib fractures; however, mechanical ventilation >3 weeks is often associated with several ventilation related complications. In patient with flail chest who are not treated surgically, pneumonia develops in 27 to 70% of cases and carries a mortality rate of 51%. Morbidity and mortality increase with age and the number of ribs that are fractured. Patients older than 45 years and with more than four rib fractures are at significantly greater risk for poorer outcomes compared to the average patient (4). In selected patients, operative fixation of fractured ribs within 72 h post injury may lead to better results (5). More randomized control trials are needed to further determine who may benefit from surgical fixation of rib fractures. Intravenous analgesia is often use for pain relief, but is associated with significant adverse effects. Epidural analgesia offers the advantage of superior analgesia with the absence of the adverse effects of parenteral narcotic.

Despite many reports of blunt chest trauma management, the impact of chest injury severity on the outcome of patients with multiple trauma has been rarely described. Significant differences in mortality and morbidity have been recently reported between different health care institutions.

Epidural analgesia provides superior pain relief compared to other analgesic techniques and improves the pulmonary function tests of injured patients. Its use has been associated with an increase in tidal volume, functional residual capacity (FRC), lung compliance, vital capacity and PaO2 with reductions in airway resistance and the paradoxical movement of flail chest wall segments (6).

MATERIALS AND METHODS

We conducted a retrospective analysis of nine cases of patients who developed flail chest following blunt trauma, and were treated with osteofixation of the chest wall and postoperative epidural analgesia at the University Clinical Center of the Republic of Srpska (UCC RS) in Banjaluka from January 2015 to December 2016. All patients received a thoracic computed tomography (CT) scan upon admission to assess the severity of thoracic trauma. Osteofixation was performed under general endotracheal anesthesia with postoperative epidural analgesia. Thoracic epidural analgesia was located to a site corresponding to the level of the rib fracture as that technique has demonstrated superior analgesia in patients with blunt thoracic trauma (5). A solution of 0, 25 % bupivacaine with 0, 01% morphine was delivered by continuous infusion. The surgical osteofixation involved a posterolateral thoracotomy with pleural exploration in order to simultaneously treat lesions of the parenchymal lung and bronchus, control intrathoracic hemorrhage, and remove intrapleural clot.

RESULTS

The analysis included nine patients. All patients were male, aged 34–76 years, mean age 50 years. Four patients (44.4%) were motor vehicle accident victims, while five patients (55.5%) were injured at work. All patients underwent a posterolateral thoracotomy with osteofixation of the chest wall using an osteosynthesis plate. All patients had contusions of the lung parenchyma, and four patients had pulmonary parenchyma lacerations. Two patients had trauma to the chest only.

All patients had fractures of at least four ribs (range 4–8) and one patient had a bilateral flail chest. Seven patients had other major non-chest injuries: one had fractured mandible, 3 had intra-abdominal injuries (1 patient had a liver laceration and 2 patients had a splenic rupture), 1 patient had an L3 compression fracture, and one patient had fractures of the pelvis and lower extremities. All patients were transfused with a minimum of two units of packed RBCs (440 ml) and two units of fresh frozen plasma (360 ml). All the patients received epidural analgesia with 0,25% bupivacaine and 0,01% morphine at a rate 5–10 ml/ h-1 to keep pain score at less than 5 (on a visual analog pain scale of 0–10). Intravenous multimodal analgesia with additional non-narcotic analgesics were started within 6 h after thoracotomy. In the majority of patients (77.7%), surgical stabilization of the chest was performed on the second day of the injury, on average within 2.33 days of the injury, and no later than 5 days after the admission. The average duration of hospitalization was 25.4 days. The average length of stay of patients in the ICU was 14.7 days (range 2–36), while the average number of days on mechanical ventilation was 8.1 (range 2–16). Tracheostomy was performed in 33.3% of study patients. The overall mortality in the observed group was 44.4%.

DISCUSSION

Recently there has been renewed interest in surgical stabilization of ribs fracture in patients with flail chest (5). However, conservative treatment is still preferred in most surgical centers. Nishiumi et al. reported on the treatment of anterior flail chest with internal pneumatic stabilization in 42 patients. Continuous positive pressure ventilation was needed for 12.5 days and mechanical ventilation for 15.6 days (7). The goal of operative chest wall stabilization is to shorten the period of mechanical ventilation and thus reduce complications from its use.

Only three randomized controlled trials have compared operative vs. nonoperative treatment of multiple rib fractures (5). Leinicke et al., in a systematic review and meta-analysis of studies totaling 538 patients with flail chest, showed that operative management of flail chest was associated with a shorter duration of mechanical ventilation [pooled reduction: −4.52

days; 95% confidence interval (CI): −5.54 to −3.50], shorter ICU length of stay (−3.40 days; 95% CI: −6.01 to −0.79), decreased hospital length of stay (−3.82 days; 95% CI: −7.12 to −0.54), and decreased mortality (pooled Relative Risk (RR): 0.44; 95% CI: 0.28–0.69). A reduction in pneumonia (RR:0.45; 95% CI: 0.30–0.69), and tracheostomy (RR:0.25; 95% CI: 0.13–0.47) were also noted (8). In our study the average number of days on mechanical ventilation was 8.1 days, similar to that reported in the above meta-analysis. In our series the average patient age was 50 years (range 34–76 years), higher than the average reported in other studies. Several studies have described increased morbidity and mortality in elderly patients with traumatic rib fractures, and the increased death rate of our study may be explained by this. An age of 45 years or greater and more than four rib fractures is associated with significantly poorer patient outcome (8). Mortality in patients over 65 years with rib fractures compared with a younger population is 20.1 vs. 11.4% (9). In one retrospective study which analyzed data from the US National Trauma Data Bank, Kent et al. reported that 56 % of the mortality in patients greater than 65 years with thoracic trauma was due to rib fractures and no other injuries (4).

Contusion of the lung parenchyma was present in all patients in our case series and is an independent risk factor for the development of respiratory dysfunction, pneumonia, and acute respiratory distress syndrome. Pneumonia and prolonged respiratory dysfunction occurs in the 25–30% of patients with blunt trauma to the chest (4). Alveolar capillaries are injured, which results in an accumulation of blood and other fluids within lung tissue and interfere with gas exchange and leading to hypoxemia. The consequences of pulmonary contusion include ventilation/perfusion mismatching, increased arterio-venous shunting and loss of compliance of lung parenchyma. These physiological consequences occur within few hours after injury and usually resolve in 7 days. In one study of 139 patients with blunt thoracic trauma and pulmonary contusion, Novakon et al. reported a mortality rate of 17% (9).

All patients in our series received postoperative epidural analgesia via a thoracic epidural catheter. In addition to epidural analgesia, all patients received intravenous multimodal analgesia beginning 6 hours after chest wall ostefixation. Our goal was to achieve a pain score of 5 or less on a visual analog scale pain, which would provide good analgesia. Neuraxial blockade offers superior analgesia to systemically administered medications, although small supplementation of opioids is often required. In patients with one or two rib fractures, treatment with a systemic NSAID and modest amounts of systemic opioids often provides sufficient analgesia. However, such analgesic techniques are often not sufficient to provide satisfactory pain relief in patients with a greater number of fractured ribs who require physiotherapy or to allow effective coughing. Thoracic epidural analgesia with a catheter sited at the mean dermatomal level of the broken ribs provides superior analgesia when measured by subjective pain scale and objective respiratory parameters. Despite better pain relief, a recent meta-analysis which compared thoracic epidural analgesia to intravenous opioid therapy showed no statistically significant difference in mortality, duration of mechanical ventilation, or length of stay in the ICU and hospital (6). There is increasing evidence that multimodal analgesia combined with regional analgesia techniques other than thoracic neuraxial blockade reduces the severity of acute pain after thoracic surgery with yet unknown impact on the incidence and severity of chronic thoracic pain. As an alternative to epidural analgesia, continuous intercostal nerve blockade with local anesthetic may be used in a large number of patients. Paravertebral blockade may provide analgesia similar to thoracic epidural in patients with thoracic trauma and may have with fewer side effects.

The selection of patients and the timing of surgical intervention play an important role in the success of surgical osteofixation. Surgical stabilization of rib fractures is currently used in less than 1% of patients with multiple rib fractures (8). In our case series 77.7% of surgical stabilizations were done on the second day following the injury. Early vs. later intervention may improve outcomes as inflammation and callus formation increase between 3 and 5 days after the injury may complicate management. Most authors recommend early operative treatment within 72 h of injury. Although the combination of osteofixation and continuous thoracic epidural analgesia may reduce mortality, our mortality rate was higher than that of other studies. This is most likely due to the older patients we treated (mean age, 50 years; range 34–76 years) all of whom had significant lung parenchymal injury and numerous other non-thoracic injuries. Our study's significance is limited by the small number of subjects.

CONCLUSION

Early surgical fixation of a flail chest followed by continuous thoracic epidural analgesia may reduce the duration of mechanical ventilation, its complications and shorten the length of ICU and hospital stay in patients with flail chest following blunt thoracic trauma. Good analgesia may help to improve a patient's respiratory mechanics and to avoid intubation of the trachea for ventilatory support in some patients. This may dramatically improve the course of recovery.

AUTHOR CONTRIBUTIONS

DG: Main author, idea of writing the analysis, coordinated writing of the text and translation in English; DS: Analysis of litherature, writing of introduction, discussion, some part of translatin in english; SP: Correction of the text, correction of english version; NK: Statistical analysis, analysis of English.

REFERENCES

1. Veysi VT, Nikolau VS, Paliobeis C, Efstathopoulos N, Giannoudis PV. Prevalence of chest trauma associated injuriesand mortality; a level I trauma centre experience.*Int.Orthopaed.* (2009) 33:1425–33. doi: 10.1007/s00264-009-0746-9
2. Sirmali M, Türüt H, Topçu S, Gülhan E, Yazici U, Kaya S, et al. A comprehensive analysis of traumatic rib fractures: morbidity, mortality, and management. *Eur J Cardiothorac Surg.* (2003) 24:133–8. doi: 10.1016/S1010-7940(03)00256-2
3. Clark GC, Schecter WP, Trunkey DD. Variables affecting outcome in blunt injury chest trauma: flail chest vs. pulmonary contusion. *J Trauma.* (1988) 28:298–304. doi: 10.1097/00005373-198803000-00004
4. Kent R, Woods W, BostromO. Fatality risk and the presence of rib fractures. *Ann Adv Automot Med.* (2008) 52:73–82.
5. Jong MB, Kokke MC, Hietbrink F, Leenen LP. Surgical management of ib fractures: strategies and literature review. *Scand. J Surg.* (2010) 72:120–5. doi: 10.1177/1457496914531928
6. Moloney JT, Fowler SJ, Chany W. Anesthetic management of thoracic trauma.*Curr Opin Anesthesiol.* (2008) 21:41–6. doi: 10.1097/ACO.0b013e3282f2aadc
7. Nishiumi N, Fujimori S, Katoh N, Iwasaki M, Inokuchi S, Inoue H. Treatment with internal pneumatic stabilization for anterior flail chest. *Exp Clin Med.* (2007) 32:126–30.
8. Leinicke JA, Elmore L, Freeman BD, Colditz GA. Operative management of rib fractures in the setting of flail chest: a systematic review and meta-analysis. *Ann Surg.* (2013) 257:914–21. doi: 10.1097/SLA.0b013e3182895bb0
9. Novakov I, Novakova S, Shterev P. Pulmonary contusion – a risk factor of mortality in blunt thoracic trauma. *Europ Resp J.* (2014) 51:355–68.

14

Application Status and Prospects of Artificial Intelligence in Peptic Ulcers

Peng-yue Zhao[1†], Ke Han[2†], Ren-qi Yao[3], Chao Ren[4]* and Xiao-hui Du[1]**

[1]Department of General Surgery, First Medical Center of the Chinese PLA General Hospital, Beijing, China, [2]Department of Gastroenterology, First Medical Center of the Chinese PLA General Hospital, Beijing, China, [3]Translational Medicine Research Center, Medical Innovation Research Division and Fourth Medical Center of the Chinese PLA General Hospital, Beijing, China, [4]Department of Pulmonary and Critical Care Medicine, Beijing Chaoyang Hospital, Capital Medical University, Beijing, China

*Correspondence:
Xiao-hui Du
duxiaohui301@sina.com
Chao Ren
rc198@sina.com
Ren-qi Yao
yaorenqixx1995@163.com

†These authors have contributed equally to this work

Peptic ulcer (PU) is a common and frequently occurring disease. Although PU seriously threatens the lives and health of global residents, the applications of artificial intelligence (AI) have strongly promoted diversification and modernization in the diagnosis and treatment of PU. This minireview elaborates on the research progress of AI in the field of PU, from PU's pathogenic factor *Helicobacter pylori (Hp)* infection, diagnosis and differential diagnosis, to its management and complications (bleeding, obstruction, perforation and canceration). Finally, the challenges and prospects of AI application in PU are prospected and expounded. With the in-depth understanding of modern medical technology, AI remains a promising option in the management of PU patients and plays a more indispensable role. How to realize the robustness, versatility and diversity of multifunctional AI systems in PU and conduct multicenter prospective clinical research as soon as possible are the top priorities in the future.

Keywords: peptic ulcer, artificial intelligence, gastric ulcer, complications, convolutional neural network

INTRODUCTION

Peptic ulcer (PU) is an inflammatory reaction and necrotizing lesion of the mucosa or submucosa under the action of various pathogenic factors. It often occurs in the gastrointestinal mucosa that performs the function of gastric acid secretion, of which the stomach and duodenum are the most common. It is estimated that the incidence of PU is 0.1%–0.3% per year, while its lifetime prevalence reaches as high as 5%–10% in the general population (1). Therefore, early diagnosis and prevention of PU is crucial to reduce the economic burden on global health.

Artificial intelligence (AI) refers to a modern technology that imitates human behavior and thinking through computer networks and is an interdisciplinary subject developed on the basis of computer science, information theory, determinism, neuropsychology, philosophy, linguistics, etc. (2). With the advent of the era of big data, AI has achieved rapid development in the field

Abbreviations: PU, peptic ulcer; GU, gastric ulcer; DU, duodenal ulcer; AI, artificial intelligence; ML, machine learning; DL, deep learning; CNNs, convolutional neural networks; DBNs, deep belief networks; *HP, Helicobacter pylori;* RFSNN, refined feature selection with neural network; RMIS, robot-assisted minimally invasive surgery; GI, gastrointestinal; AUC, area under the curve; GBS, glasgow-blatchford score; eiPDLA, end-to-end importance perception personalized DL method; LSTM, long short-term memory; NSAIDs, non-steroidal anti-inflammatory drugs; IPU-ML, idiopathic peptic ulcer ML mode; ANN, artificial neural network; CI, confidence interval; EGC, early gastric cancer; EGD, esophagogastroduodenoscopy.

of image and speech recognition with the help of technological innovations such as machine learning (ML) and deep learning (DL). Among them, the most advanced and common one is the DL technology represented by convolutional neural network (CNN), which is currently widely used in many fields (3).

The concept of DL is inspired by the synaptic system of the human brain's neural network. It is composed of multiple layers of simple computing nodes that simulate the activities of the human visual cortex through complex connections. In terms of specific research content, DL mainly includes CNNs, self-coding neural networks and deep belief networks (DBNs) (4). DL can identify important features from a large database of images through a repeated learning process. The larger the data volume given to it, the more obvious the advantages of DL, namely, the faster and higher accuracy of recognition. In the medical field, DL-based intelligent systems can automatically extract and learn clinical data, which can not only help doctors diagnose diseases but also accurately predict prognosis. Currently, DL has been prominent in the diagnosis of lung cancer, breast cancer, brain cancer, prostate cancer, Alzheimer's disease and Parkinson's disease, and has also been widely reported in the clinical diagnosis and treatment of digestive diseases (5, 6).

The differential diagnosis of benign and malignant ulcers of the digestive tract is significantly important for subsequent treatment. However, macroscopic endoscopic diagnosis is sometimes very burdensome, since the accuracy of endoscopic diagnosis largely depends on the technical level and clinical experience of endoscopists. Moreover, massive image data also require considerable time and efforts. Fortunately, the emergence of AI can solve the above problems. This minireview elaborated on the research progress of AI in the field of PU, from its pathogenic factors, diagnosis, to management and complications (**Figure 1**). Moreover, the challenges and prospects in this field were also elaborated.

APPLICATION OF AI IN PU

AI in the Pathogenic Factors of PU

Helicobacter pylori (Hp) infection is one of the important pathogenic factors of PU. Statistics show that the positive rates of *Hp* in gastric ulcer (GU) and duodenal ulcer (DU) patients are 60%–80% and 90%, respectively (7, 8). In terms of pathogenesis, on the one hand, *Hp* can release urease to break down urea to produce NH_3, which destroys the acidic environment of the gastrointestinal tract. However, *Hp* can generate numerous toxin proteins that destroy the barrier system of the gastric mucosa. Therefore, early identification of *Hp* infection is essential in preventing PU. At present, noninvasive tests, such as urea breath and stool antigen tests, are still the first choice for the exclusion of *Hp* infection, while elderly people over 60 can select direct gastroscopy for

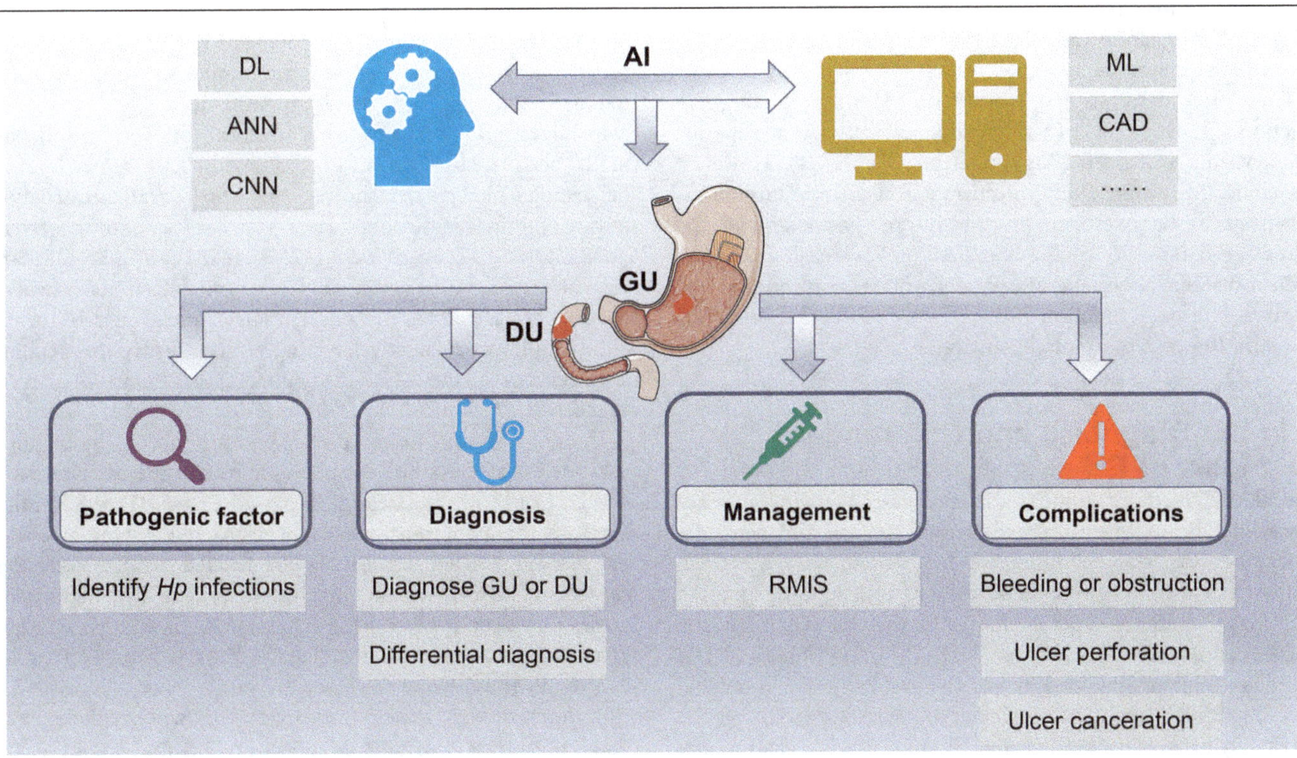

FIGURE 1 | Application of artificial intelligence in peptic ulcers. AI has achieved rapid development in the field of PU with the help of technological innovations such as ML, DL, and CNN. AI is widely applied in the field of PU, ranging from its pathogenic factors, diagnosis and differential diagnosis to management and complications. Abbreviations: AI, artificial intelligence; PU, peptic ulcer; ML, machine learning; DL, deep learning; CNN, convolutional neural network.

exclusion (9). However, most cases of subclinical *Hp* infection still rely on invasive biopsy, which takes time to avoid misdiagnosis. In addition, the severity of *Hp* infection needs to be measured by the inspector with the naked eye. This method is a subjective judgment, and there will inevitably be bias. Fortunately, the emergence of AI may shed light on the current dilemma.

The earliest application of AI technology in *Hp* infection recognition was in 2004. Huang et al. (10) first trained AI by using endoscopic images of 30 dyspeptic patients (15 *Hp* infections and 15 non-*Hp* infections) and established a refined feature selection with neural network (RFSNN) algorithm. Then, a verification test was performed on the images of the remaining 74 patients with dyspepsia. The sensitivity, specificity, and accuracy of the algorithm for identifying *Hp* infection reached 78.8%, 90.2%, and 85.1%, respectively. Since then, AI technology has developed rapidly, and CNNs have also emerged and quickly become an absolute leader in the field of medical image processing. In 2017, Shichijo et al. (11) adopted 32,208 photos from 1750 patients (735 *Hp* positive and 1,015 *Hp* negative) as a discovery cohort to train a CNN model, followed by validation of its diagnostic performance in an independent dataset. Finally, it was verified on a new data set to compare the difference between CNN and endoscopists in identifying *Hp* infections. The results showed that the sensitivity, specificity, accuracy, and diagnosis time of the CNN were 88.9%, 87.4%, 87.7% and 194 s, respectively, and these indicators were 79.0%, 83.2%, 82.4%, and 230 ± 65 min among 23 endoscopists. This showed that using a CNN to diagnose *Hp* infection has higher accuracy and costs less time than manual diagnosis by endoscopists.

There are many similar studies on AI in predicting *Hp* infection (12–16), all of which demonstrate AI's superior accuracy and sensitivity (**Supplementary Table S1**). However, AI's ability to recognize *Hp* infection still has some limitations that need to be overcome in the future. For example, the training and test sets of the above studies were all from one medical center or one country, and more continuous and rigorous external validation from various sources is necessary to ensure the credibility of conclusions.

AI in the Diagnosis and Differential Diagnosis of PU

Typical GU is more common in the gastric angle or lesser curvature. The lesions are mostly round or oval and generally solitary but can also be multiple. Most benign GUs are small in diameter and have regular edges. The surrounding mucosa often has hyperemia and edema, and the surface is mostly covered with white or yellow exudate. The morphology of DU is similar to that of GU. DU mostly occurs in the duodenal bulb, especially near the anterior or posterior wall of the gastric pylorus. Under normal circumstances, gastroscopy physicians can make corresponding clinical diagnoses based on the subject's gastrointestinal morphology or histological abnormalities, but if the situation is more complicated or the endoscopists are not fully sure, then they will take some specimens from around the lesion for pathological examination and give the final pathological diagnosis.

However, gastroscopy has two limitations: first, the sensitivity and specificity of diagnosis are closely related to the level of the examiner; if the examiner lacks clinical experience, misdiagnosis and missed diagnosis of PU can easily occur. Second, gastroenterologists need to check the abnormalities of numerous images or videos to detect the patient's lesions. However, considering the limited time and energy of clinicians, such a large number of images or videos will undoubtedly increase their workload.

The application of AI in PU diagnosis can be traced back to 2002. Saenz Bajo et al. (17) used the Neurone network to differentiate between PU and functional or idiopathic dyspepsia on the basis of clinical notes. The researchers classified and verified 81 patients who were clinically diagnosed with dyspepsia according to the presence of determined symptoms and finally found that the Neurone network successfully classified 81% of patients with negative and positive predictive values of 90% and 80%, respectively. To improve the diagnostic efficiency of GU, Al-Kasasbeh et al. (18) constructed a fuzzy logic decision-making system based on the variations in electrical resistance of acupuncture points, and the result was encouraging. The prediction error level of this decision-making system was not higher than 0.18, which once again proved the feasibility of AI application in PU.

In the past three years, with the increasingly widespread application of DL and CNN in the medical field, a body of researches on AI in PU diagnosis and differential diagnosis have emerged. To explore the ability of deep CNN to identify ulcers in wireless capsule endoscopic images, Wang et al. (19) first used 15,781 ulcer frames to train deep CNN, then used 2040 ulcer and 2,319 normal frames for verification, and finally performed it on 4,917 ulcer and 5,007 normal frames for testing. The results showed that the overall sensitivity of deep CNN in diagnosing ulcers was 89.7%, and the overall specificity and accuracy were both higher than 90%. Similarly, Alaskar et al. (20) built a CNN to detect its effect in diagnosing gastrointestinal ulcers. They trained and tested 336 and 105 photos respectively. Finally, the sensitivity, specificity and accuracy of the CNN in diagnosing gastrointestinal ulcers all reached an astonishing 100%.

In addition to its extraordinary performance in the diagnosis of PU, AI also plays an indispensable role in the discrimination of PU from other gastrointestinal diseases. To differentially diagnose the two most common stomach deformities (ulcers and bleeding), Khan et al. (21) constructed a rank-based deep features selection system that was verified by 4,000 video frames of ulcers, 4,000 video frames of bleeding and 4,000 normal ones, and found that the system only took 21.15 sec to identify all these video frames with an accuracy of 99.5%. This will undoubtedly greatly improve the work efficiency of gastroenterology clinicians. Majid et al. (22) and Xia et al. (23) established a CNN model to explore its differential diagnostic ability of four types of stomach infections (ulcer, polyp, esophagitis, and bleeding) and seven types of gastric lesions (erosion, polyp, ulcer, submucosal tumor, xanthoma, normal mucosa, and bleeding), respectively. The research results all proved the excellent differential diagnosis ability of CNN. The accuracy of the former reached 96.5%, while the sensitivity, specificity and accuracy of the latter were 96.2%, 76.2% and 77.1%, respectively. There are many similar studies (24–26), and detailed information can be seen in **Supplementary Table S2**.

AI in the Management of PU

In addition to ML and CNN, robots are also an outstanding representative of the development and application of AI in medicine. For example, the Da Vinci robot has played a crucial and irreplaceable role in multiple surgical disciplines, becoming the most representative achievement of minimally invasive surgery and intelligent medicine. The progress of robots in the field of PU is relatively slow, mainly because the proportion of surgical intervention in the treatment of PU is inherently small.

Sutures are one of the most difficult tasks in robot-assisted minimally invasive surgery (RMIS), because the surgeon needs to coordinate and control three or four tools, which will distract and consume the surgeon's energy and prolong the operation time. Gao et al. (27) proposed a robot autonomous suture task allocation method, and conducted a suture repair experiment for DU under the guidance of a surgeon. The results showed that this method obtained an optimal suture task allocation plan, which was beneficial to improve the intelligent degree of robot operation. Brungardt et al. (28) explored the feasibility of right-side robot-assisted transthoracic vagotomy for the treatment of marginal ulcers after gastric bypass surgery for the first time. The patient was a 43-year-old white female who underwent Roux-en-Y gastric bypass surgery at the age of 29. The author's team successfully ligated two vagus nerves through right-side robot-assisted thoracoscopic surgery, and the patient had a good prognosis. This successful case provides a new idea for expanding the application of robotic surgery in highly selective transabdominal vagotomy.

AI in the Complications of PU

Bleeding

When the mucosal damage of peptic ulcer has exceeded the basal layer of the mucosa, if it is further deepened, it may impair the blood vessels under the mucosa and cause bleeding. Bleeding in the digestive tract is the most common complication of PU. Nearly 20% of ulcer-related bleeding cases had no obvious alarm symptoms or signs before onset. Early recognition of the risk of bleeding and its related adverse outcomes can help doctors provide timely intervention, which may improve the prognosis.

Traditional prediction methods based on electronic health records usually do not take the correlation between static and dynamic data into consideration, but these data contain important information about the interaction effects which are important to fit the association between clinical materials and outcomes. Tan et al. paid attention to this point and developed a novel end-to-end importance perception personalized DL method (eiPDLA), which improved the accuracy of early bleeding risk at 1 year ahead with an AUC of 0.944 (29). The team also made relevant improvements in predicting mortality in patients with PU bleeding (30). The fatality rate of PU bleeding was greatly related to age, complications, severity of bleeding and recurrence of bleeding. Through the multiconvolution deep residual network (ResNet), deep fusion and long short-term memory (LSTM) methods, the AUC of the mortality prediction model for patients with PU bleeding reached 0.9353. ML models were also used to predict the risk of recurrent bleeding in idiopathic ulcers (31), which was characterized by occurring without *Hp* infection or the use of non-steroidal anti-inflammatory drugs (NSAIDs) and a high risk of recurrent bleeding and death. The idiopathic peptic ulcer ML (IPU-ML) model built in this study was trained by 22 854 patients with a diagnosis of PU disease and tested by 1,265 patients who were diagnosed with GI bleeding. It could identify patients who had 1-year recurrent ulcer bleeding, with an overall accuracy of 84.3% and an AUC of 0.775, especially idiopathic ulcer patients who were at low risk of recurrent ulcer bleeding.

AI also plays a role in guiding the practice of endoscopy. It could help identify the risk of PU bleeding under endoscopy according to the Forrest classification (32). After training on 2,378 static endoscopic images from 1,694 PU patients, the DL model had moderate to substantial consistency with advanced endoscopists on the test data set, which was higher than that of novice endoscopy. Therefore, this had certain application value for training young doctors and helping to make decisions in emergency endoscopy.

Perforation

PU perforation refers to the deep development of GU or DU, which penetrates the serosal layer and causes local flatulence and perforation. It is a severe clinical complication and a leading cause of operation-related death. Early identification of patients with perforated ulcers with poor prognosis is of great importance to patient risk stratification and identification of potential treatment. An artificial neural network (ANN) model was constructed to identify risk factors (increasing age, the presence of an active cancer, a delay from admission to surgery >24 h, hypoalbuminemia, hyperbilirubinemia and increasing creatinine values) of the 30-day mortality after surgery and their complex interactions with the mortality among patients with PU perforation (33). Among the 168 patients included in the study, the data of 117 patients were used to train the model, and 51 patients were used to test it. The mortality predicted by ANN showed an AUC of 0.90 (95% confidence interval [CI], 0.85–0.95). However, the study was restricted by its small sample size, and relied on predictor variables that were previously defined rather than extensive screening to build the model. Moreover, this research lacked true, secondary and external verification queues. Therefore, it is still necessary to enhance the accuracy of prediction to generate a more reliable model for future risk projection and clinical decision making of PU treatment.

Karargyris's team (34) developed a wireless capsule endoscope that could identify small intestinal perforated ulcers and polyps, but no similar identification method had been seen to assist in identifying PU perforations in endoscopy.

Pyloric Obstruction

Obstruction is often seen in DU and pyloric duct ulcers. The pylorus is the narrowest part of the digestive tract, with a normal diameter of approximately 1.5 cm, so it is prone to obstruction. PU may cause inflammation and swelling of the tissues around the pylorus, leading to obstruction. Temporary obstruction can be resolved after the ulcer has healed. However, pyloric ulcer scars can also cause intractable mechanical obstruction, which requires an endoscopic or surgical operation to relieve the obstruction. Unfortunately, to our knowledge, there is no relevant research report on the application of AI in pyloric obstruction.

Cancerization

DU rarely become cancerous, while GU may become cancerous, especially in those with *Hp* infection. More than 70% of early gastric cancer (EGC) patients have no obvious symptoms (35). As the disease progresses, symptoms of gastritis or gastric ulcer may gradually appear, including loss of appetite, nausea, indigestion, weight loss, upper abdominal discomfort or dull pain, and occasionally vomiting, fecal occult blood or melena, pantothenic acid deficiency, unexplained fatigue or progressive anemia. As an important basis for choosing treatment options for EGC, tumor classification and microscopic staging are very important. Esophagogastroduodenoscopy (EGD) biopsy is considered the current standard method for identifying gastric mucosal lesions. Endoscopists must have considerable experience and knowledge to correctly diagnose malignant ulcers, but this often requires long-term technical training and experience accumulation. Machines have fewer variations within and between observers, and the results are generally better than those of human endoscopists (36). The advancement of AI technology can provide higher sensitivity and specificity for the recognition and diagnosis of EGC under endoscopy.

The work of Ken Namikawa et al. proved that after training the AI-based diagnostic system with a large amount of data, the diagnostic accuracy of gastric cancer and GU classification reached a very high level, with a comprehensive diagnostic accuracy of 95.9% (37). Recently, E. Klang et al. built a CNN model aimed at distinguishing benign and malignant GU from endoscopic images in the western population (38). The study retrospectively collected endoscopic images of benign and malignant GU patients undergoing endoscopy at the Chaim Sheba Medical Center from 2011 to 2019. Every included image had a corresponding biopsy result that was sampled at the same time as endoscopic examination. Endoscope images from 2011 to 2015 and from 2016 to 2017 were used for training and validation, while the retained data from 2018 to 2019 were used to test the final model. In addition, some public pictures were obtained through the Google image search engine for pretraining the model. The final model showed an AUC of 0.91 to detect malignant ulcers. For a cut-off probability of 0.5, the model had a sensitivity of 92% and a specificity of 75%.

Moreover, a DL model based on endoscopic images to diagnose gastric mucosal lesions was developed by Joon Yeul Nam et al. (39). This model was based on a CNN algorithm to achieve the purpose of lesion detection, differential diagnosis (AI-DDx model), and depth of invasion detection (AI-ID model). A total of 1,366 patients from 2 referral centers with gastric mucosal lesions were consecutively included in this study. Representative endoscopic images of benign GU, EGC or advanced gastric cancer selected by experts for each patient were used as the training and testing sets, with the histological diagnoses as the gold standard. The results identified by the models were compared with the visual diagnosis and ultrasound endoscopy results of endoscopists with different working years. The results showed that the AI-DDx model performed better than novice and intermediate endoscopists, was comparable to expert endoscopists, and reached AUCs of 0.86 in both internal and external validation. The AUCs of the AI-ID model were 0.78 in the internal validation and 0.73 in the external validation, which were significantly better than the endoscopic ultrasonography results performed by experts. In general, there are numerous related studies on the application of AI in GU complications (40–43), and detailed information can be found in **Table 1**.

CHALLENGES AND PROSPECTS

Although significant progress has been made in the application of AI in the diagnosis, management and complication prediction of PU, there are still the following areas for improvement. First, the majority of related studies have a small sample size, and only include high-quality images for AI modeling, which cannot reflect the differences in inspection equipment covering hospitals at all levels and complex clinical scenarios. Second, most studies related to AI and GU are retrospective studies, which may overestimate the real performance of AI models due to selection bias. Moreover, few studies have evaluated the auxiliary role of AI systems for endoscopists, especially juniors. Finally, most studies only consider a certain aspect of clinical information such as imaging or biomarkers, and the integration of clinical multimodal data seems essential to further improve the performance of AI systems.

Despite the fact that AI has made major breakthroughs in the field of PU, we have more expectations for the optimization of AI systems. For instance, how can AI algorithms suitable for different scenarios be developed to achieve robust, versatile and diverse multifunctional AI systems in the PU field? How can a multifunctional AI system be integrated in the future to realize the whole process management of PU lesions from risk assessment and diagnosis to treatment? Furthermore, with the gradual improvement of residents' health awareness, an increasing number of people take health check-ups. It is hoped that in the future, different endoscopic images from healthy mucosa to severe PU can be collected to study mucosal and microvascular changes before lesions occur to identify GU lesions at an early stage. Finally, and most importantly, it is urgent to carry out multicenter and large-sample clinical research on the application of AI in PU, hoping to provide a solid theoretical basis for the

TABLE 1 | Summary of applications of AI in PU's complications.

Ref.	Year	AI technology	Research Objectives	Training and Validating set	Outcomes
Karakitsos et al. (40)	1998	ANN	To discriminate benign and malignant gastric cells	2,500 cells from 23 cancer, 19 gastritis and 58 ulcer cases for training, 8,524 cells from the same cases for testing	Correct classification of >97% benign cells and >95% malignant cells, overall accuracy of >97%
Grossi et al. (41)	2008	ANN	To recognize patients at high risk of death for nonvariceal upper GI bleeding	807 patients with nonvariceal upper GI bleeding	Average sensitivity of 89.2%, average specificity of 82.9%, average accuracy of 86%, and AUC of 0.87
Rotondano et al. (42)	2011	ANN	To predict mortality in patients with nonvariceal upper GI bleeding	2,380 patients with nonvariceal upper GI bleeding	Sensitivity of 83.8%, specificity of 97.5%, accuracy of 96.8%, and AUC of 0.95
Søreide et al. (33)	2015	ANN	To predict outcomes in patients with perforated gastroduodenal ulcers	117 patients for training and 51 patients for testing	AUC of inclusive, multifactorial ANN model is 0.90
Tan et al. (30)	2018	Deep residual network	To predict PU bleeding mortality	6,367 patients diagnosed with PU bleeding	AUC of 0.94 for PU bleeding mortality prediction
Wong et al. (31)	2019	ML	To identify patients at high risk for recurrent ulcer bleeding	22 854 patients with PU for training and 1,265 patients with PU for testing	Overall accuracy of 84.3% and AUC of 0.78
Lee et al. (43)	2019	Deep neural network and transfer-learning approach	To discriminate benign ulcer and cancer	180 normal, 200 benign ulcer, and 337 cancer images for training and 20, 30, 20 images for testing	Accuracies of discriminating Normal vs cancer, Normal vs ulcer, and Cancer vs ulcer were 96.5%, 92.6% and 77.1%
Nakashima et al. (37)	2020	Advanced CNN	To discriminate gastric cancers and gastric ulcers	13,584 gastric cancer and 4,826 gastric ulcer images for training, 739 gastric cancer images and 720 gastric ulcer images for validation	Sensitivity of 93,3%, specificity of 99.0% and positive predictive value of 99.1% for gastric ulcer
Tan et al. (29)	2021	A novel end-to-end importance perception personalized deep learning method	To predict bleeding risk	6,367 patients with peptic ulcer bleeding	AUC of 0.944 at 1 year ahead of risk prediction
Klang et al. (38)	2021	CNN	To discriminate benign and malignant GU	1,299 images for training, 364 images for validation and 315 images for testing	Sensitivity of 92%, specificity of 75% and AUC of 0.91 for detecting malignant ulcers
Nam et al. (39)	2021	AI-differential diagnosis	To diagnose gastric mucosal lesions (GU, EGC, AGC)	1,009 patients for training, 112 patients for internal validation and 245 patients for external validation	AUC of 0.86 in diagnostic performance for both internal and external validation

AI, Artificial intelligence; PU, Peptic Ulcer; ANN, Artificial Neural Networks; CNN, Convolutional Neural Network; GI, Gastrointestinal; DL, Deep Learning; EGC, Early Gastric Cancer; AGC, Advanced Gastric Cancer; AUC, Area Under the Curve; Hp, Helicobacter pylori.

transformation and application of AI systems (**Supplementary Figure S1**).

CONCLUSION

This minireview elaborates on the research progress of AI in the field of PU, from PU's pathogenic factor *Helicobacter pylori (Hp)* infection, diagnosis and differential diagnosis, to its management and complications (bleeding, obstruction, perforation and canceration). Finally, the challenges and prospects of AI application in PU are prospected and expounded. It provides us with an in-depth understanding of the research status of AI in the PU field. Numerous preclinical and clinical studies have clearly demonstrated the feasibility and safety of AI, which not only ensures the diagnostic accuracy but also greatly improves diagnostic efficiency. AI unquestionably makes a significant contribution to reducing the workload of gastrointestinal endoscopists. At the same time, AI still has some limitations in the field of PU, such as an insufficient research sample size, and existing conclusions are mainly based on retrospective research. How to realize the robustness, versatility and diversity of multifunctional AI systems in PU and conduct multicenter prospective clinical research as soon as possible are the top priorities in the future.

AUTHOR CONTRIBUTIONS

P-yZ and KH performed the majority of the writing, prepared the figures and tables. R-qY and CR edited and revised the manuscript. X-hD designed the study; all authors approved the final version to be published. All authors contributed to the article and approved the submitted version.

REFERENCES

1. Lanas A, Chan FKL. Peptic ulcer disease. *Lancet.* (2017) 390(10094):613–24. doi: 10.1016/s0140-6736(16)32404-7
2. Elemento O, Leslie C, Lundin J, Tourassi G. Artificial intelligence in cancer research, diagnosis and therapy. *Nat Rev Cancer.* (2021) 21(12):747–52. doi: 10.1038/s41568-021-00399-1
3. Hezaveh YD, Levasseur LP, Marshall PJ. Fast automated analysis of strong gravitational lenses with convolutional neural networks. *Nature.* (2017) 548 (7669):555–7. doi: 10.1038/nature23463
4. van der Laak J, Litjens G, Ciompi F. Deep learning in histopathology: the path to the clinic. *Nat Med.* (2021) 27(5):775–84. doi: 10.1038/s41591-021-01343-4
5. Kröner PT, Engels MM, Glicksberg BS, Johnson KW, Mzaik O, van Hooft JE, et al. Artificial intelligence in gastroenterology: a state-of-the-art review. *World J Gastroenterol.* (2021) 27(40):6794–824. doi: 10.3748/wjg.v27.i40.6794
6. Joseph J, LePage EM, Cheney CP, Pawa R. Artificial intelligence in colonoscopy. *World J Gastroenterol.* (2021) 27(29):4802–17. doi: 10.3748/wjg.v27.i29.4802
7. Zhang W, Liang X, Chen X, Ge Z, Lu H. Time trends in the prevalence of Helicobacter pylori infection in patients with peptic ulcer disease: a single-center retrospective study in Shanghai. *J Int Med Res.* (2021) 49 (10):3000605211051167. doi: 10.1177/03000605211051167
8. Kuipers EJ, Thijs JC, Festen HP. The prevalence of Helicobacter pylori in peptic ulcer disease. *Aliment Pharmacol Ther.* (1995) 9(Suppl 2):59–69. PMID: 8547530
9. Crowe SE. Helicobacter pylori Infection. *N Engl J Med.* (2019) 380 (12):1158–65. doi: 10.1056/NEJMcp1710945
10. Huang CR, Sheu BS, Chung PC, Yang HB. Computerized diagnosis of Helicobacter pylori infection and associated gastric inflammation from endoscopic images by refined feature selection using a neural network. *Endoscopy.* (2004) 36(7):601–8. doi: 10.1055/s-2004-814519
11. Shichijo S, Nomura S, Aoyama K, Nishikawa Y, Miura M, Shinagawa T, et al. Application of convolutional neural networks in the diagnosis of helicobacter pylori infection based on endoscopic images. *EBioMedicine.* (2017) 25:106–11. doi: 10.1016/j.ebiom.2017.10.014
12. Itoh T, Kawahira H, Nakashima H, Yata N. Deep learning analyzes Helicobacter pylori infection by upper gastrointestinal endoscopy images. *Endosc Int Open.* (2018) 6(2):E139–e44. doi: 10.1055/s-0043-120830
13. Nakashima H, Kawahira H, Kawachi H, Sakaki N. Artificial intelligence diagnosis of Helicobacter pylori infection using blue laser imaging-bright and linked color imaging: a single-center prospective study. *Ann Gastroenterol.* (2018) 31(4):462–8. doi: 10.20524/aog.2018.0269
14. Shichijo S, Endo Y, Aoyama K, Takeuchi Y, Ozawa T, Takiyama H, et al. Application of convolutional neural networks for evaluating Helicobacter pylori infection status on the basis of endoscopic images. *Scand J Gastroenterol.* (2019) 54(2):158–63. doi: 10.1080/00365521.2019.1577486
15. Zheng W, Zhang X, Kim JJ, Zhu X, Ye G, Ye B, et al. High accuracy of convolutional neural network for evaluation of Helicobacter pylori infection based on endoscopic images: preliminary experience. *Clin Transl Gastroenterol.* (2019) 10(12):e00109. doi: 10.14309/ctg.0000000000000109
16. Nakashima H, Kawahira H, Kawachi H, Sakaki N. Endoscopic three-categorical diagnosis of Helicobacter pylori infection using linked color imaging and deep learning: a single-center prospective study (with video). *Gastric Cancer.* (2020) 23(6):1033–40. doi: 10.1007/s10120-020-01077-1
17. Sáenz Bajo N, Barrios Rueda E, Conde Gómez M, Domínguez Macías I, López Carabaño A, Méndez Díez C. [Use of neural networks in medicine: concerning dyspeptic pathology]. *Aten Primaria.* (2002) 30(2):99–102. doi: 10.1016/s0212-6567(02)78978-6
18. Al-Kasasbeh R, Korenevskiy N, Alshamasin M, Ionescou F, Smith A. Prediction of gastric ulcers based on the change in electrical resistance of acupuncture points using fuzzy logic decision-making. *Comput Methods Biomech Biomed Engin.* (2013) 16(3):302–13. doi: 10.1080/10255842.2011.618926
19. Wang S, Xing Y, Zhang L, Gao H, Zhang H. A systematic evaluation and optimization of automatic detection of ulcers in wireless capsule endoscopy on a large dataset using deep convolutional neural networks. *Phys Med Biol.* (2019) 64(23):235014. doi: 10.1088/1361-6560/ab5086
20. Alaskar H, Hussain A, Al-Aseem N, Liatsis P, Al-Jumeily D. Application of convolutional neural networks for automated ulcer detection in wireless capsule endoscopy images. *Sensors (Basel).* (2019) 19(6):1265. doi: 10.3390/s19061265
21. Khan MA, Sharif M, Akram T, Yasmin M, Nayak RS. Stomach deformities recognition using rank-based deep features selection. *J Med Syst.* (2019) 43 (12):329. doi: 10.1007/s10916-019-1466-3
22. Majid A, Khan MA, Yasmin M, Rehman A, Yousafzai A, Tariq U. Classification of stomach infections: a paradigm of convolutional neural network along with classical features fusion and selection. *Microsc Res Tech.* (2020) 83(5):562–76. doi: 10.1002/jemt.23447
23. Xia J, Xia T, Pan J, Gao F, Wang S, Qian YY, et al. Use of artificial intelligence for detection of gastric lesions by magnetically controlled capsule endoscopy. *Gastrointest Endosc.* (2021) 93(1):133–9.e4. doi: 10.1016/j.gie.2020.05.027
24. Wang S, Xing Y, Zhang L, Gao H, Zhang H. Deep convolutional neural network for ulcer recognition in wireless capsule endoscopy: experimental feasibility and optimization. *Comput Math Methods Med.* (2019) 2019:7546215. doi: 10.1155/2019/7546215
25. Guo L, Gong H, Wang Q, Zhang Q, Tong H, Li J, et al. Detection of multiple lesions of gastrointestinal tract for endoscopy using artificial intelligence model: a pilot study. *Surg Endosc.* (2021) 35(12):6532–8. doi: 10.1007/s00464-020-08150-x
26. Zhang L, Zhang Y, Wang L, Wang J, Liu Y. Diagnosis of gastric lesions through a deep convolutional neural network. *Dig Endosc.* (2021) 33:788–96. doi: 10.1111/den.13844
27. Gao S, Ji S, Feng M, Lu X, Tong W. A study on autonomous suturing task assignment in robot-assisted minimally invasive surgery. *Int J Med Robot.* (2021) 17(1):1–10. doi: 10.1002/rcs.2180
28. Brungardt J, Tracy B, McBride K, Standiford D, Bailey BM. Right robotic-assisted transthoracic truncal vagotomy for marginal ulcer disease after gastric bypass surgery. *Am Surg.* (2018) 84(8):e340–2. doi: 10.1177/000313481808400828
29. Tan Q, Ye M, Ma AJ, Yip TC, Wong GL, Yuen PC. Importance-aware personalized learning for early risk prediction using static and dynamic health data. *J Am Med Inform Assoc.* (2021) 28(4):713–26. doi: 10.1093/jamia/ocaa306
30. Tan Q, Ma AJ, Deng H, Wong VW, Tse YK, Yip TC, et al. A hybrid residual network and long short-term memory method for peptic ulcer bleeding mortality prediction. *AMIA Annu Symp Proc.* (2018) 2018:998–1007.
31. Wong GL, Ma AJ, Deng H, Ching JY, Wong VW, Tse YK, et al. Machine learning model to predict recurrent ulcer bleeding in patients with history of idiopathic gastroduodenal ulcer bleeding. *Aliment Pharmacol Ther.* (2019) 49(7):912–8. doi: 10.1111/apt.15145
32. Yen HH, Wu PY, Su PY, Yang CW, Chen YY, Chen MF, et al. Performance comparison of the deep learning and the human endoscopist for bleeding peptic ulcer disease. *J Med Biol Eng.* (2021) 41(4):504–13. doi: 10.1007/s40846-021-00608-0
33. Søreide K, Thorsen K, Søreide JA. Predicting outcomes in patients with perforated gastroduodenal ulcers: artificial neural network modelling indicates a highly complex disease. *Eur J Trauma Emerg Surg.* (2015) 41 (1):91–8. doi: 10.1007/s00068-014-0417-4
34. Karargyris A, Bourbakis N. Detection of small bowel polyps and ulcers in wireless capsule endoscopy videos. *IEEE Trans Biomed Eng.* (2011) 58 (10):2777–86. doi: 10.1109/tbme.2011.2155064
35. Axon A. Symptoms and diagnosis of gastric cancer at early curable stage. *Best Pract Res Clin Gastroenterol.* (2006) 20(4):697–708. doi: 10.1016/j.bpg.2006.03.015
36. Sung JJ, Poon NC. Artificial intelligence in gastroenterology: where are we heading? *Front Med.* (2020) 14(4):511–7. doi: 10.1007/s11684-020-0742-4
37. Namikawa K, Hirasawa T, Nakano K, Ikenoyama Y, Ishioka M, Shiroma S, et al. Artificial intelligence-based diagnostic system classifying gastric cancers and ulcers: comparison between the original and newly developed systems. *Endoscopy.* (2020) 52(12):1077–83. doi: 10.1055/a-1194-8771
38. Klang E, Barash Y, Levartovsky A, Barkin Lederer N, Lahat A. Differentiation between malignant and benign endoscopic images of gastric ulcers using deep learning. *Clin Exp gastroenterol.* (2021) 14:155–62. doi: 10.2147/ceg.S292857
39. Nam JY, Chung HJ, Choi KS, Lee H, Kim TJ, Soh H, et al. Deep learning model for diagnosing gastric mucosal lesions using endoscopic images: development, validation, and method comparison. *Gastrointest Endosc.* (2021) 95(2):258–68. doi: 10.1016/j.gie.2021.08.022

40. Karakitsos P, Ioakim-Liossi A, Pouliakis A, Botsoli-Stergiou EM, Tzivras M, Archimandritis A, et al. A comparative study of three variations of the learning vector quantizer in the discrimination of benign from malignant gastric cells. *Cytopathology.* (1998) 9(2):114–25. doi: 10.1046/j.1365-2303.1998.00063.x
41. Grossi E, Marmo R, Intraligi M, Buscema M. Artificial neural networks for early prediction of mortality in patients with non variceal upper GI bleeding (UGIB). *Biomed Inform Insights.* (2008) 1:7–19. doi: 10.4137/bii.s814
42. Rotondano G, Cipolletta L, Grossi E, Koch M, Intraligi M, Buscema M, et al. Artificial neural networks accurately predict mortality in patients with nonvariceal upper GI bleeding. *Gastrointest Endosc.* (2011) 73(2):218–26, 26.e1-2. doi: 10.1016/j.gie.2010.10.006
43. Lee JH, Kim YJ, Kim YW, Park S, Choi YI, Kim YJ, et al. Spotting malignancies from gastric endoscopic images using deep learning. *Surg Endosc.* (2019) 33(11):3790–7. doi: 10.1007/s00464-019-06677-2

15

Enhanced Recovery in Thoracic Surgery

*Vesna D. Dinic[1], Milena Dragisa Stojanovic[1], Danica Markovic[1], Vladan Cvetanovic[1], Anita Zoran Vukovic[1] and Radmilo J. Jankovic[1,2]**

[1] Center for Anesthesiology and Reanimatology, Clinical Center of Niš, Niš, Serbia, [2] School of Medicine, University of Niš, Niš, Serbia

***Correspondence:**
Radmilo J. Jankovic
jankovic.radmilo@gmail.com

The main goal of enhanced recovery program after thoracic surgery is to minimize stress response, reduce postoperative pulmonary complications, and improve patient outcome, which will in addition decrease hospital stay and reduce hospital costs. As minimally invasive technique, video-assisted thoracoscopic surgery represents an important element of enhanced recovery program in thoracic surgery. Anesthetic management during preoperative, intraoperative and postoperative period is essential for the enhanced recovery. In the era of enhanced recovery protocols, non-intubated thoracoscopic procedures present a step forward. This article focuses on the key elements of the enhanced recovery program in thoracic surgery. Having reviewed recent literature, the authors highlight potential procedures and techniques that might be incorporated into the program.

Keywords: enhanced recovery, thoracic surgery, video-assisted thoracoscopic surgery, enhanced recovery after surgery, thoracic anesthesia

INTRODUCTION

Despite of the advances in surgical and anesthetic techniques as well as improvements in perioperative care, major surgery is still associated with high rate of complications (1, 2). Postoperative complications are associated with prolonged hospitalization, delayed recovery, increased healthcare costs, and poor postoperative quality of life (3, 4). The concept of enhanced recovery after surgery (ERAS), also known as "fast-track," was derived from the need to minimize hospital length of stay and reduce hospital costs.

Enhanced recovery after surgery program is a multimodal plan of care aimed at optimizing patient before surgery, minimizing patient's intraoperative stress response, consequently reducing complications, decreasing hospital length of stay and accelerating recovery (5, 6).

The concept of ERAS was introduced in 1990s by Kehlet (7), and it was primarily intended for patients undergoing elective colorectal surgery (8). Afterward, it has spread to other surgical specialties, showing improvements in terms of clinical outcomes and costs (9). Many of the principles of enhanced recovery in colorectal surgery are adjusted to enhanced recovery protocols (ERP) in thoracic surgery. Although there are variations in care protocols among institutions, the goal of ERP in thoracic surgery is prevention of pulmonary complications as they are the main cause of increased morbidity and mortality in thoracic surgical population (10). The protocol presents an evidence-based approach to patient care which begins in the preoperative period, extends to entire intraoperative period, and ends until hospital discharge. Therefore, it consists of three phases: preoperative, intraoperative, and postoperative (**Figure 1**).

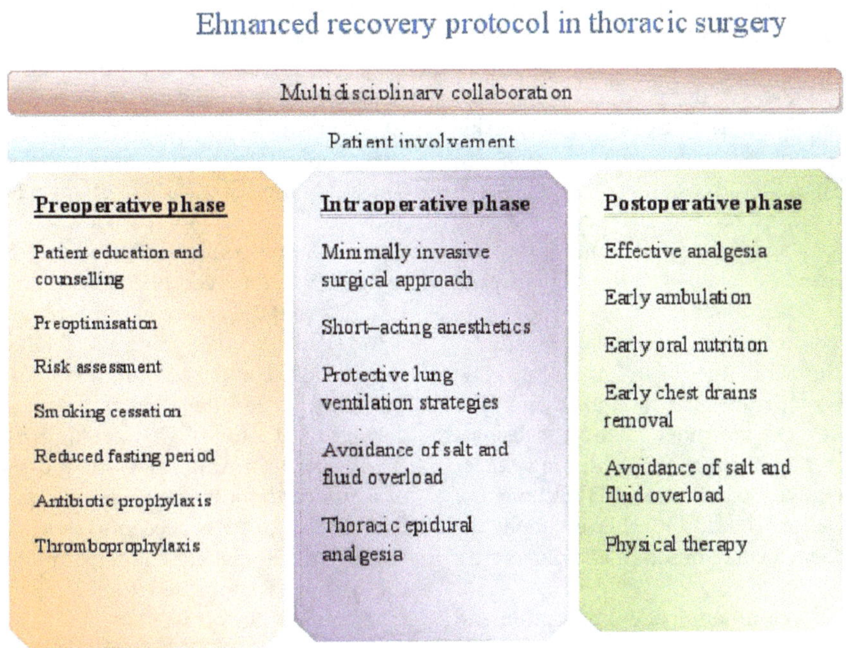

FIGURE 1 | The elements of enhanced recovery protocol in thoracic surgery.

In this article, we have reviewed the recent literature about ER in thoracic surgery. The PubMed and MEDLINE databases were searched using terms "enhanced recovery," "thoracic surgery," "anesthesia," "fast track," and "VATS." Publications from 2000 to 2017 were examined by the authors. To achieve better sensitivity, a search of references of review articles, systematic reviews, and meta-analysis were performed. The search results were limited to English language studies.

PREOPERATIVE PHASE

The main goal of preoperative assessment is to identify patients at higher risk, to address modifiable risk factors, and to optimize organ function before the surgery, so the patient could be in the best possible condition for the operation. Therefore, during preoperative phase, attention is focused on the risk assessment and optimization of patient's medical condition.

Anemia, malnutrition, and chronic obstructive pulmonary disease (COPD) are frequent in patients undergoing thoracic surgery and should be treated before the surgery. Malnutrition is common in cancer patients. It is associated with impaired wound healing, muscle weakness, immune dysfunction, leading to delayed recovery, prolonged length of stay, and costs (11). According to the European Society for Nutrition and Metabolism Guidelines, patients should be screened for malnutrition preoperatively, and those with increased risk should receive nutritional support for 10–14 days before the major surgery (12). Preoperative fasting from midnight is not necessary, as it was proven that patients given fluids 2–3 h preoperatively are not at greater risk of aspiration than those fasted for 12 h (13). Preoperative carbohydrate loading (the night before and 2 h before surgery) is recommended (12). There is evidence that preoperative administration of oral carbohydrate liquids is associated with faster recovery and reduced length of hospital stay (14).

Most of the patients undergoing thoracic surgery are high-risk patients. Preoperative risk assessment is essential for identification of higher-risk patients as they can require more intensive post-operative care and preoptimization. There are still controversies whether these patients should be included in ERAS programme.

Poor preoperative lung function, smoking, and physical inactivity are considered to be the risk factors for complications following thoracic surgery (15, 16).

It has been estimated that active smoking at the time of resection increases the risk of postoperative complications such as pneumonia, myocardial infarction, and stroke. It is also associated with a higher likelihood of death within 30 days after surgery (17). There are still controversies about the optimal time for smoking cessation. One study even reported an increase in perioperative pulmonary complications when smoking cessation occurred just before the surgery (18). Nevertheless, patients should be advised to stop smoking irrespective of timing of operation.

Improving lung function should be one of the main preoperative management strategies. With the aim to improve tolerance to the surgical procedure and enhance postoperative recovery, the concept of preoperative pulmonary rehabilitation was introduced. It integrates exercise training and self-management education. Some studies have shown that preoperative pulmonary rehabilitation can optimize functional state, decrease symptoms, and improve quality of life in patients with COPD (19). The interventions of pulmonary rehabilitation, including exercise training and smoking cessation, were also examined in patients with lung cancer and COPD undergoing lung resection. It has been shown that pulmonary rehabilitation, both before and after surgery significantly improves forced expiratory volume in 1 s (FEV_1), forced vital capacity, and quality of life (16, 20). Data from a meta-analysis and two systematic reviews have shown that preoperative exercise and smoking cessation in patients undergoing lung resection due to lung cancer, significantly improve pulmonary function and functional capacity, reduce postoperative morbidity and hospital length of stay. However, when exercises were performed only postoperatively, length of stay and postoperative morbidity did not reduce (21–23), which can be explained by the differences in the training programs among the studies.

Available data suggest that preoperative pulmonary rehabilitation, as the part of ERP in thoracic surgery, can improve exercise capacity, as well as reduce postoperative morbidity and mortality in patients with lung cancer. On the other hand, it is recommended not to delay an operation in patients with lung cancer in order to perform preoperative rehabilitation. In the context of aforementioned facts, consensus should be achieved about the training programs, as well as adequate duration of preoperative pulmonary rehabilitation.

Current ERAS guidelines recommend patient education and counseling (24). Patients should be given information about the surgical procedure, anesthesia, and recovery course. They should be encouraged to actively participate in their care as it can contribute to enhanced recovery.

Patient education, preoperative anesthetic assessment, and optimization of patient's medical condition present an essential part of preoperative phase of ERP in thoracic surgery.

During preoperative phase, special attention should be paid to the airway assessment. One—lung ventilation in patients with difficult airway can be very challenging. Chest radiography and computed tomography are important for airway assessment and selection of an appropriate double-lumen endotracheal tube (DLT). Identification of patients with difficult airway is essential for airway management planning and selection of an appropriate lung isolation device. In patients with already known or anticipated difficult airway the best option to establish an airway is by a single-lumen tube (SLT) while lung isolation can be achieved by bronchial blocker, or an SLT can be substituted with a DLT using an airway catheter technique (25).

INTRAOPERATIVE PHASE

During intraoperative period, many strategies and techniques can be applied to prevent pulmonary complications.

Surgical Techniques

The posterolateral thoracotomy (PLT), which is the traditional approach to lung resection, implies muscle-cutting incision. It provides good surgical access, but is associated with increased postoperative pain and reduced respiratory effort (26). With the aim to overcome disadvantages of PLT, muscle—sparing thoracotomy using anterolateral approach and video-assisted thoracoscopic surgery (VATS) were introduced.

Recent studies, including a meta-analysis (27), systematic review (28), and propensity-matched analysis, from Society of Thoracic Surgeons database (29) have shown significantly lower morbidity rate and shorter hospital stay in patients undergoing VATS lobectomy compared with open thoracotomy. The results from these studies are in line with recent findings from the database study from the European Society of Thoracic Surgeon Registry, which compared the outcome following VATS lobectomy versus open lobectomy in case-matched groups of patients (30). The study included 28,771 patients; 26,050 having thoracotomy and 2,721 having thoracoscopy. Compared with thoracotomy, patients undergoing VATS lobectomy had significantly lower incidence of total complications (29.1 vs. 31.7%), wound infection (0.2 vs. 0.6%), and atelectasis requiring bronchoscopy (2.4 vs. 5.5%). Patients undergoing VATS lobectomy had 2 days shorter hospital stay compared with those undergoing thoracotomy, and mortality at hospital discharge was significantly lower in this group (1.0 vs. 1.9%). Concerning patients older than 70 years, the results from this study showed significantly lower number of major cardiopulmonary complications and atelectasis, shorter length of stay, and reduced mortality in the VATS group of patients compared with patients undergoing thoracotomy. The data from these studies confirmed that in comparison to thoracotomy, lobectomies performed *via* VATS are associated with lower incidence of complications, shorter length of stay, and decreased mortality, even in high-risk patients (31). The benefits of VATS on long-term outcomes were also reported. A recent meta-analysis of 20 observational studies reported that compared with open lobectomies, VATS lobectomies were associated with improved long-term outcomes (32).

Due to its beneficial effects on patient recovery, VATS represent one of the main elements of an enhanced recovery in thoracic surgery. To minimize the injury during VATS, the idea of uniportal thoracoscopic surgery has risen. The perioperative outcomes of a single-port, two-port, and three-port approaches were studied. Recent study has shown that VATS single-port and two-port pulmonary resection were associated with decreased volume of drainage, shorter length of stay, and shorter duration of chest drainage (33). However, further randomized controlled trials with larger number of patients are needed to confirm the beneficial effects of single-port compared to three-port VATS pulmonary resections.

Anesthetic Management

Anesthetic management directed at improving patients' recovery includes maintenance of normothermia, the use of short-acting agents, protective lung ventilation (PLV), avoidance of fluid overload, and effective analgesia (34). Unlike intravenous anesthetics, volatile anesthetics inhibit hypoxic pulmonary vasoconstriction. However, some data suggest that there is no significant effect of volatile anesthetics on shunt when used in clinically relevant concentrations (35). Recent studies report the suppressive effect of volatile anesthetics and propofol on the alveolar inflammatory response during one-lung ventilation (OLV) (36).

Perioperative Fluid Management

One of the most severe pulmonary complications in thoracic surgery is an acute lung injury (ALI), presenting the main cause of mortality in patients undergoing lung resection (37). The main task of anesthesiologists is to prevent the development of

ALI focusing on the optimal fluid management, by balancing the risks for complications of fluid overload against the risks of hypovolemia and hypoperfusion. Fluid management in thoracic surgery is still controversial topic. There are disadvantages at both sides of regimes—liberal and restrictive. Numerous studies have demonstrated that excessive fluid administration can lead to postresection ALI (38–40).

It has been shown that administration of fluid >2l during pneumonectomy has negative effects on postoperative outcome (41, 42). Similar results are obtained in the studies that evaluated outcome in patients undergoing lesser pulmonary resections managed with high fluid loads (42, 43). On the other hand, there is concern that restrictive regimen can contribute to organ hypoperfusion leading to an acute kidney injury (AKI). In a retrospective study that included 1,442 patients undergoing thoracic surgery with crystalloid restriction <3 ml/kg/h, it was found that the incidence of AKI was 5.1%. The study concluded that fluid restriction neither increased nor was a risk factor for AKI (44). Recent data suggest that crystalloid administration should be <2 l intraoperatively, and <3 l during first 24 h with total fluid balance less than 20 ml/kg during the first 24 h postoperatively (42). Fluid restriction is not just important in prevention of ALI. It has been shown that fluid restrictive therapy leads to earlier resolution of already developed ALI without increasing the risk of AKI (45).

Considering the risk of AKI in a restrictive fluid management, normovolemic and goal-directed therapy protocols were examined. A prospective observational study examined the effects of normovolemia and protective lung ventilation on the development of ALI and found no increase in extravacular lung water (46). However, further studies are needed to find the optimal fluid regimen in patients undergoing pulmonary resections.

Protective Lung Ventilation

Tissue trauma during surgical intervention, lung hyperinflation, repetitive reexpansion of already collapsed alveoli, and reperfusion during OLV induce cytokine release leading to pulmonary inflammatory response (47).

It has been shown that despite potential hypoxemia, PLV reduces inflammatory response during OLV and consequently the incidence of ALI and postoperative atelectasis (48, 49). The aim of PLV is to minimize pulmonary trauma and avoid respiratory complications including lung injury. It can be achieved by avoiding overdistension and elevated plateau pressure, while providing adequate oxygenation and recruitment of alveoli (50). Although high tidal volumes (10 ml/kg/min) improve oxygenation during OLV, data from animal and human studies suggest that high tidal volumes and high pressures during ventilation are associated with lung injury (43).

Recommendations for OLV suggest that tidal volume of 4–6 ml/kg is protective (50). Protective OLV with low tidal volume is associated with increase in $PaCO_2$. Increase of respiratory rate decreases $PaCO_2$, but is associated with alveolar collapse–reexpansion cycles leading to atelectotrauma (50). Therefore, permissive hypercapnia is acceptable during protective OLV, while an adequate PEEP applied to the dependent lung keeps the alveoli open, provides oxygenation, and decreases lung injury. In patients with decreased functional residual capacity (FRC), PEEP applied to the dependent lung recruits alveoli and improves oxygenation. However, in patients with increased FRC, PEEP will decrease cardiac output and increase alveolar pressure, which will consequently increase vascular resistance in the dependent lung and increase hypoxemia by diverting blood flow to the nondependent lung (51).

The value of PEEP should be adjusted according to the respiratory mechanics of the patient, as on the one hand it should prevent lung overdistension, and on the other hand, it should recruit alveoli without hemodynamic impairment.

POSTOPERATIVE PHASE

During postoperative period, the main goal of ERP is to promote early recovery. Early mobilization, adequate pain control, and postoperative pulmonary rehabilitation present the key elements of the postoperative ERP.

Pain Management

Pain after thoracic surgery impairs effective chest expansion, coughing, and breathing leading to postoperative atelectasis and pneumonia (52). Therefore, the main goal during postoperative period is to provide effective pain relief as it improves respiratory function and reduces postoperative complications. Regional anesthetic blockade in combination with systemic nonopioid analgesia present the basis of opioid sparing multimodal analgesia in thoracic surgery.

Thoracic epidural analgesia (TEA) is considered the gold standard technique for pain control after thoracic surgery and an essential part of ERAS protocols. In comparison with conventional analgesia techniques, TEA provides superior analgesia for post-thoracotomy pain (53), attenuates surgical stress response, having a positive impact on postoperative recovery. However, TEA has several disadvantages including hypotension, urinary retention, and muscular weakness. It can be overcome by performing thoracic paravertebral block (PVB). Recent meta-analysis and systematic reviews confirmed that PVB provides comparable analgesia to the TEA, but with statistically significant lower incidence of side effects, suggesting PVB as analgesic technique for major thoracic surgery (54, 55).

Although negative effects of morphine on respiratory function are described, intravenous patient-controlled analgesia (PCA) with morphine is widely used for pain control following thoracic procedures. To reduce the dose of morphine, ketamin was added to PCA morphine. It was reported that addition of low dose of ketamin to PCA morphine provides better analgesia than PCA morphine alone, reduces morphine consumption, and improves respiratory function (56).

Chest Drain Management

Chest tubes impair patient mobilization, exacerbate pain, and impose the risk of infection. Early chest tube removal improves forced expiratory volume in 1 s and enhances recovery of vital capacity after thoracic procedures (57). It also reduces pain, allows early mobilization of the patient, and results in shorter hospital stay. Therefore, early chest drain removal represents an important element of fast-tracking protocol in thoracic surgery.

Removal of drains is determined by the volume of fluid drainage. Majority of thoracic surgeons prefer leaving the chest tube until fluid drainage decreases to 250 ml/day or less, which prolongs hospital length of stay and delays discharge. Numerous studies have demonstrated that higher threshold for chest drain removal is safe. Nevertheless, there is still debate about the fluid threshold before chest drain removal. Recently, Bjerregaard et al. reported that chest drain removal after VATS lobectomy is safe despite volumes of serous fluid production up to 500 ml/day (58). Unlike these data, data from other studies suggest that 450 ml/day volume threshold for chest tube removal increases the risk for complications (59). However, the consensus on the fluid threshold before tubes removal should be achieved.

FUTURE DIRECTIONS

In the era of ERAS protocols, steps forward were made in the field of thoracoscopic surgery. With the aim to avoid complications related to tracheal intubation and to enhance postoperative recovery, efforts have been made to perform VATS procedures without tracheal intubation. The anesthetic technique consists of regional anesthesia and sedation in spontaneously single-lung breathing patient after performing an iatrogenic open pneumothorax (60). The inhibition of cough reflex is achieved by ipsilateral vagal blockade or stellate ganglion block (61, 62). However, open pneumothorax can compromise ventilation and oxygenation in a non-intubated patient leading to hypoxemia and hypercapnia due to carbon dioxide rebreathing from non-dependent lung. Hypercapnia is often mild and well-tolerated, while satisfactory oxygenation is usually maintained *via* face-mask (60). Recently, the first reports about the use of transnasal humidified rapid-insufflation ventilatory exchange (THRIVE) in non-intubated VATS have appeared. It has been shown that in comparison to conventional oxygen masks, THRIVE with a flow rate at 20 l/min of oxygen, significantly improves oxygenation during non-intubated VATS, without expanding collapsed lung (63). Growing body of evidence suggests that non-intubated VATS procedures are safe and feasible to various thoracic procedures including pneumothorax management, wedge pulmonary resections, segmentectomy, lobectomy, as well as excision of mediastinal tumors (60). Recent studies reported that in comparison with double-lumen intubated general anesthesia, non-intubated thoracoscopic procedures were superior in terms of complication rate, overall hospital stay, and need for nursing care (62, 64, 65). Data from these studies suggest that non-intubated VATS could become an important element of ERP in the future.

CONCLUSION

Enhanced recovery protocol presents an evidence-based approach to patient care. Although there are variations in ERP among the institutions, the evidence suggests that implementation of ERPs in thoracic surgery significantly reduces postoperative complications and length of hospital stay. The role of anesthesiologists is very important during all the three phases of ERP. Minimally invasive surgical technique, adequate perioperative fluid management, protective ventilation, effective pain control, and patient's active collaboration are essential elements of ERP in thoracic surgery. In the era of fast-tracking, the results of studies regarding non-intubated VATS are promising.

AUTHOR CONTRIBUTIONS

All aforementioned authors contributed significantly to the final design of manuscript.

REFERENCES

1. Jakobson T, Karjagin J, Vipp L, Padar M, Parik AH, Starkopf L. Postoperative complications and mortality after major gastrointestinal surgery. *Medicina (Kaunas)* (2014) 50(2):111–7. doi:10.1016/j.medici.2014.06.002
2. Laursen LØ, Petersen RH, Hansen HJ, Jensen TK, Ravn J, Konge L. Videoassisted thoracoscopic surgery lobectomy for lung cancer is associated with a lower 30-day morbidity compared with lobectomy by thoracotomy. *Eur J Cardiothorac Surg* (2016) 49(3):870–5. doi:10.1093/ejcts/ezv205
3. Handy JJR, Asaph JW, Skokan L, Reed CE, Koh S, Brooks G, et al. What happens to patients undergoing lung cancer surgery? Outcomes and quality of life before and after surgery. *Chest* (2002) 122(1):21–30. doi:10.1378/chest.122.1.21
4. Patel AS, Bergman A, Moore BW, Haglund U. The economic burden of complications occurring in major surgical procedures: a systematic review. *Appl Health Econ Health Policy* (2013) 11(6):577–92. doi:10.1007/s40258-013-0060-y
5. Brunelli A. Enhanced recovery after surgery in thoracic surgery: the past, the present and the future. *Video Assist Thorac Surg* (2017) 2:37. doi:10.21037/vats.2017.07.02
6. Melnyk M, Casey RG, Black P, Koupparis AJ. Enhanced recovery after surgery (ERAS) protocols: time to change practice? *Can Urol Assoc J* (2011) 5(5): 342–8. doi:10.5489/cuaj.11002
7. Kehlet H. Multimodal approach to control postoperative pathophysiology and rehabilitation. *Br J Anaesth* (1997) 78(5):606–606. doi:10.1093/bja/78.5.606
8. Kehlet H. Fast-track colorectal surgery. *Lancet* (2008) 371(9615):791–3. doi:10.1016/S0140-6736(08)60357-8
9. Ljungqvist O, Scott M, Fearon KC. Enhanced recovery after surgery: a review. *JAMA Surg* (2017) 152(3):292–8. doi:10.1001/jamasurg.2016.4952
10. Lawrence VA, Cornell JE, Smetana GW, American College of Physicians. Strategies to reduce postoperative pulmonary complications after non-cardiothoracic surgery: systematic review for the American College of Physicians. *Ann Intern Med* (2006) 144(8):596–608. doi:10.7326/0003-4819-144-8-200604180-00011
11. Kuzu MA, Terzioglu H, Genc V, Erkek AB, Ozban M, Sonyürek P, et al. Preoperative nutritional risk assessment in predicting postoperative outcome in patients undergoing major surgery. *World J Surg* (2006) 30(3):378–90. doi:10.1007/s00268-005-0163-1
12. Weimann A, Braga M, Harsanyi L, Laviano A, Ljungqvist O, Soeters P, et al. ESPEN Guidelines on Enteral Nutrition: surgery including organ transplantation. *Clin Nutr* (2006) 25(2):224–44. doi:10.1016/j.clnu.2006.01.015
13. Brady M, Kinn S, Stuart P. Preoperative fasting for adults to prevent perioperative complications. *Cochrane Database Syst Rev* (2003) (4):CD004423. doi:10.1002/14651858.CD004423
14. Noblett SE, Watson DS, Huong H, Davison B, Hainsworth PJ, Horgan AF. Pre-operative oral carbohydrate loading in colorectal surgery: a randomized controlled trial. *Colorectal Dis* (2006) 8(7):563–9. doi:10.1111/j.1463-1318.2006.00965.x
15. Wright CD, Gaissert HA, Grab JD, O'Brien SM, Peterson ED, Allen MS. Predictors of prolonged length of stay after lobectomy for lung cancer: a Society of Thoracic Surgeons General Thoracic Surgery Database risk-adjustment model. *Ann Thorac Surg* (2008) 85(6):1857–65. doi:10.1016/j.athoracsur.2008.03.024
16. Vagvolgyi A, Rozgonyi Z, Kerti M, Vadasz P, Varga J. Effectiveness of perioperative pulmonary rehabilitation in thoracic surgery. *J Thorac Dis* (2017) 9(6):1584–91. doi:10.21037/jtd.2017.05.49

17. Turan A, Mascha E, Roberman D, Turner PL, You J, Kurz A, et al. Smoking and perioperative outcomes. *Anesthesiology* (2011) 114(4):837–46. doi:10.1097/ALN.0b013e318210f560
18. Bluman LG, Mosca L, Newman N, Simon DG. Preoperative smoking habits and postoperative pulmonary complications. *Chest* (1998) 113(4):883–9. doi:10.1378/chest.113.4.883
19. Spruit MA, Singh SJ, Garvey C, ZuWallack R, Nici L, Rochester C, et al. An official American Thoracic Society/European Respiratory Society statement: key concepts and advances in pulmonary rehabilitation. *Am J Respir Crit Care Med* (2013) 188(8):e13–64. doi:10.1164/rccm.201309-1634ST
20. Bobbio A, Chetta A, Ampollini L, Primomo GL, Internullo E, Carbognani P, et al. Preoperative pulmonary rehabilitation in patients undergoing lung resection for non-small cell lung cancer. *Eur J Cardiothorac Surg* (2008) 33(1):95–8. doi:10.1016/j.ejcts.2007.10.003
21. Mainini C, Rebelo PF, Bardelli R, Kopliku B, Tenconi S, Costi S, et al. Perioperative physical exercise interventions for patients undergoing lung cancer surgery: what is the evidence? *SAGE Open Med* (2016) 4:1–19. doi:10.1177/2050312116673855
22. Rodriguez-Larrad A, Lascurain-Aguirrebena I, Abecia-Inchaurregui LC, Seco J. Perioperative physiotherapy in patients undergoing lung cancer resection. *Interact Cardiovasc Thorac Surg* (2014) 19(2):269–81. doi:10.1093/icvts/ivu126
23. Sebio Garcia R, Yanez Brage MI, Gimenez Moolhuyzen E, Granger CL, Denehy L. Functional and postoperative outcomes after preoperative exercise training in patients with lung cancer: a systematic review and meta-analysis. *Interact Cardiovasc Thorac Surg* (2016) 23(3):486–97. doi:10.1093/icvts/ivw152
24. Jankowski CJ. Preparing the patient for enhanced recovery after surgery. *Int Anesthesiol Clin* (2017) 55(4):12–20. doi:10.1097/AIA.0000000000000157
25. Campos JH. Lung isolation techniques for patients with difficult airway. *Curr Opin Anaesthesiol* (2010) 23(1):12–7. doi:10.1097/ACO.0b013e328331e8a7
26. Loscertales J, Congregado M, Moreno S, Jimenez-Merchan R. Posterolateral thoracotomy without muscle division: a new approach to complex procedures. *Interact Cardiovasc Thorac Surg* (2012) 14(1):2–4. doi:10.1093/icvts/ivr059
27. Cao C, Zhu ZH, Yan TD, Wang Q, Jiang G, Liu L, et al. Video-assisted thoracic surgery versus open thoracotomy for nonsmall-cell lung cancer: a propensity score analysis based on a multiinstitutional registry. *Eur J Cardiothorac Surg* (2013) 44(5):849–54. doi:10.1093/ejcts/ezt406
28. Whitson BA, Groth SS, Duval SJ, Swanson SJ, Maddaus MA. Surgery for early-stage non-small cell lung cancer: a systematic review of the video-assisted thoracoscopic surgery versus thoracotomy approaches to lobectomy. *Ann Thorac Surg* (2008) 86(6):2008–18. doi:10.1016/j.athoracsur.2008.07.009
29. Paul S, Altorki NK, Sheng S, Lee PC, Harpole DH, Onaitis MW, et al. Thoracoscopic lobectomy is associated with lower morbidity than open lobectomy: a propensity-matched analysis from the STS database. *J Thorac Cardiovasc Surg* (2010) 139(2):366–78. doi:10.1016/j.jtcvs.2009.08.026
30. Falcoz PE, Puyraveau M, Thomas PA, Decaluwe H, Hürtgen M, Petersen RH, et al. Video-assisted thoracoscopic surgery versus open lobectomy for primary non-small-cell lung cancer: a propensity-matched analysis of outcome from the European Society of Thoracic Surgeon database. *Eur J Cardiothorac Surg* (2016) 49(2):602–9. doi:10.1093/ejcts/ezv154
31. Burt BM, Kosinski AS, Shrager JB, Onaitis MW, Weigel T. Thoracoscopic lobectomy is associated with acceptable morbidity and mortality in patients with predicted postoperative forced expiratory volume in 1 second or diffusing capacity for carbon monoxide less than 40% of normal. *J Thorac Cardiovasc Surg* (2014) 148(1):19–28. doi:10.1016/j.jtcvs.2014.03.007
32. Taioli E, Lee DS, Lesser M, Flores R. Long-term survival in video-assisted thoracoscopic lobectomy vs open lobectomy in lung-cancer patients: a meta-analysis. *Eur J Cardiothorac Surg* (2013) 44(4):591–7. doi:10.1093/ejcts/ezt051
33. Mu JW, Gao SG, Xue Q, Mao YS, Wang DL, Zhao J, et al. A propensity matched comparison of effects between video assisted thoracoscopic single-port, two-port and three-port pulmonary resection on lung cancer. *J Thorac Dis* (2016) 8(7):1469–76. doi:10.21037/jtd.2016.05.64
34. Jones NL, Edmonds L, Ghosh S, Klein AA. A review of enhanced recovery for thoracic anaesthesia and surgery. *Anaesthesia* (2013) 68(2):179–89. doi:10.1111/anae.12067
35. Beck DH, Doepfmer UR, Sinemus C, Bloch A, Schenk MR, Kox WJ. Effects of sevoflurane and propofol on pulmonary shunt fraction during one-lung ventilation for thoracic surgery. *Br J Anaesth* (2001) 86:38–43. doi:10.1093/bja/86.1.38
36. Schilling T, Kozian A, Senturk M, Huth C, Reinhold A, Hedenstierna G, et al. Effects of volatile and intravenous anesthesia on the alveolar and systemic inflammatory response in thoracic surgical patients. *Anesthesiology* (2011) 115(1):65–74. doi:10.1097/ALN.0b013e318214b9de
37. Licker M, Fauconnet P, Villiger Y, Tschopp JM. Acute lung injury and outcomes after thoracic surgery. *Curr Opin Anaesth* (2009) 22(1):61–7. doi:10.1097/ACO.0b013e32831b466c
38. Arslantas M, Kara H, Tuncer B, Yildizeli B, Yuksel M, Bostanci K. Effect of the amount of intraoperative fluid administration on postoperative pulmonary complications following anatomic lung resections. *J Thorac Cardiovasc Surg* (2015) 149(1):314–21. doi:10.1016/j.jtcvs.2014.08.071
39. Evans R, Naidu B. Does a conservative fluid management strategy in the perioperative management of lung resection patients reduce the risk of acute lung injury? *Interact Cardiovasc Thorac Surg* (2012) 15(3):498–504. doi:10.1093/icvts/ivs175
40. Alam N, Park B, Wilton A. Incidence and risk factors for lung injury after lung cancer resection. *Ann Thorac Surg* (2007) 84(4):1085–91. doi:10.1016/j.athoracsur.2007.05.053
41. Marret E, Miled F, Bazelly B, El Metaoua S, de Montblanc J, Quesnel C, et al. Risk and protective factors for major complications after pneumonectomy for lung cancer. *Interact Cardiovasc Thorac Surg* (2010) 10(6):936–9. doi:10.1510/icvts.2009.231621
42. Chau EHL, Slinger P. Perioperative fluid management for pulmonary resection surgery and esophagectomy. *Semin Cardiothorac Vasc Anesth* (2014) 18(1):36–44. doi:10.1177/1089253213491014
43. Licker M, de Perrot M, Spiliopoulos A, Robert J, Diaper J, Chevalley C, et al. Risk factors for acute lung injury after thoracic surgery for lung cancer. *Anesth Analg* (2003) 97(6):1558–65. doi:10.1213/01.ANE.0000087799.85495.8A
44. Ahn HJ, Kim JA, Lee AR, Yang M, Jung HJ, Heo B. The risk of acute kidney injury from fluid restriction and hydroxyethyl starch in thoracic surgery. *Anesth Analg* (2016) 122(1):186–93. doi:10.1213/ANE.0000000000000974
45. Wiedemann HP, Wheeler AP, Bernard GR, Thompson BT, Hayden D, deBoisblanc B, et al. Comparison of two fluid-management strategies in acute lung injury. *N Engl J Med* (2006) 354(24):2564–75. doi:10.1056/NEJMoa062200
46. Assaad S, Kyriakides T, Tellides G, Kim AW, Perkal M, Perrino A. Extravascular lung water and tissue perfusion biomarkers after lung resection surgery under a normovolemic fluid protocol. *J Cardiothorac Vasc Anesth* (2015) 29(4):977–83. doi:10.1053/j.jvca.2014.12.020
47. Sugasawa Y, Yamaguchi K, Kumakura S, Murakami T, Kugimiya T, Suzuki K, et al. The effect of one-lung ventilation upon pulmonary inflammatory responses during lung resection. *J Anesth* (2011) 25(2):170–7. doi:10.1007/s00540-011-1100-0
48. Tugrul M, Camci E, Karadeniz H, Senturk M, Pembeci K, Akpir K. Comparison of volume controlled with pressure controlled ventilation during one-lung anaesthesia. *Br J Anaesth* (1997) 79(3):306–10. doi:10.1093/bja/79.3.306
49. Yang M, Ahn HJ, Kim K, Kim JA, Yi CA, Kim MJ, et al. Does a protective ventilation strategy reduce the risk of pulmonary complications after lung cancer surgery? A randomized controlled trial. *Chest* (2011) 139(3):530–7. doi:10.1378/chest.09-2293
50. Della Rocca G, Coccia C. Acute lung injury in thoracic surgery. *Curr Opin Anaesthesiol* (2013) 26(1):40–6. doi:10.1097/ACO.0b013e32835c4ea2
51. Katz JA, Laverne RG, Fairley HB, Thomas AN. Pulmonary oxygen exchange during endobronchial anesthesia: effects of tidal volume and PEEP. *Anesthesiology* (1982) 56:164–71. doi:10.1097/00000542-198203000-00002
52. Silomon M, Claus T, Huwer H, Biedler A, Larsen R, Molter G. Interpleural analgesia does not influence postthoracotomy pain. *Anesth Analg* (2000) 91(1):44–50. doi:10.1213/00000539-200007000-00009
53. Ling XM, Fang F, Zhang XG, Ding M, Liu QA, Cang J. Effect of parecoxib combined with thoracic epidural analgesia on pain after thoracotomy. *J Thorac Dis* (2016) 8(5):880–7. doi:10.21037/jtd.2016.03.45
54. Davies RG, Myles PS, Graham JM. A comparison of the analgesic efficacy and side-effects of paravertebral vs. epidural blockade for thoracotomy – a systematic review and meta-analysis of randomized trials. *Br J Anaesth* (2006) 96(4):418–26. doi:10.1093/bja/ael020
55. Joshi GP, Bonnet F, Shah R, Wilkinson RC, Camu F, Fischer B, et al. A systematic review of randomized trials evaluating regional techniques

for postthoracotomy analgesia. *Anesth Analg* (2008) 107(3):1026–40. doi:10.1213/01.ane.0000333274.63501.ff

56. Michelet P, Guervilly C, Hélaine A, Avaro JP, Blayac D, Gaillat F, et al. Adding ketamine to morphine for patient-controlled analgesia after thoracic surgery: influence on morphine consumption, respiratory function, and nocturnal desaturation. *Br J Anaesth* (2007) 99(3):396–403. doi:10.1093/bja/aem168
57. Refai M, Brunelli A, Salati M, Xiumè F, Pompili C, Sabbatini A. The impact of chest tube removal on pain and pulmonary function after pulmonary resection. *Eur J Cardiothorac Surg* (2012) 41(4):820–2. doi:10.1093/ejcts/ezr126
58. Bjerregaard LS, Jensen K, Petersen RH, Hansen HJ. Early chest tube removal after video-assisted thoracic surgery lobectomy with serous fluid production up to 500 ml/day. *Eur J Cardiothorac Surg* (2014) 45(2):241–6. doi:10.1093/ejcts/ezt376
59. Xie HY, Xu K, Tang JX, Bian W, Ma HT, Zhao J, et al. A prospective randomized, controlled trial deems a drainage of 300 ml/day safe before removal of the last chest drain after video-assisted thoracoscopic surgery lobectomy. *Interact Cardiovasc Thorac Surg* (2015) 21:200–5. doi:10.1093/icvts/ivv115
60. Hung MH, Hsu HH, Cheng YJ, Chen JS. Nonintubated thoracoscopic surgery: state of the art and future directions. *J Thorac Dis* (2014) 6(1):2–9. doi:10.3978/j.issn.2072-1439.2014.01.16
61. Al-Abdullatief M, Wahood A, Al-Shirawi N, Arabi Y, Wahba M, Al-Jumah M, et al. Awake anaesthesia for major thoracic surgical procedures: an observational study. *Eur J Cardiothorac Surg* (2007) 32(2):346–50. doi:10.1016/j.ejcts.2007.04.029
62. Chen KC, Cheng YJ, Hung MH, Tseng YD, Chen JS. Nonintubated thoracoscopic lung resection: a 3-year experience with 285 cases in a single institution. *J Thorac Dis* (2012) 4(4):347–51. doi:10.3978/j.issn.2072-1439.2012.08.07
63. Wang ML, Hung MH, Chen JS, Hsu HH, Cheng YJ. Nasal high-flow oxygen therapy improves arterial oxygenation during one-lung ventilation in non-intubated thoracoscopic surgery. *Eur J Cardiothorac Surg* (2017):1–6. doi:10.1093/ejcts/ezx450
64. Pompeo E, Tacconi F, Mineo TC. Comparative results of non-resectional lung volume reduction performed by awake or non-awake anesthesia. *Eur J Cardiothorac Surg* (2011) 39(4):e51–8. doi:10.1016/j.ejcts.2010.11.071
65. Pompeo E, Mineo D, Rogliani P, Sabato AF, Mineo TC. Feasibility and results of awake thoracoscopic resection of solitary pulmonary nodules. *Ann Thorac Surg* (2004) 78(5):1761–8. doi:10.1016/j.athoracsur.2004.05.083

16

Laparoscopic Subtotal Gastrectomy and Sigmoidectomy Combined with Natural Orifice Specimen Extraction Surgery (NOSES) for Synchronous Gastric Cancer and Sigmoid Colon Cancer

*Qingshun Zhu[1], Lei Yu[1], Guangxu Zhu[2], Xuguang Jiao[2], Bowen Li[1] and Jianjun Qu[2]**

[1]Department of Clinical Medical College, Weifang Medical University, Weifang, China, [2]Department of General Surgery, The First Affiliated Hospital of Weifang Medical College, Weifang People's Hospital, Weifang, China

***Correspondence:**
Jianjun Qu
urodoc@163.com

Background: Gastric cancer and colon cancer are rarely seen in clinic, but there are still related reports. For gastric cancer and simultaneous colon cancer, surgical resection is the main treatment. Traditional surgery requires an incision from xiphoid process to pubic symphysis. With the progress of minimally invasive technology, laparoscopic surgery is also used in the treatment of gastric cancer, but also in the abdominal incision to remove specimens and in vitro anastomosis of digestive tract. Taking specimens through the natural cavity as a new surgical method can not only reduce the abdominal incision, but also reduce the occurrence of wound-related complications. Here, we report a patient with gastric cancer and colon cancer who was treated in our hospital.

Case Summary: We report a series of patients with gastric cancer and colon cancer. upper abdominal pain was treated in our hospital for 6 months. electronic gastroscopy showed large irregular ulcers on the lesser curvature of the gastric antrum and biopsy showed poorly differentiated adenocarcinoma of the gastric antrum. The enhanced CT of abdomen and pelvis showed irregular thickening of gastric antrum wall, irregular thickening of sigmoid colon wall and no obvious enlarged lymph nodes around. Further electronic enteroscopy showed that the sigmoid colon showed cauliflower protuberance, the intestinal cavity was slightly narrow, the intestinal wall was stiff, and the biopsy pathology showed moderately differentiated adenocarcinoma of the sigmoid colon. No obvious abnormality was found in serological tumor indexes. We diagnosed gastric cancer with sigmoid colon cancer and the patient received Laparoscopic subtotal gastrectomy and sigmoidectomy combined with natural orifice specimen extraction surgery. At present, 12 months after operation, no clear tumor recurrence was found in the metastasis.

Conclusion: We should improve the understanding of gastric cancer and sigmoid cancer and combine examination with pathology to avoid misdiagnosis as metastatic cancer. Laparoscopic subtotal gastrectomy should be performed for tumors with no serosa invasion, body mass index <30 and tumor diameter <6.5 cm. Sigmoidectomy combined with natural nostril sampling is feasible.

Keywords: gastric cancer, sigmoid colon cancer, natural orifice specimen extraction surgery, laparoscopic surgery, case report

INTRODUCTION

With the popularity of gastroscopy and colonoscopy, gastric cancer and sigmoid colon cancer are often diagnosed at the same time. Surgical resection is still the main treatment method for gastric synchronous sigmoid colon cancer. Studies have shown that laparoscopic surgery is similar to open surgery in terms of safety, efficacy, and completeness of tumor resection (1–3). In recent years, specimen collection through the natural orifice has gradually been used in clinical practice as a new surgical method, which can reduce the incidence of wound-related complications while reducing abdominal incisions (4). For gastric cancer with sigmoid colon cancer, there have been reports of laparoscopic synchronous resection (5), but laparoscopic radical gastrectomy combined with radical sigmoid resection for sigmoid cancer combined with natural orifice specimens for the treatment of gastric cancer with sigmoid colon cancer is rarely reported. Recently, we treated a patient with gastric cancer with sigmoid colon cancer, and performed laparoscopic radical operation for gastric cancer and sigmoid colon cancer with specimens taken from the natural orifice. The report is as follows.

CASE PRESENTATION

Clinical History and Diagnosis

A 73-year-old male patient was admitted to our hospital for 6 months with epigastric pain. Physical examination revealed a soft abdomen, mild upper abdominal tenderness without rebound tenderness, and no obvious mass palpable throughout the abdomen. There was tympanic sound on percussion, negative mobile dullness, no percussion pain in the liver and kidney areas, and no enlarged lymph nodes were palpated in the bilateral supraclavicular areas. Laboratory tests showed no significant increase in tumor markers. Electronic gastroscopy: Huge irregular ulcers with irregular hyperplasia around the lesser curvature of the gastric antrum, surface erosions, and a little oozing blood were seen (**Supplementary Figure S1A**). Gastric biopsy pathology: poorly differentiated adenocarcinoma. Electronic colonoscopy showed that the sigmoid colon was 20–26 cm away from the anus with a cauliflower-like bulge, with hyperemia, edema and erosion on the surface, around the circumference, the intestinal lumen was slightly narrow, and the intestinal wall was rigid (**Supplementary Figure S1B**). Enhanced computed tomography (CT) of the abdomen showed irregular thickening of the gastric antrum wall, enhanced enhancement, no obvious surrounding lymph nodes (**Supplementary Figure S1C**), and the sigmoid colon had local wall thickness and no obvious surrounding swelling. Lymph nodes (**Supplementary Figure S1D**). Because the patients and their families requested surgical treatment, they signed the informed consent form for surgery. We conducted a multidisciplinary oncology consultation for the patient. After evaluating the patient's cardiopulmonary function and no obvious surgical contraindications, we decided to perform Laparoscopic subtotal gastrectomy and sigmoidectomy combined with natural orifice specimen extraction (NOSE) under general anesthesia with tracheal intubation.

Treatment

After successful anesthesia, take the lithotomy position, routinely sterilize the drape, take an incision of about 1 cm above the umbilicus, incision on the skin and all layers of the abdominal wall, insert a 10 mm trocar, establish a pneumoperitoneum, and the carbon dioxide pneumoperitoneum pressure is 10–12 mmHg, and then enter the abdominal cavity. Microscopic examination: no ascites, no metastasis to liver, peritoneum and pelvis. According to the results of preoperative examination and intraoperative exploration, we decided to perform complete laparoscopic radical resection of gastric cancer and sigmoid colon cancer with specimens taken through the natural orifice. We first underwent subtotal gastrectomy. 12 mm trocar was placed as the main operation hole above the midline of the right clavicle and below the costal edge of the left anterior axillary line, and 5 mm trocar was placed above the midline of the left clavicle and below the costal edge of the right anterior axillary line as an auxiliary operation hole. Distal subtotal gastrectomy and standard lymph node dissection were performed under laparoscopy. Digestive tract reconstruction was performed with Billroth II + Braun anastomosis.

To perform sigmoidectomy, 12 mm trocar was placed as the main operating hole at the medial 2 cm of the right anterior superior iliac spine and 5 mm trocar was placed at the left lower abdominal McDonnell's point (**Supplementary Figure S2**). Cut the sigmoid colon at the upper and lower 5 cm of the tumor, Cut open the distal intestine, disinfect with iodophor gauze, and remove the gauze through the rectum to prevent abdominal infection. Put the sterile protective bag into the abdominal cavity from the right 12 mm trocar, put the oval forceps through the anus, pull out one end of the sterile protective bag from the anus, and first put the nail head of the tubular stapler into the abdominal cavity by aseptic protective bag. Then the oval forceps were used to remove the stomach and sigmoid colon specimens successively through the anus. After the specimen was removed, the aseptic protective bag was closed and protruded through the anus (**Supplementary Figure S3**). Close the broken end of the rectum, insert the nail anvil head of the tubular stapler in the proximal colon by reverse puncture, and insert the tubular anastomosis through the anus for end-to-side anastomosis of the rectosigmoid colon, and the anastomosis can be strengthened with absorbable sutures. The abdominal cavity and pelvic cavity were washed, no active bleeding was examined. Abdominal drainage was placed in the splenic fossa, under the gallbladder and in the pelvis and suture the abdominal incision (**Supplementary Figure S4A**).

The operation time was 365 min, the blood loss was 50 mL, specimens of subtotal gastrectomy and sigmoid colon in **Supplementary Figure S4B**. The patient got out of bed 36 h after the operation and was discharged from the hospital 10 days later. Postoperative pathology: (1) Gastric poorly differentiated adenocarcinoma, with an area of 4.5 cm × 3.5 cm, invading the full thickness of the gastric wall, no clear nerve invasion and intravascular tumor thrombus, positive serosal surface, and 48 lymph nodes were detected, none of which were found. See cancer metastasis, no cancer metastasis in omentum tissue, mouth, anus clean margins. (2) Moderately differentiated adenocarcinoma of the sigmoid colon, with an area of 3.5 cm × 2 cm, invading the entire thickness of the intestinal wall and reaching the fat, with tumor thrombi in the vessels, no clear nerve invasion, clean serosa, and 17 lymph nodes were detected around the intestine, all of which were No cancer metastasis was found, the mesenteric resection margin and the surrounding near incision margin were clean, and the mouth and anal incision margins were clean.

Outcome and Follow-Up

There were no complications after the operation, and the patient was discharged smoothly. As of 12 months after operation, no tumor recurrence or metastasis was found.

DISCUSSION

Multiple primary cancer (MPC), also known as compound cancer or repeat cancer, refers to the occurrence of two or more independent primary cancers in the same individual at the same time or in succession. We can understand that (1) every tumor is malignant; (2) the tumor is not the recurrence or metastasis of other tumors; for multiple primary cancers of the digestive system, with the popularization of endoscopy and CT examination, its detection The incidence rate continues to increase, and pathological diagnosis is still the gold standard for the diagnosis of multiple primary cancers. In this case, gastric cancer was first diagnosed by electronic gastroscopy, and sigmoid colon was found to occupy the sigmoid colon during preoperative CT examination, and sigmoid colon cancer was confirmed by colonoscopy. It was a double primary cancer of gastric cancer combined with sigmoid colon cancer. Pre-evaluation is particularly important for the diagnosis of multiple primary cancers. If this patient was misdiagnosed as gastric cancer with colonic metastases, the opportunity for surgery may be missed. Although gastric cancer with colon cancer is rare in clinical practice, there are still 1.3%–3.9% of patients with gastric cancer and colon cancer at the same time. Therefore, it is necessary to use colonoscopy as a routine preoperative examination item for gastric cancer (6–8).

In laparoscopic surgery, whether the placement of trocar is reasonable or not is an important factor affecting the operation. The basic principle is that the operation is convenient, the instruments do not interfere with each other, generally the focus as the center into a fan or diamond distribution is the best. In this case, we first selected the umbilical 1 cm to place the first trocar as the observation hole. In gastric surgery, placing the observation hole above the navel can obtain a good surgical field of vision and is more conducive to the clearance of the upper edge of the pancreas. In sigmoid surgery, because the inferior mesenteric blood vessel is located at the umbilical level, if the observation hole is placed in the umbilical part or too close to the operation site, it is easy to cause lens contamination. Placing the observation hole above the umbilical can avoid this problem. At the same time, the auxiliary operation hole during subtotal gastrectomy can be used as an auxiliary operation hole for sigmoidectomy without additional incision, which reduces the postoperative pain and reduces the incidence of postoperative complications such as trocar hole infection and incision hernia.

For gastric cancer with colon cancer, the conventional surgical method requires an incision from the xiphoid process to the pubic symphysis, because such an incision can ensure thorough lymph node dissection at the same time as tumor resection, severe postoperative pain, and many wound complications. With the advancement of minimally invasive technology, laparoscopy can obtain clearer images and dissect more lymph nodes, but for gastric cancer with colon cancer, laparoscopic surgery also requires a small incision in the abdominal wall to facilitate removal of specimens and anastomosis outside the body. In this case, no additional abdominal incision is required, and rectosigmoid anastomosis can be performed through the anus. Yamamot et al. (9) believe that rectosigmoid end-to-side anastomosis is simple and convenient, and does not increase the risk of anastomotic leakage, and the stool is not in the rectosigmoid blind pouch, which indicates that the channel is well preserved. Pironi et al.

(10) believe that the use of tubular stapler for colorectal anastomosis is a valuable choice. Ikeda et al. (11) believe that manual suture can increase the strength of the anastomosis and reduce the incidence of anastomotic leakage. The operation of rectosigmoid double purse end-to-side anastomosis is simple and economical, and the anastomosis can be strengthened under laparoscope, but it should be noted that if the distal intestinal tube is too long and thin, it is difficult for the stapler to reach the closed end. Violent operation will cause intestinal wall tear or bleeding, resulting in postoperative anastomotic leakage, abdominal infection and other complications. Before anastomosis, we should dilate the anus properly, and then wipe the tubular stapler with iodophor, which can not only prevent infection but also increase the degree of lubrication. This tip can better deal with this problem. Secondly, after the completion of the anastomosis, it is necessary to check the patency of the distal and proximal intestines.

At present, NOSES is gradually used in clinical practice because of its few wound complications and quick postoperative recovery, especially in sigmoid resection. Sumer et al. (12) reported for the first time NOSES total laparoscopic palliative subtotal gastrectomy with colon cancer. The patient had advanced gastric cancer combined with colon cancer, gastrointestinal bleeding and obstruction occurred before surgery, and died of cachexia 3 months after surgery. After the patient was diagnosed with dual primary cancers, after multidisciplinary oncology consultation, it was decided to undergo complete laparoscopic radical resection of gastric cancer and sigmoid colon cancer with specimens taken through the natural orifice. Laparoscopic surgery on the stomach and colon is performed at the same time, both specimens can be pulled out through the rectum, no additional abdominal incision is required, avoiding incision-related complications (incision infection, fat liquefaction, incisional hernia), reducing pain and bringing better Beauty results, faster return to normal work and life. At present, the patient is still alive and healthy 12 months after the operation, and the weight has increased by 2 Kg compared with that before the operation.

However, not all patients are suitable for NOSES, and Izquierdo et al. (13) suggested that the tumor diameter <6.5 cm and the body mass index <30 could improve the prognosis of patients by implementing NOSES. In addition, the aseptic principle and the tumor-free principle are the basic principles that must be adhered to in all gastrointestinal surgical operations. At present, some scholars worry that NOSES will increase the probability of abdominal infection. In this case, the specimen was first placed in the rectal cavity before the specimen was pulled out through the natural orifice. Put the sterile plastic protective sleeve into the protective sleeve, first put the stapler into the abdominal cavity through the protective sleeve, and then drag the specimen out of the body through the protective sleeve, the tumor tissue does not fall off due to extrusion. Up to now, no tumor recurrence or metastasis has been found in the patient.

CONCLUSION

We should improve our understanding of MPC, and combine the examination and pathology to avoid misdiagnosing it as metastatic cancer. Secondly, for tumors that do not invade the serosa, body mass index <30, and tumor diameter <6.5 cm, laparoscopic subtotal gastrectomy should be performed. and sigmoidectomy combined with natural orifice specimen extraction surgery (NOSES) is feasible.

ETHICS STATEMENT

The studies involving human participants were reviewed and approved by Medical Research Ethics Committee of Weifang people's Hospital. The patients/participants provided their written informed consent to participate in this study.

Written informed consent was obtained from the individual(s) for the publication of any potentially identifiable images or data included in this article.

AUTHOR CONTRIBUTIONS

JQ: guarantees the integrity of the entire study and edited the manuscript. QZ and LY: prepared and edited the manuscript. GZ, XJ, and BL: performed the literature research, data analysis, and text proofreading. All authors contributed to the article and approved the submitted version.

ACKNOWLEDGMENTS

I would like to express my gratitude to all those who helped me during the writing of this manuscript and their efforts in the management of this patient.

REFERENCES

1. Best LM, Mughal M, Gurusamy KS. Laparoscopic versus open gastrectomy for gastric cancer. *Cochrane Database Syst Rev.* (2016) 3:CD011389. doi: 10.1002/14651858.CD011389.pub2
2. Morneau M, Boulanger J, Charlebois P, Latulippe JF, Lougnarath R, Thibault C, et al. Laparoscopic versus open surgery for the treatment of colorectal cancer: a literature review and recommendations from the Comité de l'évolution des pratiques en oncologie. *Can J Surg.* (2013) 56:297–310. doi: 10.1503/cjs.005512
3. Hyung WJ, Yang HK, Park YK, Lee HJ, An JY, Kim W, et al. Long-term outcomes of laparoscopic distal gastrectomy for locally advanced gastric cancer: the KLASS-02-RCT randomized clinical trial. *J Clin Oncol.* (2020) 38:3304–13. doi: 10.1200/JCO.20.01210
4. Masubuchi S, Okuda J, Yamamoto M, Inoue Y, Tanaka K, Uchiyama K. Natural orifice specimen extraction in laparoscopic colorectal cancer surgery: a case series study. *Int J Surg Case Rep.* (2021) 78:204–9. doi: 10.1016/j.ijscr.2020.12.059

5. Mederos R, Lamas JR, Ramos A, Farooq A, Farooq SK. Simultaneous subtotal gastrectomy and right colectomy for synchronous gastric and colon cancer: a case report. *Cureus.* (2019) 11(1):e3892. doi: 10.7759/cureus.3892
6. Saito S, Hosoya Y, Togashi K, Kurashina K, Haruta H, Hyodo M, et al. Prevalence of synchronous colorectal neoplasms detected by colonoscopy in patients with gastric cancer. *Surg Today.* (2008) 38:20–5. doi: 10.1007/s00595-007-3567-8
7. Suzuki A, Koide N, Takeuchi D, Okumura M, Ishizone S, Suga T, et al. Prevalence of synchronous colorectal neoplasms in surgically treated gastric cancer patients and significance of screening colonoscopy. *Dig Endosc.* (2014) 26:396–402. doi: 10.1111/den.12156
8. Lee JH, Bae JS, Ryu KW, Lee JS, Park SR, Kim CG, et al. Gastric cancer patients at high-risk of having synchronous cancer. *World J Gastroenterol.* (2006) 12:2588–92. doi: 10.3748/wjg.v12.i16.2588
9. Yamamoto H, Sekimoto M, Uemura M, Miyoshi N, Haraguchi N, Takemasa I, et al. Feasibility of end-to-anterior wall anastomosis in conversion of the double-stapling technique during laparoscopically assisted surgery. *Surg Endosc.* (2010) 24(9):2178–81. doi: 10.1007/s00464-010-0921-5
10. Pironi D, Vendettuoli M, Pontone S, Panarese A, Arcieri S, Filippini A, et al. Use of the circular compression stapler and circular mechanical stapler in the end-to-side transanal colorectal anastomosis after left colon and rectal resections A single center experience. *Ann Ital Chir.* (2016) 87:23–30.
11. Ikeda T, Kumashiro R, Oki E, Taketani K, Ando K, Aishima S, et al. Evaluation of techniques to prevent colorectal anastomotic leakage. *J Surg Res.* (2015) 194:450–7. doi: 10.1016/j.jss.2014.11.045
12. Sumer F, Karakas S, Gundogan E, Sahin T, Kayaalp C. Totally laparoscopic resection and extraction of specimens via transanal route in synchronous colon and gastric cancer. *G Chir.* (2018) 39:82–6.
13. Izquierdo KM, Unal E, Marks JH. Natural orifice specimen extraction in colorectal surgery: patient selection and perspectives. *Clin Exp Gastroenterol.* (2018) 11:265–79. doi: 10.2147/CEG.S135331

17

Different Surgical Approaches for Early-Stage Ovarian Cancer Staging: A Large Monocentric Experience

Stefano Cianci [1†], Vito Andrea Capozzi [2†], Andrea Rosati [3], Valerio Rumolo [3], Giacomo Corrado [3], Stefano Uccella [4], Salvatore Gueli Alletti [3], Matteo Riccò [5], Anna Fagotti [3], Giovanni Scambia [3] and Francesco Cosentino [6,7]*

[1] Unit of Gynecology, Department of Human Pathology of Adult and Childood 'G. Barresi', University of Messina, Messina, Italy, [2] Department of Medicine and Surgery, University Hospital of Parma, Parma, Italy, [3] Dipartimento Scienze Della Salute Della Donna e del Bambino, Fondazione Policlinico Universitario A. Gemelli IRCCS, Rome, Italy, [4] Department of Obstetrics and Gynecology, AOUI Verona, University of Verona, Verona, Italy, [5] Department of Public Health, Service for Health and Safety in the Workplace, Reggio Emilia, Italy, [6] Department of Medicine and Health Science, "V.Tiberio" Università Degli Studi del Molise, Campobasso, Italy, [7] Department of Gynecologic Onocology, Gemelli Molise SpA, Campobasso, Italy

***Correspondence:**
Vito Andrea Capozzi
capozzivitoandrea@gmail.com

† These authors share first authorship

Introduction: Ovarian cancer is the third most frequent gynecological cancer. In early stage ovarian cancer (ESOC) comprehensive surgical staging is recommended. Surgical staging is traditionally approached by laparotomy, although minimally invasive surgery can be a valid alternative in selected patients. This study aims to analyze the surgical and oncological outcomes of three different surgical approaches in a large series of patients.

Methods: We retrospectively included all histologically proven ESOC cases treated between January 2014 and December 2017. ESOC was defined as stage IA to IIB according to the 2018 FIGO staging system. Subjects were divided into groups 1, 2, and 3, based on the surgical approach (open abdominal, laparoscopic, or robotic, respectively).

Results: Within patients enrolled during the study period, 455 met the inclusion criteria. No difference in intraoperative complications was recorded in the three groups ($p = 0.709$). Conversely, a significant difference occurred in postoperative complications (16.2 vs. 3.8 vs. 11.1%, in groups 1, 2, and 3 respectively, $p = 0.004$). No difference was found in overall survival (OS) (32 vs. 31 vs. 25 months, $p = 0.481$) and disease-free survival (DFS) (26 vs. 29 vs. 24 months, $p = 0.178$) in groups 1, 2, and 3, respectively. At univariate analysis FIGO stage I ($p = 0.004$) showed a lower recurrence rate compared to FIGO stage II.

Conclusion: No significant difference was found in OS and DFS among the three groups (open, laparoscopic, and robotic). The minimally invasive approach showed lower rate of complications than the laparotomic approach.

Keywords: laparoscopy, robotic, laparotomy, ovarian cancer (OC), early-stage

INTRODUCTION

Ovarian cancer (OC) is the third most frequent gynecological cancer worldwide (1). More than 70% of patients are diagnosed at an advanced stage because of the disease aggressiveness and the absence of early symptoms and adequate screening (2, 3).

The diagnosis of early-stage ovarian cancer (ESOC) (stage I-II disease) is usually incidental and associated with better survival, compared to advanced stages (4). In patients with ESOC, a radical surgical staging (RSS) including total abdominal hysterectomy, bilateral salpingo-oophorectomy, systematic pelvic and para-aortic lymphadenectomy, and radical omentectomy is recommended (4). RSS is traditionally performed by large midline laparotomies; however, due to the progressive technological improvements, minimally invasive surgery (MIS) has been increasingly adopted in the setting of ESOC (5, 6). Different studies showed that the MIS approach is associated with reduced hospitalization, fewer intra and post-operative complications, better cosmetic results, and superimposable oncological outcomes when compared to open surgery (7–12).

Given the rarity of ESOC, only few studies comparing laparotomy, laparoscopy, and robotics are currently available in the literature (13, 14). These studies have the major bias represented by small sample size, inadequate follow-up, and wide patient heterogeneity thus reducing the generalizability of the reported results.

The present study aims to analyze the surgical and oncological outcomes of the three different surgical approaches (open abdominal, laparoscopic, and robotic) for ESOC treatment in a large series of patients with a long-term follow-up.

MATERIALS AND METHODS

This is a retrospective monocentric study conducted at the "Dipartimento Scienze della Salute della Donna e del Bambino, Fondazione Policlinico Universitario A. Gemelli IRCCS, Roma, Italy" between January 2014 and December 2017. The IRB n. CICOG-31-10-18/212 was obtained. All patients provided written informed consent for their data to be collected and analyzed for scientific purposes. Data were extracted from the Research Electronic Data Capture (REDcap) database (Vanderbilt University in Nashville, Tennessee, USA) (15).

All ESOC cases, from IA to IIB International Federation of Gynecology and Obstetrics (FIGO) stage 2018 (2), were included. Age, FIGO stage, histologic subtype, American Society of Anesthesiologists (ASA) performance status, intra and postoperative complications, operative time, rate of conversion to standard laparoscopy or laparotomy, hospital stay, disease-free survival (DFS), overall survival (OS), recurrence rate, and time to chemotherapy, were collected for all patients. Histological slides were evaluated by dedicated pathologists with an extensive background in ovarian malignancies. The surgical approach was chosen based on patient BMI, previous surgery, ovarian lesion diameter, surgeon skill, and preoperative apparent FIGO stage. In the case of MIS approach, a laparoscopic endobag was used for ovarian lesion removal avoiding abdominal tumor spillage. Postoperative complications were categorized according to the Clavien-Dindo classification (16). Operative time was recorded from skin incision to skin closure. In the robotic group, the docking time was excluded. DFS was considered from the date of the histological diagnosis to the date of recurrence. OS was considered from the day of the diagnosis to death or last follow-up. Relapse and response to chemotherapy were evaluated following the response evaluation criteria in solid tumors (RECIST) (17).

Patients with FIGO stage> IIB, with missing pathological data, and those who did not provide informed consent for the enrollment in the present study were excluded.

All patients included in the analysis were divided into group 1, group 2, and group 3, based on the surgical approach as open abdominal, laparoscopic, and robotic, respectively. In addition, a comparative subanalysis between open abdominal and minimally invasive surgery (MIS) (robotic plus laparoscopic) was performed. All patients underwent RSS or fertility-sparing surgery (FSS). RSS was defined as standard staging surgery including (hysterectomy, bilateral salpingo-oophorectomy, omentectomy, systematic pelvic and para-aortic lymphadenectomy, and random peritoneal biopsies); FSS was performed in young women with IA stage disease and strong, motivated wish of conceiving, in accordance to international guidelines (4). Restaging surgery (i.e. complete lymphadenectomy, omentectomy, and possibly hysterectomy/salpingo-oophorectomy) was accomplished in all cases in which the diagnosis of ESOC was not performed intraoperatively and the malignancy was discovered only at final pathological examination.

Statistical Analysis

Continuous variables were initially described using mean and standard deviation (SD), while categorical ones were reported as absolute numbers (%). The distribution of the variables by the surgical approach was initially assessed through a chi-squared test or analysis of variance (ANOVA) when appropriate, according to the surgical approach (open abdominal, laparoscopy, robot) and eventual relapses (yes/no). Survival analyses (i.e. overall survival and disease-free survival) were initially assessed through Kaplan Meier statistics, including overall survival/disease-free survival by eventual status (death/relapse) with and without the stratum of the surgical approach (Tarone-Ware for comparisons). Next, the exact log-rank test to standardize the follow-up medians in the survival analysis was used.

RESULTS

Among patients who had access to the Department of gynecology oncology at the University Hospital Fondazione Policlinico Gemelli, IRCCS during the study period, 455 met the inclusion criteria. Patients' characteristics are summarized in **Table 1**. Specifically, 197 (43.3%), 213 (46.8%), and 45 (9.9%) patients have been allocated to group 1 (open abdominal), group 2 (laparoscopy), and group 3 (robotic surgery), respectively, according to the surgical approach. Of the overall population

TABLE 1 | Patients' characteristics.

	Total series (*n*;%) 455;100	Open abdominal (*n*;%) 197;43.3	Laparoscopy (*n*;%) 213; 46.8	Robot (*n*;%) 45, 9.9	*p* value
Age (years, mean ± sd)	52.8 ± 13.1	55.4 ± 12.8	51.0 ± 13.4	50.0 ± 10.7	**0.001**
BMI (kg/m^2, mean ± sd)	24.9 ± 5.8	25.5 ± 5.5	24.5 ± 5.8	24.8 ± 6.6	0.303
ASA status > 2	9, 5.6%	6, 9.0%	2, 2.7%	1, 5.0%	**0.030**
FIGO Stage					
IA	210; 46.2	78; 17.1	108; 23.7	24; 5.3	**0.042**
IB	53; 11.6	23; 11.7	25; 11.7	5; 11.1	0.993
IC	53; 11.6	20; 10.2	24; 11.3	9; 20.0	0.199
II	139; 30.5	76; 38.6	56; 26.3	7; 15.6	**0.002**
IIA	51; 11.2	30; 15.2	21; 9.9	-	**0.014**
IIB	88; 19.3	46; 23.4	35; 16.4	7; 15.6	0.174
Histology					
Serous carcinoma, high grade	144; 31.6	69; 35.0	59; 27.7	16; 35.6	0.248
Serous carcinoma, low grade	23; 5.1	6; 3.0%	16; 7.5	1; 2.2	0.077
Mucinous carcinoma	54; 1.9	25; 12.7	22; 10.3	7; 15.6	0.513
Clear cell carcinoma	82; 18.0	38; 19.3	38; 17.8	6; 13.3	0.651
Endometroid carcinoma	142; 31.2	53; 26.9	74; 34.7	15; 33.3	0.207
Other	10; 2.2	6; 3.0	4; 1.9	0; -	0.416
Grading					
G1	76; 16.9	24; 12.2	45; 21.4	7; 16.3	**0.041**
G2	94; 20.9	40; 20.3	46; 21.9	8; 18.6	0.925
G3	272; 60.4	131; 66.5	116; 55.2	25; 58.1	0.083
N/A	8; 1.8	2; 1.0	3; 1.4	3; 7.0	-
Chemotherapy	341, 74.9	157, 79.7	153, 71.8	31, 68.9	0.114
Time to chemotherapy (days; mean ± sd)	41.1 ± 14.0	41.8 ± 11.7	41.1 ± 16.6	36.4 ± 7.4	0.352

BMI, Body Mass Index; ASA, American Society of Anesthesiologists; SD, Standard deviation. Significant values were reported in bold.

of 455 patients, 316 (69.5%) subjects were diagnosed at stage I, and 139 (30.5%) at stage II. Within the group of FIGO stage II patients, 38.6% underwent open abdominal surgery while 26.3 and 15.6% of cases respectively underwent laparoscopic and robotic approaches ($p = 0.002$).

Seventy-six patients showed a grade 1 tumor (16.9%), 95 (20.9%) a grade 2, and 272 (60.4%) a grade 3. The most frequent histotype was high-grade serous (31.6%), followed by endometrioid (31.1%), clear cells (18.0%), low-grade serous (5.1%), and mucinous (1.9%).

No difference in adjuvant chemotherapy (79.7 vs. 71.8 vs. 68.9%, in group 1, 2, and 3, respectively, $p = 0.114$) or mean time to chemotherapy (41.8 days ± 11.7 vs. 41.1 days ± 16.6 vs. 36.4 days ± 7.4, in group 1, 2, and 3, respectively, $p = 0.352$) was observed in the three different groups.

The median age at diagnosis was 52.8 years. Patients in the open abdominal group showed a higher mean age (55.4 years) than in the laparoscopic (51.0) and robotic (50.0) groups. Most of FIGO stage IA patients were clustered in group 2 (108 cases, $p = 0.042$), while FIGO stage II patients were more represented in group 1 (76 cases, $p = 0.002$).

Surgical Outcomes

Ninety-seven (21.3%) patients underwent FSS, 358 (78.7%) underwent RSS, and 171 (37.6%) were subjected to restaging surgery after accidental OC diagnosis during previous salpingo-oophorectomy or cystectomy.

As shown in **Table 2**, no difference in intraoperative complications was recorded in the three groups ($p = 0.709$); conversely, a significant difference occurred in postoperative complications (16.2% in group 1 vs. 3.8% group 2 vs. 11.1% group 3, $p = 0.004$). In particular, postoperative anemia (9 cases vs. 0 vs. 0, $p = 0.002$), and abdominal effusion (5 cases vs. 0 vs. 0, $p = 0.036$), occurred more often in the open abdominal group, while lymphocele (3 cases vs. 0 vs. 2, $p = 0.026$) was more frequent in the robotic one. Finally, grade 1/2 Claiven-Dindo complications were more often reported in group 1 than in group 2 or 3 (28 cases vs. 8 cases vs. 5 cases, $p = 0.008$). Complications according to Claiven-Dindo classification in the different surgical approaches are shown in **Table 3**. No statistically significant difference compared to the other groups ($p = 0.112$) was observed, but four (2%) patients required reintervention for postoperative bowel perforation in the open abdominal group. Furthermore, these differences remained even when grouping laparoscopic and robotic patients into the MIS vs. the laparotomic approach.

As shown in **Table 4**, a higher estimated blood loss (EBL) (274.5 vs. 142.2 vs. 79.3 ml, $p < 0.001$), longer hospital stay (5.8 vs. 2.6 vs. 2.8 days, $p < 0.001$), and longer operative time (243.0 vs. 224.1 vs. 197.2 min, $p = 0.004$) were recorded in group 1 vs.

TABLE 2 | Intraoperative and postoperative complications.

	Total (n;%) 455;100	Open abdominal (n;%) 197;43.3	Laparoscopy (n;%) 213; 46.8	Robot (n;%) 45, 9.9	*p* value	MIS (*n*;%) 258, 56.7	*p* value LPT vs. MIS
Intraoperative	8;1.8	5;2.5	2;0.9	1; 2.2	0.709	3; 1.2	0.338
Pleural effusion	0;-	0;-	0;-	0;-	-	-	-
Pulmonary embolism	0;-	0;-	0;-	0;-	-	-	-
Hemorrhage	0;-	0;-	0;-	0;-	-	-	-
Vascular lesions	2; 0.4	1; 0.5	1; 0.5	0; -	0.894	1; 0.4	0.679
Ureteral lesions	4; 0.9	2; 1.0	1; 0.5	1; 2.2	0.501	2; 0.8	0.581
Intestinal lesions	2; 0.4	2; 1.0	0; -	0; -	0.621	-	0.268
Laparotomic conversions	-	-	8; 3.8	1; 2.2	0.358	9; 3.5	-
Postoperative	45;8.9	32;16.2	8;3.8	5;11.1	**0.004**	**13; 5.0**	**0.022**
Ureteral lesions	4; 0.9	2; 1.0	1; 0.5	1; 2.2	0.501	2; 0.8	0.723
Intestinal lesions	2; 0.4	2; 1.0	0; -	0; -	0.621		
Pleural effusion	1; 0.2	1; 0.5	0; -	0; -	0.519	0;-	0.433
Pulmonary embolism	1; 0.2	1; 0.5	0; -	0; -	0.519	0;-	0.433
Hemorrhage	1; 0.2	0; -	1; 0.5	0; -	0.566	1; 0.4	0.567
Pneumonia	3;0.7	2; 1.0	0; -	1; 2.2	0.176	1; 0.4	0.400
Sepsis	7;1.5	5;2.5	2;0.9	0; -	0.285	2; 0.8	0.130
Anemia	9	9; 4.6	0; -	0; -	**0.002**	**0;-**	**<0.001**
Abdominal effusion	5	5;2.5	0; -	0; -	**0.036**	**0;-**	**0.015**
Urinary tract infections	1; 0.2	0; -	1; 0.5	0; -	0.566	1; 0.4	0.567
Intestinal Pseudo-Obstruction	3;0.7	0; -	2;0.9	1; 2.2	0.198	3; 1.2	0.181
Lymphocele	5;1.1	3;1.5	0; -	2;4.4	**0.026**	2; 0.8	0.375
Fistula	1; 0.2	0; -	1; 0.5	0; -	0.566	1; 0.4	0.567
Wound infection	2; 0.4	2; 1.0	0; -	0; -	0.268	0; -	0.187

LPS, Laparoscopy; LPT, Laparotomy; MIS, Minimally invasive. Significant values were reported in bold.

TABLE 3 | Complications according to Claiven-Dindo classification in the different kinds of surgeries.

General population	Total	Open abdominal	Laparoscopy	Robot	*p* value	MIS	*p* value (LPT vs. MIS)
G1-G2 *	41	28	8	5	**$p = 0.008$**	**13**	**<0.001**
G3-G4**	4	4	0	0	$p = 0.112$	**0**	**0.035**
Fertility sparing							
G1-G2	6	2	2	2	$p = 0.318$	4	0.264
G3-G4**	1	2	0	0	$p = 0.139$	0	0.607
Radical surgical staging							
G1-G2	35	26	6	3	$p = 0.076$	9	0.190
G3-G4**	3	2	1	0	$p = 0.156$	1	0.072

**Vascular lesions, ureteral lesions, pulmonary embolism, pneumonia, sepsis, anemia, urinary tract infection, ileus, lymphocele, fistula, surgical site infection. ** Intestinal lesions requiring reintervention. LPS, Laparoscopy; LPT, Laparotomy; MIS, Minimally invasive. Significant values were reported in bold.*

group 2 vs. group 3, respectively. Conversely, these differences were nullified by pooling MIS patients vs. the laparotomic group (**Table 4**).

Finally, no significant difference in the number of pelvic ($p = 0.197$) and lumboortic ($p = 0.195$) lymph nodes removed was observed among the three groups.

Survival Analysis

Twenty total deaths occurred in the entire population, 12 (2.6%) in group 1, 6 (1.3%) in group 2, and 2 (0.4%) in group 3 ($p = 0.267$). Sixty total relapses (13.2%) were found in the whole series; of them, 54 occurred in patients who underwent RSS, and 24 were patients at FIGO stage II.

In the entire population, after applying the exact log-rank test, to smooth out the follow-up discrepancies, no statistically significant differences in median OS (32 months in group 1 vs. 31 in group 2 vs. 25 in group 3, $p = 0.481$) and DFS (26 months in group 1 vs. 29 in group 2 vs. 24 in group 3, $p = 0.178$) were found in the three groups. Oncological outcomes are displayed in **Table 5** and Kaplan-Meier analysis after the exact log-rank

TABLE 4 | Surgical outcomes.

	Total (*n*;%) 455;100	Open abdominal (*n*;%) 197;43.3	Laparoscopy (*n*;%) 213; 46.8	Robot (*n*;%) 45, 9.9	*p* value	MIS (n;%)	*p* value LPT vs. LPS
Type of surgery							
Fertility sparing	97; 21.3	19; 9.6	62; 29.1	16; 35.6	**<0.001**	78; 17.1	**<0.001**
Radical surgical staging	358; 78.7	178; 39.1	151; 33.2	29; 6.4	**<0.001**	**180; 39.6**	**<0.001**
Restaging	171; 37.6	19; 0.2	110; 24.2	42; 9.2	**<0.001**	**152; 33.4**	**0.374**
Aortic lymph nodes removed Number (mean ± sd)	9 ± 8.4	8 ± 9.9	8.5 ± 7.3	9 ± 6.9	0.197	10.8 ± 7.2	0.735
Pelvic lymph nodes removed Number (mean ± sd)	10 ± 8.0	10 ± 8.3	9 ± 7.5	12.5 ± 8.6	0.195	12.7 ± 9.1	0.930
Estimated blood loss (mL; mean ± sd)	179.0 ± 209.8	274.5 ± 229.3	142.2 ± 201.6	79.3 ± 47.3	**<0.001**	127.3 ±178.5	0.632
Operative time (minutes; mean ± sd)	227.5 ± 81.7	243.0 ± 83.6	224.1 ± 78.9	197.2 ± 79.4	**0.004**	245 ± 79.1	0.842
Hospital stay (days; mean ± sd)	3.9 ± 5.3	5.8 ± 7.8	2.6 ± 1.1	2.8 ± 1.7	**<0.001**	2.6± 1.2	0.610

LPS, Laparoscopy; LPT, Laparotomy; MIS, Minimally invasive. Significant values were reported in bold.

TABLE 5 | Survival analysis.

	Total median (range) 455;100%	Open abdominal median (range) 197;43.3%	Laparoscopy median (range) 213; 46.8%	Robot median (range) 45, 9.9%	*p* value	MIS	*p* value (LPT vs. MIS)
General population							
DFS (months)	28 (10–44)	26 (8–43.5)	29 (10.8–48)	24 (12–31.5)	0.178	28 (10.8–31.5)	0.067
OS (months)	30 (12–47)	32 (11.5–52.5)	31 (13–48)	25 (12–33)	0.481	29 (12–33)	0.441
Relapse (*n*; %)	60; 13.2	39; 19.8	19; 8.9	2; 4.4	0.072	21; 8.1	0.064

DFS, Disease-Free Survival; OS, Overall survival; LPS, Laparoscopy; LPT, Laparotomy; MIS, Minimally invasive.

test is shown in **Figures 1, 2**. Furthermore, these differences remained non-statistically significant even when comparing MIS with laparotomic group (DFS 28 vs. 26 months, $p = 0.067$, and, OS 29 vs. 32 months, $p = 0.441$, respectively). Kaplan Meier analysis showed 1-year OS of 100 vs. 100%, 3-years OS of 100 vs. 100%, and 5-years OS of 99.2 vs. 99.5% in the laparotomic vs. MIS approach (95% Confidence Interval 26.37–31.75).

As reported in **Table 6**, at univariate analysis FIGO stage I patients ($p = 0.004$) showed lower recurrence rates when compared to FIGO stage II patients. Furthermore, the subanalysis of patients undergoing complete surgical staging showed a higher relapse rate in the laparotomic than the MIS group, 68.5 vs. 31.5% ($p = 0.002$).

DISCUSSION

The present study showed that minimally invasive comprehensive surgical staging for ESOC was safe and associated with a lower rate of postoperative morbidity, compared to the traditional open abdominal approach. Furthermore, there was no statistically significant difference in patients' survival among the laparotomic, laparoscopic, and robotic groups.

In line with our results, Magrina et al. (14) reported an overlapping OS between these three different surgical approaches in a series of both early and advanced epithelial ovarian cancer. In the sub-analysis of early-stage cases, the same authors reported superimposable results in terms of oncological outcomes with fewer surgical complications in the MIS group (laparoscopic and robotic) when compared to the traditional open abdominal surgery. Several authors confirmed these findings: in particular, Liu et al. (18), analyzing the most relevant studies in the literature, demonstrated a comparable survival between the minimally invasive and the open approach in both early and advanced FIGO stage (19–21).

An important hurdle we faced to obtain a meaningful survival analysis was related to the wide heterogeneity of the population enrolled. As recently reported by Shi et al. (13), the heterogeneity of OC population in the different trials can afflict survival outcomes making comparisons unreliable. Furthermore, Falcetta et al. (22) stressed that trouble for data analysis of ESOC patients was related to the variety of the treatments proposed, ranging from fertility-sparing to radical surgery. Trying to overcome these limitations, we enrolled a large single-center series and we focused the survival analysis on the comprehensive surgically staged patients. Furthermore, an exact log-rank test for survival

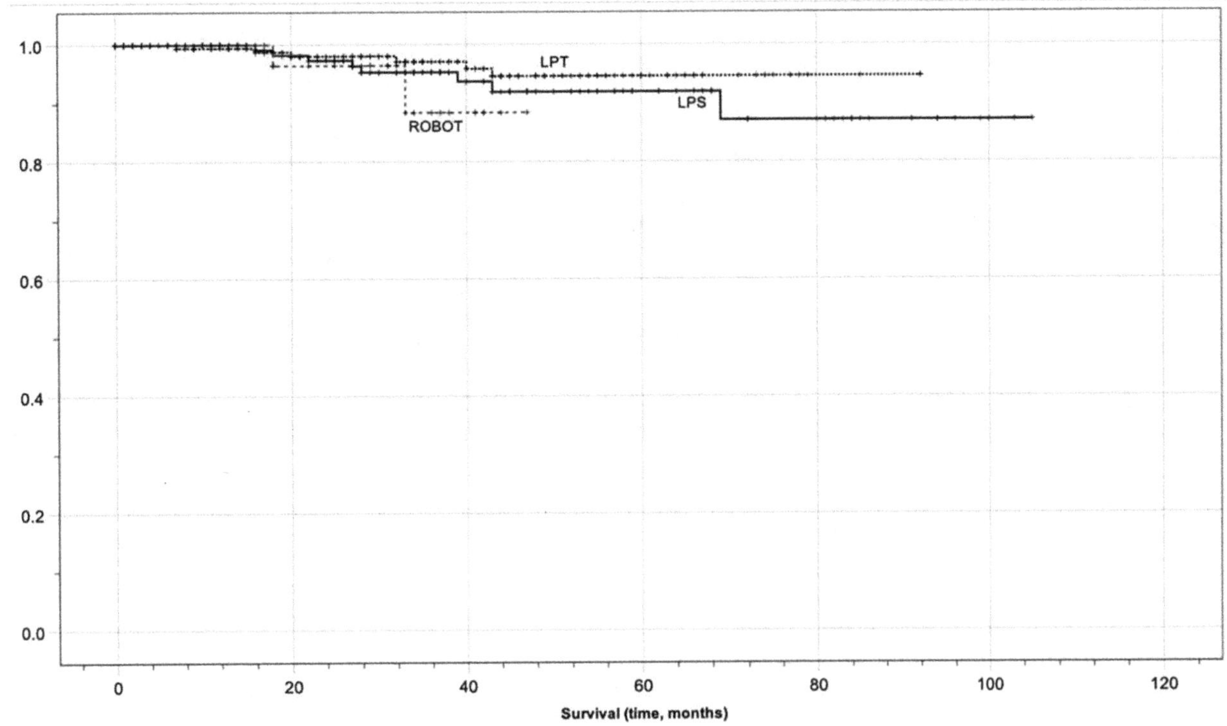

FIGURE 1 | Kaplan meier survival analysis (overall survival).

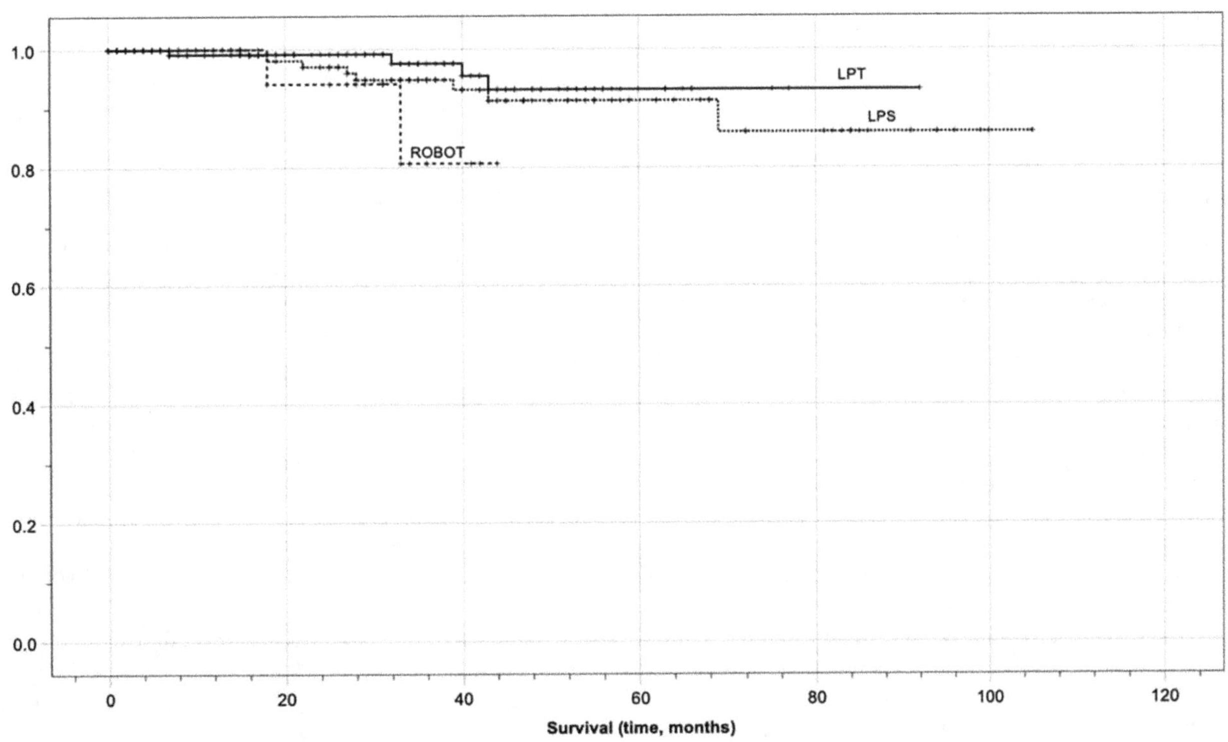

FIGURE 2 | Kaplan meier survival analysis (disease-free survival).

TABLE 6 | Univariate analysis.

Patients underwent complete surgical staging	Recurrence 54 number %		No recurrence 304 number %		*p* value
Age > 50 years	36	66.7%	200	65.8%	0.9
BMI > 30 kg/m^2	7	13.0%	36	11.8%	0.815
ASA > 2	2	3.7%	7	2.3%	0.544
Hystotype					0.178
Serous. high grade	24	44.4%	105	34.5%	
Serous. low grade	1	1.9%	16	5.3%	
Mucinous	3	5.6%	33	10.9%	
Clear cells	14	25.9%	50	16.4%	
Endometrioid	11	20.4%	92	30.3%	
Others	1	1.9%	8	2.6%	
Grading					0.053
G1	4	7.4%	48	15.8%	
G2	6	11.1%	62	20.4%	
G3	44	81.5%	188	61.8%	
FIGO stage					0.156
I	13	24.1%	115	37.8%	
IA	2	3.7%	24	7.9%	
IB	6	11.1%	34	11.2%	
IC	9	16.7%	38	12.5%	
IIA	7	13.0%	37	12.2%	
IIB	17	31.5%	56	18.4%	
II vs. I	24	44.4%	93	30.6%	**0.046**
Surgical approach					**0.002**
Laparotomy	37	68.5%	141	46.4%	
MIS	17	31.5%	163	53.6%	
Introperative complication	3	5.6%	5	1.6%	0.073
Postoperative complication	3	5.6%	30	9.9%	0.293
Chemiotherapy	47	87.0%	227	74.7%	0.072

G, Grading; LPT, Laparotomy; LPS, Laparoscopy; ASA, American Society of Anesthesiologists; MIS, Minimally invasive surgery. Significant values were reported in bold.

analysis was used to reduce the consequent bias and to adequately match the patients.

It is well established that the main prognostic factor affecting OC recurrence is the FIGO stage (23). In our series, group 1 showed a greater proportion of FIGO stage II cases ($p = 0.014$) than the two minimally invasive groups and, as expected, the relapse rate appeared higher in this group when compared to the other approaches. However, after standardization of follow-up with exact log-rank test, no significant difference was found in DFS within the three approaches ($p = 0.178$). In line with our results, Zhang et al. (24), in a meta-analysis including 8 studies, reported no significant difference in DFS of ESOC patients subjected to laparotomy vs. laparoscopy with fewer complication rates and shorter hospital stay in the latter group.

In contrast with previously reported studies, we found that patients undergoing robotic surgery had a shorter operative time (8, 25). This finding may be due to the very precise three-dimensional movement of the robotic arms that could be useful and time-saving, especially when facing complex procedures such as lumboortic lymphadenectomy (26). Furthermore, the greater number of complete surgical staging procedures in the open abdominal and laparoscopic groups compared to the robotic one could justify this result.

Compared to previous retrospective studies and clinical trials, our series showed a higher rate of mild complications (G1-G2 according to Claiven Dindo classification) in the open abdominal group (27, 28). In addition, these differences in G1-G2 complications not only remained when comparing the MIS group with the laparotomic approach but also included the G3-G4 complications. This finding could be related to the mean age ($p = 0.001$), ASA status ($p = 0.030$), and FIGO stage II ($p = 0.002$) which were higher in group 1. As reported by Patankar et al., all these demographic factors are associated with worse surgical outcomes (29).

We know that this study has several possible limitations due to its retrospective nature. Given the rarity and the good prognosis of ESOC, only 20 death events were observed in the entire population, and this may have influenced the survival analysis.

Furthermore, the different complications rate reported could be influenced by the heterogeneity of the interventions performed in the three groups. Therefore, prospective studies with standardization of interventions performed in the various approaches are needed to confirm our results.

On the other hand, we emphasize that this study has important strengths such as the size of the sample analyzed, the long follow-up time, the close selection of the patients analyzed, and the single oncological tertiary center experience reported.

CONCLUSIONS

After follow-up standardization, we observed no statistically significant difference in OS and DFS among the three groups analyzed (open abdominal, laparoscopic, and robotic).

The open abdominal approach in ESOC was associated with a higher mild complication rate than the laparoscopic and robotic ones. Based on these findings, the minimally invasive approach should be preferred in selected patients and in tertiary cancer centers.

ETHICS STATEMENT

The studies involving human participants were reviewed and approved by Dipartimento Scienze della Salute della Donna e del Bambino, Fondazione Policlinico Universitario A. Gemelli IRCCS, Roma, Italy. IRB code n. CICOG-31-10-18/212. The patients/participants provided their written informed consent to participate in this study.

AUTHOR CONTRIBUTIONS

SC, VC, and AR: conceptualization, methodology, and writing-original draft preparation. MR and VR: software and data curation. SU, GC, and SG: visualization and investigation. AF, GS, and FC: supervision, validation, reviewing, and editing. All authors contributed to the article and approved the submitted version.

REFERENCES

1. Bray F, Ferlay J, Soerjomataram I, Siegel RL, Torre LA, Jemal A. Global cancer statistics 2018 : GLOBOCAN estimates of incidence and mortality worldwide for 36 cancers in 185 countries. *CA Cancer J Clin.* (2018) 68:394–424. doi: 10.3322/caac.21492
2. Berek JS, Kehoe ST, Kumar L, Friedlander M. Cancer of the ovary, fallopian tube, and peritoneum. *Int J Gynaecol Obs.* (2018) 143:259–78. doi: 10.1002/ijgo.12614
3. Giampaolino P, Della Corte L, Foreste V, Vitale SG, Chiofalo B, Cianci S, et al. Unraveling a difficult diagnosis: the tricks for early recognition of ovarian cancer. *Minerva Med.* (2019) 110:279–91. doi: 10.23736/S0026-4806.19.06086-5
4. National Comprehensive Cancer Network. Ovarian cancer. (Version 12021) https://www.nccn.org/professionals/physician_gls/pdf/ovarian.pdf (accessed Jenuary 29, 2021).
5. Park J, Kim D, Suh D. Comparison of laparoscopy and laparotomy in surgical staging of early-stage ovarian and fallopian tubal cancer. *Am J Obs Gynecol.* (2005) 192:1614–9. doi: 10.1245/s10434-008-9893-2
6. Gueli Alletti S, Capozzi VA, Rosati A, De Blasis I, Cianci S, Vizzielli G, et al. Laparoscopy vs laparotomy for advanced ovarian cancer: a systematic review of the literature. *Minerva Med.* (2019). doi: 10.23736/S0026-4806.19.06132-9
7. Cianci S, Tarascio M, Rosati A, Caruso S, Uccella S, Cosentino F, et al. Sexual function and quality of life of patients affected by ovarian cancer: review of literature. *Minerva Med.* (2019) 110:320–9. doi: 10.23736/S0026-4806.19.06080-4
8. Minig L, Padilla Iserte P, Zorrero C, Zanagnolo V. Robotic surgery in women with ovarian cancer: surgical technique and evidence of clinical outcomes. *J Minim Invasive Gynecol.* (2016) 23:309–16. doi: 10.1016/j.jmig.2015.10.014
9. Cianci S, Rosati A, Rumolo V, Gueli Alletti S, Gallotta V, Turco LC, et al. Robotic single-port platform in general, urologic, and gynecologic surgeries: a systematic review of the literature and meta-analysis. *World J Surg.* (2019) 43:2401–19. doi: 10.1007/s00268-019-05049-0
10. Gueli Alletti S, Vizzielli G, Lafuenti L, Costantini B, Fagotti A, Fedele C, et al. Single-institution propensity-matched study to evaluate the psychological effect of minimally invasive interval debulking surgery versus standard laparotomic treatment: from body to mind and back. *J Minim Invasive Gynecol.* (2018) 25:816–22. doi: 10.1016/j.jmig.2017.12.007
11. Fagotti A, Vizzielli G, Fanfani F, Costantini B, Ferrandina G, Gallotta V, et al. Introduction of staging laparoscopy in the management of advanced epithelial ovarian, tubal and peritoneal cancer: impact on prognosis in a single institution experience. *Gynecol Oncol.* (2013) 131:341–6. doi: 10.1016/j.ygyno.2013.08.005
12. Siddiqi NN, Abuawwad M, Halls M, Rawashdeh A, Giovinazzo F, Aljaiuossi A, et al. Laparoscopic right posterior sectionectomy (LRPS): surgical techniques and clinical outcomes. *Surg Endosc.* (2018) 32:2525–32. doi: 10.1007/s00464-017-5958-2
13. Shi C, Gao Y, Yang Y, Zhang L, Yu J, Zhang T. Comparison of efficacy of robotic surgery, laparoscopy, and laparotomy in the treatment of ovarian cancer : a meta-analysis. *World J Surg Oncol.* (2019) 17:162. doi: 10.1186/s12957-019-1702-9
14. Magrina JF, Zanagnolo V, Noble BN, Kho RM, Magtibay P. Robotic approach for ovarian cancer: perioperative and survival results and comparison with laparoscopy and laparotomy. *Gynecol Oncol.* (2011) 121:100–5. doi: 10.1016/j.ygyno.2010.11.045
15. Harris PA, Taylor R, Thielke R, Payne J, Gonzalez N, Conde JG. Research electronic data capture (REDCap)–a metadata-driven methodology and workflow process for providing translational research informatics support. *J Biomed Inform.* (2009) 42:377–81. doi: 10.1016/j.jbi.2008.08.010
16. Clavien PA, Barkun J, de Oliveira ML, Vauthey JN, Dindo D, Schulick RD, et al. The clavien-dindo classification of surgical complications: five-year experience. *Ann Surg.* (2009) 250:187–96. doi: 10.1097/SLA.0b013e3181b13ca2
17. Schwartz LH, Litière S, de Vries E, Ford R, Gwyther S, Mandrekar S, et al. RECIST 1. 1-Update and clarification: From the RECIST committee. *Eur J Cancer.* (2016) 62:132–7. doi: 10.1016/j.ejca.2016.03.081
18. Liu CS, Nagarsheth NP, Nezhat FR. Laparoscopy and ovarian cancer : a paradigm change in the management of ovarian cancer? *J Minim Invasive Gynecol.* 16:250–62. doi: 10.1016/j.jmig.2009.01.007
19. Lu Q, Qu H, Liu C, Wang S, Zhang Z, Zhang Z. Comparison of laparoscopy and laparotomy in surgical staging of apparent early ovarian cancer. *Med.* (2016) 95:1–7. doi: 10.1097/MD.0000000000003655
20. Lu Y, Yao DS, Xu JH. Systematic review of laparoscopic comprehensive staging surgery in early stage ovarian cancer: a meta-analysis. *Taiwan J Obs Gynecol.* (2015) 54:29–38. doi: 10.1016/j.tjog.2014.10.003
21. Gallotta V, Petrillo M, Conte C, Vizzielli G, Fagotti A, Ferrandina G, et al. Laparoscopic versus laparotomic surgical staging for early-stage ovarian cancer: a case-control study. *J Minim Invasive Gynecol Jul-Aug.* (2016) 23:769–74. doi: 10.1016/j.jmig.2016.03.006
22. Falcetta FS, Lawrie TA, Medeiros LR, da Rosa MI, Edelweiss MI, Stein AT, et al. Laparoscopy versus laparotomy for FIGO stage I ovarian cancer. *Cochrane Database Syst Rev.* (2016) 2016:CD005344. doi: 10.1002/14651858.CD005344.pub4

23. Torre LA, Trabert B, DeSantis CE, Miller KD, Samimi G, Runowicz CD, et al. Ovarian cancer statistics, 2018. *CA Cancer J Clin.* (2018) 68:284–96. doi: 10.3322/caac.21456
24. Zhang Y, Fan S, Xiang Y, Duan H, Sun L. Comparison of the prognosis and recurrence of apparent early-stage ovarian tumors treated with laparoscopy and laparotomy: a meta-analysis of clinical studies. *BMC Cancer.* (2015) 15:597. doi: 10.1186/s12885-015-1604-3
25. Lucidi A, Chiantera V, Gallotta V, Ercoli A, Scambia G, Fagotti A. Role of robotic surgery in ovarian malignancy. *Best Pr Res Clin Obs Gynaecol.* (2017) 45:74–82. doi: 10.1016/j.bpobgyn.2017.05.005
26. Nick AM, Ramirez PT. The impact of robotic surgery on gynecologic oncology. *J Gynecol Oncol.* (2011) 22:196–202. doi: 10.3802/jgo.2011.22.3.196
27. Fagotti A, Gueli Alletti S, Corrado G, Cola E, Vizza E, Vieira M, et al. The INTERNATIONAL MISSION study: minimally invasive surgery in ovarian neoplasms after neoadjuvant chemotherapy. *Int J Gynecol Cancer.* (2019) 29:5–9. doi: 10.1136/ijgc-2018-000012
28. Tantitamit T, Lee CL. Is it the time for laparoscopic management of early-stage ovarian malignancies? *Gynecol Minim Invasive Ther.* (2018) 7:93–103. doi: 10.4103/GMIT.GMIT_59_18
29. Patankar S, Burke WM, Hou JY, Tergas AI, Huang Y, Ananth CV, et al. Risk stratification and outcomes of women undergoing surgery for ovarian cancer. *Gynecol Oncol.* (2015) 138:62–9. doi: 10.1016/j.ygyno.2015.04.037

18

Enhanced Recovery After Surgery Protocols in Major Urologic Surgery

Natalija Vukovic[1] and Ljubomir Dinic[2]*

[1] *Anesthesiology and Reanimation Center, Clinical Center Nis, Nis, Serbia,* [2] *Urology Clinic, Clinical Center Nis, Nis, Serbia*

***Correspondence:**
Natalija Vukovic
massha.vukovic@gmail.com

The purpose of the review: The analysis of the components of enhanced recovery after surgery (ERAS) protocols in urologic surgery.

Recent findings: ERAS protocols has been studied for over 20 years in different surgical procedures, mostly in colorectal surgery. The concept of improving patient care and reducing postoperative complications was also applied to major urologic surgery and especially procedure of radical cystectomy. This procedure is technically challenging, due to a major surgical resection and high postoperative complication rate that may reach 65%. Several clinical pathways were introduced to improve perioperative course and reduce the length of hospital stay. These protocols differ from ERAS modalities in other surgeries. The reasons for this are longer operative time, increased risk of perioperative transfusion and infection, and urinary diversion achieved using transposed intestinal segments. Previous studies in this area analyzed the need for mechanical bowel preparation, postoperative nasogastric tube decompression, as well as the duration of urinary drainage. Furthermore, the attention has also been drawn to perioperative fluid optimization, pain management, and bowel function.

Summary: Notwithstanding partial resemblance between the pathways in major urologic surgery and other pelvic surgeries, there are still scarce guidelines for ERAS protocols in urology, which is why further studies should assess the importance of preoperative medical optimization, implementation of thoracic epidural anesthesia and analgesia, and perioperative nutritional management.

Keywords: urology, recovery, radical cystectomy, enhanced recovery after surgery, fast-track pathway

INTRODUCTION

The new era in perioperative medicine, defined as enhanced recovery after surgery (ERAS) protocols, started with the increase of the importance of a multimodal approach to surgical patients. The most important aims of the multimodal approach are the improvement of patients' preoperative status and the perioperative maintenance of homeostasis, by minimizing stress response and inflammation. This new approach was first used in colorectal surgery (1) and then started spreading to all other types of surgeries (2–4).

There is an increased interest in ERAS protocols in urology. Radical cystectomy (RC) and radical prostatectomy (RP) are predominantly studied urologic procedures. These procedures have major surgical resection, increased risk of bleeding and perioperative transfusion, and in case of cystectomy, urinary diversion and high frequency of postoperative complications. Furthermore, patients undergoing major urologic surgery are usually the elderly, with cardiovascular and other comorbidities, anemia, possible infection, and malnutrition.

PREOPERATIVE PERIOD

The ERAS preoperative period consists of several important elements, which are described below.

Preadmission Counseling and Education

When it comes to ERAS guidelines, the initial phase of different surgeries is preadmission counseling (4–6). It has been determined that the reduction of anxiety by means of sharing details of admission, as well as surgical and anesthetic procedures, may improve pain control (7), early mobilization, and perioperative feeding and hence reduce postoperative complications (8, 9).

Even before first studies of ERAS in urology, Hobisch et al. (10) found out that 65–71% of the patients scheduled for different types of urinary diversion RC had received no information about various therapy options before being admitted to the Department of Urology. After admission, 78.8% of ileal conduit patients and 91.3% of neobladder RC patients were completely satisfied with the information given. Most of the studies from this period (10, 11) mainly examine the need to explain different types of RC urinary diversions to patients and the impact they will have on everyday care after hospitalization. The importance of preadmission counseling and patient education, along with a precise and detailed clarification of the immediate perioperative pathway was not emphasized. To the best of our knowledge, there are no specific studies dealing exclusively with preadmission counseling and education. This issue has so far been analyzed only as a part of the study of ERAS elements.

Dutton et al. (12) examined 165 patients undergoing open RC with urinary diversion implementing ERAS protocol. Patients in this study went through three stages of patient education and counseling. The first stage involved pre-referral by patient's family doctor, the second one was outpatient assessment by a nurse specialist, and the third one included preoperative patient education (both written and verbal) explaining ERAS, as well as stoma or neobladder care before hospital admission. The authors pointed out that the patients were informed at earliest opportunity. Taking everything into account, it can be concluded that the implementation of ERAS elements in this study was safe, coupled with early feeding of patients, early mobilization, and rapid discharge from hospital.

In the following years, more researchers (13, 14) have included preadmission counseling as an obligatory element of ERAS protocols in urology. In the prospective study of Pang et al. (14), preoperative counseling included detailed 30–40 min description of the treatment, provided by a surgeon, a nurse, a stoma therapist, and an anesthesiologist, if necessary. In this study, the patients were additionally preoperatively provided with an information booklet.

Matulewicz et al. (15) also suggested the use of multimedia tools (websites and videos) and intensive verbal and written counseling regarding the expectations and the goals of RC. The authors furthermore proposed the implementation of "Urostomy Education Scale" (16) as an important tool for patient education in patients with urostomy after RC. Moreover, within the systematic review (17), the importance of RC patients' participation in advocacy networks was also stressed, with the aim of improving perioperative care, both before and after surgery.

Preoperative Optimization

Preoperative optimization involves assessment and improvement of medical conditions, as well as the reduction of risks that affect perioperative homeostasis. The guidelines provided by the European Society of Anaesthesiology on preoperative evaluation (18) recommend different strategies that should be used for reducing perioperative risks.

Current or former smokers comprise 80% of RC patients (15). Preoperative smoking cessation might reduce the risk of pneumonia, mechanical ventilation longer than 48 h, and unplanned tracheal intubation. According to the study of Turan et al. (19), active smokers have higher rates of myocardial infarction, postoperative cardiac arrest and stroke, deep vein thrombosis, and sepsis. Systematic review (20), which included urological and genitourinary patients, revealed that intensive smoking cessation intervention with individual counseling and included pharmacotherapy, 4–8 weeks before surgery, reduced the risk of postoperative complications. Meta-analysis (21) of different surgical patients showed that quitting smoking 8 weeks before surgery has no negative impact on postoperative outcome. The guidelines for ERAS pathways in urology (6, 22) recommend smoking cessation 4–8 weeks before surgery.

Daily intake of more than two to three drinks decreases the immune response, prolongs bleeding time and increases endocrine stress response to surgery (23). More importantly, the preoperative 4-week-long abstinence from alcohol reduces exaggerated surgical stress response of alcohol abusers (24).

Perioperative Nutritional Therapy

It has been shown (25) that the patients undergoing RC are at risk of malnutrition due to advanced age and prolonged hospital stay with high frequency of postoperative complications. In addition, these patients already have some degree of inflammation as a part of malnutrition. In a retrospective cohort study of 538 patients with RC (26), nutritional deficiency measured by preoperative weight loss, body mass index and also serum albumin, strongly predicts a 90-day survival, as well as poor overall survival.

Therefore, nutritional risk screening before a surgical procedure (27) is a highly recommended screening tool for establishing a possible risk of malnutrition. When it comes to establishing perioperative nutritional status, dietician referral 1 day before RC, represents yet another step forward in this whole process, just as it was already shown in the study of Arumainayagam et al. (28).

Perioperative nutritional therapy should be initiated before surgery if the patient is at nutritional risk or has malnutrition (29). The indication for preoperative nutritional therapy also exists if there is a trend of less than 50% of recommended oral food intake for more than 7 days, or food abstinence for more than 5 days.

In a randomized trial of Hamilton-Reeves et al., cystectomy patients showed different immune response to surgery and late infection (30) if perioperatively fed with specialized immunonutrition in intervention group. In accordance with the guidelines (29), perioperative or at least postoperative administration of specific formula enriched with immunonutritents should be given to malnourished patients undergoing major cancer surgery. However, the potential role, specific type, and financial aspects of preoperative nutritional therapy in RC patients are yet unknown.

Bowel Preparation

The need for oral bowel preparation has been examined especially for ileum diversions of RC. Reduced bowel preparation in patients with mainly ileal conduit diversion of RC produced no detrimental effect on morbidity or mortality (28). In the study of Tabibi et al. (31), spillage was observed in all studied patients, in both bowel prepared ones and in those who had no preparation. The infection complications did not increase in the group without bowel preparation for cystectomy. In the randomized trial of Xu et al. (32), patients were randomized to a preoperative bowel preparation group and to another one with no preparation. It has been concluded that bowel preparation did not present any advantages in RC, neither with regard to patient recovery nor to complication occurrence.

The colorectal surgery meta-analysis (33) showed no clinical benefit from mechanical bowel preparation. This study also pointed out that inadequate bowel preparation with the presence of liquid content increases the risk of infections.

ERAS guidelines for RC (6) recommend that preoperative bowel preparation can be safely omitted.

Thromboembolic Prophylaxis

Patients undergoing RC and RP are considered to be high risk of venous thromboembolism (VTE) because of the cancer disease and the surgery procedure lasting more than 120 min (34). Novotny et al. (35) revealed about 5% incidence of clinically significant deep vein thrombosis in RC patients, while according to Vukina et al. (36) incidence in open RP is 1–5% and just 0.5% in robotic RP. Despite importance of prevention of VTE in major urologic surgery, variations in utilization of prevention treatment are demonstrated and criticized (37).

European guidelines on perioperative VTE prophylaxis for fast-track surgery (34) recommend the first dose of LMWH 12 h before the procedure or 6–8 h after the procedure. In case of a planned neuraxial anesthesia, postoperative administration might be a preferred option. Furthermore, according to Sachdeva et al. (38), adding graduated compression stockings or compressive stockings enables more effective thromboprophylaxis.

ERAS Society guidelines for rectal/pelvic surgery (5) recommend taking into consideration extended prophylaxis for 4 weeks in patients with the increased risk of VTE. These recommendations are in accordance with the American College of Chest Physician guideline (39) and refer to high risk patients with cancer.

Preoperative Fasting

It has been demonstrated (40) that long food and water abstinence produce stress and deteriorate surgical patient wellbeing. The European Society of Anaesthesiology fasting guidelines encourage patients to drink clear liquids (tea, coffee without milk and water) up to 2 h before the elective surgery. With the highest level of evidence, they recommend the prohibition of solid food 6 h before the elective operation. Patients with conditions such as gastro-esophageal reflux, obesity, diabetes, and pregnant women, who are not in labor, may have delayed gastric empting. More evidence is needed for fasting recommendations regarding these groups of patients.

In major urologic surgery, Rege et al. (41) reduced preoperative fasting period introducing clear liquids to 2 h before laparoscopic live kidney donor surgery in ERAS group of patients. They pointed out that the reduction of preoperative fasting period enhances patient's comfort, reduces thirst and anxiety, thus facilitating faster recovery. In their study, patients with ERAS perioperative pathway had shorter length of hospital stay. On the other hand, in some early fast-track studies (42) of patients undergoing laparoscopic RP, liquid drinks were allowed only until midnight of the preoperative day. The only difference between the conventional and the ERAS group of patients in this study was that the ERAS group of patients was allowed to have lunch and soup for dinner, whereas the patients in the conventional group were not allowed to consume any food whatsoever after breakfast on the day before the surgery. Even without this preoperative element of ERAS pathway, the authors observed shorter length of hospital stay in the ERAS group.

According to previous discrepancies more evidence is needed about impact of shortening of fasting before major urologic surgery procedures.

Preoperative Carbohydrate Loading

One of the main goals of ERAS protocols is the reduction of perioperative insulin resistance. Meta-analysis (43) of randomized controlled trials investigating preoperative oral carbohydrate treatment before elective surgery revealed significant reduction in the length of hospital stay of the patients receiving the treatment when compared with control groups. However, the authors pointed out that this was valid for patients undergoing major abdominal surgery, and they also emphasized that there was significant heterogenicity among different studies.

The extent of insulin resistance after surgery is proportional to the magnitude of the surgery (44) and blood loss (45). Both risk factors are present in RC (32) and other major urologic procedures. Several studies (40, 46, 47) of open RC conducted after the year 2010, used carbohydrate loading liquids 2 h before surgery with the aim of reducing postoperative insulin resistance. In the study of robotic-assisted laparoscopic cystectomy (48), 31 patients received carbohydrate loading at 6:00 p.m. the day before the surgery and at 5:00 a.m. on the day of the surgery. Patients within the study group showed significant differences in terms of mobilization within the room, the time to regular diet, and lower use of postoperative opioid analgesia. In other major urologic procedures, the reduction of insulin resistance was also found to be an important part of ERAS pathways. In the retrospective analysis (41) of patients undergoing laparoscopic live kidney donor surgery, preoperative carbohydrate loading liquids were used for ERAS pathway group. Further studies are needed to evaluate CHO loading for patients undergoing major urologic surgery.

Antimicrobial Prophylaxis

European Association of Urology guidelines (49) suggested optional use of antimicrobial prophylaxis in RP and nephrectomy, since there are no studies on this issue. In RC patients, prophylaxis for both aerobic and anaerobic pathogens is recommended. The combination of cefuroxime and aminopenicillin/betalaktamase inhibitor plus metronidazole is recommended. In case of prolonged operation or important morbidity factors, antimicrobial prophylaxis might be prolonged to <72 h.

Prolongation of antibiotic prophylaxis is not recommended if urinary drainage is left in place after surgery.

Prevention of Postoperative Nausea and Vomiting (PONV)

There is insufficient evidence regarding the incidence of PONV after urologic surgery. Shabsigh et al. (50) reported 29% of gastrointestinal complications from the overall number of complications, among which just 1.5% of patients were the ones with emesis. Nevertheless, PONV may intensify postoperative pain, wound dehiscence and hematoma and hence increase patient distress (51). With the aim of reducing the incidence of PONV, patient baseline risk should be assessed using validated score (52). Recommended risk scores are Apfel et al. (53) and Koivuranta et al. (54).

After establishing baseline risk, PONV is considered through all three parts of ERAS pathway, preoperative, intraoperative and postoperative. Prevention of PONV is accentuated especially in laparoscopic urologic surgery. In this way in the non-randomized retrospective analysis (43) of laparoscopic nephrectomy, antiemetics were started preoperatively with scopolamine patch, dexamethason and ondansetron were given intraoperatively and scopolamine and ondansetron postoperatively. For preoperative and postoperative phases, rescue antiemetics were also suggested. In conclusion, the rate of postoperative PONV was not analyzed albeit patients from intervention group had reduced length of hospitalization.

In the prospective randomized study (55) of RC patients, a guided intraoperative fluid therapy reduced the incidence of PONV (11 vs 3, $p < 0.01$ and 13 vs 1, $p < 0.0001$).

Yoo et al. (56) studied the incidence of PONV between group of patients with propofol total intravenous anesthesia (TIVA) and the group of patients with desflurane anesthesia for robot-assisted laparoscopic RP. The incidence of PONV was significantly lower in TIVA group both in post-anesthetic care unit and 1–6 h after the surgery.

INTRAOPERATIVE PERIOD

This section reviews several important components of the intraoperative period (**Table 1**).

Perioperative Analgesia

The use of neuraxial anesthesia in RC and in RP patients is widely applied as one of the crucial elements of fast-track pathways (42, 59, 60). The American Pain Society (61) points out the importance of using neuraxial anesthesia in major thoracic and abdominal surgery, especially in patients with cardiologic and pulmonary morbidity or in those at risk of postoperative ileus (POI).

The epidural provides different positive effects on the general perioperative status of patients. Several studies reveal decrease in mortality (61, 62) as well as decrease in the risk of cardiovascular and respiratory (63) events in abdominal surgery. In RP and in RC patients, the epidural is related with reduced intraoperative blood loss (64, 65), earlier recovery of gastrointestinal peristalsis (66), and postoperative pain control (64). Still, Doiron et al. (67) observed no difference in length of stay, 30- and 90-day readmission rate, nor any influence on 30-day mortality among cystectomy patients with or without perioperative epidural. This is consistent with other studies (68, 69) in which the epidural was compared with intravenous patient-controlled analgesia.

It is extremely important to determine the aspects of using epidural in major urologic surgeries in the future. The level of epidural insertion for different urologic procedures is not precisely defined. For example, in some studies (60, 66) authors used Th9–11 for RC patients; however, in the study of Autran et al. (69) Th11-L2 was used. In RP studies, Shir et al. (64) used L3–L5, but Hong et al. (65) used Th12-L2. ERAS guidelines for RC (6) strongly recommend the use of thoracic epidural for 72 h, by extrapolating results from rectal surgery.

There are, however, other ways of administering perioperative analgesia in urology, which showed promising results. For example, in the study of Dutton et al. (12), out of 165 cystectomy patients that entered an enhanced recovery pathway, 140 patients had rectus sheath catheter (RSC) analgesia (**Table 1**). The authors switched from regional anesthesia to RSC blocks because of their numerous benefits. The advantages of RSC blocks have previously been studied (70, 71), and they include highly successful placement, patient safety, the possibility to use in patients taking antiplatelet medications, as well as the reliability during postoperative care.

Intraoperative Fluid Therapy

The optimization of fluid therapy, as a part of fast-track pathways, aims at "zero balance," maintaining preoperative fluid composition and weight (72). According to Gupta and Gan (73), maintenance fluid therapy in adult patients during major abdominal surgery should be accomplished with 1–3 ml/kg/h.

Intraoperative fluid therapy in RC was studied in the prospective study of Pillai et al. (55). Patients were randomized to receive standard intraoperative or esophageal Doppler guided fluid therapy. The study demonstrated improvements in gastrointestinal function with significant reduction of ileus, PONV and also wound infection in the intervention group. The trial patients received significantly greater volumes of intravenous fluid during the first operative hour. Authors postulated that this was the underlying reason for avoidance of occult splanchnic hypoperfusion and lowering of postoperative complications. It was also pointed out that timing of fluid administration may be the goal for tissue perfusion, rather than volume. The major limitations of this study were small number of patients and inclusion just of ASA1 and ASA2 patients.

In another randomized trial (74), patients were allocated to receive low volume of fluid therapy (1–3 ml/kg/h) with preemptive

TABLE 1 | Summary of intraoperative elements from published trials of enhanced recovery after surgery (ERAS) protocols for RC.

Authors	Arumainayagam et al.	Mukhtar et al.	Dutton et al.	Smith et al.	Daneshmand et al.	Persson et al.	Pang et al.
Reference/(*n*)	(28)/(112)	(46)/(77)	(12)/(165)	(57)/(133)	(58)/(110)	(13)/(70)	(14)/(453)
Non-ERAS *n*/ERAS *n*	56/56	26/51	0/165	69/37 ERAS 1, 27 ERAS 2	0/110	39/31	60/393
Surgery type	Open RC	Open RC	Open RC	Open RC	Open RC	Open RC	Open and robotic RC (425/28 ptc.)
Ileal condui/Neobl./Con. cu.div.	47/9/0	48/3/0	131/34/0	133/0/0	35/70/5	52/18/0	368/25/0
Antibiotic prophylaxis	Not specified	Not specified	Single dose cefuroxime, metronidazole	Not specified	+ Continued for 24 h	+ (100% ptc.)	Coamoxiclav 24 h in men 48 h in women
Analgesic method, *n* (%)							
Epidural	+	+	+ 25 ptc.	– ERAS 1 – ERAS 2	–	+	–
RSC	–	–	+ 140 ptc.	+ ERAS 1 + ERAS 2	– Subfascial LA	–	+ (53% ptc.)
Other	–	–	–	–	iv. Acetaminophen	–	–
Avoiding of							
NGT	Not specified	+	+	+ ERAS 1 + ERAS 2	–	+	+ (84% ptc.)
Drains	–	+	–	–	–	+ (32% ptc.)	Consider omitting pelvic drain
Fluid/sodium management	Not specified	+	+ (GDFT)	+ ERAS 1, ERAS 2 (GDFT)	+ Monitored by SV and CVP	Not specified	+ (Limited fluid targeted to losses)
Intraoperative warming	Not specified	+	+	–	Not specified	+	+
Small incisions	Not specified	+	+	Change in surgical technique	Not specified	Not specified	+ (83% ptc.)
PONV prevention	Metoclopramide from day 1	+	Metoclopramide, omeprazole	Not specified	Not specified	+ (29% ptc.)	Antiemetics as needed
$MgSO_4$ replacement	–	–	–	Infusion in ERAS 2	–	–	–

RC, radical cystectomy; ptc., patients; Neobl., neobladder; Con.cu.div., continent cutaneous diversion; RSC, rectus sheath catheter; LA, local anesthetics; NGT, nasogastric tube; GDFT, goal directed fluid therapy; SV, stroke volume; CVP, central venous pressure; PONV, postoperative nausea and vomiting.

norepinephrine of 6 μg/kg/h intraoperatively. The intervention group had reduced complication rate and hospitalization time. Furthermore, in another study the authors (75) showed zero fluid balance and zero weight gain on the first postoperative day with the same intraoperative intervention.

In multivariate logistic regressions of Bazargani et al. (76), there was no significant link between higher intraoperative fluid intake and complications on the 30th and 90th days in 180 patients who underwent RC. It should be emphasized that this was ERAS pathway study for RC, *vice versa* to previously mentioned studies (55, 74). It was suggested that various measures of ERAS protocol attenuated possible negative effects of high fluid administration volumes. The controversy of fluid management in RC continues. Fluid restriction with possible silent or evident splanchnic ischemia and hypotension must be compared with fluid overload and interstitial and gut edema. Possible better monitoring of bowel perfusion and standardized protocols of intraoperative fluid administration in ERAS pathways in RC and other major urologic procedures is needed.

Preventing Intraoperative Hypothermia

The maintenance of normothermia during surgery prevents high oxygen consumption, wound infection, bleeding, and pain. China's national cross-sectional study (77) on 3,132 patients under general anesthesia showed increased ICU admissions and prolonged hospital stay in patients with intraoperative hypothermia.

The active warming strategies, such as the use of warm fluids and forced air warming (78), were more effective than passive warming in maintaining stable intraoperative hemodynamics and core temperature.

Surgery Type

Compared with open surgery (79), minimally invasive surgery enhances patients' recovery, due to less stress, and it also significantly lowers opioid requirements (80). According to systematic reviews (81, 82), the implementation of robotic RC has reduced blood loss and transfusion, inpatient narcotic requirements, time to regular diet, and length of hospital stay. In the prospective randomized study of Nix et al. (80), there was lower estimated blood loss and there were fewer narcotic requirements during robotic RC. Postoperative return of bowel function was more rapid in patients who underwent robotic RC. The authors believe that the probable reasons for the previously stated findings were lower degree of bowel manipulation, less fluid imbalance and lower overall opioid consumption. However, in addition to the benefits, it should also be stated that, according to some studies (79, 80), robotic cystectomy lasts significantly more and has similar rate of postoperative complications when compared with open RC.

Robot-assisted RP has gained popularity due to its benefits which are similar to those of robotic RC (56). Nevertheless, studies mainly investigate disease control and functional sequel. Maurice et al. (83) listed increased travel burden and limiting access to surgical care as disadvantages of RP. Further studies on the implementation of fast-track pathways in robotic prostatectomy are needed.

Studies of laparoscopic RC state different benefits. In the study (84) of 47 patients undergoing laparoscopic RC, before and after the implementation of the ERAS protocol, ERAS group had lower frequency of central vein catheter infection and paralytic ileus. Guan et al. (85) showed that patients with fast-track laparoscopic RC had shorter time to first flatus and regular diet, lower serum C-reactive protein and white blood count on the fifth and seventh day after surgery, as well as lower frequency of complications.

POSTOPERATIVE PERIOD

Several elements related to postoperative period are reviewed here.

Nasogastric Tube (NGT)

Early NGT removal was introduced in the study of Pruthi et al. (86) as a fast-track element for RC. The NGT was removed on the first day, and clear liquid was introduced on the second postoperative day. The main improvement was seen in postoperative morbidity. Park et al. (87) found out that early NGT removal after RC is not correlated with POI. In the prospective study (88), the authors examined the combination of metoclopramide and early nasogastric suction removal in RC patients and revealed reduction of postoperative atelectasis and earlier tolerance of solid food without complications, regarding bowel anastomosis. Retrospective analyses of RC patients (12) in the enhanced recovery program introduce "no routine NGT" as one step forward. The authors reserved the use of nasogastric suction only for patients with a POI. Outcomes of this study revealed no adverse effects on readmission and complications. It can be concluded that further studies will have objective to determine if the routine use of NGT in RC is necessary.

Postoperative Analgesia

Epidural analgesia given during the period of 2–3 days after surgery, preferably without opioids, provides more efficient analgesia, compared with patient-controlled analgesia (89) in colorectal surgery. As far as urologic surgery is concerned, according to the study of Hong et al. (65), postoperative pain scores were lower in patients with combined general and epidural anesthesia, compared with RP patients with general anesthesia only. The authors concluded that this may be important for the reduction of the incidence of postoperative chronic pelvic pain. In the prospective, randomized double-blinded study (90), it was shown that continuous epidural infusion of local anesthetics and sufentanil alone or combined produced adequate analgesia for RP and nephrectomy. The authors found out that ropivacaine, combined with sufentanil, was the most preferable combination because of low incidence of motor block.

As it was mentioned before, RSC analgesia (12) for RC and transverses abdominis plane block (91) in RP are getting attention as alternatives to neuraxial anesthesia for perioperative analgesia. The idea of combining motor blocks with oral paracetamol/nonsteroidal anti-inflammatory drugs (91) may potentially eliminate opioids from postoperative analgesia.

Optimal postoperative analgesia for major urologic surgery includes different techniques and different drugs. The introduction of new minimally invasive surgical techniques implies the use of different modalities; therefore, the specific role of certain combinations of analgesia regimens needs to be investigated in future.

Prevention of POI

Postoperative ileus is a frequent gastrointestinal complication especially after RC. The incidence of POI in RC has been between 4 and 31% (13, 35). With the aim to define early postoperative morbidity after RC, Shabsig et al. (50) proposed the definition of ileus as "Inability to tolerate solid food by postoperative day five, the need to place NGT or the need to stop oral intake due to abdominal distension, nausea or emesis." Proposed mechanisms for POI after RC (92) are fluid overload, electrolyte shifts, bowel manipulation, and opioid use. It has been theorized that the presence of urine in the operative field during RC delays resumption of the bowel motility (47).

It has been shown (13) that patients guided with ERAS pathway have significant reduction in the average time of the first passage of stool compared with pre-ERAS group. The prevention of POI involves a sum of benefits of ERAS elements. These are epidural perioperative analgesia (66, 92), optimization of intraoperative fluid therapy (55), minimally invasive approach to surgery, early NGT removal with early oral intake (13), and early mobilization.

Other measures used with the aim of promoting bowel function and ileus prevention are chewing gum and using alvimopan. In the study of robotic RC (93), patients that chewed gum had shorter time to first flatus in comparison with the standard ones.

In a retrospective study of Hamilton et al. (94), the alvimopan group of patients undergoing RC had significantly shorter average time of resuming a regular diet (5.3 vs 4.1 days, $p < 0.01$).

Finally, regardless of the great importance of POI regarding postoperative morbidity in ERAS for RC, its significance in other major urologic surgeries is still to be evaluated.

Early Oral Intake and Postoperative Nutrition

The safety of early oral intake after bowel anastomosis was shown in several studies (95, 96). The guidelines for perioperative care in elective rectal/pelvic surgery recommend oral diet "*ad libitum*" 4 h after rectal surgery (5). Pruthi et al. (86) showed improvement in perioperative care in patients with RC by reducing time to clear liquid and regular diet. Early oral nutrition, as a part of multimodal approach (97), revealed reduced time to first flatus. Arumainayagam et al. (28) restarted clear fluids on the day of RC with other perioperative ERAS elements in 56 out of 112 patients. This study showed reduced total and postoperative hospital stay.

ESPEN guidelines for surgery (29) recommend that oral intake, including clear liquids, should be initiated within hours after surgery in most patients. ERAS society guidelines (6) for perioperative care after RC suggest that normal diet should be reestablished as soon as possible.

In the case of impaired oral or enteral tolerance for more than seven days, ESPEN guidelines (29) recommend adding parenteral nutrition. According to EPaNIC study (98) withholding of parenteral nutrition until day eighth appears to be superior strategy than early addition of parenteral nutrition. According to authors, early administration of parenteral nutrition suppresses autophagy thus preventing clearance of damaged cells and microorganisms. The study population was low severity critical care group of patients among which major surgical patients too. Moreover in the study of Roth et al. (99) in patients after RC with urinary diversion, immediate postoperative parenteral nutrition is associated with higher incidence of infection complications vs oral nutrition alone.

Early parenteral nutrition is beneficial in malnourished patients in whom oral or enteral nutrition is not feasible (29).

Early Mobilization

Prolonged bed rest causes respiratory, musculoskeletal, and neuropsychological changes (100).

Primary conditions that have to be fulfilled before patient mobilization are the following ones: the gaining of patient's motivation, postoperative pain relief, and the prevention of orthostatic intolerance (17). Furthermore, in the randomized study of Gatt et al. (101) on colonic surgery, the implementation of structured mobility plan with an active intervention of a physiotherapist resulted in longer period of time out of bed and in increased grip strength.

In the study of Pang et al. (14), the implementation of early mobilization of patients after RC along with other perioperative elements of the ERAS protocol reduces the length of hospital stay and the frequency of readmission. In this prospective study, on the first postoperative day, patients stayed out of bed for 6 h and walked 10–20 m, while on the second postoperative day they walked 100 m. Other authors (12, 13) also enlist early mobilization of patients into local ERAS protocol for cystectomy with similar results.

Early mobilization is emphasized in perioperative care of patients after RP as well. In the prospective randomized study of Gralla et al. (42), patients walked around their room and around the ward on the very day of the surgery. Patients from the conventional group were allowed only upright position on the same day.

Already defined as part of "proactive de-medicalization" (14), patient mobilization represents important prerequisite for stoma self-management and for the decrease in length of hospital stay.

Urinary Drainage

Urinary bladder drainage is a routine procedure in major and urologic surgery. Optimal duration of catheter drainage is 1 day after colonic resections (102) and after pelvic surgery in patients with low risk of urinary retention (5, 6). Catheter removal on the first postoperative day after thoracic and abdominal surgery reduces the incidence of urinary tract infections.

The time period of urinary drainage in radical RC patients is vaguely defined in scientific literature. According to the study of Mattei et al. (102), the stenting of ureteroileal anastomosis resulted in decreased postoperative upper urinary tract dilatation; it improved postoperative bowel function and also decreased metabolic acidosis. The consensus statement about the exact timing of the stent removal in ileal conduit patients varies from 5 to 14 days. The urinary catheter in orthotopic neobladder is left for, at least, 14 days (103) after surgery.

Bearing in mind insufficient evidence (6) analyzed so far, this particular field of ERAS protocol needs to be studied in the future.

CONCLUSION

Multimodal perioperative approach involves many evidence-based interventions with the aim of helping without doing any harm. Major urologic procedures, especially RC, represent a special challenge for future investigation in the ERAS era. Important fields for future investigation, regarding preoperative phase of surgery, are the following ones: the importance of nutritional therapy with the emphases on immune formulas, the omitting of preoperative bowel preparation, and the impact it will have on postoperative outcome, possible advantage of prolonged thromboprophylaxis regarding decreasing risk of VTE and further consideration of lowering insulin resistance. Intraoperative period studies will have to distinguish between the patients with possible risks of fluid overload and the need for guided fluid therapy and the patients who need special surgical techniques. New modalities of opioid sparing postoperative analgesia, the importance of implementing new drugs and special ERAS elements with the aim of preventing POI and the defining of optimal duration of urinary drainage, will be interesting issues to be studied in future, related with postoperative period in major urology. The main prerequisite for everything stated above is the increase of ERAS implementation in major urologic surgery.

AUTHOR CONTRIBUTIONS

NV conceived, designed, and wrote the manuscript. LD helped in analyzing the data.

REFERENCES

1. Kehlet H. Multimodal approach to control postoperative pathophysiology and rehabilitation. *Br J Anaesth* (1997) 78:606–17. doi:10.1093/bja/78.5.606
2. Place K, Scott NB. Enhanced recovery for lower limb arthroplasty. *Crit Care Pain* (2014) 14:95–9. doi:10.1093/bjaceaccp/mkt037
3. Shepherd SJ, Klein AA, Martinez G. Enhanced recovery for thoracic surgery in the elderly. *Curr Opin Anaesthesiol* (2017) 30:1–9. doi:10.1097/ACO.0000000000000537

4. Scott MJ, Baldini G, Fearon KCH, Feldheiser A, Feldman LS, Gan TJ, et al. Enhanced Recovery after Surgery (ERAS) for gastrointestinal surgery, part 1: pathophysiological considerations. *Acta Anaesthesiol Scand* (2015) 59:1212–31. doi:10.1111/aas.12601
5. Nygren J, Thacker J, Carli F, Fearon KC, Norderval S, Lobo DN, et al. Guidelines for perioperative care in elective rectal/pelvic surgery: enhanced recovery after surgery (ERAS®) society recommendations. *World J Surg* (2013) 37:285–305. doi:10.1007/s00268-012-1787-6
6. Cerantola Y, Valerio M, Persson B, Jichlinski P, Ljungqvist O, Hubner M, et al. Guidelines for perioperative care after radical cystectomy for bladder cancer: enhanced recovery after surgery (ERAS®) society recommendations. *Clin Nutr* (2013) 32:879–87. doi:10.1016/j.clnu.2013.09.014
7. Thompson T, Keogh E, French CC, Davis R. Anxiety sensitivity and pain: generalisability across noxious stimuli. *Pain* (2008) 134:187–96. doi:10.1016/j.pain.2007.04.018
8. Carli F, Charlebois P, Baldini G, Cachero O, Stein B. An integrated multidisciplinary approach to implementation of a fast-track program for laparoscopic colorectal surgery. *Can J Anaesth* (2009) 56:837–42. doi:10.1007/s12630-009-9159-x
9. Clarke HD, Timm VL, Goldberg BR, Hattrup SJ. Preoperative patient education reduces in-hospital falls after total knee arthroplasty. *Clin Orthop Relat Res* (2012) 470:244–9. doi:10.1007/s11999-011-1951-6
10. Hobisch A, Tosun K, Kinzl J, Kemmler G, Bartsch G, Höltl L, et al. Quality of life after cystectomy and orthotopic neobladder versus ileal conduit urinary diversion. *World J Urol* (2000) 18:338–44. doi:10.1007/s003450000147
11. Schwartz J, Schneider F, Lataillade L, Beyeler S, Mayer F, Iselin C. Radical cystectomy and urinary diversion: assistance to patient choice. *Rev Med Suisse* (2008) 4:2614–7.
12. Dutton TJ, Daugherty MO, Mason RG, McGrath JS. Implementation of the exeter enhanced recovery programme for patients undergoing radical cystectomy. *BJU Int* (2014) 113:719–25. doi:10.1111/bju.12533
13. Persson B, Carringer M, Andre O, Andersson S, Carlsson J, Ljungqvist O. Initial experiences with the enhanced recovery after surgery (ERAS) protocol in open radical cystectomy. *Scand J Urol* (2015) 49:302–7. doi:10.3109/21681805.2015.1004641
14. Pang KH, Groves R, Venugopal S, Noon AP, Catto JWF, Novara G, et al. Prospective implementation of enhanced recovery after surgery protocols to radical cystectomy. *Eur Urol* (2017) 73(3):363–71. doi:10.1016/j.eururo.2017.07.031
15. Matulewicz RS, Brennan J, Pruthi RS, Kundu SD, Gonzalez CM, Meeks JJ. Radical cystectomy perioperative care redesign. *Urology* (2015) 86:1076–86. doi:10.1016/j.urology.2015.09.001
16. Jensen BT, de Blok W, Kiesbye B, Kristensen SA. Validation of the urostomy education scale: the European experience. *Urol Nurs* (2013) 33:219–29.
17. Maloney I, Parker DC, Cookson MS, Patel S. Bladder cancer recovery pathways : a systematic review. *Bladder Cancer* (2017) 3:269–81. doi:10.3233/BLC-170136
18. De Hert S, Imberger G, Carlisle J, Diemunsch P, Fritsch G, Moppett I, et al. Preoperative evaluation of the adult patient undergoing non-cardiac surgery: guidelines from the European Society of Anaesthesiology. *Eur J Anaesthesiol* (2011) 28:684–722. doi:10.1097/EJA.0b013e3283499e3b
19. Turan A, Mascha EJ, Roberman D, Turner PL, You J, Kurz A, et al. Smoking and perioperative outcomes. *Anesthesiology* (2011) 114:837–46. doi:10.1097/ALN.0b013e318210f560
20. Thomsen T, Tønnesen H, Møller AM. Effect of preoperative smoking cessation interventions on postoperative complications and smoking cessation. *Br J Surg* (2009) 96:451–61. doi:10.1002/bjs.6591
21. Myers K, Hajek P, Hinds C, McRobbie H. Stopping smoking shortly before surgery and postoperative complications. *Arch Intern Med* (2011) 171:983–9. doi:10.1001/archinternmed.2011.97
22. Azhar RA, Bochner B, Catto J, Goh AC, Kelly J, Patel HD, et al. Enhanced Recovery after Urological Surgery : a contemporary systematic review of outcomes, key elements, and research needs. *Eur Urol* (2016) 70:176–87. doi:10.1016/j.eururo.2016.02.051
23. Tønnesen H, Nielsen PR, Lauritzen JB, Møller AM. Smoking and alcohol intervention before surgery: evidence for best practice. *Br J Anaesth* (2009) 102:297–306. doi:10.1093/bja/aen401
24. Tønnesen H, Rosenberg J, Nielsen HJ, Rasmussen V, Hauge C, Pedersen IK, et al. Outcome in alcohol misusers: randomized controlled trial. *BMJ* (1999) 318:1311–6. doi:10.1136/bmj.318.7194.1311
25. Stojanović N, Pavlović S, Nikolić M, Nikolic J. Nutrition screening importance for patients that underwent radical cystectomy. *Acta Fac Med Naiss* (2007) 4:195–9.
26. Gregg JR, Cookson MS, Phillips S, Salem S, Chang SS, Clark PE, et al. Effect of preoperative nutritional deficiency on mortality after radical cystectomy for bladder cancer. *J Urol* (2011) 185:90–6. doi:10.1016/j.juro.2010.09.021
27. Kondrup J, Rasmussen HH, Hamberg O, Stanga Z, Ad Hoc Espen Working Group. Nutritional risk screening (NRS 2002): a new method based on an analysis of controlled clinical trials. *Clin Nutr* (2003) 22:321–36. doi:10.1016/S0261-5614(02)00214-5
28. Arumainayagam N, McGrath J, Jefferson KP, Gillatt DA. Introduction of an enhanced recovery protocol for radical cystectomy. *BJU Int* (2008) 101:698–701. doi:10.1111/j.1464-410X.2007.07319.x
29. Weimann A, Braga M, Carli F, Higashiguchi T, Hübner M, Klek S, et al. ESPEN guideline : clinical nutrition in surgery. *Clin Nutr* (2017) 36:623–50. doi:10.1016/j.clnu.2017.02.013
30. Hamilton-Reeves JM, Yankee TM, Chalise P, Lee EK, Mirza M, Wyre H, et al. Effects of immunonutrition for cystectomy on immune response and infection rates : a pilot randomized controlled clinical trial. *Eur Urol* (2016) 69:389–92. doi:10.1016/j.eururo.2015.11.019
31. Tabibi A, Simforoosh N, Basiri A, Ezzatnejad M, Abdi H, Farrokhi F. Bowel preparation versus no preparation before ileal urinary diversion. *Urology* (2007) 70:654–8. doi:10.1016/j.urology.2007.06.1107
32. Xu R, Zhao X, Zhong Z, Zhang L. No advantage is gained by preoperative bowel preparation in radical cystectomy and ileal conduit: a randomized controlled trial of 86 patients. *Int Urol Nephrol* (2010) 42:947–50. doi:10.1007/s11255-010-9732-9
33. Güenaga KF, Matos D, Wille-Jørgensen P. Preoperative mechanical bowel preparation in elective colorectal surgery. An update of systematic review of the literature and meta-analysis. *J Coloproctol* (2012) 32:7–17. doi:10.1590/S2237-93632012000100002
34. Venclauskas L, Llau JV, Jenny JY, Kjaersgaard-Andersen P. European guidelines on perioperative venous thromboembolism prophylaxis: day surgery and fast-track surgery. *Eur J Anaesthesiol* (2017) 34:1–5. doi:10.1097/EJA.0000000000000706
35. Novotny V, Hakenberg OW, Wiessner D, Heberling U, Litz RJ, Oehlschlaeger S, et al. Perioperative complications of radical cystectomy in a contemporary series. *Eur Urol* (2007) 51:397–402. doi:10.1016/j.eururo.2006.06.014
36. Vukina J, McKibben MJ, McBride A, Matthews J, Pruthi R, Wallen E, et al. Identifying incidence and risk factors for venous thromboembolism (VTE) among radical prostatectomy patients for prostate cancer. *J Am Coll Surg* (2014) 219(3):S145. doi:10.1016/j.jamcollsurg.2014.07.349
37. Weinberg A, Wright J, Deibert C, Lu Y-S, Hershman D, Neugut A, et al. Nationwide practice patterns for the use of venous thromboembolism prophylaxis among men undergoing radical prostatectomy. *World J Urol* (2014) 32:1313–21. doi:10.1007/s00345-013-1212-2
38. Sachdeva A, Dalton M, Amaragiri SV, Lees T. Elastic compression stockings for prevention of deep vein thrombosis. *Cochrane Database Syst Rev* (2010) 7(7):CD001484. doi:10.1002/14651858.CD001484.pub2
39. Guyatt GH, Akl EA, Crowther M, Gutterman DD, Schuunemann HJ. Executive summary: antithrombotic therapy and prevention of thrombosis, 9th ed: American College of Chest Physicians evidence-based clinical practice guidelines. *Chest* (2012) 141:7–47. doi:10.1378/chest.1412S3
40. Smith I, Kranke P, Murat I, Smith A, O'Sullivan G, Sreide E, et al. Perioperative fasting in adults and children. *Eur J Anaesthesiol* (2011) 28:556–69. doi:10.1097/EJA.0b013e3283495ba1
41. Rege A, Leraas H, Vikraman D, Ravindra K, Brennan T, Miller T, et al. Could the use of an enhanced recovery protocol in laparoscopic donor nephrectomy be an incentive for live kidney donation? *Cureus* (2016) 8(11):e889. doi:10.7759/cureus.889
42. Gralla O, Haas F, Knoll N, Hadzidiakos D, Tullmann M, Romer A, et al. Fast-track surgery in laparoscopic radical prostatectomy : basic principles. *World J Urol* (2007) 25:185–91. doi:10.1007/s00345-006-0139-2
43. Awad S, Varadhan KK, Ljungqvist O, Lobo DN. A meta-analysis of randomised controlled trials on preoperative oral carbohydrate treatment in elective surgery. *Clin Nutr* (2013) 32:34–44. doi:10.1016/j.clnu.2012.10.011
44. Thorell A, Nygren J, Ljungqvist O. Insulin resistance: a marker of surgical stress. *Curr Opin Clin Nutr Metab Care* (1999) 2:69–78. doi:10.1097/00075197-199901000-00012

45. Ljungqvist O, Nygren J, Thorell A. Modulation of post-operative insulin resistance by pre-operative carbohydrate loading. *Proc Nutr Soc* (2002) 61:329–35. doi:10.1079/PNS2002168
46. Mukhtar S, Ayres BE, Issa R, Swinn MJ, Perry MJA. Challenging boundaries: an enhanced recovery programme for radical cystectomy. *Ann R Coll Surg Engl* (2013) 95:200–6. doi:10.1308/003588413X13511609957579
47. Kulkarni J. Perioperative morbidity of radical cystectomy: a review. *Indian J Urol* (2011) 27:226–32. doi:10.4103/0970-1591.82842
48. Saar M, Ohlmann C, Siemer S, Lehmann J, Becker F, Stöckle M, et al. Fast-track rehabilitation after robot-assisted laparoscopic cystectomy accelerates postoperative recovery. *BJU Int* (2012) 112:99–106. doi:10.1111/j.1464-410X.2012.11473.x
49. Bonkat G, Pickard R, Bartoletti R, Bruyers F, Geerlings SE, Wagelehner F, et al. *EAU Guidelines on Urological Infections*. Arnhem: EAU Guidelines Office (2018). Available from: http://uroweb.org/guidelines/compilations-of-all-guidelines/
50. Shabsigh A, Korets R, Vora KC, Brooks CM, Cronin AM, Savage C, et al. Defining early morbidity of radical cystectomy for patients with bladder cancer using a standardized reporting methodology. *Eur Urol* (2009) 55:164–76. doi:10.1016/j.eururo.2008.07.031
51. Sinclair DR, Chung F, Mezei G. Can postoperative nausea and vomiting be predicted? *Anesthesiology* (1999) 91:109–18. doi:10.1097/00000542-199907000-00018
52. Pierre S. A risk score-dependent antiemetic approach effectively reduces postoperative nausea and vomiting – a continuous quality improvement initiative. *Can J Anesth* (2004) 51:320–5. doi:10.1007/BF03018235
53. Apfel CC, Laara E, Koivuranta E, Greim CA, Roewer N. A simplified risk score for predicting postoperative conclusions from cross-validations between two centers. *Anesthesiology* (1999) 91:693–700. doi:10.1097/00000542-199909000-00022
54. Koivuranta M, Laara E, Snare L, Alahuta S. A survey of postoperative nausea and vomiting. *Anaesthesia* (1997) 52:443–9. doi:10.1111/j.1365-2044.1997.117-az0113.x
55. Pillai P, McEleavy I, Gaughan M, Snowden C, Nesbitt I, Durkan G, et al. A double-blind randomized controlled clinical trial to assess the effect of Doppler optimized intraoperative fluid management on outcome following radical cystectomy. *J Urol* (2011) 186:2201–6. doi:10.1016/j.juro.2011.07.093
56. Yoo Y-C, Bai S-J, Lee K-Y, Shin S, Choi EK, Lee JW. Total intravenous anesthesia with propofol reduces postoperative nausea and vomiting in patients undergoing robot-assisted laparoscopic radical prostatectomy: a prospective randomized trial. *Yonsei Med J* (2012) 53:1197. doi:10.3349/ymj.2012.53.6.1197
57. Smith J, Meng ZW, Lockyer R, Dudderidge T, McGrath J, Hayes M, et al. Evolution of the Southampton Enhanced Recovery Programme for radical cystectomy and the aggregation of marginal gains. *BJU Int* (2014) 114:375–83. doi:10.1111/bju.12644
58. Daneshmand S, Ahmadi H, Schuckman AK, Mitra AP, Cai J, Miranda G, et al. Enhanced recovery protocol after radical cystectomy for bladder cancer. *J Urol* (2014) 192:50–5. doi:10.1016/j.juro.2014.01.097
59. Maffezzini M, Campodonico F, Canepa G, Gerbi G, Parodi D. Current perioperative management of radical cystectomy with intestinal urinary reconstruction for muscle-invasive bladder cancer and reduction of the incidence of postoperative ileus. *Surg Oncol* (2008) 17:41–8. doi:10.1016/j.suronc.2007.09.003
60. Maffezzini M, Campodonico F, Capponi G, Manuputty E, Gerbi G. Fast-track surgery and technical nuances to reduce complications after radical cystectomy and intestinal urinary diversion with the modified Indiana pouch. *Surg Oncol* (2012) 21:191–5. doi:10.1016/j.suronc.2012.02.001
61. Chou R, Gordon DB, de Leon-Casasola OA, Rosenberg JM, Bickler S, Brennan T, et al. Management of postoperative pain: a clinical practice guideline from the American Pain Society, the American Society of Regional Anesthesia and Pain Medicine, and the American Society of Anesthesiologists' Committee on Regional Anesthesia, Executive Committee, and Administrative Council. *J Pain* (2016) 17:131–57. doi:10.1016/j.jpain.2015.12.008
62. Popping DM, Elia N, Marret E, Remy C, Tramer MR. Protective effects of epidural analgesia on pulmonary complications after abdominal and thoracic surgery: a meta-analysis. *Arch Surg* (2008) 143:990–9. doi:10.1001/archsurg.143.10.990
63. Popping DM, Elia N, Van Aken H, Marret E, Schug SA, Kranke P, et al. Impact of epidural analgesia on mortality and morbidity after surgery: systematic review and meta-analysis of randomized controlled trials. *Ann Surg* (2014) 259:1056–67. doi:10.1097/SLA.0000000000000237
64. Shir Y, Raja SN, Frank SM, Brendler CB. Intraoperative blood loss during radical retropubic prostatectomy: epidural versus general anesthesia. *Urology* (1995) 45:993–9. doi:10.1016/S0090-4295(99)80120-4
65. Hong JY, Yang SC, Yr J, Kil HK. Epidural ropivacaine and sufentanil and the perioperative stress response after a radical retropubic prostatectomy. *Acta Anaesthesiol Scand* (2011) 55:282–9. doi:10.1111/j.1399-6576.2010.02360.x
66. Mazul-Sunko B, Gilja I, Jelisavac M, Kozul I, Troha D, Osmancevic N, et al. Thoracic epidural analgesia for radical cystectomy improves bowel function even in traditional perioperative care: a retrospective study in eighty-five patients. *Acta Clin Croat* (2014) 53:319–25.
67. Doiron RC, Jaeger M, Booth CM, Wei X, Siemens DR. Is there a measurable association of epidural use at cystectomy and postoperative outcomes? A population-based study. *Can Urol Assoc J* (2016) 10:321. doi:10.5489/cuaj.3856
68. Toren P, Ladak S, Ma C, McCluskey S, Flesner N. Comparison of epidural and intravenous patient controlled analgesia in patients undergoing radical cystectomy. *Can J Urol* (2009) 16:4716–20.
69. Autran AM, Clarke C, Smith D, Yutkin V, Alzahrani A, Izawa JI. Is postoperative epidural analgesia better than patient-controlled analgesia for radical cystectomy? *J Clin Urol* (2014) 7:190–7. doi:10.1177/2051415813500954
70. Parsons BA, Aning J, Daugherty MO, McGrath JS. The use of rectus sheath catheters as an analgesic technique for patients undergoing radical cystectomy. *Br J Med Surg Urol* (2011) 4:24–30. doi:10.1016/j.bjmsu.2010.05.003
71. Dutton TJ, McGrath JS, Daugherty MO. Use of rectus sheath catheters for pain relief in patients undergoing major pelvic urological surgery. *BJU Int* (2014) 113:246–53. doi:10.1111/bju.12316
72. Brandstrup B, Svendsen PE, Rasmussen M, Belhage B, Rodt SA, Hansen B, et al. Which goal for fluid therapy during colorectal surgery is followed by the best outcome: near-maximal stroke volume or zero fluid balance? *Br J Anaesth* (2012) 109:191–9. doi:10.1093/bja/aes163
73. Gupta R, Gan TJ. Peri-operative fluid management to enhance recovery. *Anaesthesia* (2016) 71:40–5. doi:10.1111/anae.13309
74. Wuetrich PY, Burkhard FC, Talmann GN, Stueber F, Studer UE. Restrictive deferred hydration combined with preemptive norepinephrine infusion during radical cystectomy reduces postoperative complications and hospitalization time: a randomized clinical trial. *Anesthesiology* (2014) 120:365–77. doi:10.1097/ALN.0b013e3182a4444
75. Wuethrich PY, Burkhard FC. Improved perioperative outcome with norepinephrine and a restrictive fluid administration during open radical cystectomy and urinary diversion. *Urol Oncol Semin Orig Investig* (2015) 33:.e21–66. doi:10.1016/j.urolonc.2014.07.018
76. Bazargani ST, Ghodoussipour S, Tse B, Miranda G, Cai J, Schuckman A, et al. The association between intraoperative fluid intake and postoperative complications in patients undergoing radical cystectomy with an enhanced recovery protocol. *World J Urol* (2018) 36(3):401–7. doi:10.1007/s00345-017-2164-8
77. Yi J, Lei Y, Xu S, Si Y, Li S, Xia Z, et al. Intraoperative hypothermia and its clinical outcomes in patients undergoing general anesthesia: national study in China. *PLoS One* (2017) 12(6):e0177221. doi:10.1371/journal.pone.0177221
78. Moola S, Lockwood C. Effectiveness of strategies for the management and/or prevention of hypothermia within the adult perioperative environment. *Int J Evid Based Healthcare* (2011) 9:337–45. doi:10.1111/j.1744-1609.2011.00227
79. Adding C, Collins JW, Laurin O, Hosseini A, Wiklund NP. Enhanced recovery protocols (ERP) in robotic cystectomy surgery review of current status and trends. *Curr Urol Rep* (2015) 16:32. doi:10.1007/s11934-015-0497-7
80. Nix J, Smith A, Kurpad R, Nielsen ME, Wallen EM, Pruthi RS. Prospective randomized controlled trial of robotic versus open radical cystectomy for bladder cancer : perioperative and pathologic results. *Eur Urol* (2010) 57:196–201. doi:10.1016/j.eururo.2009.10.024
81. Tang K, Xia D, Li H, Guan W, Guo X, Hu Z, et al. Robotic vs. open radical cystectomy in bladder cancer: a systematic review and meta-analysis. *Eur J Surg Oncol* (2014) 40:1399–411. doi:10.1016/j.ejso.2014.03.008
82. Novara G, Catto JWF, Wilson T, Annerstedt M, Chan K, Murphy DG, et al. Systematic review and cumulative analysis of perioperative outcomes and complications after robot-assisted radical cystectomy. *Eur Urol* (2015) 67:376–401. doi:10.1016/j.eururo.2014.12.007

83. Maurice MJ, Zhu H, Kim SP, Abouassaly R. Robotic prostatectomy is associated with increased patient travel and treatment delay. *Can Urol Assoc J* (2016) 10:192–201. doi:10.5489/cuaj.3628
84. Rivas J, Gregorioo S, Ledo J, Orejon R, Doslada P, Sebastian J, et al. Early recovery protocol in patients undergoing laparoscopic radical cystectomy. *Urol Sci* (2017) 28:2–5. doi:10.1016/j.urols.2015.01.006
85. Guan X, Liu L, Lei X, Zu X, Li Y, Chen M, et al. A comparative study off fast-track versus conventional surgery in patients undergoing laparoscopic radical cystectomy and ileal conduit diversion: Chinese experience. *Sci Rep* (2014) 4:6820. doi:10.1038/srep06820
86. Pruthi RS, Chun J, Richman M. Reducing time to oral diet and hospital discharge in patients undergoing radical cystectomy using a perioperative care plan. *Urology* (2003) 62:661–5. doi:10.1016/S0090-4295(03)00651-4
87. Park HK, Kwak C, Byun S-S, Lee E, Lee SE. Early removal of nasogastric tube after cystectomy with urinary diversion: does postoperative ileus risk increase? *Urology* (2005) 65:905–8. doi:10.1016/j.urology.2004.11.046
88. Donat SM, Slaton JW, Pisters LL, Swanson DA. Early nasogastric tube removal combined with metoclopramide after radical cystectomy and urinary diversion. *J Urol* (1999) 162:1599–602. doi:10.1016/S0022-5347(05)68175-X
89. Marret E, Remy C, Bonnet F, Forum P. Meta-analysis of epidural analgesia versus parenteral opioid analgesia after colorectal surgery. *Br J Surg* (2007) 94:665–73. doi:10.1002/bjs.5825
90. Hubler M, Litz R, Sengebusch K, Kreinecker I, Frank M, Hakenberg O. A comparison of five solutions of local anaesthetics and/or sufentanil for continuous, postoperative epidural analgesia after major urological surgery. *Eur J Anaesthesiol* (2001) 18:450–7. doi:10.1097/00003643-200107000-00004
91. Dudderidge TJ, Doyle P, Mayer EK, Taylor J, Agrawal S, Stolzenburg JU, et al. Evolution of care pathway for laparoscopic radical prostatectomy. *J Endourol* (2012) 26:660–5. doi:10.1089/end.2011.0427
92. Fitzgerald J, Ahmed I. Systematic review and meta-analysis of chewing-gum therapy in the reduction of postoperative paralytic ileus following gastrointestinal surgery. *World J Surg* (2009) 33:2557–66. doi:10.1007/s00268-009-0104-5
93. Choi H, Kang SH, Yoon DK, Kang SG, Ko HY, Moon du G, et al. Chewing gum has a stimulatory effect on bowel motility in patients after open or robotic radical cystectomy for bladder cancer: a prospective randomized comparative study. *Urology* (2011) 77:884–90. doi:10.1016/j.urology.2010.06.042
94. Hamilton Z, Parker W, Griffin J, Isaacson T, Mirza M, Wyre H, et al. Alvimopan in an enhanced recovery program following radical cystectomy. *Bladder Cancer* (2015) 1:137–42. doi:10.3233/BLC-150017
95. Andersen HK, Lewis SJ, Thomas S. Early enteral nutrition within 24h of colorectal surgery versus later commencement of feeding for postoperative complications. *Cochrane Database Syst Rev* (2006) 18:CD004080. doi:10.1002/14651858.CD004080.pub2
96. Basse L, HjortJakobsen D, Billesbølle P, Werner M, Kehlet H. A clinical pathway to accelerate recovery after colonic resection. *Ann Surg* (2000) 232:51–7. doi:10.1097/00000658-200007000-00008
97. Kehlet H, Wilmore DW. Multimodal strategies to improve surgical outcome. *Am J Surg* (2002) 183:630–41. doi:10.1016/S0002-9610(02)00866-8
98. Casaer MP, Mesotten D, Hermans G, Wouters PJ, Schetz M, Meyfroidt G, et al. Early versus late parenteral nutrition in critically ill adults. *N Engl J Med* (2011) 365:506–17. doi:10.1056/NEJMoa1102662
99. Roth B, Birkhäuser FD, Zehnder P, Thalmann GN, Huwyler M, Burkhard FC, et al. Parenteral nutrition does not improve postoperative recovery from radical cystectomy: results of a prospective randomised trial. *Eur Urol* (2013) 63:475–82. doi:10.1016/j.eururo.2012.05.052
100. Harper C, Lyles Y. Physiology and complications of bed rest. *J Am Geriatr Soc* (1988) 36:1047–54. doi:10.1111/j.1532-5415.1988.tb04375.x
101. Gatt M, Anderson ADG, Reddy BS, Hayward-Sampson P, Tring IC, MacFie J. Randomized clinical trial of multimodal optimization of surgical care in patients undergoing major colonic resection. *Br J Surg* (2005) 92:1354–62. doi:10.1002/bjs.5187
102. Mattei A, Birkhaeuser FD, Baermann C, Warncke SH, Studer SU. To stent or not to stent perioperatively the ureteroileal anastomosis of ileal orthotopic bladder substitutes and ileal conduits? Results of a prospective randomized trial. *J Urol* (2008) 179:582–6. doi:10.1016/j.juro.2007.09.066
103. Collins JW, Patel H, Adding C, Annerstedt M, Dasgupta P, Khan SM, et al. Enhanced recovery after robot-assisted radical cystectomy: EAU robotic urology section scientific working group consensus view. *Eur Urol* (2016) 70:649–60. doi:10.1016/j.eururo.2016.05.020

19

Gastric-Type Endocervical Adenocarcinoma Mimicking Submucosal Myoma Under Hysteroscopy

*Jiao Wang, Qing Yang, Dandan Wang, Mengyuan Li and Ningning Zhang**

Department of Obstetrics and Gynecology, Shengjing Hospital of China Medical University, Shenyang, China

Correspondence:
Ningning Zhang
18940257604@163.com

Gastric-type endocervical adenocarcinoma (GAS) is considered a distinct and clinically important entity because it is unrelated to human papillomavirus infection and has aggressive behavior and worse clinical outcomes than the usual type of endocervical adenocarcinoma (ECA). The preoperative diagnosis of GAS is often difficult because of its nonspecific clinical manifestations and special lesion location. We report the case of a 50-year-old Chinese woman who presented with intermittent left lower abdominal pain for 1 year. Preoperative images showed left hydrosalpinx and a lesion that was mainly located in the lower part of the uterine cavity. We considered the lesion to be a polyp before surgery. During hysteroscopic surgery, we suspected that it may be a submucosal myoma. However, pathology revealed that it was a GAS. GAS may be located in the upper endocervix or even reach the uterine cavity. The appearance is occasionally similar to that of submucosal myoma, resulting in difficult preoperative diagnosis and even misdiagnosis.

Keywords: endocervical adenocarcinoma, gastric-type, human papillomavirus, submucosal myoma, diagnosis

INTRODUCTION

Cervical cancer is the fourth most common gynecological malignancy worldwide (1). Most cervical cancers are related to the continuous infection of high-risk human papillomavirus (HPV). However, a few are not, such as some endocervical adenocarcinoma (ECA). ECA accounts for 20–25% of invasive cervical cancers, and its incidence is gradually increasing (2). In the 2020 World Health Organization (WHO) classification of female genital tumors, ECAs are subclassified into human papillomavirus (HPV)-associated (HPVA) and HPV-independent (HPVI) groups based on their distinct etiology and clinical behavior (3). The most common histological type of the HPVI group is gastric-type ECA (GAS) (4), which has a worse prognosis than HPVA (5). The clinical manifestations are not specific, the focus is hidden, and the positive rate of screening and biopsy is low, which brings great challenges to timely and correct diagnosis. Here, we present a patient with GAS with lower uterine cavity involvement, which was misdiagnosed as submucosal myoma during hysteroscopic surgery. However, pathology confirmed the diagnosis of GAS.

CASE REPORT

The patient was a 50-year-old premenopausal female, gravida 2, para 1. Cesarean section followed by right adnexectomy, which was performed due to a right ovarian cyst, was performed in 1995. On June 15, 2021, the patient visited our hospital for "intermittent left lower abdominal pain for 1 year." In May 2020, pelvic ultrasound was performed in another hospital because of left lower abdominal pain and fever. The results showed a cystic mass in the left adnexa, about 7.6 × 1.4 cm, with a high possibility of hydrosalpinx; an intrauterine device (IUD) and liquid dark area in the uterine cavity, and Nabothian cysts in the cervix. Her symptoms were relieved after anti-inflammatory treatment, but slight intermittent pain persisted in the lower abdomen. The patient underwent pelvic ultrasound again on May 26, 2021. The results showed left hydrosalpinx, about 7.5 × 3.4 cm, and in addition to the IUD and cervical Nabothian cysts, a slightly strong echo mass was seen in the uterine cavity. Then the patient was referred to our hospital. On gynecological examination, the vulva and vagina were normal, a small amount of secretion could be seen, the cervix was of normal size with a smooth surface, the uterus was normal, the left adnexa were thickened and accompanied by slight tenderness. Pelvic ultrasound revealed that a mass around 2.3 × 1.8 × 1.7 cm was seen in the lower part of uterine cavity. The internal echo was uneven, and the boundary was clear (**Figures 1A,B**). Color Doppler flow imaging detected blood flow signals. The size of the left ovary was normal, and a 7.7 × 3.6 × 1.6 cm cystic mass was seen in the left adnexal area, which was tortuous and tubular, with liquid inside and a clear boundary. Thinprep cytology test (TCT) revealed atypical squamous cells of undetermined significance (ASCUS); HPV: negative. The serum carbohydrate antigen (CA)-199, carcinoembryonic antigen (CEA), CA-125, and CA-724 levels were normal. Preoperative diagnoses included left hydrosalpinx and endometrial polyp. Laparoscopic left salpingectomy, removal of the IUD, and resection of the mass under hysteroscopy were performed on June 22, 2021. Laparoscopic exploration revealed a thickened left fallopian tube, with a size of about 7.0 × 2.0 cm, which surrounded the left ovary. The right adnexa were absent. The uterus was normal in size and regular in shape. After removing the left fallopian tube, the left ovary was exposed and appeared normal, and hysteroscopic surgery was subsequently performed. We first removed the T-shaped IUD. A mass with a size of about 2.5 × 2.0 cm was seen at the left anterior wall close to the internal os (**Figures 1C,D**). The texture was tough, the local shape was irregular, the surface contained thickened blood vessels (**Figure 1E**), and the mucosa of the cervical canal was smooth. The lesion was removed using a circular electrode (**Figure 1F**). All resected tissues were sent for pathology examination. The patient recovered and was discharged on the fourth postoperative day. Paraffin pathology results were as follows: well-differentiated GAS and left hydrosalpinx. We contacted the patient and asked her to return to our hospital for further treatment.

After the second admission, the patient's medical history was recorded. The patient said that she began having intermittent watery vaginal fluid approximately 1 year prior. She did not care for it or inform the doctors because she thought it was vaginitis. Gynecological examination showed that the cardinal and uterosacral ligaments were not thickened. Pelvic contrast-enhanced magnetic resonance imaging (MRI) showed that the cervix was plump, with an uneven equal T1 and slightly higher T2 signal shadow, which was mainly located in the posterior lip of the cervix. Weak enhancement was seen on contrast-enhanced scan, with a range of about 3.5 × 2.7 cm, in which there were many small circular long T1 and long T2 signal shadows (**Figures 2A,B**). No definite abnormality was found in the left ovary. Abdominal contrast-enhanced computed tomography (CT) showed that the cervix was slightly plump, and multiple low-density small nodules could be seen in it (overall range of about 2.8 × 2.5 cm), and the enhancement was not obvious (**Figures 2C,D**). Therefore, the diagnosis of stage IB2 GAS was made. Open operation was performed on July 26, 2021. During the operation, we found that the cervix was slightly plump (**Figure 2E**), the parauterine tissue was not thickened, and the appearance of the left ovary, peritoneal surface, greater omentum, and appendix were normal. First, the left ovary was removed and a tumor of approximately 1.5 × 1.3 cm was seen inside. The cut surface was yellowish white. Multiple cystic cavities were seen around (**Figure 2F**). The left ovary was subjected to frozen pathology, which suggested heterotypic glands and metastases. Therefore, radical hysterectomy, pelvic and paraaortic lymph node resection, greater omentum resection, and appendectomy were performed. There were no untoward events intraoperatively and postoperatively, and the patient was discharged on the eighth postoperative day. The paraffin pathological results were reported as follows: well-differentiated GAS, infiltrating the outer 1/3 of the cervical stroma; metastatic carcinoma of the left ovary; and no cancer at the surgical margin, parauterine, greater omentum, appendix, and lymph nodes. Microscopic examination revealed GAS (**Figures 3A,B**) and metastatic carcinoma of the left ovary (**Figure 3C**). Immunohistochemical analysis showed that the tumor was focally positive for CEA (**Figure 3D**), about 5% positive for Ki-67 (**Figure 3E**), and negative for P16, ER, and PR (**Figures 3F–H**). Four weeks after the second operation, the patient was referred to the gynecological tumor center for concurrent chemoradiotherapy (CCRT): pelvic intensity-modulated radiotherapy 50.4 Gy/28f + cisplatin concurrent chemotherapy. The patient completed the treatment, and there was no recurrence or metastasis during outpatient follow-up.

DISCUSSION

GAS, first described by Kojima et al. (6), was included as a subtype of HPVI group in the latest 2020 WHO classification of female genital tumors (3). It is an aggressive type of ECA characterized by mucinous morphology, gastric-type mucin, lack of association with HPV, and resistance to chemo/radiotherapy (7).

The incidence of GAS has obvious regional differences; GAS accounts for 10% of all ECA in an international population (4) and 20–25% of cases in Japanese women (8). Precursor lesions are essential for the prevention and early detection of cancer. Some findings suggest that atypical lobular endocervical

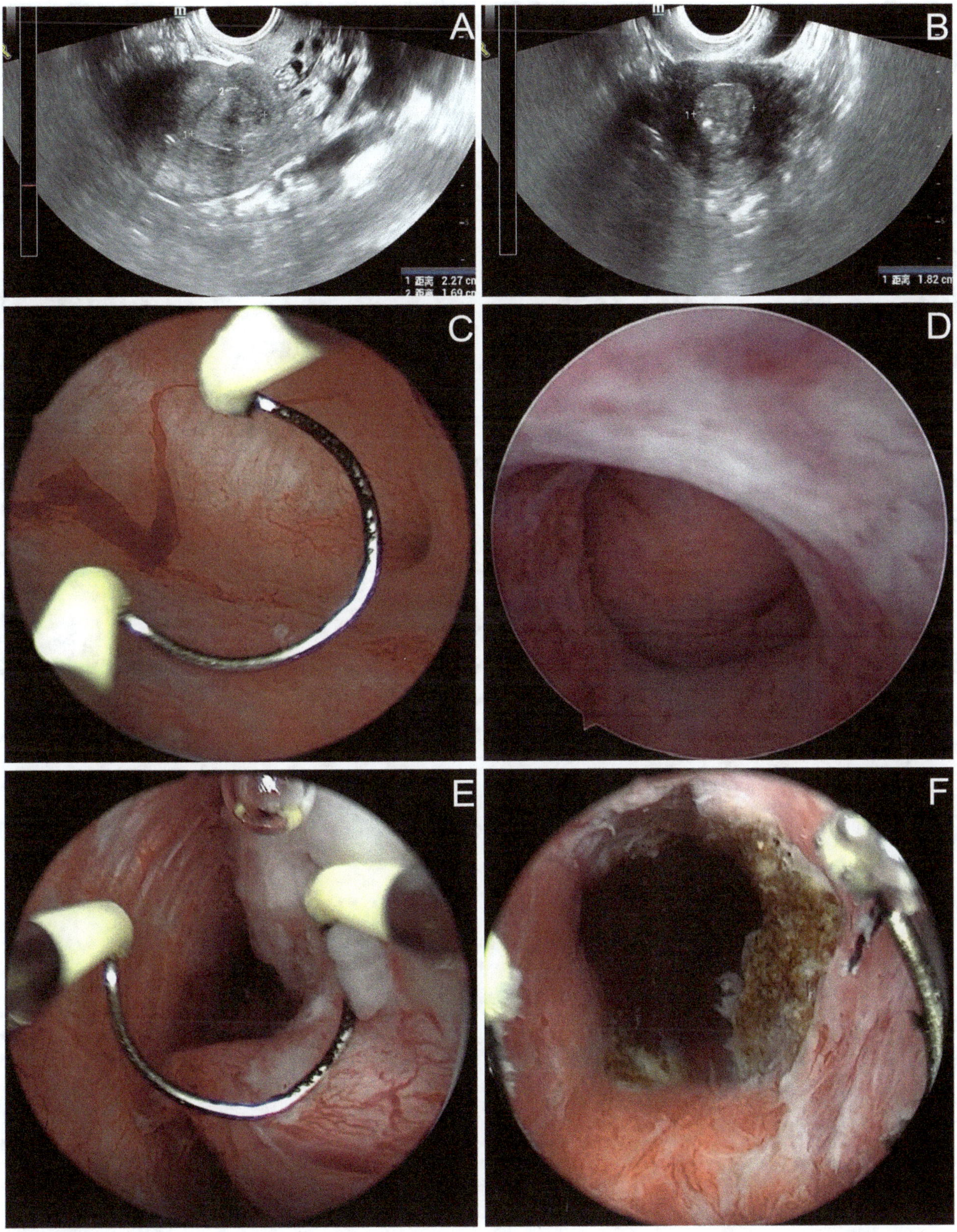

FIGURE 1 | Imaging findings of the patient before and during the first operation. **(A,B)** Pelvic ultrasound: a mass around 2.3 × 1.8 × 1.7 cm was seen in the lower part of uterine cavity. The internal echo was uneven, and the boundary was clear. **(C–F)** Hysteroscopy: a mass with a size of about 2.5 × 2.0 cm was seen at the left anterior wall close to the internal os. The local shape was irregular, the surface contained thickened blood vessels. The tumor was removed using a circular electrode, the boundary between the attachment position of tumor and cervical tissue was unclear.

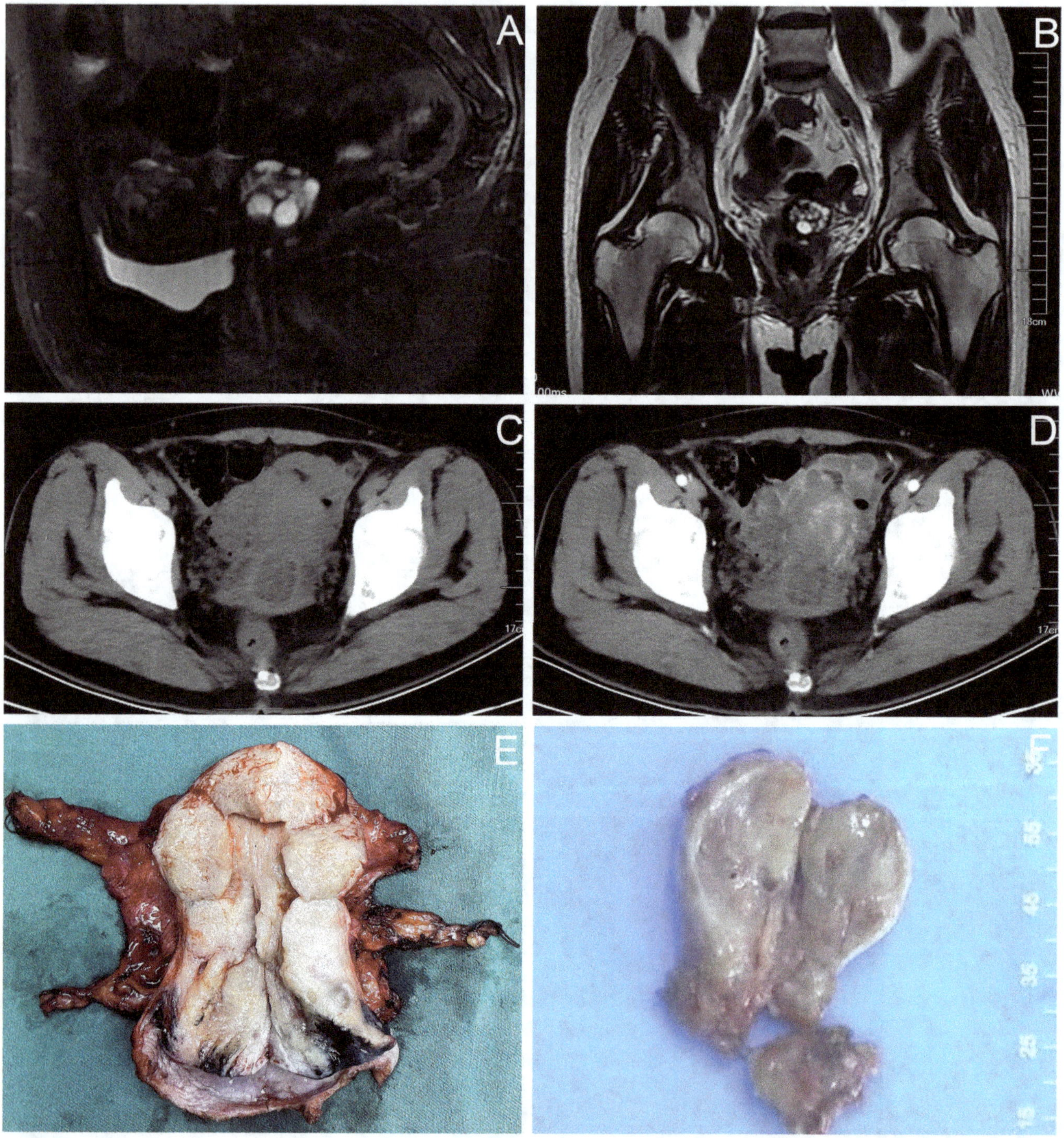

FIGURE 2 | Imaging findings of the patient before and during the second operation. **(A,B)** Pelvic MRI: the cervix was plump, with an uneven equal T1 and slightly higher T2 signal shadow, which was mainly located in the posterior lip of the cervix, about 3.5 × 2.7 cm, in which there were many small circular long T1 and long T2 signal shadows. **(C,D)** Abdominal CT: the cervical was slightly plump, and multiple low-density small nodules could be seen in it (overall range of about 2.8 × 2.5 cm), and the enhancement was not obvious. **(E)** The cervix was slightly plump. **(F)** The appearance of the left ovary was normal, a tumor of approximately 1.5 × 1.3 cm was seen inside, the cut surface was yellowish white, multiple cystic cavities were seen around.

glandular hyperplasia (LEGH) and gastric-type adenocarcinoma in *situ* are the precursors of GAS (9). D'Alessandro et al. (10) reported a case of GAS in presence of Nabothian cysts. They thought it would be interesting to evaluate the role of Nabothian cysts in the pathogenesis of GAS. The genetic underpinnings of GAS are beginning to be elucidated, as

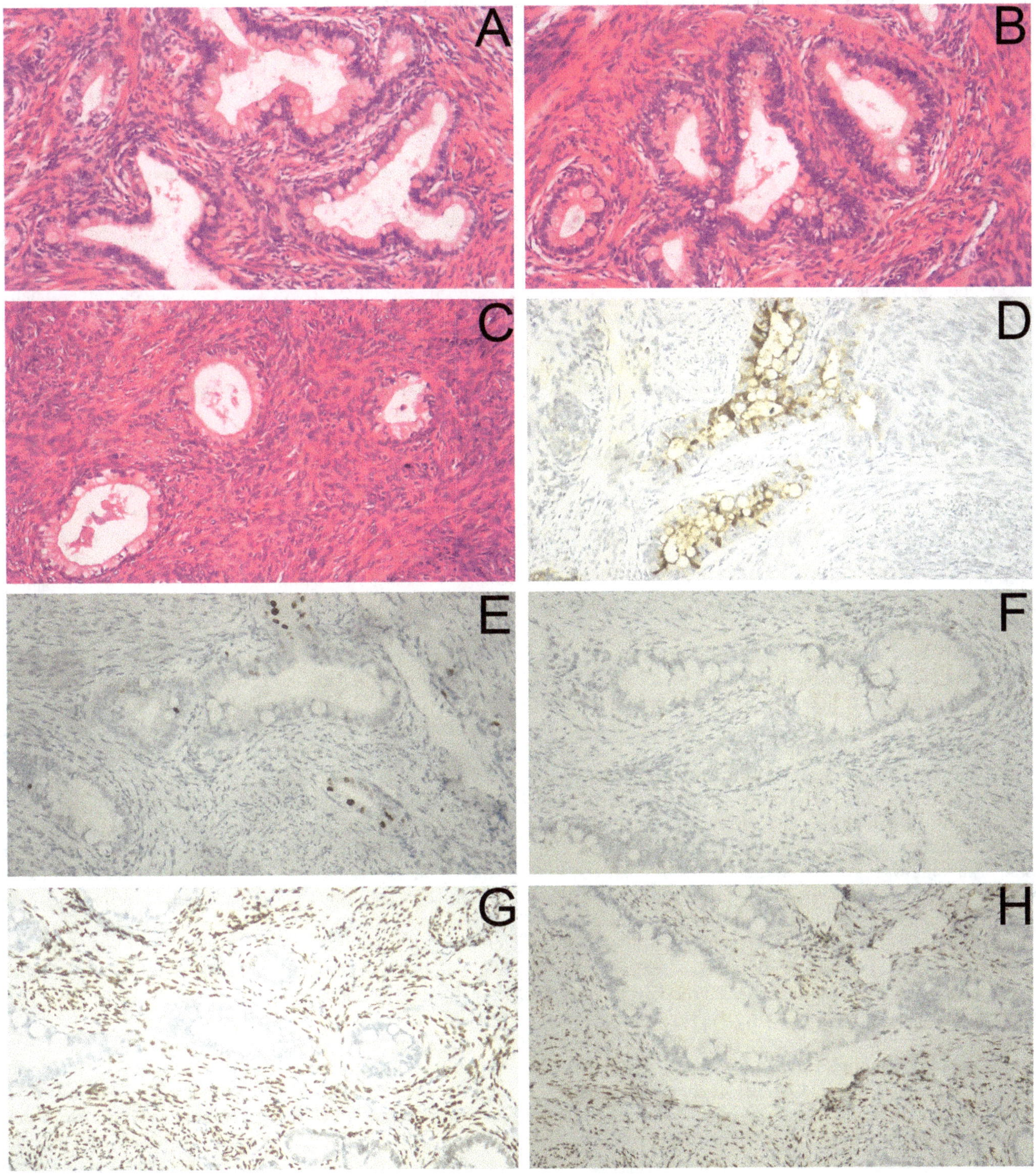

FIGURE 3 | Histopathological and immunohistochemical staining findings. **(A,B)** The cancer cells were columnar and arranged in irregular glandular tubes, some nuclei were large and deeply stained, cytoplasm was empty and bright, and intracellular mucus were seen (H&E staining, ×40). **(C)** Heterotypic glands were seen in the left ovary (H&E staining, ×40). **(D)** CEA (focally +). **(E)** Ki-67 (about 5% +). **(F)** P16 (–). **(G)** ER (–). **(H)** PR (–) **(D–H**, ×100).

illustrated by the following recent studies. In the study by Park et al. (11) next-generation sequencing was performed in 21 GAS cases, and a total of 54 nonsynonymous somatic mutations were detected, with an average mutation rate of 2.6 per lesion. The mutated genes, of which TP53 was the most frequent, were mostly involved in signal transduction, DNA damage repair, and epithelial-mesenchymal transition. Another study showed that GAS most frequently harbored somatic mutations in TP53, CDKN2A, KRAS, and STK11, and potentially targetable mutations were identified in ERBB3, ERBB2, and BRAF (7).

The average age of patients with GAS is 49–51 years (6, 12). The symptoms of patients with GAS are diverse and non-specific. They are often situated in the upper endocervix, present with bleeding or profuse watery discharge, and are associated with a clinically bulky cervix without a well-defined mass due to an infiltrative growth pattern (13). Patients with GAS often have no specific signs of cervical cancer, and the surfaces of the cervix are mostly smooth. Most patients with GAS present at an advanced stage, and pelvic, abdominal, and distant metastases are not uncommon (5). Patients with ovarian and pelvic-abdominal metastases may have signs similar to those of ovarian cancer.

Screening methods for the usual cervical cancer are ineffective for GAS, which may result in a probable delay in diagnosis. Our case was initially treated in another hospital because of lower abdominal pain and fever. Ultrasound showed a hydrosalpinx, dark area in the uterine cavity, and cervical Nabothian cysts. Considering the abdominal pain and fever caused by hydrosalpinx, the patient was given anti-inflammatory treatment, while ignoring the performance of the dark area in the uterine cavity. Until this year, the patient did not undergo pelvic ultrasound again. In addition to hydrosalpinx, an abnormal mass in the uterine cavity was observed. Although TCT showed ASCUS, all high-risk HPVs were negative, and the possibility of an endometrial polyp was considered. During hysteroscopic surgery, we found that the tumor was located in the lower part of the uterine cavity near the internal os and considered that the possibility of submucosal myoma. However, the local shape of the tumor was irregular and like a fingertip; secondly, there was local vascular proliferation of the tumor; thirdly, multiple glandular cavities were seen on the section of the tumor; fourthly, after tumor resection, the capsule of myoma was not seen, and the boundary between the attachment position of tumor and cervical tissue was unclear. Hence, the diagnosis of GAS was accidentally determined based on the pathology. The diagnosis of GAS is primarily based on pathological morphology, combined with immunohistochemical examination if necessary (8). GAS is characterized by tumor cells showing clear, foamy, or pale eosinophilic cytoplasm and well-defined cytoplasmic borders, spanning the spectrum from well-differentiated to poorly differentiated tumors (7). Hysteroscopy is of great significance in the diagnosis of endometrial lesions. Ianieri et al. (14) developed a hysteroscopic scoring system according to some morphological and hysteroscopic parameters, which helps physicians, especially those less experienced, to make a differential diagnosis among normal endometrium, endometrial hyperplasia, and endometrial carcinoma. We believe that hysteroscopy also plays an important role in the diagnosis of cervical canal lesions because we can clearly observe the atypical vessels on the lesion in addition to the location of lesions, which can be useful in suspecting malignant lesions, as described in the report by Ianieri et al. and shown in our hysteroscopic images.

Patients with GAS may have elevated tumor markers, especially serum CA19-9 levels (15). However, the results of serum tumor markers in our case were all normal. Pelvic MRI features of "cosmos pattern" (CP), which means some small cysts or solid components are present in the central part of the lesion surrounded by relatively large cysts, can help to distinguish gastric-type mucin-positive lesions (GMPL) such as LEGH and GAS from gastric-type mucin-negative lesions (GMNL) such as cervical Nabothian cyst. If CP is observed as a hypointense area compared with the cervical stroma on T1WI, GMPL should be strongly suspected (16). A combination of cytology and MRI and an assay for gastric-type mucin have been suggested to be effective for the early detection and preoperative diagnosis of GAS (17). The differential diagnosis of GAS requires the inclusion of both benign and malignant lesions because of its complex and diverse morphologic features (12).

Clinical management can be challenging due to its rare incidence rate, cognitive limitations, diagnostic dilemmas, and aggressive behavior. Currently, there are no specific treatment guideline recommendations for GAS. Surgical removal of the uterus, adnexa, pelvic and/or paraaortic lymph nodes, omentum, appendix, and gross tumor might be considered because of its tendency to spread along surfaces throughout the peritoneal cavity and the higher likelihood of presenting with advanced stage (5). Our case confirmed the diagnosis of stage IB2 GAS after the second admission. Because GAS is prone to ovarian metastasis, we first removed the left ovary and sent it to intraoperative frozen pathology. The results suggested that heterotypic glands were observed, and metastasis was considered. During the first laparoscopic surgery, we did not find any abnormalities in the appearance of the left ovary. Radiologists also did not report any left ovarian abnormalities. This suggested that the ovarian metastatic lesions were insidious, and ovarian preservation was not recommended. Combined with the preoperative staging and intraoperative pathology, we performed radical hysterectomy and removed the paraaortic lymph nodes, greater omentum, and appendix. Postoperative paraffin pathology also revealed metastatic cancer of the left ovary. Although there were no high-risk factors for positive lymph nodes, positive margins, or positive parauterine status after surgical resection, CCRT was still recommended according to pathologic moderate risk factors of adenocarcinoma and invasion of the outer 1/3 cervical stroma.

GAS prognosis is significantly worse than that of UEA: the overall 5-year disease-specific survival rate of GAS is reportedly 30–42% compared to 74–91% for UEA (18). Progression-free survival and overall survival are poorer in patients with GAS than in those with UEA (8). The prognosis is related to tumor stage, parametrial invasion, surgical margin, metastasis, and treatment. Our patient completed the treatment and is in good condition without recurrence or metastasis.

There were some deficiencies in the diagnosis and treatment of our case. Although the patient's TCT suggested ASCUS, it did not attract enough attention because all high-risk HPVs were negative. Although some differences were found between the tumor and submucosal myoma during hysteroscopic surgery, the possibility of GAS was not considered, which led to another operation and increased the physical and economic burden. Due to economic reasons, the patient did not agree to undergo genetic testing.

CONCLUSIONS

GAS is a type of HPV-independent ECA, which may be located in the upper endocervix or even reach the uterine cavity, resulting in a difficult preoperative diagnosis. Sometimes, the appearance is similar to submucosal myoma under hysteroscopy, which is easily misdiagnosed. MRI can show some characteristic changes and hysteroscopy can be used as a method to obtain pathological tissues for patients with GAS. Timely diagnosis is of great significance for the formulation of treatment plan and improving the prognosis of patients.

ETHICS STATEMENT

The studies involving human participants were reviewed and approved by the Institutional Review Board of Shengjing Hospital of China Medical University (approval number: 2021PS849K). The patients/participants provided their written informed consent to participate in this study. Written informed consent was obtained from the individual(s) for the publication of any potentially identifiable images or data included in this article.

AUTHOR CONTRIBUTIONS

JW was responsible for the data collection and drafting of the manuscript. QY and DW participated in providing knowledge of the disease. ML analyzed the literature. NZ was responsible for critical revision of the manuscript. All authors read and approved the final manuscript.

ACKNOWLEDGMENTS

We would like to thank the patient for her permission to present this case report to sensitize practitioners. We also thank all the medical staff who participated in the diagnosis and treatment of this patient.

REFERENCES

1. Koh HH, Jung YY, Kim HS. Clinicopathological characteristics of gastric-type endocervical adenocarcinoma misdiagnosed as an endometrial, ovarian or extragenital malignancy, or mistyped as usual-type endocervical adenocarcinoma. *In Vivo.* (2021) 35:2261–73. doi: 10.21873/invivo.12499
2. Smith HO, Tiffany MF, Qualls CR, Key CR. The rising incidence of adenocarcinoma relative to squamous cell carcinoma of the uterine cervix in the United States–a 24-year population-based study. *Gynecol Oncol.* (2000) 78:97–105. doi: 10.1006/gyno.2000.5826
3. WHO Classification of Tumours Editorial Board. *WHO Classification of Tumours:Female Genital Tumours.* Lyon: IARC Press (2020).
4. Stolnicu S, Barsan I, Hoang L, Patel P, Terinte C, Pesci A, et al. International endocervical adenocarcinoma criteria and classification (IECC): a new pathogenetic classification for invasive adenocarcinomas of the endocervix. *Am J Surg Pathol.* (2018) 42:214–26. doi: 10.1097/pas.0000000000000986
5. Karamurzin YS, Kiyokawa T, Parkash V, Jotwani AR, Patel P, Pike MC, et al. Gastric-type endocervical adenocarcinoma: an aggressive tumor with unusual metastatic patterns and poor prognosis. *Am J Surg Pathol.* (2015) 39:1449–57. doi: 10.1097/pas.0000000000000532
6. Kojima A, Mikami Y, Sudo T, Yamaguchi S, Kusanagi Y, Ito M, et al. Gastric morphology and immunophenotype predict poor outcome in mucinous adenocarcinoma of the uterine cervix. *Am J Surg Pathol.* (2007) 31:664–72. doi: 10.1097/01.pas.0000213434.91868.b0
7. Selenica P, Alemar B, Matrai C, Talia KL, Veras E, Hussein Y, et al. Massively parallel sequencing analysis of 68 gastric-type cervical adenocarcinomas reveals mutations in cell cycle-related genes and potentially targetable mutations. *Mod Pathol.* (2021) 34:1213–25. doi: 10.1038/s41379-020-00726-1
8. Nishio S, Mikami Y, Tokunaga H, Yaegashi N, Satoh T, Saito M, et al. Analysis of gastric-type mucinous carcinoma of the uterine cervix - AN aggressive tumor with a poor prognosis: a multi-institutional study. *Gynecol Oncol.* (2019) 153:13–9. doi: 10.1016/j.ygyno.2019.01.022
9. Mikami Y. Gastric-type mucinous carcinoma of the cervix and its precursors - historical overview. *Histopathology.* (2020) 76:102–11. doi: 10.1111/his.13993
10. D'Alessandro P, Giudicepietro A, Della Corte L, Arduino B, Saccone G, Iacobelli A, et al. A case of gastric-type mucinous endocervical adenocarcinoma in presence of nabothian cysts. *Eur J Obstet Gynecol Reprod Biol.* (2019) 236:254–5. doi: 10.1016/j.ejogrb.2019.02.024
11. Park E, Kim SW, Kim S, Kim HS, Lee JY, Kim YT, et al. Genetic characteristics of gastric-type mucinous carcinoma of the uterine cervix. *Mod Pathol.* (2021) 34:637–46. doi: 10.1038/s41379-020-0614-0
12. Lu S, Shen D, Zhao Y, Kang N, Wang X. Primary endocervical gastric-type adenocarcinoma: a clinicopathologic and immunohistochemical analysis of 23 cases. *Diagn Pathol.* (2019) 14:72. doi: 10.1186/s13000-019-0852-y
13. Kido A, Mikami Y, Koyama T, Kataoka M, Shitano F, Konishi I, et al. Magnetic resonance appearance of gastric-type adenocarcinoma of the uterine cervix in comparison with that of usual-type endocervical adenocarcinoma: a pitfall of newly described unusual subtype of endocervical adenocarcinoma. *Int J Gynecol Cancer.* (2014) 24:1474–9. doi: 10.1097/igc.0000000000000229
14. Ianieri MM, Staniscia T, Pontrelli G, Di Spiezio Sardo A, Manzi FS, Recchi M, et al. A new hysteroscopic risk scoring system for diagnosing endometrial hyperplasia and adenocarcinoma. *J Minim Invasive Gynecol.* (2016) 23:712–8. doi: 10.1016/j.jmig.2016.02.017
15. Nakamura A, Yamaguchi K, Minamiguchi S, Murakami R, Abiko K, Hamanishi J, et al. Mucinous adenocarcinoma, gastric type of the uterine cervix: clinical features and HER2 amplification. *Med Mol Morphol.* (2019) 52:52–9. doi: 10.1007/s00795-018-0202-2
16. Ohya A, Kobara H, Miyamoto T, Komatsu M, Shiozawa T, Fujinaga Y. Usefulness of the 'cosmos pattern' for differentiating between cervical gastric-type mucin-positive lesions and other benign cervical cystic lesions in magnetic resonance images. *J Obstet Gynaecol Res.* (2021) 47:745–56. doi: 10.1111/jog.14602
17. Omori M, Kondo T, Nakazawa K, Tagaya H, Ohgi M, Fukasawa H, et al. Interpretation of endocervical cells with gastric-type mucin on pap smears. *Am J Clin Pathol.* (2018) 150:259–66. doi: 10.1093/ajcp/aqy055
18. Ida K, Yamanoi K, Asaka S, Takeuchi H, Miyamoto T, Shiozawa T, et al. αGlcNAc and its catalyst α4GnT are diagnostic and prognostic markers in uterine cervical tumor, gastric type. *Sci Rep.* (2019) 9:13043. doi: 10.1038/s41598-019-49376-7

Preliminary Analysis of Safety and Feasibility of a Single-Hole Laparoscopic Myomectomy via an Abdominal Scar Approach

Huimin Tang[1†], *Zhiyong Dong*[1†], *Zhenyue Qin*[1†], *Shoufeng Zhang*[1], *Huihui Wang*[1], *Weiwei Wei*[1], *Ruxia Shi*[1], *Jiming Chen*[1]* *and Bairong Xia*[2]*

[1]*Department of Gynecology, The Affiliated Changzhou No. 2 People's Hospital of Nanjing Medical University, Changzhou, China,* [2]*Department of Gynecology, The First Affiliated Hospital of USTC, Division of Life Sciences and Medicine, University of Science and Technology of China, Hefei, China*

***Correspondence:**
Jiming Chen
cjming@126.com,
Bairong Xia
xiabairong@ustc.edu.cn

†*These authors share first authorship.*

Purpose: This paper aims to explore the safety and feasibility of a single-hole laparoscopic myomectomy through an abdominal scar approach.

Method: The clinical data of seven patients who underwent the single-hole laparoscopic myomectomy *via* the abdominal scar approach from January to November 2021 in the Department of Gynecology, the Affiliated Changzhou No. 2 People's Hospital of Nanjing Medical University, were studied retrospectively. The duration of operation, the intraoperative blood loss, the decrease of postoperative hemoglobin, and the postoperative visual analogue score (0 points: no pain, 10 points: maximum pain) were recorded.

Results: All seven patients received the operation successfully, without changing to the conventional laparoscopic operation or open appendectomy. The average blood loss was 101.42 ± 7.89 ml, the average length of hospital stay was 5 ± 0.53 days, the average operation duration was 130 ± 26.86 min, and the 24-h pain score was 1.57 ± 0.53. The seven patients had no intraoperative or postoperative complications and no damage to the ureter or bladder. All patients could urinate spontaneously without urinary retention or urinary tract infection after catheter removal. No analgesic drugs were used after the operation.

Conclusion: The single-hole laparoscopic myomectomy *via* the abdominal scar approach is a more aesthetic and feasible option for eligible patients, but more cases and studies are needed for further confirmation.

Keywords: abdominal wall scar, single hole laparoscopic surgery, hysteromyoma, minimally invasive surgery, hidden scar

INTRODUCTION

Hysteromyoma is the most common gynecological benign tumor in women, especially women of childbearing age, accounting for about 20%–25% of women (1). Epidemiological statistics are far lower than the actual incidence. Although most patients have no clinical symptoms, 30% (2) of the patients still show symptoms such as increased menstruation, prolonged menstruation, anemia, frequent urination, urgent urination, and low back pain, which seriously affect the quality of life. As uterine leiomyoma is an estrogen-dependent disease, it often occurs in women of childbearing age. It is extremely rare in non-menarche women, and some fibroids may atrophy in peri-menopausal or postmenopausal women (2). For asymptomatic patients with uterine leiomyoma, regular follow-ups and treatments are often taken. For patients with symptoms, the current treatment primarily includes drug treatment, surgical treatment, and other interventional treatments. For symptomatic patients who have uterine leiomyoma but do not want to receive an operation, drugs can be used, such as progesterone, gonadotropin-releasing hormone agonist (GnRH-a), and mifepristone. The literature shows that oral progesterone can reduce symptoms or prevalence by 25% (3). GnRH-a treatment for 3 months can reduce the myoma and uterine volume by up to 50% (4), but the treatment is not well accepted because of the accompanying "quasi-menopause" symptoms. The reverse addition theory has been proposed to make up for this defect. Surgical treatment is feasible for uterine fibroids that lead to increased menstruation, anemia, frequent urination caused by bladder compression, and changes in defecation habits caused by rectal compression. For women with submucosal leiomyoma, the change in the endometrial environment affects fertility to a certain extent, increasing the rate of spontaneous abortion, and fertility can be improved after hysteroscopic treatment (3). For intramural myoma or subserous leiomyoma, transabdominal or laparoscopic surgery can be the option. Compared with laparotomy, laparoscopy has the advantages of less trauma, faster postoperative recovery, and less intraoperative bleeding (5). Since single-hole laparoscopy was first used for myomectomy (6), the operation has become increasingly mature after improvements. With people's aesthetic requirements increasing, single-hole laparoscopic myomectomy has been selected by more and more patients. Based on the successful fallopian tube recanalization by an abdominal scar approach (7), our hospital has combined the advantages of the two methods and completed the single-hole laparoscopic myomectomy through the abdominal scar approach, with achieving satisfactory results.

DATA AND METHODS

General Data

Seven patients who underwent single-hole laparoscopic myomectomy *via* the abdominal scar approach from January to November 2021 were selected from Changzhou No. 2 People's Hospital Affiliated to Nanjing Medical University. The patients were 33–46 years old, with the average age being 38.71 ± 4.89 years, and the BMI was 22.52 ± 2.62 kg/m^2 (**Table 1**). One of the patient cases was subserosal myoma, four cases were anterior intramural myoma, one case was multiple uterine myomas, and one case was broad ligament myoma. Among the seven patients, one had bilateral tubal ligation history and six had cesarean section history (two cases were a transverse scar of the cesarean section and four cases were a vertical scar of the cesarean section), including two with a vertical scar of the cesarean section combined with myomectomy history (**Table 2**).

TABLE 1 | Statistical data of the seven patients.

Characteristics	Mean ± standard deviation (n = 7)
Age (years)	38.71 ± 4.89
BMI (kg/m^2)	22.52 ± 2.62
Intraoperative bleeding volume (ml)	101.42 ± 7.89
Operation duration (min)	130 ± 26.86
Postoperative hospital stay (days)	5 ± 0.53
Preoperative HB (g/L)	125.42 ± 14.63
Postoperative HB (g/L)	111.86 ± 16.10
VAS	1.57 ± 0.53

BMI, body mass index; HB, hemoglobin; VAS, visual analogue score.

(1) *Inclusion criteria:* (1) Previous history of abdominal incision; (2) indication of hysteromyoma surgery (4); and (3) patient's voluntary choice of the abdominal scar approach and signing the informed consent of the operation.
(2) *Exclusion criteria:* (1) Possibility of a malignant tumor; (2) body mass index (BMI) ≥ 30 kg/m^2; and (3) patient with an underlying disease that is unsuitable for operation.

Operation Method

Preoperative Preparation

All seven patients underwent general anesthesia; fasting and water deprivation 10 h before the operation to prepare for anesthesia; skin preparation and vaginal cleaning; diet preparation 3 days before the operation to improve the intestinal environment and reduce the impact of the intestinal tract on operation; disinfection of the scar to reduce postoperative infection; and preoperative education by nurses to patients before the operation to reduce their tension.

Equipment Preparation

A complete set of digital systems for laparoscopy (such as lens, display, pneumoperitoneum system, light source system, and recorder), instrument set for conventional gynecological transabdominal surgery, and the items required for single-hole laparoscopy (such as the port and protective ring required for access, as well as the lens, operating instruments, and suture required for laparoscopy) were kept ready.

Surgical Procedures

The patient took the bladder lithotomy position (kept the head low and foot height ≥30° and the abduction of both legs <90°). After the general anesthesia was satisfactory, the patient received routine disinfection and was draped, and the assistant placed the uterine lifting device and retained the catheterization. The transabdominal scar approach was adopted. Taking the scar after a cesarean section as an example, first, an incision of 2.0 cm was made in the lower part of the scar of the original cesarean section (**Figure 1A**) layer by layer into the abdomen. Then, the incision protection ring and the single-hole

TABLE 2 | General information of patients.

Case	Age (years)	BMI (kg/m^2)	Reproductive history	Surgical history	Scar site of the abdominal wall
1	37	26.44	G5P2	History of cesarean section, history of myomectomy	Vertical scar of the abdominal wall during cesarean section
2	34	26.51	G5P3	History of cesarean section	Vertical scar of the abdominal wall during cesarean section
3	37	20.88	G5P1	History of cesarean section	Vertical scar of the abdominal wall during cesarean section
4	46	20.81	G1P1	History of cesarean section	Transverse scar of the abdominal wall during cesarean section
5	46	22.67	G3P1	History of tubal ligation	Abdominal tubal ligation scar
6	33	20.32	G3P1	History of cesarean section	Transverse scar of the abdominal wall during cesarean section
7	38	20	G2P1	History of cesarean section, history of myomectomy	Vertical scar of the abdominal wall during cesarean section

Reproductive history: G, gestation; P, production.

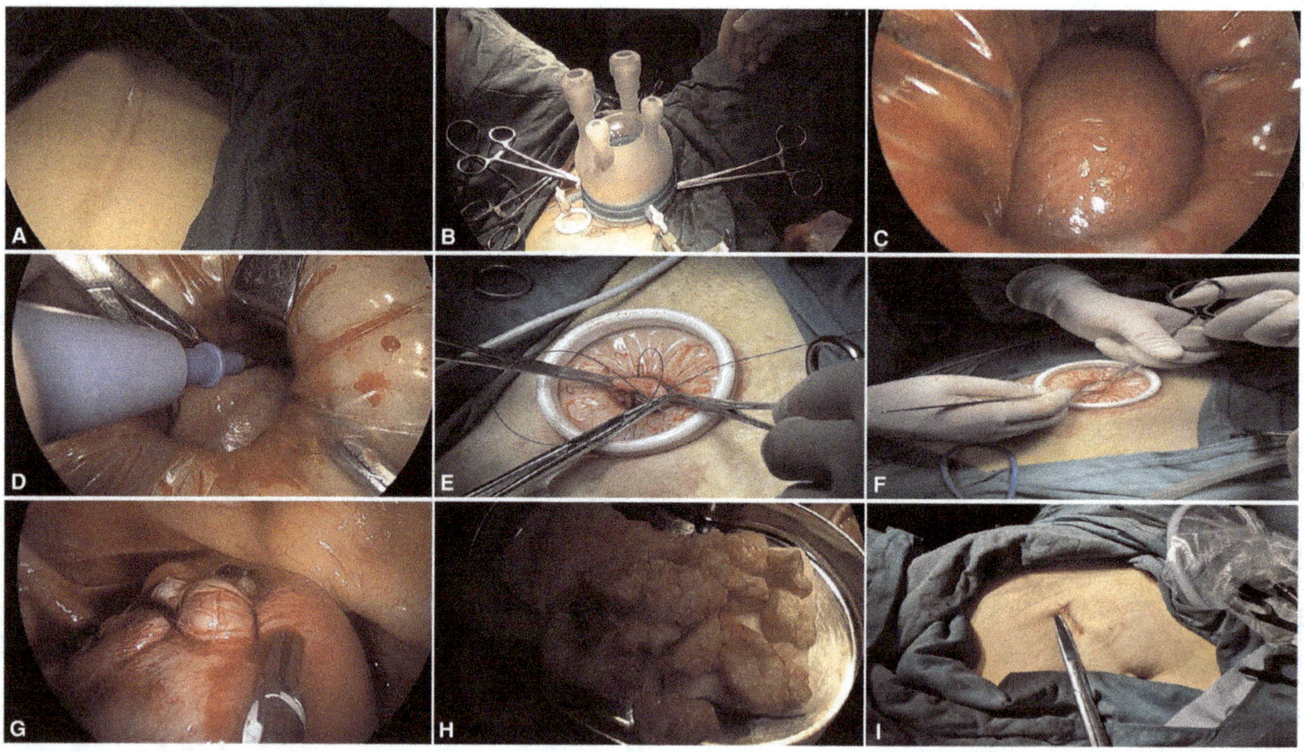

FIGURE 1 | **(A)** Incision through abdominal wall scar; **(B)** connecting the single-hole port; **(C)** using the uterine lifter to push the uterus to the incision; **(D)** dissecting the tumor with an electric knife under direct vision; **(E)** suturing the uterus under direct vision; **(F)** removing the tumor from the incision in blocks; **(G)** laparoscopic exploration and hemostasis; **(H)** stripped tumor; and **(I)** suturing abdominal incision.

laparoscopic special port was connected (**Figure 1B**), the disposable single-hole flexible sheath was fixed, the CO_2 gas was filled until the abdominal pressure reached 14 mmHg, and then the 30° laparoscopic lens and other operating instruments were placed. Single-hole laparoscopy was used to detect the abdominal adhesion and separate the adhesion with an ultrasound knife to restore the normal pelvic structure. The laparoscopic device was removed, the abdominal wall was gently lifted with a thyroid retractor, and the uterus was pushed to the abdominal wall incision by using the uterine device in conjunction (**Figure 1C**). The inject diluted vasopressin into the myometrium locally (avoiding the tumor). Under direct vision, the serous layer was cut open on the surface of the tumor with an electric knife, and the tumor was stripped bluntly and sharply with fingers or the electric knife (**Figure 1D**). The operator can extend his/her finger from the incision into the pelvic cavity and cooperate with the uterine lifter to carefully check for any other suspicious tumor tissue (for uterine leiomyoma in the posterior wall, the approach can be on the upper part of the scar and laparoscopy can be used to peel off the tumor as much as possible). Under direct vision, the myometrium and serosa of the uterine wound were sutured, the wound was closed, the dead space was avoided, and the uterine body was formed (if a certain wound surface was located in the posterior wall or it was difficult to be sutured directly, the laparoscopic device can be connected for fine suture) (**Figure 1E**). Under direct vision, the tumor was cut, removed with a scalpel or scissors, and sent for pathological examination as necessary (**Figure 1F**). The single-hole laparoscopic device was connected, the pelvis was rinsed with normal saline to avoid residue, any active bleeding of the wound was checked under the microscope (**Figure 1G**), the instrument was removed to empty the gas, and the abdominal cavity was closed layer by layer.

Postoperative Treatment

All seven patients returned to the ward smoothly without intraoperative complications. Oxytocin was given to facilitate uterine contraction and rehydration, and antibiotics were given to prevent infection as necessary. The dressing was changed after the operation.

Observation Indicators

The operation duration, intraoperative bleeding, intraoperative/postoperative complications, preoperative and postoperative hemoglobin, postoperative hospital stay, postoperative visual analogue scale (pain score scale: 0–10 represents the degree of pain from painless to intolerable pain), and grade of incision healing (Grade A refers to one-time wound healing without infection after stitch removal, Grade B refers to incision infection and healing after treatment, and Grade C refers to incision rupture or infection without healing) were used.

Postoperative Follow-Ups

Six months after the operation, follow-ups were conducted to check for any long-term complications such as incision hernia and myoma with recurrence in a short time. The follow-up results showed that the seven patients had no incision hernia and no abnormality was found in vaginal ultrasound. The symptoms of patients were significantly improved and followed up on regularly.

Statistical Analysis

SPSS Statistics was used for data statistics, and the data meeting the normal distribution conditions were expressed as mean ± standard deviation ($x \pm s$).

RESULTS

All seven patients received the operation successfully, without changing to the conventional laparoscopic operation or gynecological transabdominal surgery. The ureter or bladder was not injured during the operation, and the urine was clear after the operation. The postoperative hospital stay was 4–6 days, with an average of 5 ± 0.53 days. The average postoperative blood loss was 101.42 ± 7.89 ml, and the postoperative visual analog score was 1.57 ± 0.53. All patients had exhausted, catheter removal was performed 1–2 days after the operation, and the postoperative incision healed well, without complications such as wound infection and bleeding (**Table 3**). Abdominal drainage tubes were placed in two patients and removed on the second day. The incision sites of the seven patients were original abdominal wall scars and were not changed to traditional laparoscopy or laparotomy.

DISCUSSION

Hysteromyoma is the most common gynecological benign tumor for women of childbearing age, and its etiology is not clear, which may be related to the patient's age, not having a child or late childbearing, obesity, and other factors (4). Most patients have no clinical symptoms, and only a small number of patients have symptoms such as increased menstruation, increased vaginal secretions, and abdominal pain. For women who have fertility requirements or want to retain the uterus, hysteromyoma removal is a relatively safe and feasible method. Compared with open surgery, traditional laparoscopy or single-hole laparoscopy has a better cosmetic effect, faster postoperative recovery, and shorter hospital stay (8). However, traditional laparoscopy needs to insert 3–4 puncture devices, which increases the incidence of abdominal incision hernia to a certain extent, and the injury rate of intestinal tubes and blood vessels during puncture also increases (9). With people's aesthetic requirements increases, LESS came into being. Wheelless (10) first applied single-hole laparoscopy to gynecological tubal ligation as early as 1969. However, due to the different operation modes of single-hole laparoscopy, the operation is more difficult, which often leads to a longer operation time than traditional laparoscopy. Besides, after transumbilical single-hole laparoscopy, the umbilical hole is more difficult and the umbilical hole plastic surgery is also challenging. Many beginners have encountered the conditions of red and swollen umbilical hole tissue, seepage, necrosis, and infection after suture, resulting in the limited application of single-hole laparoscopy (11). The transabdominal scar approach can avoid umbilical hole plastic surgery and the resulting risks to a certain extent. Meanwhile, the transabdominal scar approach can reduce the formation of new abdominal scars and hide new surgical scars with the original scars to form "hidden scars" (12).

Taking the cesarean scar on the abdominal wall as an example, its location is closer to the pelvic cavity and the uterus than the single-hole laparoscopy through the umbilical approach. It has the following advantages and disadvantages: (1) The operator can cooperate using a 30° laparoscopic lens, which has a wider field of vision and more convenient operation. The surgical instruments that are double curved or of different lengths can be used to avoid the "chopstick effect" of laparoscopic surgery (13), which also helps shorten the operation duration. After stripping the tumor body in the field of vision, the operator can penetrate the finger into the pelvic cavity through the

TABLE 3 | Single-hole laparoscopic myomectomy *via* the abdominal scar approach.

Case	Number of myomas (piece)	Myoma size (cm)	Myoma location	Operation duration (min)	Intraoperative bleeding volume (ml)	Preoperative hemoglobin (g/L)	Postoperative hemoglobin (g/L)	Pathology	Grade of incision healing	Postoperative visual analogue score
1	1	6.2×4.5×5.9	Left broad ligament	125	105	139	117	Cellular leiomyoma with steatosis	A	Two
2	1	7.3×6.0×5.3	Anterior wall	120	105	127	118	Leiomyoma	A	One
3	2	Front wall 1 piece: 6.5×6.0×6.0; Rear wall 1 piece: 1.8×1.0×1.0	Front wall 1 piece and Rear wall 1 piece	110	110	118	124	Leiomyoma	A	Two
4	10	Maximum myoma: 8.1×5.1×7.9	Intramural (maximum in posterior wall)	180	90	96	79	Leiomyoma with degeneration	A	Two
5	1	7.0*6.0×5.0	Posterior wall	160	110	128	108	Leiomyoma	A	One
6	1	4.5×5.0×5.0	Anterior wall	115	90	145	133	Leiomyoma	A	One
7	2	Front wall 2 pieces: 6.0×5.0×5.0 and 4.0×4.5×4.5	Anterior wall	100	100	125	104	Leiomyoma	A	Two

incision channel and scatter the small tumor body through tactile perception, the mode that helps accurately identify the scattered small tumor body of the uterus, to peel off the myoma as much as possible and reduce the recurrence of postoperative hysteromyoma and damage to the myometrium caused by blind exploration of myoma by instruments. The authors' team has also used the "finger probe method" to complete the traditional laparoscopic myomectomy (14), which is the advantage of this method. (2) For patients with hysteromyoma on the anterior wall, they can choose to cut near the scar of the uterine fundus, combine the transabdominal operation with the pneumoperitoneum-free single-hole laparoscopic operation, cooperate with the uterine lifting device, and use the laparoscopic surgical instruments under direct vision. This method can increase the surgical field, reduce intraoperative bleeding, facilitate the suture procedure of the laparoscopic operation, and simplify the operation to a certain extent. Meanwhile, the thyroid retractor is used to gently lift the skin to avoid the damage of gram steel needle to the abdominal wall. For patients with uterine fibroids in the anterior wall, this is a more feasible scheme with a higher aesthetic value. The authors' team also completed several cases of pneumoperitoneum-free single-hole laparoscopic ovarian cyst stripping (15). For patients with posterior wall hysteromyoma, the upper abdominal scar approach can be selected, combined with laparoscopic assistance, which can address the disadvantage of small pelvic operation space through the abdominal scar approach and improve the safety of the operation. (3) The scar of the cesarean section is closer to the uterus, the operation space of laparoscopic instruments is small, and the operation is difficult. In comparison, the transumbilical approach is easier to lead to the "conflict" of surgical instruments, and the "chopstick effect" is more serious. Therefore, the operator is required to have better operation skills. Especially for patients with the transverse scar of cesarean section, because their transverse scar is close to the bladder, the operation may easily damage the bladder, and the operator is required to pay more attention to the anatomical level when entering the abdomen layer by layer. Patients should be evaluated before the operation, and other operation methods should be chosen for patients not suitable for this operation. (4) Compared with laparoscopy-assisted mini-laparotomy, the transabdominal scar approach can reduce the number of abdominal wall puncture holes. This operation is based on the abdominal wall scar; the incision is smaller, without creating a new abdominal wall scar and is more aesthetically pleasing. Meanwhile, it can fine-suture the uterus and reduce the bleeding of uterine wounds. If the position of uterine leiomyoma is difficult to suture directly, the laparoscopy can be used without adding new puncture holes. (5) For patients with a history of abdominal wall scar, the most noticeable problem is abdominal adhesion. According to research, the risk of postoperative adhesion can reach 90% regardless of the operation method adopted (16, 17), which greatly increases the difficulty of laparoscopic operation, as well as the probability of damaging pelvic and abdominal organs and the incidence of a change to transabdominal operation (18). For abdominal organ adhesion, due to the lower local heat generated by the ultrasonic scalpel and less thermal damage to the tissue, the ultrasonic scalpel is the best choice for separating adhesion (19). Because the patient has a history of surgery, the intestinal canal may adhere to the original surgical incision, which requires the operator to pay attention to the layers when entering the abdomen and be more cautious in the operation. After the incision protective ring is placed, the laparoscopic lens can be used to detect the adhesion of the abdominal wall and intestinal canal, and the patient should be changed to transabdominal operation as necessary to ensure safety.

In general, the single-hole laparoscopic myomectomy *via* abdominal scar approach is more in line with the aesthetic requirements of patients. It is a safe and feasible scheme for patients who meet the inclusion criteria of surgery. However, if it is widely used, more randomized controlled studies are needed to further validate its effectiveness and feasibility.

AUTHOR CONTRIBUTIONS

All authors contributed to the article and approved the submitted version.

REFERENCES

1. Puchar A, Feyeux C, Luton D, Koskas M. Therapeutic management of uterine fibroid tumors. *Minerva Ginecol.* (2016) 68:466–76. PMID: 26698838
2. Giuliani E, As-Sanie S, Marsh EE. Epidemiology and management of uterine fibroids. *Int J Gynaecol Obstet.* (2020) 149(1):3–9. doi: 10.1002/ijgo.13102
3. Marret H, Fritel X, Ouldamer L, CNGOF (French College of Gynecology and Obstetrics). Therapeutic management of uterine fibroid tumors: updated French guidelines. *Eur J Obstet Gynecol Reprod Biol.* (2012) 165(2):156–64. doi: 10.1016/j.ejogrb.2012.07.030
4. Pavone D, Clemenza S, Sorbi F, Fambrini M. Epidemiology and risk factors of uterine fibroids. *Best Pract Res Clin Obstet Gynaecol.* (2018) 46:3–11. doi: 10.1016/j.bpobgyn.2017.09.004
5. Csatlós E, Rigó Jr J, Laky M. Gene expression patterns of insulin-like growth factor 2 in human uterine fibroid tissues: a genetic study with clinical correlations. *Gynecol Obstet Invest.* (2013) 75(3):185–90. doi: 10.1159/000347017
6. Kim YW, Park BJ, Ro DY. Single-port laparoscopic myomectomy using a new single-port transumbilical morcellation system: initial clinical study. *J Minim Invasive Gynecol.* (2010) 17(5):587–92. doi: 10.1016/j.jmig.2010.04.009
7. Qin Z, Bao M, Chen J. Single hole laparoscopic fallopian tube recanalization via abdominal scar approach. *Chin J Mod Surg.* (2021) 25(1):55–9. doi: 10.16260/j.cnki.1009-2188.2021.01.011
8. Angioni S, Pontis A, Pisanu A. Single-port access subtotal laparoscopic hysterectomy: a prospective case-control study. *J Minim Invasive Gynecol.* (2015) 22(5):807–12. doi: 10.1016/j.jmig.2015.03.011
9. Boruta DM. Laparoendoscopic single-site surgery in gynecologic oncology: an update. *Gynecol Oncol.* (2016) 141(3):616–23. doi: 10.1016/j.ygyno.2016.03.014
10. Wheeless Cr. A rapid, inexpensive, and effective method of surgical sterilization by laparoscopy. *J Reprod Med.* (1969) 3:65–9.
11. Sun HD, Horng HC, Liu CH. Comparison of single-port and three-port laparoscopic salpingectomy in the management for tubal pregnancy. *J Chin Med Assoc.* (2018) 81(5):469–74. doi: 10.1016/j.jcma.2017.11.005
12. Takeda A, Imoto S, Mori M, Yamada J, Nakamura H. Isobaric two-port laparoscopic-assisted myomectomy by combined approach through umbilical and suprapubic mini-incisions with hidden scar: a technique and initial experience. *Eur J Obstet Gynecol Reprod Biol.* (2012) 160:88–92. doi: 10.1016/j.ejogrb.2011.09.050
13. Wang Y, Yao Y, Dou Y, Tang S, Chen C, Li Y, et al. Chopstick technique used in laparoendoscopic single site radical hysterectomy for early stage cervical cancer. *Sci Rep.* (2021) 11(1):6882. doi: 10.1038/s41598-021-85783-5
14. Zhong A, Liu W, Liu J, Chen J. Finger probe assisted transumbilical single hole laparoscopic multiple myomectomy: a case report. *Chin J Mod Surg.* (2020) 24(4):318–9. doi: 10.16260/j.cnki.1009-2188.2020.04.016
15. Qin Z, Wang H, Bao M. A case report of simple suspension airless abdominal micro incision single hole laparoscopic exploration combined with extracorporeal operation mode in the treatment of huge ovarian tumors in mid pregnancy. *J Laparosc Surg.* (2021) 26(4):316–8. doi: 10.13499/j.cnki.fqjwkzz.2021.04.316
16. Lee SY, Kim CH, Kim YJ. Laparoscopic surgery for colorectal cancer patients who underwent previous abdominal surgery. *Surg Endosc.* (2016) 30(12):5472–80. doi: 10.1007/s00464-016-4908-8
17. Strik C, Stommel MW, Schipper LJ. Risk factors for future repeat abdominal surgery. *Langenbecks Arch Surg.* (2016) 401(6):829–37. doi: 10.1007/s00423-016-1414-3
18. Aytac E, Stocchi L, De Long J. Impact of previous midline laparotomy on the outcomes of laparoscopic intestinal resections: a case-matched study. *Surg Endosc.* (2015) 29(3):537–42. doi: 10.1007/s00464-014-3719-z
19. Tulandi T, Bugnah M. Operative laparoscopy: surgical modalities. *Fertil Steril.* (1995) 63(2):237–45. doi: 10.1016/S0015-0282(16)57347-6

21

Enhanced Recovery after Vascular Surgery

*Milena D. Stojanovic[1], Danica Z. Markovic[1], Anita Z. Vukovic[1], Vesna D. Dinic[1], Aleksandar N. Nikolic[1], Tijana G. Maricic[1] and Radmilo J. Janković[1,2]**

[1] Center for Anesthesiology, Reanimatology and Intensive Care, Clinical Center Nis, Nis, Serbia, [2] School of Medicine, University of Nis, Nis, Serbia

***Correspondence:**
Radmilo J. Janković
jankovic.radmilo@gmail.com

The beginnings of the enhanced recovery after surgery (ERAS) program were first developed for patients in colorectal surgery, and after it was established as the standard of care in this surgical field, it began to be applied in many others surgical areas. This is multimodal, evidence-based approach program and includes simultaneous optimization of preoperative status of patients, adequate selection of surgical procedure and postoperative management. The aim of this program is to reduce complications, the length of hospital stay and to improve the patients outcome. Over the past decades, special attention was directed to the postoperative management in vascular surgery, especially after major vascular surgery because of the great risk of multiorgan failure, such as: respiratory failure, myocardial infarction, hemodynamic instability, coagulopathy, renal failure, neurological disorders, and intra-abdominal complications. Although a lot of effort was put into it, there is no unique acceptable program for ERAS in this surgical field, and there is still a need to point out the factors responsible for postoperative outcomes of these patients. So far, it is known that special attention should be paid to already existing diseases, type and the duration of the surgical intervention, hemodynamic and fluid management, nutrition, pain management, and early mobilization of patients.

Keywords: vascular surgery, recovery, postoperative management, intensive care, preoperative care

INTRODUCTION

Enhanced recovery after surgery (ERAS) program or a "fast-track surgery" was first developed and successfully implemented in colorectal surgery (1), and was later reported in orthopedic (2, 3), cardiac (4), and vascular surgery (5, 6). The aims of this program are to improve the perioperative care of patients, avoid complications, accelerate recovery, shorten hospital stays and improve the patient's prognosis. Introduced by Danish surgeon Dr. Henrick Kehlet, this multimodal evidence-based approach program starts in the preoperative period and extends to the patient's release (1, 2).

It is possible to accelerate the patient's recovery, reduce complications and the length of hospital stay by changing factors which are responsible for prolonged recovery (1, 7, 8). Previous studies have shown the safety and efficiency of ERAS program, and they emphasize that for early recovery after surgery following factors are important: patient education, short-acting anesthetics, pain

---

Abbreviations: ERAS, enhanced recovery after surgery; ICU, intensive care unit; DVT, deep vein thrombosis; AAA, abdominal aortic aneurysm; AKI, acute kidney injury; NTG, nitrloglycerine; MAP, mean arterial pressure; ND, nasogastric drainage; PCA, patient-controlled analgesia; PCEA, patient-controlled epidural analgesia; CO, cardiac output.

management, fluid therapy, oral nutrition, and early mobilization (9, 10).

It is already proved in several studies that application of ERAS program reduces the length of hospital stay (11), decreases the surgical and non-surgical complications in postoperative period (12), and improves the outcome (13).

So far, the fields of interest in vascular surgery are ERAS in aortic (5) and carotid (6) surgery, but there are still not enough solid evidence to form a unique acceptable program.

PREOPERATIVE PERIOD

Preoperative assessment is as important as the intraoperative and postoperative period. It allows evaluation of risk and provides an opportunity to stabilize already existing disease and optimize organ dysfunction before surgery, as it is well known that postoperative organic dysfunction is undoubtfully associated with preoperative comorbidities. This period provides an opportunity for patient education, which refers to obtaining information about surgery itself, anticipated postoperative course, analgesia, and discharge. It is thought that in this way anxiety, the need for analgesics and the length of hospital stay can be reduced (1). The recommendations for ERAS in vascular surgery (including preoperative, intraoperative, and postoperative period) are shown in **Table 1**.

Special attention should be paid to premedication with an aim to reduce the stress response to surgery. Beta-blockers reduce the catecholamine level and thus reduce the perioperative and postoperative cardiovascular complications. Since surgical intervention is a stress that leads to activation of the sympathetic nervous system and catabolism, these medications with their anti-catabolic effect could have a positive impact on postoperative course. It is considered that alpha-2 adrenergic agonists, such as clonidine and dexmedetomidin, reduce myocardial ischemia, intraoperative blood loss, and postoperative nausea and vomiting (1).

Preoperative overnight fasting can lead to dehydration, and its avoidance reduces the risk of postoperative pain and nausea. It has even been proved that clear carbohydrate fluids given during this period can reduce the postoperative anxiety and endocrine response (1, 14).

INTRAOPERATIVE PERIOD

One of the major interventions in vascular surgery is an aortic surgery. Today available surgical techniques are endovascular and open repair. Study form Hertzer et al. showed that after elective open infrarenal aortic repair median length of stay in intensive care unit (ICU) is about 3 days and mortality rates are between 1.2 and 10.5% (15). Postoperative complications such as aneurysm rupture, thrombosis and graft migration are same after both surgical techniques, while endovascular repair has advantages in terms of length of intervention, blood loss, shorter length of mechanical ventilation, less malnutrition, and shorter hospital stay (16–18).

Special attention should be directed to intraoperative heat loss in order to avoid hypothermia and patient warming system should be strongly considered (16).

TABLE 1 | Recommendations for enhanced recovery program in vascular surgery.

Respiratory
Preoperative antibiotics use
Early extubation
Protective modes of ventilation
Prevention of ventilator-associated pneumonia
High-flow oxygen therapy or intermittent nasal continuous positive airway pressure after extubation
Breathing exercises
Cardiovascular
Monitoring for signs of myocardial ischemia
Goal directed fluid therapy
Maintaining the MAP above 80–90 mmHg
Renal
Monitoring of the amount of urine and creatinine clearance
Maintaining the normovolemia and electrolyte balance
Use diuretics with caution
Avoid fluid overload and dopamine
Nutrition
Without preoperative mechanical bowel preparation
Maintenance the glucose level < 215 mg/dl
Oral nutrition within the first 24–48 h after operation
Use prokinetics (metoclopramid and erithromycin)
Avoidance of nasogastric drainage or early removal
Monitoring of IAP
Pain management
PCEA 48 h before and 48 h after intervention
Avoid systemic opioid use
Other
Stabilize already existing disease and optimize organ dysfunction before surgery
Oral carbohydrate drinks before surgery
Minimize the time for surgical intervention
Patient education
Consider thromboprophylaxis
Avoid hypothermia
Early mobilization

POSTOPERATIVE PERIOD

A postoperative period in vascular surgery plays a pivotal role in the patient's recovery. The quality of postoperative care is essential for the successful recovery. Following the interventions in vascular surgery the most significant are considered to be: optimization of microcirculation after ischemic–reperfusion syndrome and inflammatory reaction caused by the operation itself, adequate fluid resuscitation, maintenance of satisfactory aerobic metabolism, stable blood glucose levels and adequate oxygen delivery, flow directed hemodynamic support, and use of vasodilators and vasoconstrictors with the goal of achieving adequate blood flow (19).

The spectrum of complications depends on the disease itself, its urgency and the surgical procedure (16). Some of these complications can appear in the early postoperative phase, but some of them can be manifested in the late postoperative period.

Immediately after operation, Crimi and Hill in their study point out the importance of resolving hemodynamic, pulmonary, renal, neurological, hematological, and gastrointestinal complications (20). The disorders of these organ systems are the result of ischemic–reperfusion injury.

Managing in the first postoperative day, mainly depends on the type of surgical intervention, the length of operation and the condition of the patient. During this period, it is important to be cautious about.

Hemodynamic Stability

Hemodynamic instability often occurs after major and complicated surgery. It is preferable to avoid hypertension, yet allowing adequate perfusion of vital organs. For this purpose, a combination of nitrloglycerine (NTG) and labetalol with some inodilators such as dobutamine is mostly recommended (19). The patients are often vasoplegic and hyperdynamic and require vasoconstrictors in the form of noradrenaline or vasopressin. This requires adequate invasive monitoring or the placement of pulmonary catheter. Oxygen delivery markers such as SvO_2 and serum lactate levels should also be monitored. Transesophageal ultrasound should be available, especially during the periods of hemodynamic instability (19).

Respiratory Failure

Respiratory failure, most commonly caused by infection and pulmonary pathology, is still the most common complication after surgery of thoracoabdominal aorta and occurs in about 30% of patients (20). Respiratory function is often most stable shortly after surgery and patients can usually be extubated within 6–12 h or even earlier. Only in rare cases of transfusion-related acute lung injury, or pulmonary infection exacerbation in high-risk patients, gas exchange remains compromised and requires prolonged ventilatory support. Additionally, major surgery and preexisted kidney disease can lead to significant pulmonary complications (21). If there is a risk of volotrauma, low tidal volumes can be used. Hypercapnia and respiratory acidosis are logical consequence of this ventilation mode, but if the patient does not have cerebral edema, this permissive hypercapnia is generally well tolerated with pH > 7.2 (22). If there is a need for lung recruitment and after separating from the ventilator, it is preferable to use high-flow oxygen therapy or intermittent nasal continuous positive airway pressure (19).

Factors such as: extreme age, comorbidities, extensive surgery, prolonged use of muscle relaxants and sedatives, preexisting pulmonary disease, postoperative hypothermia and fluid overload can lead to V/Q mismatch, hypoxia, and respiratory failure. Prevention of respiratory complications should start in the preoperative period using antibiotics and breathing exercises (22).

Myocardial Ischemia

Study of Landesberg et al. showed that transient myocardial ischemia developed among 21% of patients and myocardial infarction in 6.5% of cases (23). Combination of two precordial leads are more than 95% sensitive than troponin level for postoperative ischemia monitoring. If myocardial ischemic event occurs, supplemental oxygen, beta-blockers, afterload reduction agents, anticoagulants and antiplatelets should be administered. Percutaneous coronary intervention is also recommended, while postoperative fibrinolysis is a relative contraindication (22). If ischemic events are associated with signs of myocardial impairments, manifested by an increased need for inotropic use, reduced cardiac output (CO), cardiac arrhythmias or disorders of wall motility, urgent angiography can be indicated (19).

Bleeding and Coagulopathy

A typical consequence of aortic surgery is coagulopathy with subsequent bleeding. Early stabilization of coagulopathy is important in prevention of further complications. Special point-of-care laboratory tests such as thromboelastography or activated clotting time allow the treatment of such disorders (19). Preoperative administration of antifibrinolytics can be continued in the short postoperative period.

Liberal blood transfusions for treatment of massive bleeding are no longer in use because of high 30 days' adverse events among these patients. It is recommended that if hemoglobin is above 9 g/dl, transfusion should be avoided. When there is a need for correction of clotting factors deficiency, the dose of fresh frozen plasma should be 10–15 ml/kg of body weight, with a maximum dose of 30 ml/kg, and most important is that fresh frozen plasma should not be used as a volume expander (22).

Temperature Management

Immediately after surgery patients are often hypothermic, especially after long interventions. Maintaining an adequate body temperature in postoperative period is important for adequate oxygen supply, functioning of the coagulation system, hemodynamic stability, and neurocognitive integrity (19).

Neurologic Disorders

Typical complications following aortic surgery are stroke, spinal cord ischemia or generalized cognitive dysfunctions presented as delirium or confusion/agitation (19, 20). Study from Beydon et al. showed that lorazepam in premedication was associated with prolonged extubation time and a lower rate of cognitive recovery (24). But Scavee et al. showed that fear and anxiety increase the incidence of postoperative complications and that use of anxiolytics can be desirable (25).

Deep Vein Thrombosis (DVT)

The risk of DVT after open abdominal aortic aneurysm repair (AAA) is 2–33% without chemoprophylaxis, and 1–10.2% in patients who received postoperative enoxaparin (26). Previous studies, which had some limitations, have shown that because of low incidence of postoperative DVT or high risk of bleeding, there is no need for postoperative thromboprophylaxis (26).

Scarborough et al. in their study (6,000 patients) showed that the incidence of DVT after AAA is only 2.4%, but the limitation in this study was that they did not know which patient received thromboprophylaxis. They emphasize that the risk factors for DVT after open surgery are: length of surgery more than 5 h, obesity and ruptured aneurysmal disease (27).

For the time being, there are no unique guidelines for thromboprophylaxis. Although many studies in this field were conducted, they included small number of patients, so their conclusions cannot be considered as relevant.

Based on available data, the majority of vascular surgeons consider that the use of thromboprophylaxis should become a routine for patients undergoing AAA repair (27).

Special attention should be paid to patients with carotid surgery, especially those who develop some neurological deficit. Due to uncontrolled hypertension, cerebral hyperperfusion syndrome can develop, and this should be controlled with IV labetalol. Hypotension should be treated with volume infusion and phenylephrine (22).

In the late postoperative period the focus should be put on acute kidney injury (AKI) and intra-abdominal complications.

Acute Kidney Injury

The most common predictor factors for AKI are physiological reserve as well as the severity of atherosclerotic disease (28, 29). The incidence of postoperative AKI requiring dialysis ranges from 5 to 15%, and its occurrence is associated with a worse prognosis (30). Monitoring the amount of urine as well as creatinine clearance in postoperative period is crucial. Diuretics and dopamine can promote urine output, but integrity or functional reserve of glomerular function may be compromised (31). Patients with intra-abdominal pressure >25 mmHg are at risk for compartment syndrome development, which may cause AKI. In this group of patients it is important to maintain higher values of blood pressure and better oxygen delivery (22).

Intra-Abdominal Complications

Some of these complications are rare, such as mesenteric ischemia (2–5%), but the mortality rate is high (55–60%) (32). Cross-clamping the aorta may cause mesenteric ischemia with consequent reperfusion injury, translocation of the bacteria and systemic inflammatory response. After cardiopulmonary bypass, low CO can cause gut ischemia (where local vasodilatators, such as nitric oxide and papaverine, can be helpful) and colonic infarction with high mortality rate (89%) (33).

GUIDELINES FOR MANAGEMENT IN POSTOPERATIVE PERIOD

Hemodynamic Management

Hypoxia and hypertension in postoperative period can be harmful for patients. Hypertension is associated with increased incidence of strokes or aorta dissection. On the other hand, hypotension is associated with graft thrombosis and multiorgan failure, therefore, maintenance of adequate oxygen supply is crucial for kidneys, CNS, and spinal cord (22). The recommendations are to keep mean arterial pressure above 80–90 mmHg, as well as maintenance the systolic blood pressure above 130 mmHg. Achieving these values of blood pressure is not always easy in practice and often requires the use of vasodilatatotors—NTG and labetalol, vasoconstrictors—noradrenaline and vasopressin, and even inotropes such as dobutamin. Even with this support, fluid replacement can be a real challenge (19). Recent recommendations are based not only on the satisfactory pressure maintenance but also on tissue perfusion which is equally important (34). Among various types of arrhythmias, bradiarrythmias should not be treated if they are not associated with hemodynamic instability (35, 36).

Hemodynamic management is now directed not only toward the maintenance of satisfactory tissue perfusion but also toward flow directed approach, with clinical assessment of urine output and oxygen extraction index (19, 37). Recently, it has been showed that diuretics can improve venous drainage from the microcirculation, increase the oxygen extraction at cellular level and improve mitochondrial function (37).

Fluid Management

Many patients after operation do not have the ability to excrete fluids and sodium; on the other side, many of them are hypovolemic in this period (38). Crystalloid solutions like Ringer-lactate should be favourized during this period. Normal saline should be avoided due to hyperchloremic metabolic acidosis, which can reduce tissue perfusion and worsen the final outcome (19). In general, colloids are better in raising the blood pressure and improving the tissue perfusion, but they should be used with great caution due to renal toxicity and unfavorable effects on coagulation system (19). With limited evidence, it is advised to avoid them in patients with an already impaired kidney function (39).

Nutrition

Postoperative insulin therapy with the goal of maintenance the glucose level < 215 mg/dl (11.9 mmol/l) is mandatory for diabetic and non-diabetic patients (40). The relationship between high glucose levels and worse outcomes is a well-known concept. Study from Krinsley et al. showed that the mortality is twice as high when glucose level is above 140–150 mg/dl (41). An increase of glucose level for every 40 mg/dl carries a 30% higher risk of infection, graft failure, and longer ICU stay (42). Achieving these values is significant for wound healing, integrity of gastrointestinal system, and inflammatory response reduction (43).

Malnutrition in preoperative period is associated with muscle weakness, fatigue, immunological dysfunction, and slower wound healing. Some studies have proven that adequate nutrition even in the preoperative period can improve surgical outcome (44, 45). Restoration of bowel motility plays a very important role in the ERAS program since the beginning of food intake depends on it. Enteral feeding has fewer metabolic complications than parenteral nutrition (22), and it should be started as soon as possible in the postoperative period (6–8 h) (46). On the contrary, Ksienski et al. showed in their study that early oral nutrition should start within the first 24–48 h while gastric emptying occurs within 18 h after elective aortic aneurysm repair (47). If there is a postoperative disturbance in bowel motility, first-line choice therapy for prokinetic medications are metoclopramid and erythromycin (18).

The use of nasogastric drainage (ND) is not recommended and can even be harmful. It has been shown that in patients without ND bowel function returns earlier and that they have fewer pulmonary complications (18, 48).

Pain Management

Pain management in postoperative period is very important and one Cohrane review showed that use of epidural analgesia has fewer cardiovascular and renal complications compared with systemic opioid use with no difference in mortality (20). Patient-controlled epidural analgesia (PCEA) with local anesthetics provides better analgesic effect than patient-controlled analgesia (PCA) with intraveonous opioids, but there is no statistical difference in hospital stay and its outcome when these two techniques are compared (49). Additionally, based on available evidences for ERAS protocol, the PCA epidural analgesia is highly recommended (50). PCEA should begin 48 h before intervention and continue 48 h after operation (51). Criteria for discharge are: hemodynamic stability, urine output >0.5 ml/kg/h, adequate analgesia to make patients active, ability to consume solid fluid, and no indications for further surgical interventions (23, 49).

CONCLUSION

Although ERAS program was most studied and applied in colorectal surgery, recent studies suggest that it can be successfully applied in vascular surgery, too. The most important is establishing the guidelines and form a team whose members (surgeons, anesthesiologists, nurses, rehabilitation members, and nutritionists) should be familiar with ERAS program and must be motivated to carry out the program.

Since the field of vascular surgery is too broad, one cannot even expect that the conceptualization of just one program is sufficient for all areas in vascular surgery. For the moment, some acceptable guidelines for the postoperative management already exist, therefore, it is necessary to direct the attention to the preoperative status of a patient and improvements in surgical techniques.

AUTHOR CONTRIBUTIONS

RJ conceived of the presented idea. MS, AV, VD, and DM wrote the beginning version of the manuscript. MS, AV, RJ, VD, DM, AN, and TG contributed to the design of the research and the writing of the final version of the manuscript. RJ supervised the manuscript.

REFERENCES

1. Kitching AJ, O'Neill SS. Fast-track surgery and anesthesia. *Contin Educ Anesth Crit Care Pain* (2009) 9(2):39–43. doi:10.1093/bjaceaccp/mkp006
2. Husted H, Troelsen A, Otte KS, Kristensen BB, Holm G, Kehlet H. Fast track surgery for bilateral total knee replacement. *J Bone Joint Surg Br* (2011) 93:351–6. doi:10.1302/0301-620X.93B3.25296
3. Holm B, Kristensen MT, Myhrmann L, Husted A, Andersen LO, Kristensen B, et al. The role of pain for early rehabilitation in fast track total knee arthroplasty. *Disabil Rehabil* (2010) 32:300–6. doi:10.3109/09638280903095965
4. Salhiyyah K, Elsobaky S, Raja S, Attia R, Brazler J, Cooper GJ. A clinical and economic of fast-track recovery after cardiac surgery. *Heart Surg Forum* (2011) 14:E330–4. doi:10.1532/HSF98.20111029
5. Muehling MB, Schelzig H, Steffen P, Meierhenrich R, Sunder-Plassmann L, Orend KH. A prospective randomized trial comparing traditional and fast-track patient care in elective open infra renal aneurysm repair. *World J Surg* (2009) 33:577–85. doi:10.1007/s00268-008-9892-2
6. Guay J. Regional or general anesthesia for carotid endarterectomy? Evidence from published prospective and retrospective studies. *J Cardiothorac Vasc Anesth* (2007) 21:127–32. doi:10.1053/j.jvca.2006.07.022
7. Kehlet H, Slim K. The future of fast-track surgery. *Br J Surg* (2012) 99:1025–6. doi:10.1002/bjs.8832
8. Ansari D, Gianotti L, Schroder J, Andersson R. Fast-track surgery: procedure-specific aspects and future direction. *Langenbecks Arch Surg* (2013) 398:29–37. doi:10.1007/s00423-012-1006-9
9. Fagevik Olsen M, Wennberg E. Fast-track concept in major open upper abdominal and thoracoabdominal surgery: a review. *World J Surg* (2011) 35:2586–93. doi:10.1007/s00268-011-1241-1
10. Basse L, Raskov HH, Hjort Jakobsen D, Sonne E, Billesbolle P, Hendeel HW, et al. Accelerated postoperative recovery programme after colonic resection improves physical performance, pulmonary function and body composition. *Br J Surg* (2002) 89(4):446–53. doi:10.1046/j.0007-1323.2001.02044
11. Wind J, Polle SW, Fung Kon Jin PH, Dejong CH, von Mayenfeldt MF, Ubbinik DT, et al. Systematic review of enhanced recovery programmes in colonic surgery. *Br J Surg* (2006) 93:800–9. doi:10.1002/bjs.5384
12. Muller S, Zalunardo MP, Hubner M, Clavien PA, Demartines N; Zurich Fast Track Study Group. A fast-track program reduces complications and length of hospital stay after open colonic surgery. *Gastroentrology* (2009) 136:842–7. doi:10.1053/j.gastro.2008.10.030
13. Kremer M, Ulrich A, Buchler MW, Uhl W. Fast-track surgery: the Heidelberg experience. *Recent Results Cancer Res* (2005) 165:14–20. doi:10.1007/3-540-27449-9_3
14. Svanfeldt M, Thorell A, Hausel J, Soop M, Nygren J, Ljungqvist O. Effect of "preoperative" oral carbohydrate treatment on insulin action—a randomized cross-over unblended study in healthy subjects. *Clin Nutr* (2005) 24(5):815–21. doi:10.1016/j.clnu.2005.05.002
15. Hertzer NR, Mascha EJ, Karafa MT, Para PJ, Krajewski LP, Beven EG. Open infrarenal abdominal aortic aneurysm repair: the Cleveland clinic experience from 1989 to 1998. *Vasc Surg* (2002) 35(6):1145–54. doi:10.1067/mva.2002.123686
16. Muehling MB, Halter G, Lang G, Schelzig H, Steffen P, Wagner F, et al. Prospective randomized controlled trial to evaluate "fast-track" elective open infrarenal aneurysm repair. *Langenbecks Arch Surg* (2008) 393:281–7. doi:10.1007/s00423-008-0284-8
17. Chaar CI, Fitzgerald TN, Dewan M, Huddle M, Schlosser FJ, Perkal M, et al. Endovascular aneurysm repair is associated with less malnutrition than open abdominal aortic aneurysm repair. *Am J Surg* (2009) 198:623–7. doi:10.1016/j.amjsurg.2009.07.022
18. van Zanten ARH. Nutrition barriers in abdominal aortic surgery: a multimodal approach for gastrointestinal dysfunction. *J Parenter Enteral Nutr* (2013) 37(2):172–7. doi:10.1177/0148607112464499
19. Shraag S. Postoperative management. *Best Pract Res Clin Anaesthesiol* (2016) 30:381–93. doi:10.1016/j.bpa.2016.06.001
20. Crimi E, Hill CC. Postoperative ICU management of vascular surgery patients. *Anesthesiol Clin* (2014) 32(3):735–57. doi:10.1016/j.anclin.2014.05.001
21. Etz CD, Luozzo G, Bello R, Luehr M, Khan MZ, Bodian CA, et al. Pulmonary complications after descending thoracic and thoracoabdominal aneurysm repair: prediction, prevention and treatment. *Ann Thorac Surg* (2007) 83(2):S870–6. doi:10.1016/j.athoracsur.2006.10.099
22. Choudhury M. Postoperative management of vascular surgery patients: a brief review. *Clin Surg* (2017) 2:1584.
23. Landesberg G, Shatz V, Akopnik I, Wolf YG, Mayer M, Berlatzky Y, et al. Association of cardiac troponin, CK-MB and postoperative myocardial ischemia with long term survival after major vascular surgery. *J Am Coll Cardiol* (2003) 42(9):1547–54. doi:10.1016/j.jacc.2003.05.001
24. Beydon L, Rouxel A, Camut N, Schinkel N, Malinovsky JM, Aveline C, et al. Sedative premedication before surgery – a multicentre randomized study versus placebo. *Anaesth Crit Care Pain Med* (2015) 34(3):165–71. doi:10.1016/j.accpm.2015.01.005
25. Scavee V, Dehullu JP, Scavee JP, Michel I. Impact of anxiety in ambulatory superficial venous surgery: a prospective study using the HADS-A scale. *Acta Chir Belg* (2015) 115(1):42–8. doi:10.1080/00015458.2015.11681065
26. Killewich LA, Aswad MA, Sandager GP, Flinn WR. A randomized, prospective trial of deep venous thrombosis prophylaxis in aortic surgery. *Arch Surg* (1997) 132:499–504. doi:10.1001/archsurg.1997.01430290045007
27. Scarborough JE, Cox MW, Mureebe L, Pappas TN, Shortell CK. A novel scoring system for predicting postoperative venous thromboembolic complications in patients after open aortic surgery. *J Am Coll Surg* (2012) 214:620–8. doi:10.1016/j.jamcollsurg.2011.12.031

28. Sear JW. Kidney dysfunction in the postoperative period. *Br J Anaesth* (2005) 95(1):20–32. doi:10.1093/bja/aei018
29. Sawhney S, Mitchell M, Marks A, Fluck N, Black C. Long-term prognosis after acute kidney injury (AKI): what is the role of baseline kidney function and recovery? A systematic review. *BMJ Open* (2015) 4:e006497. doi:10.1136/bmjopen-2014-006497
30. Palevsky PM, Liu KD, Brophy PD, Chawla LS, Parikh CR, Thakar CV, et al. KDOQI US commentary on the 2012 KDIGO clinical practice guideline for acute kidney injury. *Am J Kidney Dis* (2013) 61(5):649–72. doi:10.1053/j.ajkd.2013.02.349
31. Kellum JA, Decker JM. Use of dopamine in acute renal failure: a meta-analysis. *Crit Care Med* (2001) 29(8):1526–31. doi:10.1097/00003246-200108000-00005
32. Achouh PE, Madsen K, Miller CC, Erstrera AL, Azizzadeh A, Dhareshwar J, et al. Gastrointestinal complications after descending thoracic and thoracoabdominal aortic repairs: a 14-year experience. *J Vasc Surg* (2006) 44(3):442–6. doi:10.1016/j.jvs.2006.05.018
33. Lee ES, Pevec WC, Link DP, Dawson DL. Use of T-stat to predict colonic ischemia during and after endovascular aneurysm repair: a case report. *J Vasc Surg* (2008) 47(3):632–4. doi:10.1016/j.jvs.2007.09.037
34. Moore JPR, Dyson A, Singer M, Fraser J. Microcirculatory dysfunction and resuscitation: why, when, and how. *Br J Anaesth* (2015) 115(3):366–75. doi:10.1093/bja/aev163
35. Singh A, Antognini JF. Perioperative hypotension and myocardial ischemia: diagnostic and therapeutic approaches. *Ann Card Anaesth* (2011) 14(2): 127–32. doi:10.4103/0971-9784.81569
36. Heintz KM, Hollenberg SM. Perioperative cardiac issues: postoperative arrhythmias. *Surg Clin North Am* (2005) 85(6):1103–14. doi:10.1016/j.suc.2005.09.003
37. Dunser MV, Takala J, Braunauer A, Bakker J. Re-thinking resuscitation: leaving blood pressure cosmetics behind and moving forward to permissive hypotension and tissue perfusion-based approach. *Crit Care* (2013) 17(5):326. doi:10.1186/cc12727
38. Gupta R, Gan TJ. Peri-operative fluid management to enhance recovery. *Anaesthesia* (2015) 71:40–5. doi:10.1111/anae.13309
39. Hoste EA, Maitland K, Brudney CS, Mehta R, Vincent JL, Yates D, et al. Four phases on intravenous fluid therapy: a conceptual model. *Br J Anaesth* (2014) 113(5):740–7. doi:10.1093/bja/aeu300
40. Van den Berghe G, Wouters P, Weekers F, Verwaest C, Bruyninckx F, Schetz M, et al. Intensive insulin therapy in critical ill patients. *N Engl J Med* (2001) 345:1359–67. doi:10.1056/NEJMoa011300
41. Krinsley JS. Association between hyperglycemia and increased hospital mortality in a heterogenous population of critically ill patients. *Mayo Clin Proc* (2003) 78(12):1471–8. doi:10.4065/78.12.1471
42. Serio S, Clements JM, Grauf D, Merchant AM. Outcomes of diabetic and nondiabetic patients undergoing general and vascular surgery. *ISRN Surg* (2013) 2013:963930. doi:10.1155/2013/963930
43. Nair BG, Horibe M, Neradilek MB, Newman SF, Peterson GN. The effect of intraoperative blood glucose levels in noncardiac surgery patients. *Anesth Analg* (2016) 122(3):893–902. doi:10.1213/ANE.0000000000001100
44. Kratzing C. Pre-operative nutrition and carbohydrate loading. *Proc Nutr Soc* (2011) 70:311–5. doi:10.1017/S0029665111000450
45. Hegazi RA, Wischmeyer PE. Clinical review: optimizing enteral nutrition for critically ill patients—a simple data-driven formula. *Crit Care* (2011) 15:234. doi:10.1186/cc10430
46. Boelens P, Heesakkers F, Luyer M, van Bernevald KW, de Hingh IH, Nieuwenhuijzen GA, et al. Reduction of postoperative ileus by early enteral nutrition in patients undergoing major rectal surgery. *Ann Surg* (2014) 259:649–55. doi:10.1097/SLA.0000000000000288
47. Ksienski MR, Fenton TR, Eliasziw M, Zuege DJ, Petrasek P, Shahpori R, et al. A cohort study of nutrition practices in the intensive care unit following abdominal aortic aneurysm repair. *JPEN J Parenter Enteral Nutr* (2013) 37:261–7. doi:10.1177/0148607112464654
48. Nelson RL, Edwards S, Tse B. Prophylactic nasogastric decompression after abdominal surgery. *Cochrane Database Syst Rev* (2005) 25(3):CD004929. doi:10.1002/14651858.CD004929.pub2
49. Fearon KC, Ljungqvist O, Von Meyenfeldt M, Revhaug A, Dejon CH, Lassen K, et al. Enhanced recovery after surgery: a consensus review of clinical care for patients undergo colonic resection. *Clin Nutr* (2005) 24:466–77. doi:10.1016/j.clnu.2005.02.002
50. Norris EJ, Beattie C, Perler PA, Martinez EA, Meinert CL, Anderson GF, et al. Double-masked randomized trial comparing alternate combinations of intra-operative anesthesia and postoperative analgesia in abdominal aortic surgery. *Anesthesiology* (2001) 95:1054–67. doi:10.1097/00000542-200111000-00006
51. Boric K, Boric M, Boric T, Puljak L. Analysis of perioperative pain management in vascular surgery indicates that practice does not adhere with guidelines: a retrospective cross-sectional study. *J Pain Res* (2017) 10:203–9. doi:10.2147/JPR.S123894

22

Toward Exempting from Sentinel Lymph Node Biopsy in T1 Breast Cancer Patients

Guozheng Li[1†], Jiyun Zhao[2†], Xingda Zhang[1†], Xin Ma[1], Hui Li[1], Yihai Chen[1], Lei Zhang[1], Xin Zhang[1], Jiale Wu[1], Xinheng Wang[1], Yan Zhang[2]* and Shouping Xu[1]*

[1]Department ofs Breast Surgery, Harbin Medical University Cancer Hospital, Harbin, China, [2]School of Life Science and Technology, Computational Biology Research Center, Harbin Institute of Technology, Harbin, China

*Correspondence:
Shouping Xu
Shoupingxu@hrbmu.edu.cn
Yan Zhang
zhangtyo@hit.edu.cn

Background and Objective: Sentinel lymph node biopsy (SLNB) is used to assess the status of axillary lymph node (ALN), but it causes many adverse reactions. Considering the low rate of sentinel lymph node (SLN) metastasis in T1 breast cancer, this study aims to identify the characteristics of T1 breast cancer without SLN metastasis and to select T1 breast cancer patients who avoid SLNB through constructing a nomogram.
Methods: A total of 1,619 T1 breast cancer patients with SLNB in our hospital were enrolled in this study. Through univariate and multivariate logistic regression analysis, we analyzed the tumor anatomical and clinicopathological factors and constructed the Heilongjiang Medical University (HMU) nomogram. We selected the patients exempt from SLNB by using the nomogram.
Results: In the training cohort of 1,000 cases, the SLN metastasis rate was 23.8%. Tumor volume, swollen axillary lymph nodes, pathological types, and molecular subtypes were found to be independent predictors for SLN metastasis in multivariate regression analysis. Distance from nipple or surface and position of tumor have no effect on SLN metastasis. A regression model based on the results of the multivariate analysis was developed to predict the risk of SLN metastasis, indicating an AUC of 0.798. It showed excellent diagnostic performance (AUC = 0.773) in the validation cohort.
Conclusion: The HMU nomogram for predicting SLN metastasis incorporates four variables, including tumor volume, swollen axillary lymph nodes, pathological types, and molecular subtypes. The SLN metastasis rates of intraductal carcinoma and HER2 enriched are 2.05% and 6.67%. These patients could be included in trials investigating the SLNB exemption.

Keywords: T1 breast cancer, SLNB, exempting, axillary surgery, molecular subtypes

INTRODUCTION

Breast cancer has the highest incidence rate among female malignant tumors, accounting for 24.2% of all new cases each year (1). Breast cancer treatment drugs are constantly evolving, as is the concept of surgery. From the initial "expanded radical treatment" to "modified radical treatment," and to the current "breast-conserving surgery," all of them reflect that breast cancer surgery focuses not only on effective treatment, but also on maximizing aesthetics and minimizing trauma.

SLN is the first regional lymph node from the primary tumor metastasis and the first lymph node capable of receiving lymph fluid from a specific organ and region (2). It can be used as a treatment and prognostic factor for breast cancers (3–5). Therefore, SLNB can predict the metastasis status of ALNs with a low false-negative rate, allowing more patients to avoid upper limb pain, sensory loss, and lymphedema caused by axillary lymph node dissection (6, 7). However, approximately 65%–70% of patients have suffered from unnecessary invasive axilla surgery (8, 9). This raises the question of whether we can pinpoint who might avoid SLNB.

Several studies have found a strong association between the molecular subtypes and the axillary status in breast cancer patients (10, 11). Furthermore, whether SLNB should be performed for luminal A breast cancer is still controversial (12). At the same time, the reports verified that tumor size was positively correlated with the SLN metastasis rate (13). T1 patients with small tumors and lower SLN metastasis rates (14) are more likely to be exempt from SLNB. So we enrolled 1,619 T1 breast cancer patients in this study and identified predictors for SLN metastasis in T1 breast cancers, especially the relationship between SLN metastasis and molecular subtypes.

The goal of this retrospective study was to establish a predictive model that includes tumor volume, swollen axillary lymph nodes, pathological types, and risk subtypes for SLN metastasis in T1 breast cancers. In addition, patients with a low risk of SLN metastasis could be exempt from SLNB.

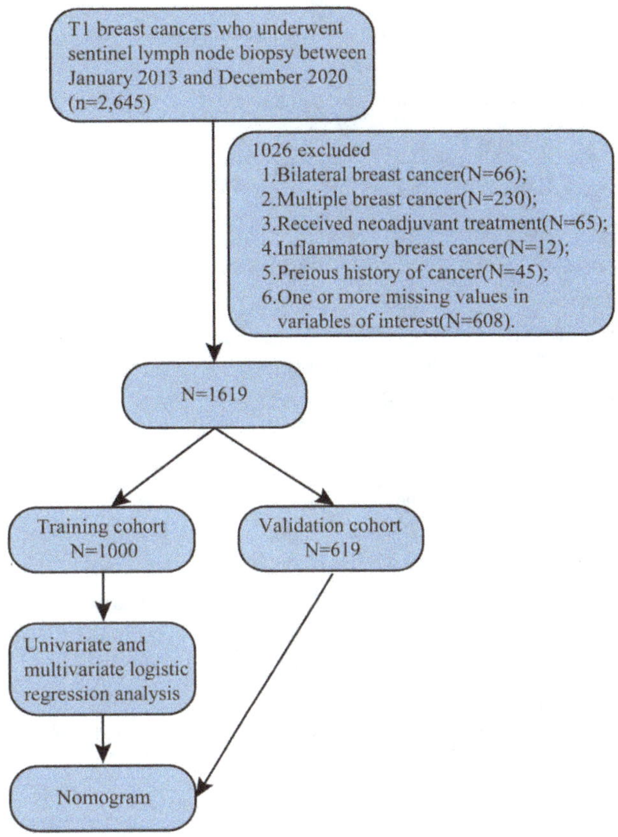

FIGURE 1 | The process for selecting patients for model development.

PATIENTS AND METHODS

Patients

We reviewed the clinicopathologic data of breast cancer patients with SLN metastasis who underwent SLNB during surgery at Harbin Medical University Cancer Hospital between January 1, 2013 and December 31, 2020. Patients with SLN metastasis were examined by SLNB during surgery. **Figure 1** depicts the selection of patients for model development.

Molecular Typing

Estrogen receptor (ER), progesterone receptor (PR) and ki67 were determined using immunohistochemistry and HER2 by immunohistochemistry or fluorescent *in situ* hybridization (FISH). Based on ER, PR, and HER2 status, patients were categorized into five molecular subtypes: luminal A[ER(+) and/or PR(+), HER2(−), ki67 ≤ 14%]; luminal B HER2(−)[ER (+) and/or PR(+), HER2(−), ki67>14%]; luminal B HER2(+) [ER(+) and/or PR(+), HER2(+)]; HER2 enriched [ER(−) and PR(−), HER2(+)] and triple negative[ER(−) and PR(−), HER2 (−)]. Based on univariate analysis results, we regrouped molecular subtypes, and defined them as risk subtypes: low-risk subtype[HER2 enriched]; median risk subtype[Luminal B HER(+) and TNBC]; high-risk subtype[Luminal A and Luminal B HER(−)].

Statistical Analysis

Univariate analysis was performed to detect predictors for SLN metastasis. Then, multivariate analysis, including all variables from the univariate analysis that were related to SLN status, was performed to test the factors' independence. Statistical significance was defined as $p < 0.05$; odds ratio (OR) and 95% confidence intervals (CI) were also calculated. Statistical tests were two-sided, and analyses were performed using SPSS v.19.0 Software (SPSS, Chicago, IL, http://www.spss.com).

RESULTS

Clinicopathological and Tumor Anatomical Factors of the Study Population

1,619 female patients with T1 breast cancer were enrolled. 1,000 patients between January 1, 2013 and April 10, 2018 were classified as a training cohort. The remaining 619 patients from April 10, 2018 to December 31, 2020 were classified as a validation cohort. The training cohort and the validation cohort were comparable in clinicopathological and tumor anatomical factors (**Table 1**). The median patient age was 55 years. The median tumor volume (length × width × width × 0.5) was 936 cm^3. The SLN metastasis rate of the training cohort was 23.8% (n = 1,000), and that of validation was 24.4% (n = 619).

TABLE 1 | Demographic and baseline characteristics of the study population.

Variables	Total	Training, *N* (%)	Validation, *N* (%)	*P*
No. of cases	1,619	1,000	619	
Age				
>55	774	472(47.2)	269(43.5)	0.142
≤55	905	528(52.8)	350(56.5)	
Tumor volume				
>936 cm^3	611	370(37.0)	234(37.8)	0.745
≤936 cm^3	1,068	630(63.0)	385(62.2)	
Distance from nipple				
>3 cm	714	418(41.8)	264(42.6)	0.737
≤3 cm	965	582(58.2)	355(57.4)	
Distance from surface				
>6 mm	718	409(40.8)	277(44.7)	0.128
≤6 mm	961	591(59.1)	342(55.3)	
Position of tumor				
Outer upper	710	416(41.6)	271(43.8)	0.502
Upper inner	486	296(29.6)	166(26.8)	
Lower inner	182	115(11.5)	65(10.5)	
Outer upper	301	173(17.3)	117(18.9)	
Swollen lymph nodes				
Positive	454	276(27.6)	170(27.5)	0.952
Negative	1,225	724(72.4)	449(72.5)	
ER				
Positive	1,341	774(77.4)	501(80.9)	0.091
Negative	338	226(22.6)	118(19.1)	
PR				
Positive	1,264	732(73.2)	472(76.3)	0.172
Negative	415	268(26.8)	147(23.7)	
HER2				
Positive	288	190(19.0)	98(15.8)	0.105
Negative	1,391	810(81.0)	521(84.2)	
Ki67				
>14%	752	442(44.2)	278(44.9)	0.780
≤14%	927	558(55.8)	341(55.1)	
Pathological types				
Invasive breast cancer	1,452	854(85.4)	546(88.2)	0.109
Intraductal carcinoma	227	146(14.6)	73(11.8)	

The bold values of P values means a significant difference.

TABLE 2 | Univariate analysis of tumor anatomical factors.

Variables	No. of positive SLN (%)	OR	95% CI	*P*
Age				
>55	108(22.9)	0.908	0.678–1.217	0.519
≤55	130(24.6)			
Tumor volume				
>936 cm^3	139(37.6)	3.227	2.390–4.359	**<0.001**
≤936 cm^3	99(15.7)			
Distance from nipple				
>3 cm	104(24.9)	1.107	0.825–1.486	0.497
≤3 cm	134(23.0)			
Distance from surface				
>6 mm	88(21.5)	0.806	0.597–1.088	0.159
≤6 mm	150(25.4)			
Position of tumor				
Outer upper	99(23.8)			
Upper inner	65(22.0)	0.566	0.631–1.286	0.901
Lower inner	27(23.5)	0.943	0.604–1.598	0.982
Outer upper	47(27.2)	0.389	0.798–1.789	1.194
Swollen lymph nodes				
Positive	116(42.0)	3.577	2.629--4.869	**<0.001**
Negative	122(16.9)			

The bold values of P values means a significant difference.

TABLE 3 | Univariate analysis of clinicopathological factors.

Variables	No. of positive SLN (%)	OR	95% CI	*P*
ER				
Positive	214(27.6)	3.216	2.048–5.052	**<0.001**
Negative	24(10.6)			
PR				
Positive	205(28.0)	2.770	1.860–4.126	**<0.001**
Negative	33(12.3)			
HER2				
Positive	15(7.9)	0.226	0.130–0.391	**<0.001**
Negative	223(27.5)			
Ki67				
>14%	108(24.4)	1.065	0.795–1.426	0.675
≤14%	130(23.3)			
Pathological types				
Invasive breast cancer	235(27.5)	18.096	5.712–57.336	**<0.001**
Intraductal carcinoma	3(2.1)			
Molecular subtypes				
Luminal A	114(24.1)	4.433	2.002–9.819	**<0.001**
Luminal B(HER+)	8(12.3)	1.965	0.677–5.703	*0.214*
Luminal B(HER-)	98(39.0)	8.967	3.999–20.110	**<0.001**
TNBC	11(10.5)	1.638	0.609–4.405	*0.328*
HER2 enriched	7(6.7)			

The bold values of P values means a significant difference.

The Identification of Independent Prognostic Factors for SLN Metastasis

To determine the independent predictors for SLN metastasis in the training cohort, a univariate analysis was first performed. Only tumor volume and swollen axillary lymph nodes, among tumor anatomical factors, were significantly associated with SLN metastasis (**Table 2**). Among clinicopathological factors, ER, PR, HER2, pathological types and molecular subtypes were significantly associated with SLN metastasis (**Table 3**).

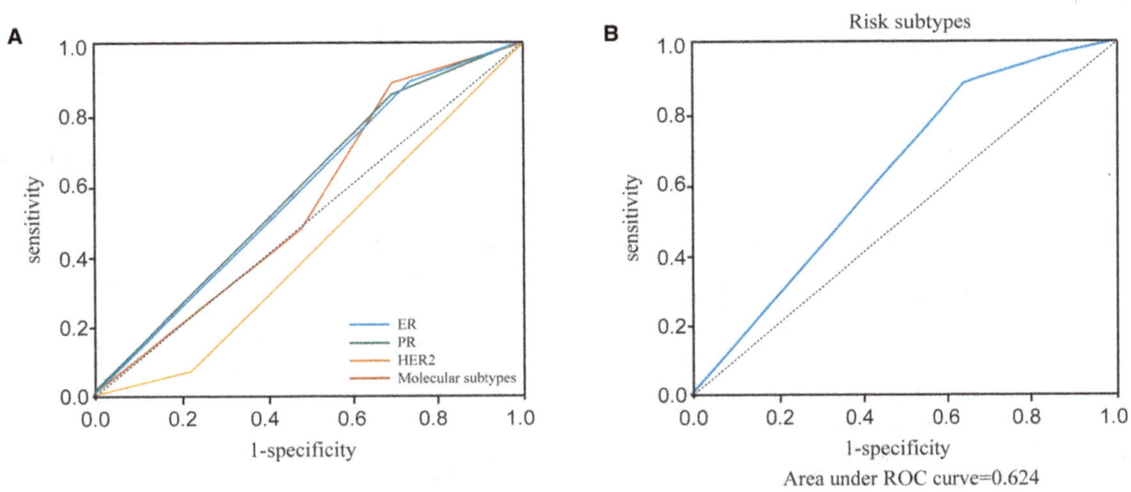

FIGURE 2 | ROC curves of ER, PR, HER2, molecular subtypes and risk subtypes. **(A)** ROC curves of ER, PR, HER2, molecular subtypes. **(B)** ROC curves of risk subtypes.

TABLE 4 | AUC curves of ER, PR, HER2, molecular subtypes and risk subtypes.

Variables	AUC	95% CI	*P*
ER	0.582	0.543–0.621	**<0.001**
PR	0.585	0.546–0.624	**<0.001**
HER2	0.417	0.378–0.455	**<0.001**
Molecular subtypes	0.562	0.524–0.600	**<0.001**
Risk subtypes	0.624	0.586–0.661	**<0.001**

The bold values of P values means a significant difference.

Therefore, breast cancer patients of ER positive, PR positive, and HER2 negative are more likely to develop SLN metastasis.

Before performing multivariate analysis, we analyzed the value of ER, PR, HER2, and molecular subtypes and compared their AUC values through Receiver-operating characteristic (ROC) analysis. The results are shown in **Figure 2A** and **Table 4**. The four variables have low AUC values. To improve their AUC, we retyped breast cancer based on the status of ER, PR, and HER2 and defined them as risk subtypes. The AUC value was 0.624 (**Figure 2B** and **Table 4**). Furthermore, the univariate analysis also showed that risk subtypes were related to SLN metastasis (**Table 5**).

Then multivariate analysis indicated that tumor volume, swollen axillary lymph nodes and pathological types were independent statistically significant predictors for SLN metastasis (**Table 6**). Furthermore, luminal A and luminal B HER2 (−), as the high-risk subtypes, were also independent statistically predictors for SLN metastasis. The SLN metastasis rates of these four variables are shown in **Figure 3**.

TABLE 5 | Univariate analysis of risk subtypes.

Variables	No. of positive SLN (%)	OR	95% CI	*P*
Risk subtypes				
Low risk				
HER2 enriched	7(6.7)			
Median risk				
Luminal B(HER+)	19(10)	1.556	0.632–3.832	*0.337*
TNBC				
High risk				
Luminal A	212(30.1)	6.020	2.750–13.179	**<0.001**
Luminal B(HER-)				

The bold values of P values means a significant difference.

TABLE 6 | Multivariate analysis of tumor anatomical location and clinicopathologic variables.

Variables	OR	95% CI	*P*
Tumor volume	5.574	3.382–8.107	**<0.001**
Swollen lymph nodes	6.423	4.365–9.453	**<0.001**
Pathological types	11.393	3.516–36.917	**<0.001**
Risk subtypes			**<0.001**
Low risk			**<0.001**
Median risk	2.231	0.823–6.048	*0.115*
High risk	11.349	4.622–27.868	**<0.001**

The bold values of P values means a significant difference.

Construction and Validation of the SLN Metastasis Nomogram

The four independent variables, including tumor volume, swollen axillary lymph nodes, pathological types, and risk subtypes, were incorporated to construct the HMU nomogram for estimating the SLN metastasis (**Figure 4A**). Each factor could be assigned a score by the HMU nomogram (**Table 7**). By summing the score of each factor together, the total score corresponded to an estimated SLN metastasis rate (**Figure 4A**).

The constructed HMU nomogram was then validated internally and externally. In the training cohort, ROC analysis showed that the AUC was 0.798 (**Figure 5A**). When fitted into the validation cohort, the AUC of the prediction model derived from the training cohort was 0.773 (**Figure 5B**). The calibration curves also revealed that the predictive model could accurately match the SLN metastasis rate (**Figure 4B**). These results demonstrated that the predictive model performs well in SLN metastasis. For example, the SLN metastasis rate in HER-type intraductal carcinoma, with tumor volume ≤936 cm^3 and without swollen axillary lymph nodes, is less than 0.1%. We believe that such patients do not require SLNB. If the tumor volume of HER2-invasive breast cancer is ≤936 cm^3, there is no swollen axillary lymph node. If the SLN metastasis rate is less than 1%, the clinician may not perform SLNB after considering the patient's wishes and clinical experience. Therefore, by calculating the patient's SLN metastasis rate according to the above four variables incorporated into the nomogram, we could provide a reference for the patient to decide whether to perform SLNB.

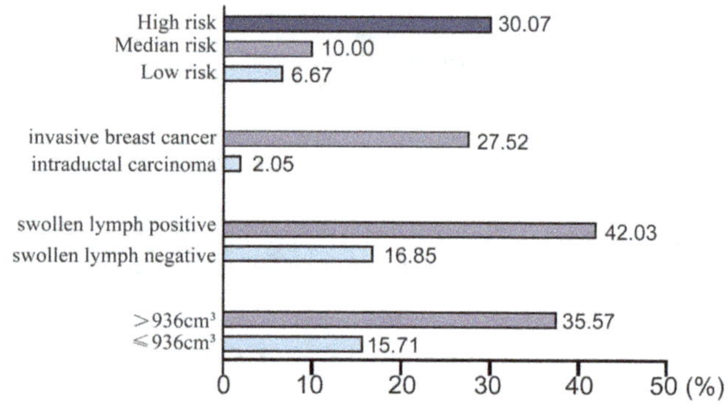

FIGURE 3 | SLN metastasis rate of four independent variables.

Patients Exempted from Sentinel Lymph Node Biopsy

According to the four variables in the HMU nomogram, we presented the SLN metastasis rate of patients with different characteristics (**Figure 6**). Patients with low metastasis rates are characterized by intraductal carcinoma (2.05%), low risk (6.67%), and median risk subtypes (10.00%). Therefore, those with HER2 enriched (group A) and intraductal carcinoma (group B) could be included in trials investigating the SLNB exemption. Patients with other characteristics would have lower metastasis rates, such as those with HER2 enriched associated tumor volume smaller than 936 cm^3 or without axillary lymphadenopathy, so they also could be included in this study.

DISCUSSION

The SLN metastasis is the gold standard for assessing ALN metastasis, but SLNB still has the following problems: positive SLN exemption, false negative rate, and complications after SLNB (6–9). Therefore, patients could avoid SLNB if some screening criteria can be defined to correctly assess the sentinel metastasis.

TABLE 7 | Detailed scores of each variable in HMU nomogram.

Variables		Nomogram scores
Tumor volume	>936 cm^3	62
	≤936 cm^3	0
Swollen lymph nodes	Positive	68
	Negative	0
Pathological types	Invasive breast cancer	88
	Intraductal carcinoma	0
Risk subtypes	Low risk	0
	Median risk	50
	High risk	100

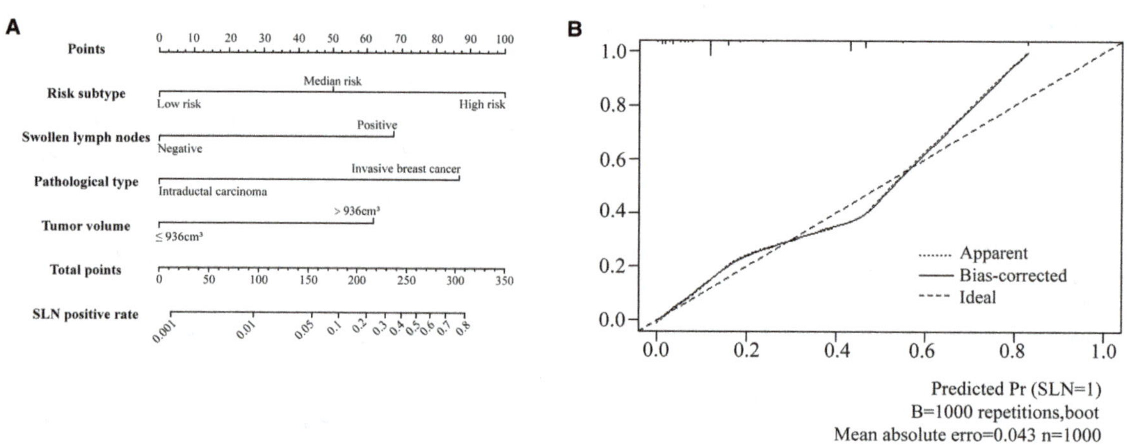

FIGURE 4 | Nomogram to predict the probability of SLN metastases in T1 breast cancer patients and calibration plot. **(A)** The nomogram of SLN metastases rate. **(B)** The calibration plot of nomogram.

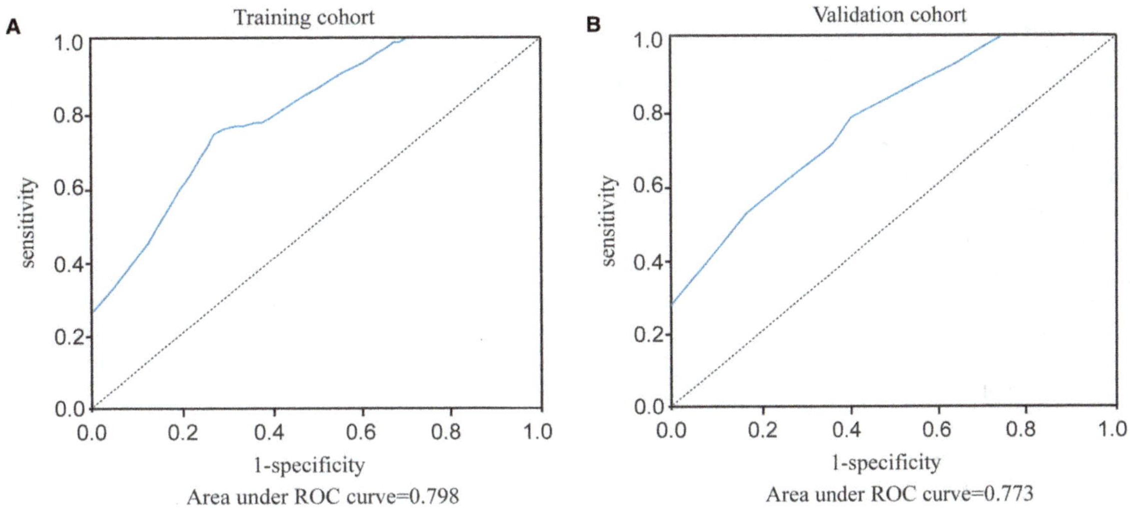

FIGURE 5 | ROC curves of our prediction model in the training cohort and validation cohort. **(A)** Area under ROC curve of training cohort. **(B)** Area under ROC curve of validation cohort.

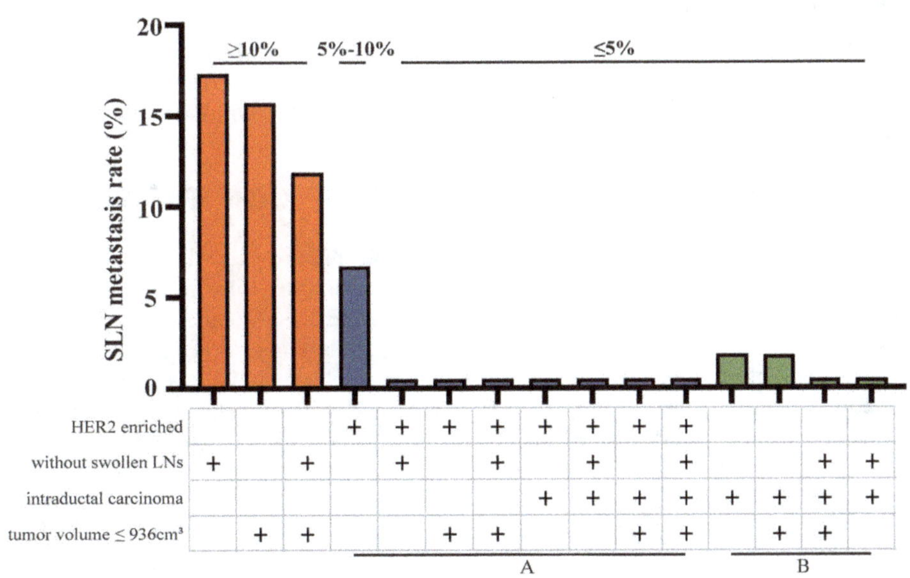

FIGURE 6 | The patients exempted from SLNB.

To fully evaluate the tumor size in this study, we adopted the concept of tumor volume, which took into account the tumor's long diameter and short diameter. When the tumor volume is less than or equal to 936 cm^3, the SLN metastasis rate is low (15.71%). This is consistent with previous studies that large tumors increase the risk of SLN metastasis (15–17). Swollen axillary lymph nodes are also highly suggestive of SLN metastasis (42.03%). However, some lymph node enlargement without SLN metastasis may be caused by congenital development of inflammation (18).

There is still controversy about whether SLNB should be performed in ductal carcinoma of breast cancer (19, 20). According to a meta-analysis, the incidence of SLN metastasis was 7.4 in patients with a preoperative diagnosis of intraductal carcinoma (21). Another study suggested that the only criterion for recommending SLNB in intraductal carcinoma should be any uncertainty about the presence of invasive lesions (22). Therefore, considering the risk of missed detection of microinvasion in some intraductal carcinomas and the high risk of intraductal carcinomas, we included intraductal carcinomas in the study. Intraductal carcinoma of the high-risk subtype has a tumor volume greater than 936 cm^3, accompanied by swollen axillary lymph nodes, and the SLN metastasis rate is as high as 30%, so SLNB should be performed. Studies have shown that the positive rate of SLNB in patients diagnosed with intraductal carcinoma by preoperative core needle biopsy is significantly higher than that in patients diagnosed with intraductal carcinoma after surgery (23, 24). If the preoperative diagnosis of intraductal carcinoma with swollen axillary lymph nodes is associated with undetected microinvasion, core needle biopsy should be performed to confirm the status of the swollen axillary lymph nodes (25–27).

Moreover, among the five molecular types of breast cancer, luminal A and luminal B HER2(−) have the highest SLN metastasis rate (30.07%). In other words, patients with ER (+)/PR(+)/HER2(−) T1 breast cancer are more likely to develop SLN metastasis. This is also consistent with previous studies, which confirm that triple-positive breast cancer is more prone to SLN metastasis (28), and that triple-negative breast cancer has a lower SLN metastasis rate (29). Our study demonstrated that ki67 has no effect on SLN metastasis of T1 breast cancer, which is consistent with Fabinshy's finding (30). However, another study found that ki67 was positively correlated with SLN metastasis (31). T1 breast cancer may be smaller, on the other hand, so ki67 is more likely to reflect the proliferation state rather than metastasis.

According to the study on an American breast cancer patient conducted by Memorial Sloan Kettering Cancer Center (MSKCC), age, tumor size, tumor type, lymphovascular invasion, tumor location, multifocality, ER and PR were all associated with SLN metastasis (32). The nomogram's AUC is 0.754. The Fudan University Shanghai Cancer Center in China, with an AUC value of 0.7649, included age, tumor size, tumor location, tumor type, and lymphovascular invasion (33). Two studies predicted the risk factors of SLN metastasis, but they ignored the impact of molecular subtypes on SLN metastasis. More importantly, our study focused on patients with low SLN metastasis rate. We thought that T1 breast cancer patients reduced the implementation of SLNB with less risk. The AUC value is 0.798 in the HMU nomogram, indicating that SLNB could be avoided more safely and effectively.

In conclusion, we developed and validated a nomogram for predicting SLN metastasis by adopting clinicopathological and tumor anatomical factors location from 1,000 T1 breast cancer patients. The remaining 619 T1 breast cancer patients were classified as validation cohort for external validation. The HMU nomogram provides comprehensive SLN metastasis information to optimize surgical procedures and benefit breast cancer patients. We focused on patients included in the SLNB exemption study, including intraductal carcinoma, HER2-enriched. Those with HER2-enriched and other low-risk factors may also be included in the study.

The potential limitations should be considered. First, more patients' information from other hospitals will be more useful for validating HMU nomograms. Second, the SLNB exemption only applies to T1 breast cancer patients, and additional and refined HMU nomograms should be further studied for various types of breast cancer patients.

ETHICS STATEMENT

The studies involving human participants were reviewed and approved by Changhong Zhao Harbin Medical University Cancer Hospital. The patients/participants provided their written informed consent to participate in this study.

AUTHOR CONTRIBUTIONS

SX and YZ provided direction and guidance throughout the preparation of this manuscript. GL, XM analyzed and interpreted the patient, tumor, and risk factor data as well as drafted the manuscript. JZ, XZ, YC generated the figures and made significant revisions to the manuscript. HL, LZ and XZ provided patient data and clinical information. All authors contributed to the article and approved the submitted version.

REFERENCES

1. Bray F, Ferlay J, Soerjomataram I, Siegel RL, Torre LA, Jemal A. Global cancer statistics 2018: globocan estimates of incidence and mortality worldwide for 36 cancers in 185 Countries. *CA Cancer J Clin.* (2018) 68 (6):394–424. doi: 10.3322/caac.21492
2. Nieweg OE, Tanis PJ, Kroon BB. The definition of a sentinel node. *Ann Surg Oncol.* (2001) 8(6):538–41. doi: 10.1007/s10434-001-0538-y
3. Carter CL, Allen C, Henson DE. Relation of tumor size, lymph node status, and survival in 24,740 breast cancer cases. *Cancer.* (1989) 63(1):181–7. doi: 10.1002/1097-0142(19890101)63:1<181::aid-cncr2820630129>3.0.co;2-h
4. Silverstein MJ, Skinner KA, Lomis TJ. Predicting axillary nodal positivity in 2282 patients with breast carcinoma. *World J Surg.* (2001) 25(6):767–72. doi: 10.1007/s00268-001-0003-x
5. Fowble B, Solin LJ, Schultz DJ, Frequency GR, Relapse So. And outcome of regional node failures following conservative surgery and radiation for early breast cancer. *Int J Radiat Oncol Biol Phys.* (1989) 17(4):703–10. doi: 10.1016/0360-3016(89)90055-2
6. Cody HS 3rd. Sentinel lymph node mapping in breast cancer. *Breast Cancer.* (1999) 6(1):13–22. doi: 10.1007/BF02966901
7. Ashikaga T, Krag DN, Land SR, Julian TB, Anderson SJ, Brown AM, et al. Morbidity results from the nsabp B-32 trial comparing sentinel lymph node dissection versus axillary dissection. *J Surg Oncol.* (2010) 102(2):111–8. doi: 10.1002/jso.21535
8. Viale G, Zurrida S, Maiorano E, Mazzarol G, Pruneri G, Paganelli G, et al. Predicting the Status of axillary sentinel lymph nodes in 4351 patients with invasive breast carcinoma treated in a single institution. *Cancer.* (2005) 103 (3):492–500. doi: 10.1002/cncr.20809
9. Nos C, Harding-MacKean C, Freneaux P, Trie A, Falcou MC, Sastre-Garau X, et al. Prediction of tumour involvement in remaining axillary lymph nodes when the sentinel node in a woman with breast cancer contains metastases. *Br J Surg.* (2003) 90(11):1354–60. doi: 10.1002/bjs.4325
10. Nakagawa T, Huang SK, Martinez SR, Tran AN, Elashoff D, Ye X, et al. Proteomic profiling of primary breast cancer predicts axillary lymph node metastasis. *Cancer Res.* (2006) 66(24):11825–30. doi: 10.1158/0008-5472.CAN-06-2337
11. Zhang J, Pei J, Liu H. Clinical risk analysis of non-visualized sentinel lymph node in breast cancer. *Cancer Biomark.* (2018) 23(2):179–83. doi: 10.3233/CBM-170958

12. Fragomeni SM, Sciallis A, Jeruss JS. Molecular subtypes and local-regional control of breast cancer. *Surg Oncol Clin N Am.* (2018) 27(1):95–120. doi: 10.1016/j.soc.2017.08.005
13. Chua B, Ung O, Taylor R, Boyages J. Frequency and predictors of axillary lymph node metastases in invasive breast cancer. *ANZ J Surg.* (2001) 71 (12):723–8. doi: 10.1046/j.1445-1433.2001.02266.x
14. Ding J, Jiang L, Wu W. Predictive value of clinicopathological characteristics for sentinel lymph node metastasis in early breast cancer. *Med Sci Monit.* (2017) 23:4102–8. doi: 10.12659/msm.902795
15. Atkinson EN, Brown BW, Montague ED. Tumor volume, nodal status, and metastasis in breast cancer in women. *J Natl Cancer Inst.* (1986) 76(2):171–8.
16. Sopik V, Narod SA. The relationship between tumour size, nodal status and distant metastases: on the origins of breast cancer. *Breast Cancer Res Treat.* (2018) 170(3):647–56. doi: 10.1007/s10549-018-4796-9
17. Yen TW, Hunt KK, Ross MI, Mirza NQ, Babiera GV. Predictors of invasive breast cancer in patients with an initial diagnosis of ductal carcinoma in situ: a guide to selective use of sentinel lymph node biopsy in management of ductal carcinoma in situ. *J Am Coll Surg.* (2005) 200(4):516–26. doi: 10.1016/j.jamcollsurg.2004.11.012
18. Dimcic M, Stevanovic O, Jakovljevic B. [Metastasis in axillary lymph nodes in breast carcinoma–possibilities of mammographic diagnosis]. *Srp Arh Celok Lek.* (1997) 125(3–4):124–6. Epub 1997/03/01.
19. Garganese G, Fragomeni SM, Bove S, Fabbri C, D'Alba P, Chiesa F, et al. Current controversies in the treatment of ductal carcinoma in situ of the breast. *Transl Cancer Res.* (2017):S307–18.
20. Terribile DA, Accetta C, d'Archi S, Paris I, Di Giorgio D, Garganese G, et al. Axillary lymph node surgical treatment. *Transl Cancer Res.* (2017): S390–S404.
21. Ansari B, Ogston SA, Purdie CA, Adamson DJ, Brown DC, Thompson AM. Meta-analysis of sentinel node biopsy in ductal carcinoma in situ of the breast. *Br J Surg.* (2008) 95(5):547–54. doi: 10.1002/bjs.6162
22. Moore KH, Sweeney KJ, Wilson ME, Goldberg JI, Buchanan CL, Tan LK, et al. Outcomes for women with ductal carcinoma-in-situ and a positive sentinel node: a multi-institutional audit. *Ann Surg Oncol.* (2007) 14 (10):2911–7. doi: 10.1245/s10434-007-9414-8
23. Schneider C, Trocha S, Mckinley B, Shaw J, Bielby S, Blackhurst D, et al. The use of sentinel lymph node biopsy in ductal carcinoma in situ. *Am Surg.* (2010) 76(9):943–6. doi: 10.1177/000313481007600925
24. van la Parra RF, Ernst MF, Barneveld PC, Broekman JM, Rutten MJ, Bosscha K. The value of sentinel lymph node biopsy in ductal carcinoma in situ (DCIS) and DCIS with microinvasion of the breast. *Eur J Surg Oncol.* (2008) 34(6):631–5. doi: 10.1016/j.ejso.2007.08.003
25. Klauber-Demore N, Tan LK, Liberman L, Kaptain S, Fey J, Borgen P, et al. Sentinel lymph node biopsy: is it indicated in patients with high-risk ductal carcinoma-in-situ and ductal carcinoma-in-situ with microinvasion? *Ann Surg Oncol.* (2000) 7(9):636–42. doi: 10.1007/s10434-000-0636-2
26. Pendas S, Dauway E, Giuliano R, Ku N, Cox CE, Reintgen DS. Sentinel node biopsy in ductal carcinoma in situ patients. *Ann Surg Oncol.* (2000) 7 (1):15–20. doi: 10.1007/s10434-000-0015-z
27. Kelly TA, Kim JA, Patrick R, Grundfest S, Crowe JP. Axillary lymph node metastases in patients with a final diagnosis of ductal carcinoma in situ. *Am J Surg.* (2003) 186(4):368–70. doi: 10.1016/S0002-9610(03)00276-9
28. Crabb SJ, Cheang MC, Leung S, Immonen T, Nielsen TO, Huntsman DD, et al. Basal breast cancer molecular subtype predicts for lower incidence of axillary lymph node metastases in primary breast cancer. *Clin Breast Cancer.* (2008) 8(3):249–56. doi: 10.3816/CBC.2008.n.028
29. Nguyen PL, Taghian AG, Katz MS, Niemierko A, Abi Raad RF, Boon WL, et al. Breast cancer subtype approximated by estrogen receptor, progesterone receptor, and Her-2 is associated with local and distant recurrence after breast-conserving therapy. *J Clin Oncol.* (2008) 26 (14):2373–8. doi: 10.1200/JCO.2007.14.4287
30. Thangarajah F, Malter W, Hamacher S, Schmidt M, Kramer S, Mallmann P, et al. Predictors of sentinel lymph node metastases in breast cancer-radioactivity and Ki-67. *Breast.* (2016) 30:87–91. doi: 10.1016/j.breast.2016.09.003
31. Ozemir IA, Orhun K, Eren T, Baysal H, Sagiroglu J, Leblebici M, et al. Factors affecting sentinel lymph node metastasis in Turkish breast cancer patients: predictive value of Ki-67 and the size of lymph node. *Bratisl Lek Listy.* (2016) 117(8):436–41. doi: 10.4149/bll_2016_085
32. Bevilacqua JL, Kattan MW, Fey JV, Cody 3rd HS, Borgen PI, Van Zee KJ. Doctor, what are my chances of having a positive sentinel node? A validated nomogram for risk estimation. *J Clin Oncol.* (2007) 25 (24):3670–9. doi: 10.1200/JCO.2006.08.8013
33. Chen JY, Chen JJ, Yang BL, Liu ZB, Huang XY, Liu GY, et al. Predicting sentinel lymph node metastasis in a Chinese breast cancer population: assessment of an existing nomogram and a new predictive nomogram. *Breast Cancer Res Treat.* (2012) 135(3):839–48. doi: 10.1007/s10549-012-2219-x

23

Laparoscopic High Uterosacral Ligament Suspension vs. Laparoscopic Sacral Colpopexy for Pelvic Organ Prolapse

Giuseppe Campagna [1], Lorenzo Vacca [1], Giovanni Panico [1], Giuseppe Vizzielli [2], Daniela Caramazza [1], Riccardo Zaccoletti [3], Monia Marturano [1], Roberta Granese [4], Martina Arcieri [4], Stefano Cianci [5], Giovanni Scambia [1,6] and Alfredo Ercoli [5]*

[1] Department of Woman, Child, and Public Health, Fondazione Policlinico Universitario A. Gemelli Istituto di Ricovero e Cura a Carattere Scientifico (IRCCS), Rome, Italy, [2] Department of Medicinal Area (DAME) Clinic of Obstetrics and Gynecology, Santa Maria della Misericordia Hospital, Azienda Sanitaria Universitaria Friuli Centrale, Udine, Italy, [3] Obstetrics and Gynecology Unit, P. Pederzoli Hospital, Peschiera del Garda, Verona, Italy, [4] Department of Biomedical, Dental, Morphological and Functional Imaging Science, University of Messina, Messina, Italy, [5] Department of Human Pathology in Adult and Childhood "G. Barresi," University of Messina, Messina, Italy, [6] Department of Woman, Child and Public Health, Catholic University of Sacred Heart, Rome, Italy

***Correspondence:**
Giovanni Panico
giovanni.panico@policlinicogemelli.it

Introduction: Laparoscopic sacral colpopexy is the gold standard technique for apical prolapse correction but it is a technically challenging procedure with rare but severe morbidity. Laparoscopic high uterosacral ligament suspension could be a valid technically easier alternative using native tissue.

Material and Methods: In the period from 2015 to 2018, 600 women were submitted to laparoscopic sacral colpopexy while 150 to laparoscopic high uterosacral ligament suspension in three Italian urogynecology referral centers. We enrolled women with apical prolapse stage $\geq$2 alone or multicompartment descensus. To reduce allocation bias, we performed a propensity matched analysis. Women undergoing laparoscopic high uterosacral ligament suspension surgery were matched 1:2 to women undergoing laparoscopic sacral colpopexy. The cumulative proportion of relapse-free women in time was analyzed by the Kaplan–Meier method. The primary objective of this multicenter case-control retrospective study was to compare the recurrence rate while the secondary objectives were to compare feasibility, safety, and efficacy of laparoscopic sacral colpopexy and laparoscopic high uterosacral ligament suspension in surgical treatment of pelvic organ prolapse.

Results: Three hundred and nine women were enrolled (103 laparoscopic high uterosacral ligament suspension; 206 laparoscopic sacral colpopexy). Median operatory time was significantly shorter in the laparoscopic high uterosacral ligament suspension group (P = 0.0001). No statistically significative difference was found in terms of estimated blood loss, admission time, intraoperative, and major early postoperative complications, postoperative pelvic pain, dyspareunia and *de novo* stress urinary incontinence. Surgical approach was the only independent risk factor for prolapse recurrence (RR = 6.013 [2.965–12.193], P = 0.0001). The objective cure rate was higher in the laparoscopic sacral colpopexy group (93.7 vs. 68%, 193/206 vs. 70/103, P = 0.0001) with a highly reduced risk of recurrence (RR = 5.430 [1.660–17.765]). Median follow up was 22 months.

Conclusion: Both techniques are safe, feasible, and effective. Laparoscopic sacral colpopexy remains the best choice in treatment of multicompartment and advanced pelvic organ prolapse while laparoscopic high uterosacral ligament suspension could be appropriate for moderate and isolated apical prolapse when laparoscopic sacral colpopexy is not suitable for the patient or to prevent prolapse in women at high risk at the time of the hysterectomy.

Keywords: laparoscopic high uterosacral ligament suspension, laparoscopic sacral colpopexy, pelvic organ prolapse, laparoscopic surgery, urogynecology

INTRODUCTION

Pelvic organ prolapse (POP) is a common female condition which involves the descent alone or in combination of the bladder, the rectum, the uterus (cervix) or the apex of the vagina (in case of previous hysterectomy) from their normal position in the pelvis with a consequent bulge into the vagina (1, 2). Although rarely resulting in severe morbidity or mortality, POP with is lower genital, urinary, and gastrointestinal tracts symptoms, affects the quality of life up to 40% of all women influencing daily activities, sexual function, and exercise (3). Its presence can have a negative impact on body image and sexuality (4, 5). Both the incidence and prevalence of POP surgery tend to increase with age. The estimated incidence of POP surgery ranges from 1.5 to 1.8 per 1,000 women year with the incidence peaking in women between 60 and 69 years (6).

Even though the vaginal approach continues to be the most common contributing up to 90% of surgical intervention (7), the know high rate of POP recurrence after transvaginal surgery with native tissue and the increasingly frequent reports on mesh-related complications with the consequent FDA transvaginal mesh-related litigation, have caused a decrease in the practice of this type of surgery in favor of laparoscopic abdominal procedures (8–10).

Nowadays, laparoscopic sacral colpopexy (LSCP) can be considered the gold standard technique for apical prolapse correction because of its lower recurrence and reoperation rates than a variety of vaginal procedures (vaginal sacrospinous colpopexy, uterosacral colpopexy, and transvaginal mesh) with a longer operating time as the only disadvantage (7). However, LSCP is a technically challenging procedure, because of the need of deep pelvic dissections and high skill in suturing and it is associated with rare but severe morbidity, with documented cases of vascular injuries and sacral nerve roots damage and consequent chronic constipation and pain (11, 12). For these reasons, new strategies were investigated to suspend vaginal apex in a technically easier way avoiding the most difficult and dangerous steps of LSCP.

Laparoscopic high uterosacral ligament suspension (L-HUSLS) is an alternative surgical intervention for apical prolapse correction using native tissue with feasibility, safety, and efficacy already demonstrated by several studies (13–18). When compared with the conventional vaginal approach, the laparoscopic procedure has similar objective success rates and a small number of ureteral injuries (13–16).

Despite the current state of affairs, the previously published studies able to compare the two techniques are few and characterized by a small sample of size (13, 19). For these reasons, our case-control study aimed to compare feasibility, safety, efficacy, and prolapse recurrence rates of LSCP and L-HUSLS in a high-volume urogynecology practice.

MATERIALS AND METHODS

This is a multicenter retrospective case control study including patients with apical POP (ICS) stage $\geq$ 2 (1) alone or in association with anterior and/or posterior descensus who underwent to L-HUSLS (Cases) and LSCP (Controls). The study was conducted at urogynecology referral centers of Fondazione Policlinico Universitario A. Gemelli IRCCS of Rome, Azienda Ospedaliera Universitaria Gaetano Martino of Messina and Clinica Polispecialistica Convenzionata Pederzoli of Peschiera d/G. In the period from 2015 to 2018, we enrolled 600 patients in the Control group and 150 patients in the Case Group (**Figure 1**). Both types of surgical techniques were performed in all the hospitals involved in the study.

Inclusion and Exclusion Criteria

Inclusion criteria were the following: postmenopausal patients with POP (ICS) stage $\geq$ 2 for the apical compartment; age $<$ 80 years; no uterine cervix dysplasia or endometrial disorders; no uterine size larger than conform 12 weeks' gestation; no previous longitudinal major abdominal surgery.

We excluded patients with anesthesiologic contraindications for minimally invasive approach. Cases were retrieved from our institutional database.

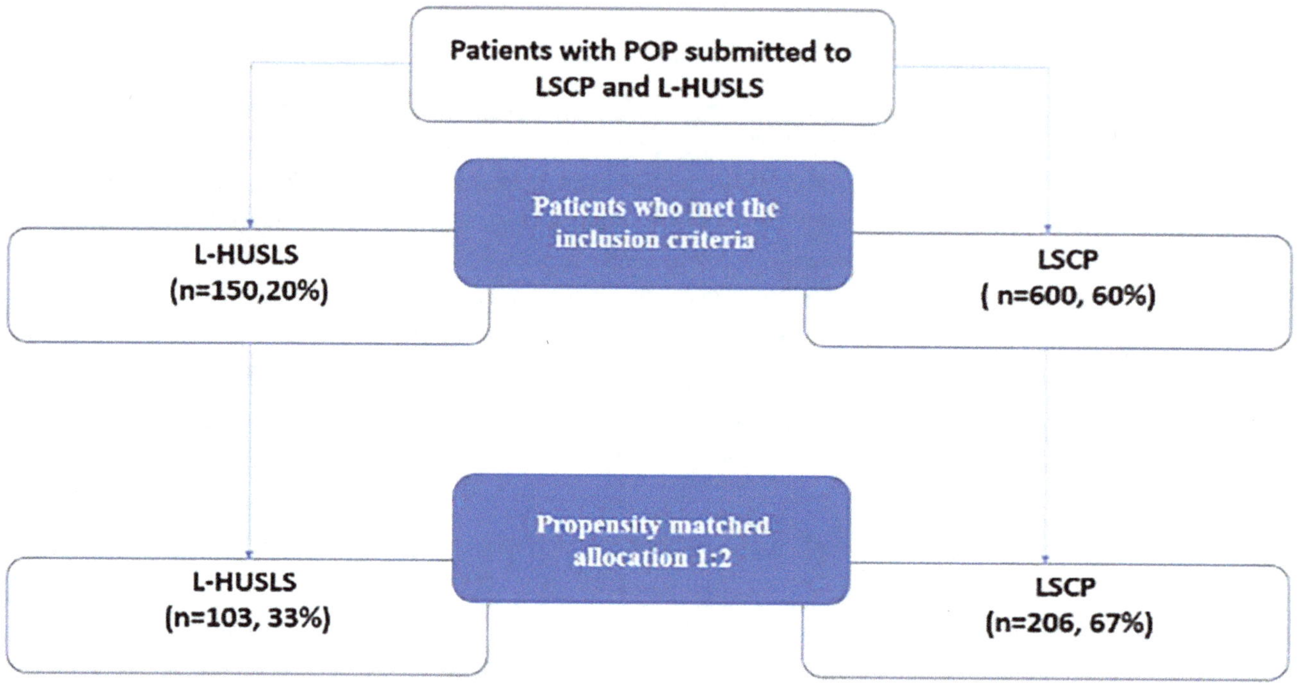

FIGURE 1 | Study design and selection process. In the period from 2015 to 2018, patients in the Control group and 150 patients in the Case Group were enrolled. Because of the nonrandomized nature of the study design and the possible allocation biases arising from the retrospective comparison between groups, we performed a propensity matched analysis. LSCP, laparoscopic sacral colpopexy; L-HUSLS, laparoscopic high uterosacral ligament suspension.

Four expert uro-gynecological surgeons (GC, GP, AE, and RZ) with a minimum of 30 LSCP and 30 L-HUSLS per year, prior to this study, performed all procedures.

The surgical selection was based on prolapse type and grade, surgeon preference, risk factors, and women history of previous surgery and preference. Additional procedures performed when indicated include total or supracervical hysterectomy, anterior colporrhaphy, and suburethral sling.

All patients received an upfront explanation of the surgical approach. Women signed written consent to undergo the described procedure and to permit data use.

The study was approved by the three hospitals institutional review boards and has been carried out in accordance with The Code of Ethics of the World Medical Association (Declaration of Helsinki) for experiments involving humans.

Preoperative and Perioperative Assessment

Preoperative assessment involving exhaustive history, physical examination, urodynamic testing, smear test and ultrasound scan was performed by an urogynecologist of each surgical team. When urogenital or ano-rectal malignant pathologies were suspected, supplementary exams and/or imaging were executed. POP was classified according to the Pelvic organ prolapse quantification (POP-Q) system published by the International Continence Society (1). Preoperatively women were questioned about urinary, bowel, and sexual function.

Surgical Technique

The three surgical teams performed all procedures using a standard technique in accordance with what we previously published (20–23).

In case of LSCP two adequately shaped polypropylene type 1 mesh fixed with non-absorbable sutures were used to correct the POP. Finally, the anterior mesh was fixed to the longitudinal vertebral ligament at L5-S1 level with 1–0 non absorbable suture on a noncutting needle.

When L-HUSLS was performed two polydioxanone 1 suture stitch (PDS®; Ethicon, Somerville, NJ, USA) were used to suspend vaginal apex. During the procedure, we mobilized and lateralized the ureters and hypogastric nerves to avoid injuries.

Follow-Up

We used Clavien–Dindo's (CD Grade) classification for grading postoperative complications during the first 30 days after surgery (24) and the ICS/IUGA joint report on the terminology for pelvic floor dysfunction (25) to describe surgical results.

We considered as an anatomic surgical failure a POP stage $\geq$ 2 in any compartment.

Patients underwent postoperative routine follow up at 1, 3, 6, and 12 months after the intervention and then yearly which were performed by an urogynecologist of each group. Urodynamic testing was repeated 12 months after the surgical treatment in all women without problems.

The Patient Global Impression of Improvement (PGI-I) questionnaire administered at 3 and 12 months (26) was used to evaluate the overall postoperative patient satisfaction. Women were asked about the changing of urinary and/or bowel and/or sexual function after the surgical procedure. During medical interview, sexually active patients were asked if they were affected by dyspareunia, defined as a perceived pain or discomfort during sexual intercourse.

Statistical Analysis

Because of the non-randomized nature of the study design and the possible allocation biases arising from the retrospective comparison between groups, we performed a propensity matched analysis (**Figure 1**). Propensity-matched comparison attempts to estimate the effect of a treatment by accounting for possible factors (e.g., constitutional variables) that predict receiving the treatment. Propensity-matched comparison aims to reduce biases arising from different covariates (27–29). A propensity score was developed through a multivariable logistic regression model. Age, body mass index, the preoperative stage of apical prolapse, were included in the model. Patients undergoing L-HUSLS surgery were matched 1:2 to patients undergoing LSCP using a caliper width $\leq$ 0.1 standard deviations of the logit odds of the estimated propensity score. Univariate analysis was performed to verify any difference between the two groups. The χ^2 analysis or Fisher's exact test were used, when appropriate, for categorical variables and the Student *t*-test and Mann–Whitney test, when appropriate, for continuous variables. Differences between the groups were considered statistically significant at $p < 0.05$ (95% confidence interval). The Kaplan–Meier method was used to analyze the cumulative proportion of relapse-free patients in time. The NCSS statistical software program, version 11.0 (NCSS Statistical Software, Kaysville, UT), was used.

RESULTS

After propensity matching, 103 patients were in the case cohort and 206 patients were in the control cohort. Patient characteristics of the two cohorts are shown in **Table 1**. No difference between groups was found in terms of age, BMI, comorbidities, previous POP surgery, parity, prior hysterectomy. Smokers were prevalent in the control group.

Even though the distribution of apical POP Q stage was similar among two groups there was a trend toward more severe (stage III/IV) anterior and posterior prolapse in the sacral colpopexy cohort (83.0 vs. 61.2% $p = 0.0001$ for the anterior descensus and 0 vs. 9% for the posterior one) Perioperative parameters are summarized in **Table 2**.

Median OT was significantly shorter in the L-HUSLS group 120 min vs. 190 min ($p = 0.0001$). No statistically significative difference was found in terms of estimated blood loss, admission time, intraoperative complication and major early postoperative complication. We registered 1 (0.5%) intraoperative complication: a bladder injury in LSCP group.

All women with uterus underwent total hysterectomy in the case group and subtotal hysterectomy in the control group.

There were no significant differences between the two cohorts in terms of postoperative pelvic pain (1% in the case group vs. 2.4% in the control group, $p = 0.382$), dyspareunia (2% in the case group vs. 6% in the control group, $p = 0.612$) and *de novo* stress urinary incontinence (6.8% in the case group vs. 13.1% in the control group, $p = 0.123$).

There was one case of LSCP mesh erosion (0.5%) managed conservatively with vaginal estrogen. There were four cases

TABLE 1 | Baseline patients characteristics.

Variables	L-HUSLS+ (N) (%)	LSCPa (N) (%)	p-value
All cases	103	206	–
Age			
<65 years	74 (71.8)	147 (71.4)	0.929
≥65 years	29 (28.2)	59 (28.6)	
Body mass index (Kg/m²)			
<25	44 (42.7)	94 (45.6)	0.716
≥25	59 (57.3)	112 (54.4)	
Diabetes			
Yes	7 (6.8)	13 (6.3)	0.870
No	96 (93.2)	193 (93.7)	
COPD°			
Yes	4 (3.9)	4 (1.9)	0.448
No	99 (96.1)	202 (98.1)	
Parity			
Yes	102 (99.0)	199 (96.6)	0.277
No	1 (1.0)	7 (3.4)	
Prior POP* surgery			
Yes	7 (6.8)	25 (12.1)	0.169
No	96 (93.2)	181 (87.9)	
Prior hysterectomy			
Yes	11 (10.7)	40 (19.4)	0.053
No	92 (89.3)	166 (80.6)	
Smoking			
Yes	5 (4.9)	28 (13.6)	**0.01**
No	98 (95.1)	178 (86.4)	
Preoperative SUI**			
Yes	25 (24.3)	55 (26.7)	0.681
No	78 (75.7)	151 (73.3)	
POP Q stage anterior			
1–2	40 (38.8)	35 (17.0)	**0.0001**
3–4	63 (61.2)	171 (83.0)	
POP Q stage apical			
2	48 (46.6)	91 (44.2)	0.717
3–4	55 (53.4)	115 (55.8)	
POP Q stage posterior			
1–2	103 (100)	187 (90.8)	**0.001**
3–4	0	19 (9.2)	

+*Laparoscopic sacral colpopexy.*
a*Laparoscopic high uterosacral ligament suspension (L-HUSLS).*
°*Chronic obstructive pulmonary disease.*
**Pelvic organ prolapse.*
***Stress urinary incontinence.*
LSCPa, aLaparoscopic sacral colpopexy; L-HUSLS+, +Laparoscopic high uterosacral ligament suspension.

TABLE 2 | Perioperative data.

Variables	L-HUSLS (*N*) (%)	LSCP (*N*) (%)	*p*-value
All cases	103	206	–
Operative time (minimum) (median) (range)	120 (60–270)	190 (110–290)	**0.0001**
Estimated blood loss (mL) (median) (range)	70 (0–130)	50 (0–110)	0.965
Concomitant procedures			
Anterior colporrhaphy	66 (64.1)	0	**0.0001**
Sub-urethral sling	12 (11.7)	1 (0.5)	**0.0001**
Intraoperative complications	–	1 (0.5)	0.479
Early (<30 days) major postoperative complications*	–	–	n.a.**
Hospital stay (days) (median) (range)	2 (1–4)	2 (1–4)	0.186

*≥3 according to Clavien-Dindo scale (xx); **n.a., not applicable.

TABLE 3 | Patient global Impression of Improvement (PGI-I).

	Very much better Much better Score 1–2	A little better No change Score 3–4
L-HUSLS (*N*) (%)	74 (72%)	29 (28%)
LSCP (*N*) (%)	194 (94%)	12 (6%)
***p*-value**	**0.0001**	**0.0001**

of urinary retention in the L-HUSLS group which all resolved spontaneously within 1 week, two cases of urinary infection in the LSCP group treated successfully with antibiotics and 1 case of Deep vein thrombosis cured with anticoagulant therapy.

PGI-I score for both groups is summarized in **Table 3**.

In the univariate and multivariate analysis surgical approach was the only independent risk factor for POP recurrence (RR = 6.013; CI: 2.965–12.193, $p = 0.0001$; **Table 4**).

Anatomic outcomes are presented in **Table 5**. The objective cure rate was higher in the LSCP group (93.7 vs. 68%, $p = 0.0001$) with a highly reduced risk of prolapse recurrence (RR = 5.430, CI: 1.660–17.765). The length of follow-up was similar with a median of 22 months in both groups.

Kaplan–Meier curves of objective recurrence in the whole population are shown in **Figure 2**.

DISCUSSION

Our study demonstrates that both laparoscopic procedures are safe with rare and minor perioperative complications and a superimposable admission time in accordance with the main principles of the mini-invasive approach. In addition, L-HUSLS showed significative lower OT than LSCP. The absence of ureteral injuries further emphasizes the safety of the L-HUSLS techniques if compared to the 11% of the ureteral damaging rate described in previous studies on V-USLS (30). One of the perceived benefits of the laparoscopic approach includes the magnified view of the operative field allowing an easier dissection, a more precise suture placement and a better visualization of vital structures. This may help to reduce the possible damage to the ureter which could be further protected by a prophylactic ureterolysis before the apical suspension. This confirms what already published studied demonstrated about the minimal ureteric injury rates during this laparoscopic procedure (14, 15, 31, 32). Mesh erosion rate in LSCP group with only in 1 case (0.5%) was lower compared to data already reported in literature (7, 12, 33, 34). This may be related to the surgical technique, to the prothesis material (polypropylene type 1 with mesh weight ranging from 16 to 65 g/m^2) (35) and to time of follow up. The use of a standard subtotal hysterectomy avoids the communication between the vaginal and the abdominal cavities and the consequent exposition of the surgical bed to the vaginal microbiota. This element, combined with the devascularization of the vaginal cuff caused by uterus removal, may play a significative role in the evolution of subsequent erosion. Even though the length of the follow up in the study is enough to detect mesh related complications, it's still too short to compare our results with those included in the study by Nygaard et al. (33) which report a rate of mesh erosion of 10.5% at 7 years. The incidence of *de novo* SUI was higher in the LSCP group but not in a significative manner. Our data don't differ from those already published in literature (13, 36).

The present study founded that LSCP has higher objective success rate than L-HUSLS in multicompartment advanced pelvic organ prolapse. Regarding LSCP our anatomic outcome was similar to those already described in literature (33, 34). The recurrence rate in patients underwent L-HUSLS were higher than those previously published (13, 15, 37, 38). This may be related to the larger sample size investigated, the longer follow up time and the highest grade of preoperative pelvic organ prolapse. Filmar et al. (13) reported an anatomic success rate for L-HUSLS of 89.7 % in only 29 patients with a preoperative POP stage 2 and a follow up of 6 months. Haj Yahya et al. reported with the same procedure an anatomic success rate of 91.3% but 54% of the population had a preoperative apical prolapse of grade I, and 22.9% of grade II with a FUP of 17.5 months (38). The PGI-I reflects the anatomical outcome with a significative higher percentage of women in the LSCP group with a score of 1–2.

TABLE 4 | Risk factors for prolapse recurrence.

Variable	Univariate analysis		Multivariate analysis*	
	Risk ratio (95% CI)	*p*-value**	Risk ratio (95% CI)	*p*-value**
Age				
≤65[§]	0.497 (0.222–1.116)	0.107	2.110 (0.897–4.964)	0.087
>65				
Body mass index (BMI)				
≤25 Kg/m^2	1.123 (0.593–2.128)	0.748	–	–
>25 Kg/m^2[§]				
Surgical approach				
L-HUSLS[§]	6.691 (3.324–13.470)	**0.0001**	6.013 (2.965–12.193)	**0.0001**
LSCP				
COPD				
Yes§	0.850 (0.811–0.892)	0.237	–	–
No				
Prior POP surgery				
Yes[§]	0.363 (0.084–1.574)	0.159	1.586 (0.336–7.491)	0.560
No				
Prior hysterectomy				
Yes[§]	0.921 (0.386–2.196)	0.853	–	–
No				
POP Q stage anterior				
1–2	1.333 (0.610–2.914)	0.574	–	–
3–4§				
POP Q stage apical				
2	0.924 (0.490 – 1.741)	0.872	–	–
3–4§				
POP Q stage posterior				
1–2	0.845 (0.804–0.888)	0.063	1.198 (0.01–8.493)	0.998
3–4§				

Multivariate analysis with method backward stepwise was performed for variable with $p < 0.2$ at univariate analysis.
**Bold cases are statistically significant: $p < 0.05$.*

TABLE 5 | Pattern of recurrent prolapse according to surgical approach.

Variable	*N* (%)	L-HUSLS (%)	LSCP (%)	*p*-value	Risk ratio (95% CI)
All cases	309	103	206	–	–
Recurrences	46 (14.9)	33 (32)	13 (6.3)	0.0001	5.430 (1.660–17.765)
Anterior	26 (56.5)	18 (54.5)	8 (61.6)	0.0001	5.743 (2.768–11.917)
Apical	4 (8.7)	4 (12.1)	0	0.0001	7.944 (2.544–24. 809)
Posterior	2 (4.3)	1 (3.0)	1 (7.7)	0.011	6.309 (1.251–31.832)
Multicompartmental	14 (30.5)	10 (30.4)	4 (30.7)	0.002	5.430 (1.660–17.765)

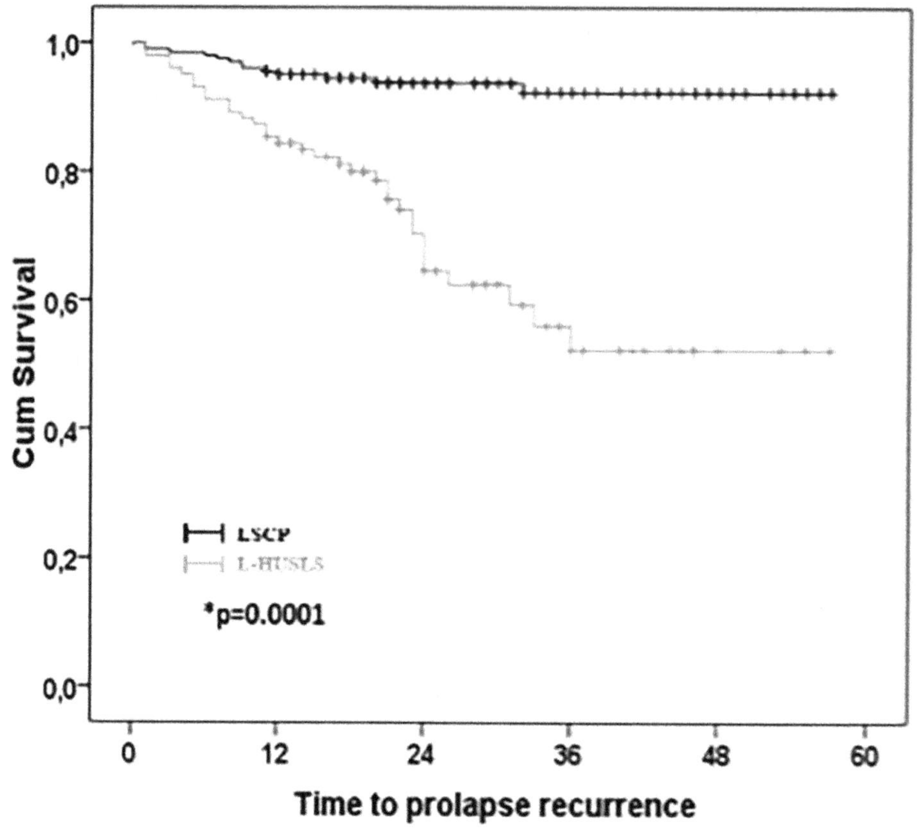

FIGURE 2 | Kaplan–Meier survival curves for anatomical recurrence. Kaplan–Meier curves of objective recurrence in the whole population.

To better evaluate the effectiveness of the two techniques, the univariate and multivariate analysis was performed to understand which could be possible confounding risk factors for surgical failure. However, none of the tested independent variables, including preoperative POP Q stage, had an influence on anatomic recurrence except for the type of surgical procedures. This may be related to the characteristics of our population characterized by multicompartmental POP. L-HUSLS is a fascial technique indicated for the correction of apical prolapse. Higher grade of apical prolapse is often associated with anterior or posterior descensus. While LSCP is often able to correct the defects in all the compartments in this clinical situation, L-HUSLS often requires an additional vaginal native tissue repair. This exposes the women to the augmented risk of surgical failure of fascial surgery. Significantly we observed that 85% of prolapse recurrence in L-HUSLS group involved the anterior compartment even though the procedure was associated with anterior colporrhaphy in 66 cases (64.1 %). The anatomical failure rate in the anterior compartment (28/103, 27%) is similar to those described by Maher's Cochrane indicating that 27–42% of women would have a recurrence after native tissue repair (39). Taking in consideration only the apical compartment we observed that, even if the LSCP remains the referral treatment with an objective success rate of 98% (202/206), the anatomical success rate for the L-HUSLS technique increases up to 87% (89/103). This demonstrates that although L-HUSLS is significantly less effective than LSCP in advanced multi- component prolapses, it remains an effective treatment for isolated and mild apical prolapses bypassing the limits of the vaginal routes (such as chronic pelvic pain, dyspareunia, ureteral obstruction) (14, 15). There are particular clinical situations such as the need for a total hysterectomy (in case of cervical pathology) and the presence of contraindications to the positioning of the prosthetic material (patients at high risk of mesh infection) in which the L-HUSLS may play a significative role. Moreover, results showed a significative shorter operative time of L-HUSLS. This would be an advantage for patients who, due to their comorbidities, cannot sustain a long surgical procedure. Thanks to its demonstrated safety and feasibility this technique should take in consideration for POP prevention in patients undergoing total hysterectomy for benign indication in which risk factors for future descensus have been recognized.

This was a pilot study before planning a multicentric prospective study with a larger sample. In the absence of specific questionnaires, women completed the PGI-I questionnaire and expressed their satisfaction with the surgical treatment in terms of sexual function and bulge symptom resolution.

In our prospective study, we plan to evaluate additional subjective outcomes.

Strengths of our study include large sample size, the multicentric setting in high volume hospitals, all participating surgeon performing both techniques and the long follow up.

Limitations of our study include those inherent to cohort studies. Because of the possibility of selection bias due to the absence of randomization we balanced the differences in patient characteristics between groups by using propensity score-matching. Although differences remained between the matched groups related to the preoperative POP Q stage anterior and posterior, we have attempted to address this discrepancy using the regression modeling.

CONCLUSION

In conclusion, both presented techniques suggest safety, feasible, and efficacy in the treatment POP. LSCP still remains (remove the extra space) to be the best choice in the treatment of multicompartment and advanced pelvic organ prolapse while L-HUSLS appears to be well-appropriate for moderate and isolated apical prolapse when LSCP is not suitable for the patient or to prevent prolapse in patients at high risk at the time of the hysterectomy.

ETHICS STATEMENT

The studies involving human participants were reviewed and approved by Comitato Etico Policlinico Universitario A. Gemelli—Largo Agostino Gemelli 8, 00168 Roma—Prot. ID 3487. The patients/participants provided their written informed consent to participate in this study.

AUTHOR CONTRIBUTIONS

GC, AE, LV, and RZ: conception and design. LV, RZ, and MM: acquisition of data. GV, SC, and GP: analysis and interpretation of data. LV, GP, MA, and DC: drafting of the manuscript. AE, GC, RG, and GS: critical revision of the manuscript. All authors contributed to the article and approved the submitted version.

REFERENCES

1. Haylen BT, Maher CF, Barber MD, Camargo S, Dandolu V, Digesu A, et al. An International Urogynecological Association (IUGA) / International Continence Society (ICS) Joint Report on the Terminology for Female Pelvic Organ Prolapse (POP): International Urogynecological Association (IUGA). *Neurourol Urodyn.* (2016) 35:137–68. doi: 10.1002/nau.22922
2. Abrams P, Cardozo L, Fall M, Griffiths D, Rosier P, Ulmsten U, et al. The standardisation of terminology of lower urinary tract function: report from the standardisation sub-committee of the international continence society. *Am J Obstetr Gynecol.* (2002) 187:116–26. doi: 10.1067/mob.2002.125704
3. Handa VL, Garrett E, Hendrix S, Gold E, Robbins J. Progression and remission of pelvic organ prolapse: a longitudinal study of menopausal women. *Am J Obstetr Gynecol.* (2004) 190:27–32. doi: 10.1016/j.ajog.2003.07.017
4. Lowder JL, Ghetti C, Nikolajski C, Oliphant SS, Zyczynski HM. Body image perceptions in women with pelvic organ prolapse: a qualitative study. *Am J Obstetr Gynecol.* (2011) 204:441.e1–e5. doi: 10.1016/j.ajog.2010.12.024
5. Jelovsek JE, Barber MD. Women seeking treatment for advanced pelvic organ prolapse have decreased body image and quality of life. *Am J Obstetr Gynecol.* (2006) 194:1455–61. doi: 10.1016/j.ajog.2006.01.060
6. Barber MD, Maher C. Epidemiology and outcome assessment of pelvic organ prolapse. *Int Urogynecol J.* (2013) 24:1783–90. doi: 10.1007/s00192-013-2169-9
7. Maher C, Feiner B, Baessler K, Schmid C. Surgical management of pelvic organ prolapse in women. *Cochrane Database Syst Rev.* (2013) 30:CD004014. doi: 10.1002/14651858.CD004014.pub5
8. Olsen A, Smith V, Bergstrom J, Colling J, Clark A. Epidemiology of surgically managed pelvic organ prolapse and urinary incontinence. *Obstetr Gynecol.* (1997) 89:501–6. doi: 10.1016/S0029-7844(97)00058-6
9. Wang LC, Al Hussein Al Awamlh B, Hu JC, Laudano MA, Davison WL, Schulster ML, et al. Trends in mesh use for pelvic organ prolapse repair from the medicare database. *Urology.* (2015) 86:885–91. doi: 10.1016/j.urology.2015.08.022
10. U.S. Food and Drug Administration. *Urogynecologic Surgical Mesh Implants.* Available online at: https://www.fda.gov/medical-devices/implants-and-prosthetics/urogynecologic-surgical-mesh-implants n.d (accessed April 16, 2019).
11. Possover M, Lemos N. Risks, symptoms, and management of pelvic nerve damage secondary to surgery for pelvic organ prolapse: a report of 95 cases. *Int Urogynecol J.* (2011) 22:1485–90. doi: 10.1007/s00192-011-1539-4
12. Nygaard IE, McCreery R, Brubaker L, Connolly A, Cundiff G, Weber AM, et al. Abdominal sacrocolpopexy: a comprehensive review. *Obstetr Gynecol.* (2004) 104:805–23. doi: 10.1097/01.AOG.0000139514.90897.07
13. Filmar GA, Fisher HW, Aranda E, Lotze PM. Laparoscopic uterosacral ligament suspension and sacral colpopexy: results and complications. *Int Urogynecol J.* (2014) 25:1645–53. doi: 10.1007/s00192-014-2407-9
14. Rardin CR, Erekson EA, Sung VW, Ward RM, Myers DL. Uterosacral colpopexy at the time of vaginal hysterectomy: comparison of laparoscopic and vaginal approaches. *J Reprod Med.* (2009) 54:273–80.
15. Turner LC, Lavelle ES, Shepherd JP. Comparison of complications and prolapse recurrence between laparoscopic and vaginal uterosacral ligament suspension for the treatment of vaginal prolapse. *Int Urogynecol J.* (2016) 27:797–803. doi: 10.1007/s00192-015-2897-0
16. Vallabh-Patel V, Saiz C, Salamon C. Subjective and objective outcomes of robotic and vaginal high uterosacral ligament suspension. *Female Pelvic Med Reconstr Surg.* (2016) 22:420–4. doi: 10.1097/SPV.0000000000000306
17. Lin LL, Phelps JY, Liu CY. Laparoscopic vaginal vault suspension using uterosacral ligaments: a review of 133 cases. *J Minim Invasive Gynecol.* (2005) 12:216–20. doi: 10.1016/j.jmig.2005.03.014
18. Wyman AM, Rodrigues AA, Hahn L, Greene KA, Bassaly R, Hart S, et al. Estimated levator ani subtended volume: a novel assay for predicting surgical failure after uterosacral ligament suspension. *Am J Obstetr Gynecol.* (2016) 214:611.e1–e6. doi: 10.1016/j.ajog.2015.11.005
19. Lavelle ES, Giugale LE, Winger DG, Wang L, Carter-Brooks CM, Shepherd JP. Prolapse recurrence following sacrocolpopexy vs uterosacral ligament suspension: a comparison stratified by Pelvic Organ Prolapse Quantification stage. *Am J Obstetr Gynecol.* (2018) 218:116.e1–e5. doi: 10.1016/j.ajog.2017.09.015
20. Lizee D, Campagna G, Morciano A, Panico G, Ercoli A, Gadonneix P. Laparoscopic sacral colpopexy: how to place the posterior mesh into rectovaginal space? *Neurourol Urodyn.* (2017) 36:1529–34. doi: 10.1002/nau.23106
21. Campagna G, Panico G, Morciano A, Vacca L, Anchora LP, Gallucci V, et al. Laparoscopic supracervical hysterectomy and sacral colpopexy for pelvic organ prolapse with percutaneous surgical system: results from a pilot study. *Eur J Obstetr Gynecol Reprod Biol.* (2018) 221:160–5. doi: 10.1016/j.ejogrb.2017.12.043

22. Ercoli A, Cosma S, Riboni F, Campagna G, Petruzzelli P, Surico D, et al. Laparoscopic nerve-preserving sacropexy. *J Minim Invasive Gynecol.* (2017) 24:1075–7. doi: 10.1016/j.jmig.2017.03.008
23. Panico G, Campagna G, Caramazza D, Amato N, Ercoli A, Scambia G, et al. Laparoscopic high uterosacral ligament suspension: an alternative route for a traditional technique. *Int Urogynecol J.* (2018) 29:1227–9. doi: 10.1007/s00192-018-3588-4
24. Dindo D, Demartines N, Clavien P-A. Classification of surgical complications: a new proposal with evaluation in a cohort of 6336 patients and results of a survey. *Ann Surg.* (2004) 240:205–13. doi: 10.1097/01.sla.0000133083.54934.ae
25. Toozs-Hobson P, Freeman R, Barber M, Maher C, Haylen B, Athanasiou S, et al. An international urogynecological association (IUGA)/international continence society (ICS) joint report on the terminology for reporting outcomes of surgical procedures for pelvic organ prolapse. *Neurourol Urodyn.* (2012) 31:415–21. doi: 10.1002/nau.22238
26. Srikrishna S, Robinson D, Cardozo L. Validation of the Patient Global Impression of Improvement (PGI-I) for urogenital prolapse. *Int Urogynecol J.* (2010) 21:523–8. doi: 10.1007/s00192-009-1069-5
27. Rosenbaum PR, Rubin DB. Reducing bias in observational studies using subclassification on the propensity score. *J Am Stat Assoc.* (1984) 79:516–24. doi: 10.1080/01621459.1984.10478078
28. Rubin DB. Estimating causal effects from large data sets using propensity scores. *Ann Intern Med.* (1997) 127:757. doi: 10.7326/0003-4819-127-8_Part_2-199710151-00064
29. Austin PC. An introduction to propensity score methods for reducing the effects of confounding in observational studies. *Multivariate Behav Res.* (2011) 46:399–424. doi: 10.1080/00273171.2011.568786
30. Barber MD, Visco AG, Weidner AC, Amundsen CL, Bump RC. Bilateral uterosacral ligament vaginal vault suspension with site-specific endopelvic fascia defect repair for treatment of pelvic organ prolapse. *Am J Obstetr Gynecol.* (2000) 183:1402–11. doi: 10.1067/mob.2000.111298
31. Houlihan S, Kim-Fine S, Birch C, Tang S, Brennand EA. Uterosacral vault suspension (USLS) at the time of hysterectomy: laparoscopic versus vaginal approach. *Int Urogynecol J.* (2019) 30:611–21. doi: 10.1007/s00192-018-3801-5
32. Barbier HM, Smith MZ, Eto CU, Welgoss JA, Von Pechmann W, Horbach N, et al. Ureteral compromise in laparoscopic versus vaginal uterosacral ligament suspension: a retrospective cohort. *Female Pelvic Med Reconstr Surg.* (2015) 21:363–8. doi: 10.1097/SPV.0000000000000202
33. Nygaard I, Brubaker L, Zyczynski HM, Cundiff G, Richter H, Gantz M, et al. Long-term outcomes following abdominal sacrocolpopexy for pelvic organ prolapse. *JAMA.* (2013) 309:2016. doi: 10.1001/jama.2013.4919
34. Brubaker L, Nygaard I, Richter HE, Visco A, Weber AM, Cundiff GW, et al. Two-year outcomes after sacrocolpopexy with and without burch to prevent stress urinary incontinence. *Obstetr Gynecol.* (2008) 112:49–55. doi: 10.1097/AOG.0b013e3181778d2a
35. Costantini E, Brubaker L, Cervigni M, Matthews CA, O'Reilly BA, Rizk D, et al. Sacrocolpopexy for pelvic organ prolapse: evidence-based review and recommendations. *Eur J Obstetr Gynecol Reprod Biol.* (2016) 205:60–5. doi: 10.1016/j.ejogrb.2016.07.503
36. Alas AN, Chinthakanan O, Espaillat L, Plowright L, Davila GW, Aguilar VC. *De novo* stress urinary incontinence after pelvic organ prolapse surgery in women without occult incontinence. *Int Urogynecol J.* (2017) 28:583–90. doi: 10.1007/s00192-016-3149-7
37. Haj Yahya R, Chill HH, Herzberg S, Asfour A, Lesser S, Shveiky D. Anatomical outcome and patient satisfaction after laparoscopic uterosacral ligament hysteropexy for anterior and apical prolapse. *Female Pelvic Med Reconstr Surg.* (2018) 24:352–5. doi: 10.1097/SPV.0000000000000446
38. Haj-Yahya R, Chill HH, Levin G, Reuveni-Salzman A, Shveiky D. Laparoscopic uterosacral ligament hysteropexy vs total vaginal hysterectomy with uterosacral ligament suspension for anterior and apical prolapse: surgical outcome and patient satisfaction. *J Minim Invasive Gynecol.* (2020) 27:88–93. doi: 10.1016/j.jmig.2019.02.012
39. Maher C, Feiner B, Baessler K, Christmann-Schmid C, Haya N, Brown J. Surgery for women with anterior compartment prolapse. *Cochrane Database Syst Rev.* (2016) 11:CD004014. doi: 10.1002/14651858.CD004014.pub6

24

Indocyanine Green Fluorescence Angiography During Laparoscopic Bariatric Surgery

Andrea Balla, Diletta Corallino, Silvia Quaresima, Livia Palmieri, Francesca Meoli, Ingrid Cordova Herencia and Alessandro M. Paganini*

Department of General Surgery and Surgical Specialties "Paride Stefanini", Sapienza University of Rome, Rome, Italy

**Correspondence:*
Diletta Corallino
diletta.corallino1989@gmail.com

Aims: Indocyanine green (ICG) fluorescence angiography (FA) is used for several purposes in general surgery, but its use in bariatric surgery is still debated. The objective of the present pilot study is to evaluate the intraoperative utility of ICG-FA during bariatric surgery in order to focus future research on a reliable tool to reduce the postoperative leak rate.

Methods: Thirteen patients (4 men, 30.8%, 9 women, 69.2%) with median age of 52 years (confidence interval, CI, 95% 46.2–58.7 years) and preoperative median body mass index of 42.6 kg/m^2 (CI, 95% 36 to 49.3 kg/m^2) underwent bariatric surgery with ICG-FA in our center. Three mL of ICG diluted with 10 cc sterile water were intravenously injected after gastric tube creation during laparoscopic sleeve gastrectomy (LSG) and after the gastric pouch and gastro-jejunal anastomosis creation during laparoscopic gastric by-pass (LGB). For the ICG-FA, Karl Storz Image 1S D-Light system (Karl Storz Endoscope GmbH & C. K., Tuttlingen, Germany) placed at a fixed distance of 5 cm from the structures of interest and zoomed vision modality were used to identify the vascular supply. The perfusion pattern was assessed by the surgical team according to a score. The score ranged from 1 (poor vascularization) to 5 (excellent vascularization) based on the intensity and timing of fluorescence of the vascularized structures.

Results: Fom January 2021 to February 2022, six patients underwent LSG (46.2%), three patients underwent LGB (23.1%), and four patients underwent re-do LGB after LSG (30.8%). No adverse effects to ICG were observed. In 11 patients (84.6%) ICG-FA score was 5. During two laparoscopic re-do LGB, the vascular supply was not satisfactory (score 2/5) and the surgical strategy was changed based on ICG-FA (15.4%). At a median follow-up of five months postoperatively, leaks did not occur in any case.

Conclusions: ICG-FA during bariatric surgery is a safe, feasible and promising procedure. It could help to reduce the ischemic leak rate, even if standardization of the procedure and objective fluorescence quantification are still missing. Further prospective studies with a larger sample of patients are required to draw definitive conclusions.

Keywords: indocyanine green (ICG), fluorescence angiography (FA), laparoscopic sleeve gastrectomy (LSG), laparoscopic gastric by-pass (LGB), bariatric surgery, leakage

INTRODUCTION

Bariatric surgery has strong evidence of efficacy and safety in the management of obesity and related comorbidities (1, 2). Laparoscopic sleeve gastrectomy (LSG) and laparoscopic gastric bypass (LGB) are among the most commonly performed bariatric procedures worldwide (1–4). Re-do laparoscopic gastric bypass (RLGB) proved to be an effective conversional procedure after LSG, in terms of total body weight loss, body mass index (BMI) loss and high remission rates of comorbidities (5).

Staple line dehiscence and leak after LSG and of the gastric pouch or gastro-jejunal anastomosis after LGB are the most severe and feared complications after bariatric surgery (6, 7), with an incidence rate ranging from 0 to 7% and from 0.1 to 8.3% for LSG and LGB, respectively (8, 9). The leak etiology is multifactorial with a sharing of mechanical and ischemic causes which has not been fully clarified yet (10, 11). In the literature, the mortality rate related to unrecognized leaks reaches 17% (7, 12). Leaks are associated with increased length of hospital stay and greater readmission rate leading to increased costs (13). The cumulative cost for complicated postoperative leak after bariatric surgery can exceed US $ 200,000 (7, 14, 15).

Several techniques have been described to prevent and to decrease the ischemic and mechanical leak incidence, including manual oversewing of the staple line or the use of sealants, or the use of staple line buttressing material (Seamguard, Gore & Associates, Inc., Newark, Delaware, USA) (16, 17). However, the effectiveness of these techniques for leak prevention is still debated (9, 17–20). Moreover, various intraoperative leak detection modalities have also been described, such as the methylene blue test and intraoperative gastroscopy with air insufflation and hydropneumatic test, but the results are not univocal (21).

Some authors have recently used the intravenous administration of indocyanine green (ICG) to evaluate the real-time tissue perfusion during LSG, without achieving definitive results (22–24). ICG is a water-soluble anionic dye with hepatic excretion through the first pass effect (25, 26). It is safe since adverse events are reported in less than 1 in 40.000 patients and mostly including hypersensitivity reactions (25, 26). It is used in surgery for various purposes: evaluation of the anastomotic blood supply, visualization of the biliary tract during cholecystectomy, identification of the sentinel lymph node in breast cancer, melanoma and gastric carcinoma (27–32), but its use in bariatric surgery is still debated (22–24).

The objective of the present pilot study is to evaluate the intraoperative utility of ICG-FA during bariatric surgery in order to focus future research on a reliable tool to reduce the postoperative leak rate.

MATERIALS AND METHODS

This is a prospective observational pilot study. Institutional review board approval (RP120172B794FE16) and informed consent from all participants were obtained.

Fom January 2021 to February 2022, thirteen consecutive patients underwent bariatric surgery with ICG-FA in our center (Department of General Surgery and Surgical Specialties "Paride Stefanini", Sapienza University of Rome, Rome, Italy).

Preoperative Workup

All patients were candidate for bariatric surgery according to the Italian Society for Obesity and Metabolic Surgery (SICOB) guidelines as well as the European Association for Endoscopic Surgery (EAES) guidelines, as previously reported (33, 34).

Preoperative endoscopy with biopsies for Helicobacter Pylori (HP) detection was performed routinely (34–36). In case of HP infection, antibiotic therapy followed by preoperative urea breath test to prove its eradication, were performed (37).

The presence of signs of gastroesophageal reflux disease (GERD) was evaluated by endoscopy and patients' symptoms were investigated by the Modified Italian Gastroesophageal reflux disease - Health-Related Quality of Life (MI-GERD-HRQL) questionnaire in all patients (38). When present at endoscopy, esophagitis was classified according to the Los Angeles Classification (39). Hiatal hernia (HH) was considered by calculating the distance between the lower edge of the palisade vessels and the diaphragmatic hiatus (40), but the definitive diagnosis was ascertained by intraoperative direct visualization of the esophageal hiatus.

Routine preoperative manometry, pH-metry and Rx-esophagogram were performed in accordance with Severe Acute Respiratory Syndrome CoronaVirus 2 (SARS-CoV-2) restrictions and patient compliance (41, 42). A De Meester score greater than 14.7 at pH-metry was considered abnormal.

Based on this preoperative workup, after multidisciplinary evaluation and after obtaining the patients' informed consent, patients without GERD underwent LSG and patients with GERD underwent LGB. Patients with GERD after LSG, with or without weight regain, underwent RLGB.

In any case, if a diagnosis of HH was made intraoperatively, this was repaired with hiatoplasty according to guidelines (43), with mesh reinforcement as previously reported (36, 41).

Surgical Techniques

Surgery was performed by the same surgeon (A.M.P.) and surgical team.

LSG was performed with a standardized technique as previously reported (34–36). Double loop technique was employed to perform both LGB and RLGB (44, 45). The bougie size was 36 F in all patients.

After gastric tube creation during LSG and after gastric pouch creation and gastro-jejunal anastomosis during LGB and RLGB, three mL of ICG (Pulsion Medical Systems SE, Feldkirchen, Germany) diluted with 10 cc of sterile water were injected intravenously. For the ICG-FA, Karl Storz Image 1S D-Light system (Karl Storz Endoscope GmbH & C. K., Tuttlingen, Germany) placed at a fixed distance of five centimeters from the structures of interest was used to identify the vascular supply.

During LSG, the rationale to ICG administration after gastric tube creation is related to the fact that to obtain sufficient weight loss, the stomach must be divided on the guide of the bougie. So ICG-FA is useful to decide the site of a manual stitch on the section line, if ischemic.

The perfusion pattern was evaluated by the surgical team in real time, immediately after ICG injection and was assessed according to a score ranging from 1 (poor vascularization) to 5 (excellent vascularization) based on the intensity and rapidity of fluorescence appearance in the observed structures (**Figure 1**).

A score of 1–2 was considered inadequate and led to a change in surgical strategy, while a score of 3–5 was considered satisfactory, and the surgical strategy did not change. A methylene blue test is routinely performed after ICG-FA during LGB and RLGB. A routine Rx-esophagogram is performed on the third postoperative day after LGB and RLGB.

Study Design

Preoperative variables (gender, age, BMI, associated comorbidities, smoking habit, American Society of Anesthesiologists - ASA - class, data obtained from endoscopy, Rx-esophagogram, MI-GERD-HRQL questionnaire, manometry, pH-metry and HP eradication), intraoperative variables (type of surgery, associated procedures, IGF-FA score, methylene blue test outcome, conversion to open surgery and operative time) and postoperative variables (complications according to Clavien-Dindo classification (46), postoperative hospital stay, mortality, follow-up data), were recorded using the Microsoft Excel program (Microsoft Corporation, Redmond, Washington, USA).

Continuous variables are expressed as median and 95% confidence interval (CI) while categorical variables are expressed as frequencies and percentages.

RESULTS

Tables 1 and **2** show patients' characteristics and surgical details, respectively.

Six (46.2%), three (23.1%) and four (30.8%) patients underwent LSG, LGB and RLGB, respectively. Ten patients underwent associated procedures (76.9%): hiatoplasty in 5 cases (38.5%), cholecystectomy in 3 (23.1%), lysis of adhesions from previous abdominal surgery in 1 (7.7%) and liver biopsy for severe hepatic steatosis in 1 (7.7%). All patients underwent preoperative multidisciplinary surgical-hepatological-radiological evaluation.

ICG-FA was performed in all patients with no adverse events, and without significant increase in operative time. In 11 patients ICG-FA score was 5/5 (84.6%). During two RLGB procedures, ICG-FA score was 2/5, and the surgical strategy was changed (15.4%).

In a 48-year-old woman with symptomatic GERD after LSG and weight regain (preoperative BMI 42.6 kg/m^2), the ICG-FA demonstrated poor blood supply of a small area of the gastro-jejunal anastomosis (score 2/5), so reinforcement stitches were placed along the staple line.

In a 64-year-old woman with mild GERD and weight regain (preoperative BMI 43.5 kg/m^2) after LSG the ICG-FA showed inadequate perfusion at the periphery of the gastric pouch (score 2/5). The gastric pouch was thus reshaped with the stapler, and the subsequent ICG-FA confirmed good perfusion of the residual gastric pouch (score 5/5).

Methylene blue test was negative in all cases. No conversion to open surgery occurred.

Postoperative complications were observed in three cases (23.1%): two patients with fever, and one with wound infection, all treated by antibiotic therapy (Clavien-Dindo grade II).

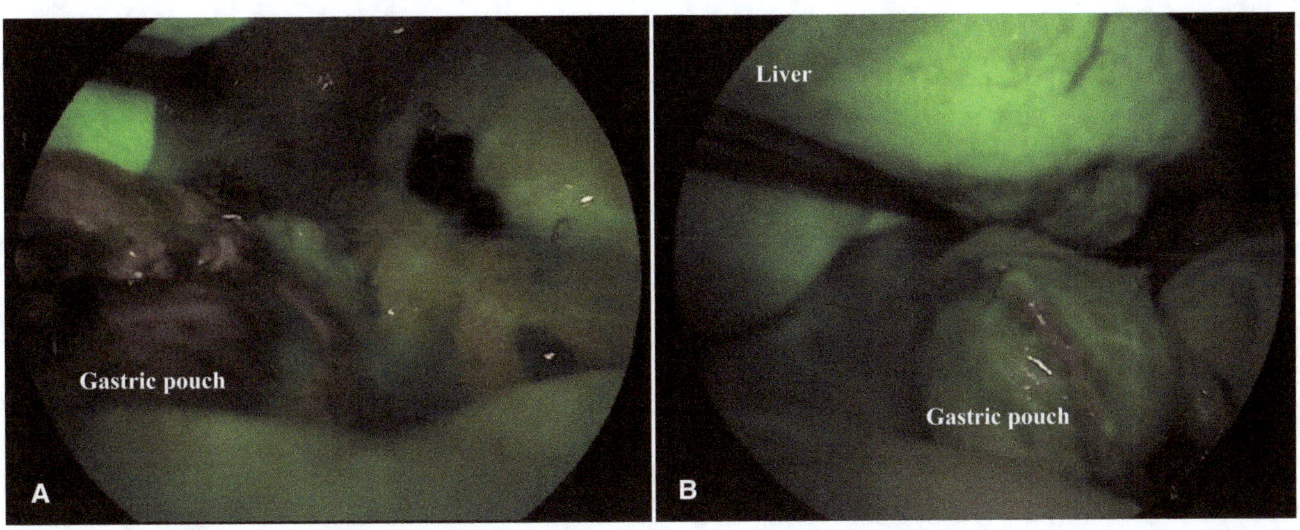

FIGURE 1 | Intraoperative satisfactory ICG-FA score. ICG-FA: Indocyanine green-fluorescence angiography. **(A)** not perfused gastric pouch. **(B)** perfused gastric pouch.

TABLE 1 | Patients' characteristics.

	Entire series, $N = 13$	LSG, $n = 6$(46.2%)	LGB, $n = 3$(23.1%)	RLGB, $n = 4$(30.8%)
Sex ratio (men : women)	4:9	3:3	0:3	1:3
Median age, years (CI 95%)	52(46.2–58.7)	51.5(37.3–57)	57(28.9–89.1)	55(42.5–68.5)
Median preoperative BMI, kg/m^2 (CI 95%)	42.6(36–49.3)	52.6(39.3–59.9)	38.5(20–57.9)	35.6(19.8–50)
Comorbidities, *n*(%)				
T2DM	3(23.1)	2(33.3)	1(33.3)	–
Hypertension	7(53.9)	5(83.3)	2(66.7)	–
Sleep apnea syndrome[a]	8(61.5)	5(83.3)	2(66.7)	1(25)
Symptomatic GERD	7(53.9)	1(16.7)	3(100)	3(75)
Smoking habit	1(7.7)	–	–	1(25)
ASA class, *n*(%)				
II	5(38.5)	3(50)	–	2(50)
III	8(61.5)	3(50)	3(100)	2(50)
Endoscopic findings, *n*(%)				
Incontinent cardias	5(38.5)	1(16.7)	2(66.7)	2(50)
Hiatal hernia	7(53.9)	3(50)	3(100)	1(25)
Esophagitis	4(30.8)	2(33.3)	1(33.3)	1(25)
Gastritis	7(53.9)	4(66.7)	–	3(75)
Eradicated Helicobacter pylori, *n*(%)	1(7.7)	1(16.7)	–	–

LSG, laparoscopic sleeve gastrectomy; LGB, laparoscopic gastric by-pass; RLGB, re-do laparoscopic gastric bypass; CI, confidence interval; BMI, body mass index; T2DM, Type 2 diabetes mellitus; GERD, Gastroesophageal reflux disease; ASA, American Society of Anesthesiologists.
[a]*Needing Continuous Positive Airway Pressure.*

TABLE 2 | Surgical details.

	Entire series, $N = 13$	LSG, $n = 6$(46.2%)	LGB, $n = 3$(23.1%)	RLGB, $n = 4$(30.8%)
Associated procedures, n(%)	10(76.9)			
Hiatoplasty	5(38.5)	2(33.3)	2(66.7)	1(25)
Cholecystectomy	3(23.1)	2(33.3)	1(33.3)	–
Lysis of adhesions	1(7.7)	1(16.7)	–	–
Liver biopsy	1(7.7)	–	1(33.3)	–
ICG-FA score, n(%)	13(100)	6(100)	3(100)	4(100)
Satisfactory	11(84.6)	6(100)	3(100)	2(50)
Not satisfactory	2(15.4)	–	–	2(50)
Methylene blue test, n(%)	7(53.9)	–	3(100)	4(100)
Negative	7(53.9)	–	3(100)	4(100)
Positive	–	–	–	–
Conversion, n(%)	–	–	–	–
Median operative time, minutes (CI 95%)	285(193.6–294.1)	167.5(124.3–204.1)	320(226.3–427)	300(278.4–324.1)
Postoperative complications,				
n(%, Clavien-Dindo classification, grade)	3(23.1)	1(16.7)	1(33.3)	1(25)
Fever	2(15.4, II)	–	1(33.3)	1(25)
Wound infection	1(7.7, II)	1(16.7)	–	–
Median postoperative hospital stay, days (CI 95%)	4(3.3–5.5)	4(2.6–4.6)	5(−0.6–12.6)	4(1.9–6.6)
Mortality, *n*(%)	–	–	–	–
Median follow-up, months (CI 95%)	5(3.9–8.2)	5(2.3–8.4)	10(0.04–18)	5(−1.6–11.6)

LSG, laparoscopic sleeve gastrectomy; LGB, laparoscopic gastric bypass; RLGB, laparoscopic re- gastric bypass; ICG-FA, Indocyanine green-fluorescence angiography; CI, confidence interval.

No leaks were observed at postoperative Rx -esophagogram. Median hospital stay was four days (CI, 95% 3.3–5.5 days) and mortality was nil. At a median follow-up of five months (CI, 95% 3.9–8.2 months) leaks did not occur.

DISCUSSION

The aim of this pilot study was to investigate if the intraoperative use of ICG-FA during bariatric surgery is a useful tool to reduce the postoperative ischemic leak rate. For this purpose, we prospectively analyzed the preliminary results of thirteen patients undergoing LSG or LGB with ICG-FA in our center. Even if leaks were not observed in any case, the use of ICG-FA changed the surgical strategy intraoperatively in two out of thirteen patients (15.4%), who underwent re-do surgery.

Leak of the staple line and of the gastric pouch or the gastro-jejunal anastomosis after LSG or LGB, respectively, are the most severe complications and the second most common cause of death after bariatric surgery (6, 7, 47). Knowing the exact pathogenesis would reduce the risk of a leak occurring after bariatric surgery. The leak etiology is multifactorial, and the causes fall into two main categories: mechanical/tissue causes and ischemic ones (10, 11, 48).

According to the mechanical theory, the intraluminal pressure due to pyloric conservation after LSG exceeds the strength of the staple-line, resulting in a leak (10). Mechanical leaks, which usually appear early after surgery (acute leaks), are usually related to the intrinsic characteristic of the long staple line (10, 49). The "weapons" described in the literature to prevent the onset of mechanical leaks have recently been re-evaluated (33). Routine staple line reinforcement (buttress, glues, suturing, clips) in LSG seems to reduce the risk of perioperative complications such as bleeding and overall mortality, but there does not appear to be a direct correlation between reinforcement and leak rate reduction (33, 50–52). Some authors describe the use of a bougie size ≥40 Fr as a leak-prevention technique (49, 53), but this has not been confirmed by the latest European Association for Endoscopic Surgery (EAES) guidelines which provide a conditional recommendation for the use of bougie sized ≤36 Fr (33, 54). Regarding the distance of the gastric transection from the pylorus, although some authors define 5–6 cm as a safety distance, this data are not confirmed by the most recent literature (49, 55–57).

On the other hand, according to the ischemic theory, leaks are due to localized ischemia which occurs most frequently in the "critical area" at the level of the angle of His after gastroepiploic and short gastric vessels ligation (10). Ischemic leaks, occurring after postoperative day 7 (early leaks), can be partially prevented by maintaining a safety distance of 1–2 cm from the gastroesophageal junction during LSG and they are also a major challenge during revisional bariatric surgery, in which tissues are more frequently hypo-perfused (10, 58, 59). In this situation, the use of ICG-FA could be useful to prevent leak.

Several modalities of intraoperative leak diagnosis (air leak test, intraoperative endoscopy, dye leak test) have been described, with discordant results (21, 53, 60). First of all, the intraoperative leak test might be useful to identify staple line disruption, but it does not allow to identify an ischemic area at risk for subsequent leak (24, 60). Furthermore, the stress of the intraoperative leak test on the newly formed staple line may itself be the cause of staple line weakness and leak (24, 53).

Some authors have recently used the intraluminal or intravenous administration of ICG to evaluate real-time tissue perfusion and to assess the integrity of the staple line during bariatric surgery, without, however, achieving definitive results yet (22–24, 27, 61).

In the literature, the use of ICG-FA during bariatric surgery is reported only in three articles (22–24), and by the results of Spota et al. which report data obtained from 129 bariatric procedures with ICG-FA retrieved from the European-Fluorescence Imaging-Guided Surgery (EURO-FIGS) registry (27). They reported that the choice of the anastomotic level was ICG-FA unrelated in almost all cases and that the ICG-FA was primarily used to assess blood perfusion of the anastomoses, with a partial or high surgeons' sense of confidence (27).

Frattini et al. used ICG-FA in 15 patients undergoing LSG (23). They reported that ICG-FA was feasible and comparable with other intraoperative or postoperative tests (including methylene blue test and Rx-esophagogram) in terms of leak detection rate, and it also allowed for a real-time assessment of gastric perfusion (23). In our opinion the latter feature gives added value to ICG-FA. In fact, although the methylene blue test was negative, in the present series, in two cases of RLGB, the ICG-FA showed that the vascular supply was lower than 3/5, underlining how the two tests are complementary to each other, highlighting one the mechanical causes of the leak and the other the ischemic ones.

Di Furia et al. performed LSG with ICG-FA in 45 patients with the aim of clarifying the exact pathogenesis of gastric leak supporting the ischemic theory and to evaluate if ICG-FA could adequately estimate the ischemic area along the staple line and to prevent leaks (24). They defined adequate perfusion as "the direct and clear visualization of fluorescence along the gastric tube, compared with the excised specimen, after an estimated time of 150–180 seconds from intravenous injection". Despite intraoperative methylene blue test and postoperative Rx-esophagogram were negative for leak in all patients and the ICG-FA score was evaluated "satisfactory and adequate" in all patients, one patient in their series developed symptomatic leak on the fifth post-operative day (24). Therefore, the leak detection rate of the various tests would seem to be comparable, but not reliable probably because the main causes of gastric leak arise not during the procedure or in the early postoperative course, but, as confirmed by the literature, later (5, 8). This data suggests the poor role of the ICG-FA, as well as other leak tests, during LSG probably because the ischemic theory alone is not able to explain the onset of the leakage, emphasizing once again its multifactorial etiology (8, 10, 11, 24).

In our opinion, although this conclusion can be applied to LSG, we do not believe it is entirely true for revisional bariatric surgery. To the best of our knowledge, this is the first study evaluating the role of ICG-FA during primary or revisional LGB. In this series the only two cases in which the

ICG-FA determined a change in surgical strategy were RLGB, suggesting how the ICG could have a higher detection rate of ischemic areas during revisional surgery.

With the same goal, Ortega et al. performed ICG-FA before the gastric division during LSG to identify the variable blood supply patterns of the gastroesophageal junction and the ICG-FA was repeated at the end of the procedure to ensure that all the pertinent blood vessels were preserved (22). They have identified three patterns of blood supply: a right-side–dominant pattern (20%), arising from the left gastric artery; a right-side–accessory pattern (36%), running in the gastrohepatic ligament and a left-side accessory pattern (34%) arising from tributaries from the left inferior phrenic artery significantly contributing to the right-side blood supply (22). Therefore ICG-FA represents a good strategy to avoid unnecessary injury to these vessels during the procedure thanks to "perfusion-preserving" dissection and checking for adequate perfusion of the sleeve product afterward (22).

Finally, another use of ICG described in the literature is the intraluminal gastric injection (61). Kalmar et al. performed intraoperative leak test using the intraluminal ICG method in 59 patients and the gastroscopy method in 196 patients who underwent bariatric surgery, proving that intraluminal ICG is an alternative for intraoperative detection of leak with comparable specificity to intraoperative endoscopy (61). The advantage of the intraluminal ICG, in comparison to intraoperative endoscopy, is that it does not require an experienced endoscopist, any personnel and material cost to resterilize the equipment and not increasing the operative time (61). It is a similar test with a reported lower false negative rate than the methylene blue test, although there are no comparative studies in the literature (21, 61, 62). This ICG using modality is different from the one employed in our experience, and it is aimed at identifying the mechanical rather than vascular causes of the onset of leaks (61). It may be useful to evaluate the feasibility of concomitant administration of ICG both orally and intravenously.

No adverse effects of ICG administration were observed in the reported series as in the present analysis, which therefore is confirmed to be a safe dye (22, 24, 27).

In the literature a wide heterogeneity regarding the doses and timing of ICG administration is reported (25), as well as the distance of the laparoscope from the target organs during visualization, and finally the mostly subjective evaluation of the vascularity which does not allow to make the interpretation of fluorescence intensity objective. Although we have tried to standardize our technique, through the administration of a standard dose of ICG, at the same time and at a fixed optic distance and with an ICG-FA score evaluated by the same surgical team, there are still several limitations of the present study, such as the small sample size, the lack of a control group and the lack of a quantitative fluorescence evaluation. During the study period, our Institute was converted into a SARS-CoV-2 hospital, partially justifying the paucity of the study cohort. With the end of the state of emergency, we hope to increase the number of bariatric procedures with ICG-FA, aiming to enlarge the patients sample size and to draw more definitive conclusions.

In the present study the use of ICG-FA allowed to identify an ischemic area leading to a change in the surgical strategy in half of the patients undergoing revisional bariatric surgery. Although this result could be influenced by the small sample size, this is not yet described in the literature, so if our preliminary results will be confirmed, the use of ICG-FA could represent a decisive weapon in the prevention of ischemic leak in revisional bariatric surgery.

In conclusion, based on the present study, ICG-FA during bariatric surgery is a safe and feasible procedure. Its use could reduce the ischemic leak rate, especially in patients undergoing revisional bariatric surgery even if standardization of the procedure and objective fluorescence quantification are still missing. Definitive data from this pilot study increasing the number of patients included, and further prospective studies with a larger number of patients are required to draw definitive conclusions.

ETHICS STATEMENT

The studies involving human participants were reviewed and approved by La Sapienza, University of Rome. The patients/ participants provided their written informed consent to participate in this study.

CONTRIBUTION TO THE FIELD STATEMENT

The intraoperative utility of ICG-FA during bariatric surgery as a tool to reduce postoperative leak rate represents a still little known and much debated topic in the literature.

The preliminary results of this pilot study, partly similar to those reported by other authors, underlined a new aspect which is the potential role of the ICG-FA in reducing the ischemic leak rate in patients undergoing revisional bariatric surgery.

AUTHOR CONTRIBUTIONS

AB: Study conception and design, Acquisition of data, Analysis, and interpretation of data, Drafting of manuscript, Critical revision of manuscript. Final approval. DC: Study conception and design, Acquisition of data, Analysis, and interpretation of data, Drafting of manuscript, Critical revision of manuscript. Final approval. LP: Study conception and design, Acquisition of data, Analysis, and interpretation of data, Drafting of manuscript, Critical revision of manuscript. Final approval. FM: Study conception and design, Acquisition of data, Analysis, and interpretation of data, Drafting of manuscript, Critical revision of manuscript. Final approval. ICH: Study conception and design, Acquisition of data, Analysis, and interpretation of data,

Drafting of manuscript, Critical revision of manuscript. Final approval. SQ: Study conception and design, Acquisition of data, Analysis, and interpretation of data, Drafting of manuscript, Critical revision of manuscript. Final approval. AMP: Study conception and design, Acquisition of data, Analysis, and interpretation of data, Drafting of manuscript, Critical revision of manuscript. Final approval. All authors contributed to the article and approved the submitted version.

REFERENCES

1. Arterburn DE, Telem DA, Kushner RF, Courcoulas AP. Benefits and risks of bariatric surgery in adults: a review. *JAMA*. (2020) 324(9):879–87. doi: 10.1001/jama.2020.12567
2. Balla A, Batista Rodríguez G, Corradetti S, Balagué C, Fernández-Ananín S, Targarona EM. Outcomes after bariatric surgery according to large databases: a systematic review. *Langenbecks Arch Surg*. (2017) 402(6):885–99. doi: 10.1007/s00423-017-1613-6
3. Golzarand M, Toolabi K, Farid R. The bariatric surgery and weight losing: a meta-analysis in the long- and very long-term effects of laparoscopic adjustable gastric banding, laparoscopic Roux-en-Y gastric bypass and laparoscopic sleeve gastrectomy on weight loss in adults. *Surg Endosc*. (2017) 31(11):4331–45. doi: 10.1007/s00464-017-5505-1
4. Brethauer SA, Aminian A, Romero-Talamás H, Batayyah E, Mackey J, Kennedy L, et al. Can diabetes be surgically cured? Long-term metabolic effects of bariatric surgery in obese patients with type 2 diabetes mellitus. *Ann Surg*. (2013) 258(4):628–37. doi: 10.1097/SLA.0b013e3182a5034b
5. Rheinwalt KP, Schipper S, Plamper A, Alizai PH, Trebicka J, Brol MJ, et al. Roux-en-Y versus one anastomosis gastric bypass as redo-operations following sleeve gastrectomy: a retrospective study. *World J Surg*. (2022) 46 (4):855–64. doi: 10.1007/s00268-021-06424-6
6. Galloro G, Ruggiero S, Russo T, Telesca DA, Musella M, Milone M, et al. Staple-line leak after sleeve gastrectomy in obese patients: a hot topic in bariatric surgery. *World J Gastrointest Endosc*. (2015) 7:843–6. doi: 10.4253/wjge.v7.i9.843
7. Fullum TM, Aluka KJ, Turner PL. Decreasing anastomotic and staple line leaks after laparoscopic Roux-en-Y gastric bypass. *Surg Endosc*. (2009) 23:1403–8. doi: 10.1007/s00464-009-0370-1
8. Aurora AR, Khaitan L, Saber AA. Sleeve gastrectomy and the risk of leak: a systematic analysis of 4888 patients. *Surg Endosc*. (2012) 26(6):1509–15. doi: 10.1007/s00464-011-2085-3
9. Kim J, Azagury D, Eisenberg D, DeMaria E, Campos GM. American Society for Metabolic and Bariatric Surgery Clinical Issues Committee ASMBS position statement on prevention, detection, and treatment of gastrointestinal leak after gastric bypass and sleeve gastrectomy, including the roles of imaging, surgical exploration, and nonoperative management. *Surg Obes Relat Dis*. (2015) 11(4):739–48. doi: 10.1016/j.soard.2015.05.001
10. Baker RS, Foote J, Kemmeter P, Brady R, Vroegop T, Serveld M. The science of stapling and leaks. *Obes Surg*. (2004) 14(10):1290–8. doi: 10.1381/0960892042583888
11. Yehoshua RT, Eidelman LA, Stein M, Fichman S, Mazor A, Chen J, et al. Laparoscopic sleeve gastrectomy–volume and pressure assessment. *Obes Surg*. (2008) 18(9):1083–8. doi: 10.1007/s11695-008-9576
12. Mohos E, Schmaldienst E, Richter D, Prager M. Examination of the efficacy and safety of intraoperative gastroscopic testing of the gastrojejunal anastomosis in laparoscopic Roux Y gastric bypass surgery. *Obes Surg*. (2011) 21(10):1592–6. doi: 10.1007/s11695-011-0428-8
13. Lee SW, Gregory D, Cool CL. Clinical and economic burden of colorectal and bariatric anastomotic leaks. *Surg Endosc*. (2020) 34(10):4374–81. doi: 10.1007/s00464-019-07210-1
14. Champion JK, Williams MD. Prospective randomized comparison of linear staplers during laparoscopic Roux-en-Y gastric bypass. *Obes Surg*. (2003) 13(6):855–9. doi: 10.1381/096089203322618641
15. Carucci L, Turner MA, Conklin RC, DeMaria EJ, Kellum JM, Surgerman HJ. Roux-en-Y gastric bypass surgery for morbid obesity: evaluation of postoperative extraluminal leaks with upper gastrointestinal series. *Radiology*. (2006) 238(1):119–27. doi: 10.1148/radiol.2381041557
16. Consten EC, Gagner M, Pomp A, Inabnet WB. Decreased bleeding after laparoscopic sleeve gastrectomy with or without duodenal switch for morbid obesity using a stapled buttressed absorbable polymer membrane. *Obes Surg*. (2004) 14(10):1360–6. doi: 10.1381/0960892042583905
17. Miller K, Pump A. Use of bioabsorbable staple reinforcement material in gastric bypass: a prospective randomized clinical trial. *Surg Obes Relat Dis*. (2007) 3:417–22. doi: 10.1016/j.soard.2007.03.244
18. Silecchia G, Boru C, Pecchia A, Rizzello M, Casella G, Leonetti F, et al. Efectiveness of laparoscopic sleeve gastrectomy (frst stage of biliopancreatic diversion with duodenal switch) on co-morbidities in super-obese high-risk patients. *Obes Surg*. (2006) 16(9):1138–44. doi: 10.1381/096089206778392275
19. Shikora SA. The use of staple-line reinforcement during laparoscopic gastric bypass. *Obes Surg*. (2011) 14(10):1313–20. doi: 10.1381/0960892042583770
20. Sapala JA, Wood MH, Schuhknecht MP. Anastomotic leak prophylaxis using a vapor-heated fbrin sealant: report on 738 gastric bypass patients. *Obes Surg*. (2004) 14(1):35–42. doi: 10.1381/096089204772787266
21. Bingham J, Lallemand M, Barron M, Kuckelman J, Carter P, Blair K, et al. Routine intraoperative leak testing for sleeve gastrectomy: is the leak test full of hot air? *Am J Surg*. (2016) 211(5):943–7. doi: 10.1016/j.amjsurg.2016.02.002
22. Ortega CB, Guerron AD, Yoo JS. The Use of Fluorescence Angiography During Laparoscopic Sleeve Gastrectomy. *JSLS*. (2018) 22(2):e2018. doi: 10.4293/JSLS.2018.00005
23. Frattini F, Lavazza M, Mangano A, Amico F, Rausei S, Rovera F, et al. Indocyanine green-enhanced fluorescence in laparoscopic sleeve gastrectomy. *Obes Surg*. (2015) 25(5):949–50. doi: 10.1007/s11695-015-1640-8
24. Di Furia M, Romano L, Salvatorelli A, Brandolin D, Lomanto D, Cianca G, et al. Indocyanine green fluorescent angiography during laparoscopic sleeve gastrectomy: preliminary results. *Obes Surg*. (2019) 29(12):3786–90. doi: 10.1007/s11695-019-04085-y
25. Morales-Conde S, Licardie E, Alarcón I, Balla A. Indocyanine green (ICG) fluorescence guide for the use and indications in general surgery: recommendations based on the descriptive review of the literature and the analysis of experience. *Cir Esp Epub*. (2022). doi: 10.1016/j.ciresp.2021.11.018
26. Van Manen L, Handgraaf HJM, Diana M, Dijkstra J, Ishizawa T, Vahrmeijer AL, et al. A practical guide for the use of indocyanine green and methylene blue in fluorescence-guided abdominal surgery. *J Surg Oncol*. (2018) 118 (2):283–300. doi: 10.1002/jso.25105
27. Spota A, Al-Taher M, Felli E, Morales Conde S, Dal Dosso I, Moretto G, et al. Fluorescence-based bowel anastomosis perfusion evaluation: results from the IHU-IRCAD-EAES EURO-FIGS registry. *Surg Endosc*. (2021) 35 (12):7142–53. doi: 10.1007/s00464-020-08234-8
28. Valsecchi ME, Silbermins D, De Rosa N, Wong SL, Lyman GH. Lymphatic mapping and sentinel lymph node biopsy in patients with melanoma: a meta-analysis. *J Clin Oncol*. (2011 10) 29(11):1479–87. doi: 10.1200/JCO.2010.33.1884
29. He PS, Li F, Li GH, Guo C, Chen TJ. The combination of blue dye and radioisotope versus radioisotope alone during sentinel lymph node biopsy for breast cancer: a systematic review. *BMC Cancer*. (2016) 16:107. doi: 10.1186/s12885-016-2137-0
30. Agnus V, Pesce A, Boni L, Van Den Bos J, Morales-Conde S, Paganini AM, et al. Fluorescence-based cholangiography: preliminary results from the IHU-IRCAD-EAES EURO-FIGS registry. *Surg Endosc*. (2020) 34(9):3888–96. doi: 10.1007/s00464-019-07157-3
31. Hayashi H, Ochiai T, Mori M, Karube T, Suzuki T, Gunji Y, et al. Sentinel lymph node mapping for gastric cancer using a dual procedure with dye- and gamma probe-guided techniques. *J Am Coll Surg*. (2003) 196(1):68–74. doi: 10.1016/s1072-7515(02)01594-6.
32. Vettoretto N, Foglia E, Ferrario L, Gerardi C, Molteni B, Nocco U, et al. Could fluorescence-guided surgery be an efficient and sustainable option? A SICE (Italian Society of Endoscopic Surgery) health technology

assessment summary. *Surg Endosc.* (2020) 34(7):3270–84. doi: 10.1007/s00464-020-07542-3

33. Di Lorenzo N, Antoniou SA, Batterham RL, Busetto L, Godoroja D, Iossa A, et al. Clinical practice guidelines of the European Association for Endoscopic Surgery (EAES) on bariatric surgery: update 2020 endorsed by IFSO-EC, EASO and ESPCOP. *Surg Endosc.* (2020) 34(6):2332–58. doi: 10.1007/s00464-020-07555-y
34. Balla A, Quaresima S, Leonetti F, Paone E, Brunori M, Messina T, et al. Laparoscopic sleeve gastrectomy changes in the last decade: differences in morbidity and weight loss. *J Laparoendosc Adv Surg Tech A.* (2017) 27 (11):1165–71. doi: 10.1089/lap.2017.0059
35. Balla A, Quaresima S, Palmieri L, Seitaj A, Pronio A, Badiali D, et al. Effects of laparoscopic sleeve gastrectomy on quality of life related to gastroesophageal reflux disease. *J Laparoendosc Adv Surg Tech A.* (2019) 29 (12):1532–8. doi: 10.1089/lap.2019.0540
36. Balla A, Quaresima S, Ursi P, Seitaj A, Palmieri L, Badiali D, et al. Hiatoplasty with crura buttressing versus hiatoplasty alone during laparoscopic sleeve gastrectomy. *Gastroenterol Res Pract.* (2017) 2017:6565403. doi: 10.1155/2017/6565403
37. O'Connor A. The urea breath test for the noninvasive detection of helicobacter pylori. *Methods Mol Biol.* (2021) 2283:15–20. doi: 10.1007/978-1-0716-1302-3_2
38. Balla A, Leone G, Ribichini E, Sacchi MC, Genco A, Pronio A, et al. Gastroesophageal reflux disease - health-related quality of life questionnaire: prospective development and validation in Italian. *Eur J Gastroenterol Hepatol.* (2020) 33(3):339–45. doi: 10.1097/MEG.0000000000001914
39. Lundell LR, Dent J, Bennett JR, Blum AL, Armstrong D, Galmiche JP, et al. Endoscopic assessment of oesophagitis: clinical and functional correlates and further validation of the Los Angeles classification. *Gut.* (1999) 45(2):172–80. doi: 10.1136/gut.45.2.172
40. Hanada Y, Hoshino S, Hoshikawa Y, Takenouchi N, Umezawa M, Kawami N, et al. Endoscopic diagnosis of hiatus hernia under deep inspiration is not consistent with esophageal manometric diagnosis. *J Gastroenterol.* (2018) 53(6):712–7. doi: 10.1007/s00535-017-1403-5
41. Balla A, Palmieri L, Corallino D, Meoli F, Carlotta Sacchi M, Ribichini E, et al. Does sleeve gastrectomy worsen gastroesophageal reflux disease in obese ptients? A prospective study. *Surg Innov.* (2021) 4:15533506211052745. doi: 10.1177/15533506211052745
42. Balla A, Meoli F, Palmieri L, Corallino D, Sacchi MC, Ribichini E, et al. Manometric and pH-monitoring changes after laparoscopic sleeve gastrectomy: a systematic review. *Langenbecks Arch Surg.* (2021) 406 (8):2591–609. doi: 10.1007/s00423-021-02171-3
43. Rosenthal RJ, International Sleeve Gastrectomy Expert Panel, Diaz AA, Arvidsson D, Baker RS, Basso N, et al. International Sleeve Gastrectomy Expert Panel Consensus Statement: best practice guidelines based on experience of >12,000 cases. *Surg Obes Relat Dis.* (2012) 8(1):8–19. doi: 10.1016/j.soard.2011.10.019
44. Palmisano S, Giuricin M, Casagranda B, de Manzini N. Zero frequency of internal hernias after laparoscopic double loop gastric bypass without closure of mesenteric defects. *Surg Today.* (2014) 44(10):1920–4. doi: 10.1007/s00595-014-0916-2
45. AlSabah S, Alsharqawi N, Almulla A, Akrof S, Alenezi K, Buhaimed W, et al. Approach to poor weight loss after laparoscopic sleeve gastrectomy: re-sleeve Vs. gastric bypass. *Obes Surg.* (2016) 26(10):2302–7. doi: 10.1007/s11695-016-2119-y
46. Clavien PA, Barkun J, de Oliveira ML, Vauthey JN, Dindo D, Schulick RD, et al. The Clavien-Dindo classification of surgical complications: five-year experience. *Ann Surg.* (2009) 250(2):187–96. doi: 10.1097/SLA.0b013e3181b13ca2
47. Jurowich C, Thalheimer A, Seyfried F, Fein M, Bender G, Germer CT, et al. Gastric leakage after sleeve gastrectomy-clinical presentation and therapeutic options. *Langenbecks Arch Surg.* (2011) 396(7):981–7. doi: 10.1007/s00423-011-0800-0
48. Chahine E, Kassir R, Dirani M, Joumaa S, Debs T, Chouillard E. Surgical management of gastrogastric fistula after roux-en-Y gastric bypass: 10-year experience. *Obes Surg.* (2018) 28(4):939–44. doi: 10.1007/s11695-017-2949-2
49. Iossa A, Abdelgawad M, Watkins BM, Silecchia G. Leaks after laparoscopic sleeve gastrectomy: overview of pathogenesis and risk factors. *Langenbecks Arch Surg.* (2016) 401(6):757–66. doi: 10.1007/s00423-016-1464-6
50. Shikora SA, Mahoney CB. Clinical beneft of gastric staple line reinforcement (SLR) in gastrointestinal surgery: a metaanalysis. *Obes Surg.* (2015) 25 (7):1133–41. doi: 10.1007/s11695-015-1703-x
51. Wang Z, Dai X, Xie H, Feng J, Li Z, Lu Q. The efficacy of staple line reinforcement during laparoscopic sleeve gastrectomy: a meta-analysis of randomized controlled trials. *Int J Surg.* (2016) 25:145–52. doi: 10.1016/j.ijsu.2015.12.007
52. Gagner M, Hutchinson C, Rosenthal R. Fifth international consensus conference: current status of sleeve gastrectomy. *Surg Obes Relat Dis.* (2016) 12(4):750–6. doi: 10.1016/j.soard.2016.01.022
53. Parikh M, Issa R, McCrillis A, Saunders JK, Ude-Welcome A, Gagner M. Surgical strategies that may decrease leak after laparoscopic sleeve gastrectomy: a systematic review and metaanalysis of 9991 cases. *Ann Surg.* (2013) 257(2):231–7. doi: 10.1097/SLA.0b013e31826cc714
54. Wang Y, Yi XY, Gong L, Li Q, Zhang J, Wang Z. The efectiveness and safety of laparoscopic sleeve gastrectomy with diferent sizes of bougie calibration: a systematic review and meta-analysis. *Int J Surg.* (2018) 49:32–8. doi: 10.1016/j.ijsu.2017.12.005
55. ElGeidie A, ElHemaly M, Hamdy E, El Sorogy M, Abdelgawad M, GadElHak N. The effect of residual gastric antrum size on the outcome of laparoscopic sleeve gastrectomy: a prospective randomized trial. *Surg Obes Relat Dis.* (2015) 11(5):997–1003. doi: 10.1016/j.soard.2014.12.025
56. Obeidat F, Shanti H, Mismar A, Albsoul N, Al-Qudah M. The magnitude of antral resection in laparoscopic sleeve gastrectomy and its relationship to excess weight loss. *Obes Surg.* (2015) 25(10):1928–32. doi: 10.1007/s11695-015-1642-6
57. McGlone ER, Gupta AK, Reddy M, Khan OA. Antral resection versus antral preservation during laparoscopic sleeve gastrectomy for severe obesity: Systematic review and meta-analysis. *Surg Obes Relat Dis.* (2018) 14 (6):857–64. doi: 10.1016/j.soard.2018.02.021
58. Bellanger DE, Greenway FL. Laparoscopic sleeve gastrectomy, 529 cases without a leak: short-term results and technical considerations. *Obes Surg.* (2011) 21(2):146–50. doi: 10.1007/s11695-010-0320-y
59. Velotti N, Vitiello A, Berardi G, Di Lauro K, Musella M. Roux-en-Y gastric bypass versus one anastomosis-mini gastric bypass as a rescue procedure following failed restrictive bariatric surgery. A systematic review of literature with metanalysis. *Updates Surg.* (2021) 73(2):639–47. doi: 10.1007/s13304-020-00938-9
60. Aggarwal S, Bhattacharjee H, Chander Misra M. Practice of routine intraoperative leak test during laparoscopic sleeve gastrectomy should not be discarded. *Surg Obes Relat Dis.* (2011) 7(5):e24–5. doi: 10.1016/j.soard.2011.03.013
61. Kalmar CL, Reed CM, Peery CL, Salzberg AD. Intraluminal indocyanine green for intraoperative staple line leak testing in bariatric surgery. *Surg Endosc.* (2020) 34(9):4194–9. doi: 10.1007/s00464-020-07606-4
62. Kirby GC, Macano CAW, Nyasavajjala SM, Sahloul M, Nijjar R, Daskalakis M, et al. The Birmingham experience of high-pressure methylene blue dye test during primary and revisional bariatric surgery: a retrospective cohort study. *Ann Med Surg (Lond).* (2017) 23:32–4. doi: 10.1016/j.amsu.2017.09.015

25

Short-Term and Long-Term Outcomes in Mid and Low Rectal Cancer with Robotic Surgery

Jingwen Chen[†], *Zhiyuan Zhang*[†], *Wenju Chang*[†], *Tuo Yi*[†], *Qingyang Feng, Dexiang Zhu, Guodong He*[*†] *and Ye Wei*[*†]

Department of General Surgery, Zhongshan Hospital, Fudan University, Shanghai, China

***Correspondence:**
Ye Wei
13818661815@126.con
Guodong He
angelhgd@163.com

[†]*These authors have contributed equally to this work*

Objective: To investigate the risk factors for postoperative complications and anastomotic leakage after robotic surgery for mid and low rectal cancer and their influence on long-term outcomes.

Methods: A total of 641 patients who underwent radical mid and low rectal cancer robotic surgery at Zhongshan Hospital Fudan University from January 2014 to December 2018 were enrolled in this study. The clinicopathological factors of the patients were collected. The risk factors for short-term outcomes of complications and anastomotic leakage were analyzed, and their influences on recurrence and overall survival were studied.

Results: Of the 641 patients, 516 (80.5%) underwent AR or LAR procedures, while 125 (19.5%) underwent the NOSES procedure. Only fifteen (2.3%) patients had stoma diversion. One hundred and seventeen patients (17.6%) experienced surgical complications. Anastomotic leakage occurred in 44 patients (6.9%). Eleven patients (1.7%) underwent reoperation within 90 days after surgery. Preoperative radiotherapy did not significantly increase anastomotic leakage in our study (7.4% vs. 6.8%, $P = 0.869$). The mean postoperative hospital stay was much longer with complication (10.4 vs. 7.1 days, $P<0.05$) and leakage (12.9 vs. 7.4 days, $P < 0.05$). Multivariate analysis showed that male sex ($OR = 1.855$, 95% CI: 1.175–2.923, $P < 0.05$), tumor distance 5 cm from the anus ($OR = 1.563$, 95% CI: 1.016–2.404, $P < 0.05$), and operation time length ($OR = 1.563$, 95% CI: 1.009–2.421, $P < 0.05$) were independent risk factors for complications in mid and low rectal cancer patients. The same results for anastomotic leakage: male sex ($OR = 2.247$, 95% CI: 1.126–4.902, $P < 0.05$), tumor distance 5 cm from the anus ($OR = 2.242$, 95% CI: 1.197–4.202, $P < 0.05$), and operation time length ($OR = 2.114$, 95% CI: 1.127–3.968, $P < 0.05$). The 3-year DFS and OS were 82.4% and 92.6% with complication, 88.4% and 94.0% without complication, 88.6% and 93.1% with leakage, and 87.0% and 93.8% without leakage, respectively. The complication and anastomotic leakage showed no significant influences on long-term outcomes.

Conclusion: Being male, having a lower tumor location, and having a prolonged operation time were independent risk factors for complications and anastomotic leakage in mid and low rectal cancer. Complications and anastomotic leakage might have no long-term impact on oncological outcomes for mid and low rectal cancer with robotic surgery.

Keywords: rectal cancer, robotic surgery, complications, anastomotic leakage, long-term outcomes

INTRODUCTION

Colorectal cancer is the world's fourth most deadly cancer, with almost 900,000 deaths annually (1). Surgical resection remains the mainstay of curative treatment. The optimal oncological operation consists of low anterior resection or abdominoperineal resection with complete total mesorectal excision (TME) based on the tumor location. A robotic approach with superior agility and precise movements of the robotic arms could provide the surgeon with better exposure and greater ergonomic comfort during the dissection of small anatomical structures, such as the pelvic cavity (2). In recent years, with the renewal of rectal cancer surgery and the advancements in equipment and surgical techniques, the anus preservation rate has been increasing. Many patients have avoided permanent stoma damage, and their quality of life has improved. There are growing anus preservation practices and new surgical methods, such as robots and natural orifice specimen extraction surgery (NOSES), in colorectal surgery. However, these new procedures could increase the risks inherent to complications, such as anastomotic leakage and damage to the autonomic nerve function of the pelvic floor, which adversely affect surgical outcomes and delayed hospital stay. Although the negative impact of complications on short-term effects is overtly clear, the impact on cancer recurrence and survival remains uncertain. A previous report indicated greater local recurrence risk and worse overall and cancer-specific survival in patients with anastomotic leakage (3). Other authors have reported alternative findings with no long-term impact on oncological outcomes in patients with complication (4). Our study retrospectively analyzed the clinical data of 641 cases of robotic rectal surgery in the mid- and low rectum in our hospital from January 2014 to December 2018. We explored the risk factors for complications and anastomotic leakage and their influence on long-term oncological outcomes.

MATERIALS AND METHODS

From January 2014 to December 2018, 641 cases of mid and low rectal cancer with robotic surgery were collected retrospectively at Zhongshan Hospital Fudan University. Inclusion criteria: a) 18–80 years old; b) preoperative biopsy confirmed adenocarcinoma; c) tumor within 10 cm from the anus; and d) standard radical surgery, including AR, LAR, and the NOSES procedure, with some undergoing stoma diversion. The exclusion criteria were as follows: a) the previous history of colorectal cancer surgery; b) tumor accompanied by distant metastases or other tumors; c) emergencies and abdominal adhesions, which precluded minimally invasive surgery; and d) combined organ resection.

The Fudan University Ethics Committee approved the study, and all patients provided informed consent. Preoperative data, pathological results, and complication information were obtained from electronic medical records, and postoperative survival information was collected during regular follow-ups.

Surgical Approach

All of the patients underwent surgery using the da Vinci Surgical System. The TME was performed robotically in all of the patients. Anterior resection, low anterior resection, and the NOSES procedure were performed using the double-stapled technique. The NOSES procedure is shown in **Supplement S1**.

Intraoperative frozen pathological diagnosis was carried out using tissue from distal margins. The pelvic peritoneum was routinely closed. The methylene blue perfusion test was used to check anastomotic integrity. If blue dye leakage was found, we sutured the leakage point with 3-0 Vicryl followed by a retest of leakage using methylene blue. In some cases, the leakage persisted; we then performed prophylactic stoma diversion. In other cases, where the anastomosis was too low to suture, or the patients had severe tissue edema, prophylactic stoma diversion was also performed. A double cannula was placed near the anastomosis. When anastomotic leakage occurred, the cannula could be used to wash and drain and, in some cases, to avoid a salvage stoma.

Complications and Anastomotic Leakage

Complications were diagnosed and categorized according to patients' symptoms, with laboratory and radiological evaluations to confirm clinical suspicions. The grading of complications was scored based on the detailed tables of the Surgical Complications Severity Scoring System proposed by Mazeh et al. (5).

Anastomotic leakage after anterior resection of the rectum was defined as a defect of the intestinal wall integrity at the colorectal or colo-anal anastomotic site (including suture and staple lines of anorectal reservoirs) leading to communication between the intra- and extraluminal compartments. A pelvic abscess close to the anastomosis is also considered anastomotic leakage. Severity grading was as follows: Grade A, requiring no active therapeutic intervention; Grade B, requiring active therapeutic intervention but manageable without relaparotomy; and Grade C, requiring relaparotomy (6). Aspiration drainage or transverse colon stoma was performed according to the severity of the infection.

Statistical Analysis

Statistical analysis was conducted using IBM SPSS Statistics software version 19 (SPSS Inc., IBM, Chicago, IL, USA). Categorical variables were analyzed using the $\chi 2$ test, and continuous variables were analyzed using the t-test. One-way analysis of variance was used for the study of quantitative differences between various groups. Logistic regression was used for multivariate analysis. The Kaplan–Meier method was used to calculate disease-free survival and overall survival. P values less than 0.05 were considered statistically significant.

RESULTS

Clinical Data

The selection of patients included in the study is illustrated in **Figure 1**. A total of 1,591 patients were admitted with rectal cancer from 2014 to 2018, and 641 patients underwent robotic treatment in the mid and low rectum enrolled in the analyses.

Among the study patients, 403 cases were males (62.9%), and the average age was 60.9 ± 10.4 years. The median body mass index (BMI) was 23.4. A total of 53 (8.3%) patients were considered to have American Society of Anesthesiologists scores (ASA) of III. Anterior resection (AR) and low anterior resection (LAR) were performed in 516 (80.5%) patients, while 125 (19.5%) patients underwent the NOSES procedure. The mean operation time was 164.5 ± 47.5 min, and the mean estimated blood loss was 66.1 ± 35.9 ml. Intraoperative methylene blue leakage was found in 41 cases (6.4%). Diverting ileostomies were performed in 15 cases (2.3%). A total of 67 (10.5%) patients with T4 or N2 mid and low rectal cancer underwent preoperative radiochemotherapy. The mean duration of hospital stay after surgery was 7.73 ± 3.24 days. The mean number of harvested lymph nodes was 17.2 ± 6.7. The positive rate of circumferential margin (CRM) was 7 (1.1%). According to the American Joint Committee on Cancer (AJCC) TNM stage, stages I, II, and III patients accounted for 180 (28.1%), 191 (29.9%), and 270 (42.1%) patients, respectively. The characteristics of all patients are shown in **Supplement S2**.

Surgical Complications

One hundred seventeen patients (17.6%) experienced surgical complications, with Grades 1–2 and Grades 3–4 complications accounting for 16.5% and 1.8%, respectively (5). There was no perioperative mortality. Anastomotic leakage occurred in

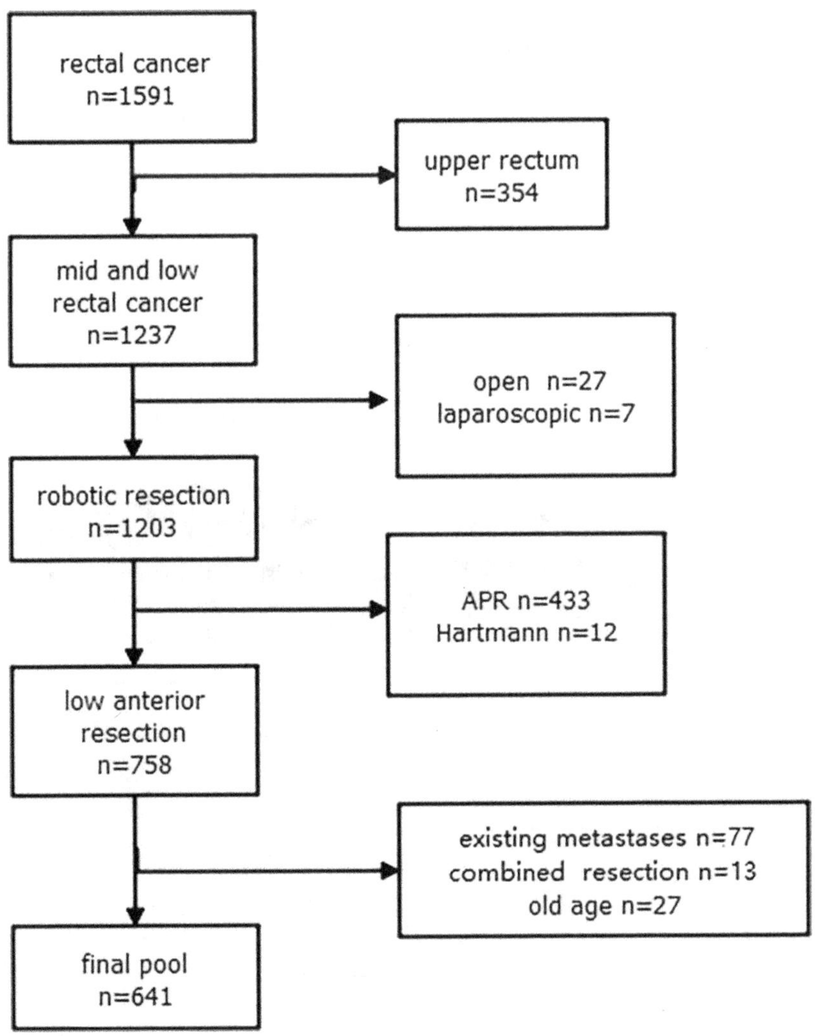

FIGURE 1 | Flow Chart of Enrollment of Mid and Low Robotic Cancer.

44 patients (6.9%), with one case of rectovaginal fistula. Based on severity grading, 16 (36.4%), 21 (47.7%), and 7 (15.9%) had Grade A, B, and C leakages, respectively. Two postoperative anastomotic leakages occurred in patients with a positive methylene blue test intraoperatively (2/41, 4.8%). Eleven cases had reoperation (1.7%), including seven cases of anastomosis leakage (1.1%), two cases of bleeding after surgery, and two cases of ileus. (**Table 1**). The mean postoperative hospital stay with complication was much longer than the hospital stay without complication (10.4 ± 5.6 vs. 7.1 ± 2.0 days, p<0.01). The mean postoperative hospital stay with leakage was much longer than that in the nonleakage group (12.5 ± 7.0 vs. 7.4 ± 2.4 days, P<0.01).

Long-Term Outcomes

The median follow-up duration from primary treatment was 39 months (25th–75th percentile 30-47). Local recurrence occurred in 13 patients (2.0%), while distant metastases occurred in 87 patients (13.6%). The most common metastatic sites were the liver (5.1%) and lung (5.0%). Complications and anastomotic leakage showed no significant influences on local recurrences and distant metastases (**Table 2**). The 3-year disease-free survival rate of all cases was 87.1%, with rates of 82.4% with complication and 88.4% without complication (p=0.198) and 88.6% with leakage and 87.0% without leakage (P=0.635). The 3-year overall survival rate was 93.7%, with rates of 92.6% with complication and 94.0% without complication (p=0.139) and 93.1% with leakage and 93.8% without leakage (P=0.934) (**Figure 2**).

TABLE 1 | Surgical complications.

Characteristics	Value; n(%)
Total complication rate[a]	117(18.3%)
Grades 1–2	106(16.5%)
Grade 3	10(1.6%)
Grade 4	1(0.2%)
Complications	
Infection events[b]	24(3.7%)
Anastomosis leakage	44(6.9%)
Urinary retention	18(2.8%)
Postoperative bleeding	5(0.8%)
Ileus	10(1.6%)
Gastric motility disorders	4(0.6%)
Organ dysfunction	4(0.6%)
Thrombotic events	2(0.3%)
Others	4(0.6%)
Mortality	0
Reoperation rate[c]	11(1.7%)

[a]*Surgical complication rate and mortality analysis within 30 days of operation following the Mazeh system.*
[b]*Infection events included intraabdominal infection or abscess, catheter-derived infection, wound infection or lung infection, excluding anastomotic leakage events.*
[c]*The rates of reoperation related to surgical complications were analyzed within 90 days of operation.*

Risk Factors Associated With Complication

Univariate analysis showed that male sex, ASA score, tumor distance within 5 cm from the anus, prolonged operation time, and prophylactic stoma diversion were associated with overall complications after robotic mid and low rectal cancer surgery (P<0.05). Preoperative radiotherapy and the NOSES procedure showed no significant effect on complications in our study.

Multivariate analyses showed that male sex (OR=1.855, 95% CI: 1.175–2.923, P<0.05), a tumor distance of 5 cm from the anus (OR=1.563, 95% CI: 1.016–2.404, P<0.05), and a prolonged operation time (OR=1.563, 95% CI: 1.009–2.421, P<0.05) were independent risk factors for complications after robotic mid and low rectal procedures (**Table 3**).

Risk Factors Associated With Anastomotic Leakage

Univariate and multivariate analyses showed similar results: being male (OR=2.247, 95% CI: 1.126–4.902, P<0.05), a tumor distance of 5 cm from the anus (OR= 2.242, 95% CI: 1.197–4.202, P<0.05), and operation time length (OR= 2.114, 95% CI: 1.127–3.968, P<0.05) were significantly associated with the occurrence of anastomotic leakage after robotic mid and low rectal cancer surgery. Preoperative radiotherapy, stoma diversion, and the NOSES procedure showed no significant effect on anastomosis leakage in our study (**Table 4**).

DISCUSSION

With the rise of minimally invasive surgery, radical resection of mid and low rectal cancer has increased, with the goal of causing less trauma and pursuing better functional preservation.

TABLE 2 | Recurrence patterns with complication and anastomotic leakage.

Outcomes	Total N=641	Complications			Leakage		
		(+)n=117	(-)n=524	P	(+)n=44	(-)n=597	P
Local recurrence	13(2.0%)	2(1.7%)	11(2.1%)	0.787	1(2.2%)	12(2.0%)	0.905
Metastases[a]	74(11.5%)	18(15.4%)	56(10.7%)	0.150	4(9.0%)	70(11.7%)	0.598
Liver	33(5.1%)						
Lung	32(5.0%)						
Bone	4(0.6%)						
Peritoneal	11(1.7%)						
Brain	2(0.3%)						
Others[b]	6(0.9%)						

[a]*Some patients had multi-site metastases.*
[b]*Others include two cases of abdominal wall, two cases of the spleen, one case of the ovary, and one case of the adrenal gland.*

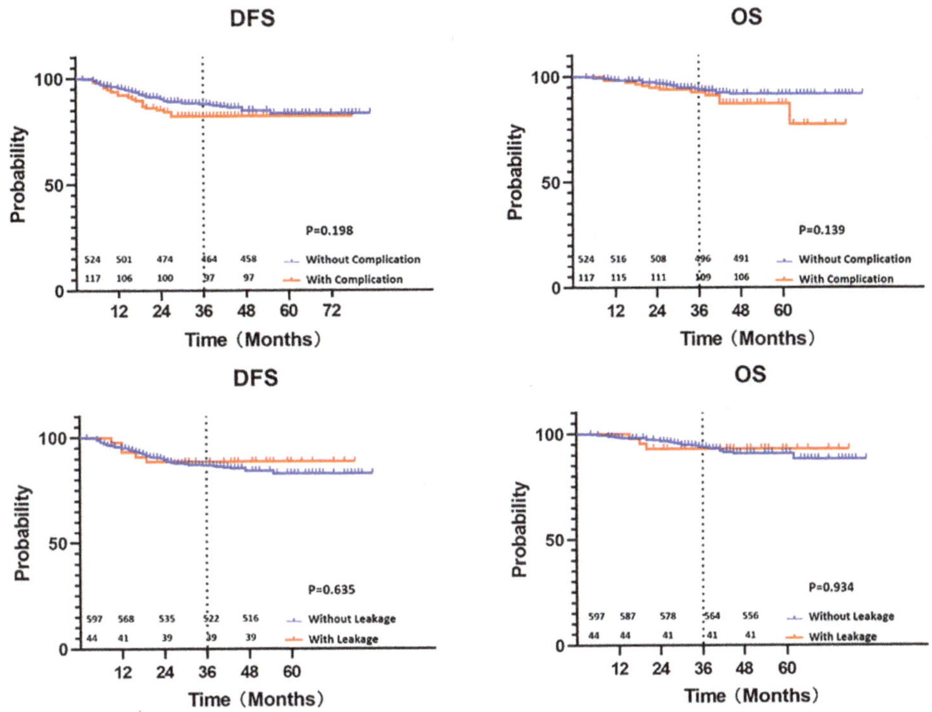

FIGURE 2 | Kaplan-Meier curves of disease-free survival and overall survival with or without complication and leakage (survival numbers were added).

Postoperative complications could prolong hospitalization, increase the medical burden, and decrease quality of life, which are among the challenging problems faced by mid and low rectal cancer surgery (7). Due to the narrow area of the pelvis and the limited operation space, traditional laparoscopic rectal cancer operations have disadvantages, such as operative difficulty, increased requirements for assistants, and a steep learning curve (8). Some studies have reported no difference in the incidence of complications between robotic surgery and traditional laparoscopic surgery (9). Since 2010, the robotic surgery system has been gradually applied to radical surgery for mid and low rectal cancer due to its capability of producing high-definition images and its stable and flexible operation (10). These features are advantageous in distinguishing pelvic nerves, dissecting the anterior and lateral tissues, and suturing.

Anastomotic leakage is one of the most critical complications postoperatively. Many factors may affect anastomotic leakage after rectal cancer surgery. Studies have shown that being male, smoking, diabetes, hypoalbuminemia, and obesity are potentially high-risk factors for anastomotic leakage (11–13). Frouws' analysis (14) showed that men are at high risk for anastomotic Grade C leakage in patients with low rectal cancer. In this study, being male was an independent risk factor for complications and leakage. Five men and two women underwent reoperations for anastomotic leakage in the cohort. One of the women suffered from a rectovaginal fistula. This could be explained by the fact that the male pelvic outlet is narrow and difficult to operate, resulting in an unsatisfactory anastomosis. The ASA score is a subjective assessment of patients' overall health. A high ASA score might lead to high risks of complications after surgery. In our study, a high score was associated with more complications but was not an independent factor. Conversely, preoperative smoking cessation, respiratory management, strict blood sugar control, and nutritional support are protective factors for reducing postoperative complications.

In our study, we observed that a short distance between the tumor and the anal margin was associated with a higher incidence of complications and anastomotic leakage. Multivariate analysis confirmed that the distance from the anal margin is an independent risk factor for complications and anastomotic leakage. The reasons could be the difficulty of dissections and anastomosis, the inability to suture in a limited space, and insufficient blood supply. Fukada's research (11) showed that tumors less than 6 cm from the anal margin were correlated with increased anastomotic leakage after rectal cancer.

Yasui et al. (15) reported that a tumor diameter larger than 4 cm was a risk factor for anastomotic leakage after rectal cancer surgery. However, there was no apparent correlation between tumor size and complications or anastomotic leakage in our study. As laparoscopic and robotic surgery for rectal cancer is associated with attenuated blood loss, this technique appears beneficial compared with an open approach (16). Leichtle (17) reported that blood loss greater than 100 ml is associated with an increased risk of complications. In our study, blood loss was not associated with higher complication or leakage rates.

Neoadjuvant chemoradiotherapy is beneficial to tumor regression and preoperative downstaging of advanced mid and low rectal cancer. With this treatment, some patients would have

TABLE 3 | Risk factors associated with complication.

Clinical factors	N	with complication (%)	Univariate analysis		Multivariate analysis	
			***OR* value (95% *CI*)**	**P-value**	**OR value (95% CI)**	**P-value**
Gender			1.812 (1.159–2.833)	0.009*	1.855 (1.175–2.923)	0.008*
Feale	238	31(13.0%)				
Male	403	86(21.3%)				
Age			0.973 (0.646–1.464)	0.894		
≥65	254	47(18.5%)				
<65	387	70(18.1%)				
BMI(kg/m^2)			1.033 (0.671–1.591)	0.881		
≥25	199	37(18.6%)				
<25	442	80(18.1%)				
ASA score			1.444 (1.057–1.973)	0.021*		
I–II	588	101 (17.2%)				
III	53	16 (18.9%)				
Diabetes			1.307 (0.742–2.302)	0.354		
yes	82	18(22.0%)				
no	559	99(17.7%)				
Hb(g/L)			1.182 (0.644–2.168)	0.590		
<110	73	15(20.5%)				
≥110	528	102(19.3%)				
ALB(g/L)			1.220 (0.791–1.884)	0.369		
<40	181	37(20.4%)				
≥40	460	80(17.4%)				
CEA (ng/ml)			1.162 (0.767–1.760)	0.479		
<5	418	73(17.5%)				
≥5	223	44(19.7%)				
Tumor location from anus(cm)			1.562 (1.025–2.387)	0.038*	1.563 (1.016–2.404)	0.042*
>5	456	74(16.2%)				
≤5	185	43(23.2%)				
Tumor size(cm)			1.242 (0.830–1.858)	0.293		
>5	268	54(20.1%)				
≤5	373	63(16.9%)				
preoperative radiotherapy			0.975 (0.504–1.884)	0.939		
yes	67	12(17.9%)				
no	574	105(18.3%)				
Operation			1.152 (0.704–1.886)	0.573		
NOSES	125	25(20.0%)				
AR or LAR	516	92(17.8%)				
Diverting stoma			3.093 (1.079–8.867)	0.036*		
yes	15	6(40.0%)				
no	626	111(17.7%)				
Estimated blood loss(ml)			1.140 (0.702–1.853)	0.597		
≥100	131	26(19.8%)				
<100	510	91(17.8%)				
Operation time(min)			1.616 (1.065–2.451)	0.024*	1.563 (1.009–2.421)	0.046*
<180	445	71(16.0%)				
≥180	196	46(23.5%)				
Pathological type			1.265 (0.731–2.189)	0.400		
adenocarcinoma	525	99(18.9%)				
Mucinous adenocarcinoma	116	18(15.5%)				
Differentiation			1.105 (0.904–1.351)	0.329		
I–II	322	54(16.8%)				
III–IV	319	63(19.7%)				
Vascular invasion			1.089 (0.687–1.727)	0.716		
yes	156	30(19.2%)				
no	485	87(17.9%)				
Perineural invasion			1.084 (0.699–1.682)	0.718		
yes	183	35(19.1%)				
no	458	82(17.9%)				

(Continued)

TABLE 3 | Continued

Clinical factors	N	with complication (%)	Univariate analysis		Multivariate analysis	
			OR value (95% *CI*)	P-value	OR value (95% CI)	P-value
N stage			0.727 (0.480–1.101)	0.132		
yes	270	42(15.6%)				
no	371	75(20.2%)				
T stage			0.906 (0.737–1.114)	0.350		
$T_{1\text{-}2}$	228	46(20.2%)				
$T_{3\text{-}4}$	413	71(17.2%)				

BMI, body mass index; ALB, albumin; ASA, American Society of Anesthesiologists; AR, anterior resection; LAR, low anterior resection; NOSES, natural orifice specimen extraction surgery.
**P < 0.05.*

the opportunity to save the anus and reduce the local recurrence rate of tumors after surgery. Schiffman et al. (18) reported that the incidence of postoperative anastomotic leakage was 26.6% in patients who received preoperative chemoradiation, while the incidence of patients who did not receive chemoradiation was only 9.7%. Neoadjuvant chemoradiotherapy may cause tissue edema, which increases the difficulty of surgery, accompanied by vascular endothelial degeneration. Moreover, it increases the probability of microthrombosis and affects the blood supply of tissues around the anastomosis, leading to increased leakage. Borstlap et al. (19) analyzed the data of 2095 patients and found that neoadjuvant chemoradiotherapy was an independent risk factor for anastomotic leakage. In Borstlap's study, anastomotic leakage was diagnosed in 13.4% of the patients within 30 days, with almost routine use of neoadjuvant radiotherapy (88.8%) in the patients. Frouws et al. (14) indicated that patients with neoadjuvant therapy were at risk for increased postoperative Grade B anastomotic leakage. However, the controversy remains. Randomized controlled studies from Sebag-Montefiore (20) suggested that neoadjuvant chemoradiation did not increase the incidence of anastomotic leakage. Salmenkylä et al. (21) also showed that the anastomotic leakage rate did not significantly differ between the surgery and radiochemotherapy groups (20.6% vs. 27.4%). In this study, neoadjuvant chemoradiation did not show a significant increase in the risk of complications and leakage. The incidence of anastomotic leakage after preoperative radiochemotherapy was 7.4%, compared with 6.8% in the surgery group.

In recent years, natural orifice specimen extraction surgery (NOSES) has been gradually applied in the treatment of colorectal cancer (22). The abdominal incision to extract the specimen is avoided, and the ultimate cosmetic effect is achieved with radical treatment. The NOSES procedure should reduce postoperative pain, surgical wound infection, and incisional hernia (23). Ding's study (24) showed that the NOSES rectal cancer procedure did not increase short-term complications and may reduce intraoperative bleeding and patient pain. Liu et al. (25) reported that the NOSES rectal cancer procedure did not increase the occurrence of short-term complications such as anastomotic leakage. In our study, 127 cases of robotic NOSES in the mid and low rectum did not increase the incidence of postoperative complications. The incidence rates of complications and anastomotic leakage were 20.0% and 7.2% in the NOSES procedure, respectively, which seemed higher than those in the LAR group but showed no significant difference.

It should be noted that this study reflects single-center data, and both the surgeon and assistant have rich experience in robotic rectal cancer surgery. A prolonged operation time might indicate that the operation is more complicated. Antonio's study (26) showed that a longer operating time was significantly associated with leakage among the operative factors. In our study, prolonged operation time was also significantly correlated with increasing incidence rates of complications and anastomotic leakage. We thus suggest that when facing difficulty in dissection or hemostasis, timely transfer of the patient to open surgery or stoma diversion could be considered.

Maeda et al. (27) reported the efficacy of intracorporeal reinforcing sutures for anastomotic leakage after laparoscopic surgery for rectal cancer. The methylene blue perfusion test was used to check the defective location. The number of linear stapler firings during rectal division is associated with anastomotic leakage. Lateral intersecting staple lines (dog-ears) are a weak point in the anastomosis (28), and intersections of staple lines after the double stapling technique tend to be associated with anastomotic leakage (29). Anastomotic reinforcing sutures were used in the defective parts and weak points. In our study, the pelvic peritoneum was routinely closed to reduce the risks of diffuse peritonitis, which made washing and drainage in the pelvic cavity possible. Seven cases (1.1%) of reoperation occurred in 44 cases of anastomotic leakage in this study.

It is still controversial whether a stoma diversion is necessary for mid and low rectal cancer operations. A meta-analysis (30) with 44.5% of patients undergoing a stoma diversion suggested that a stoma diversion could reduce the incidence of serious complications such as peritonitis caused by anastomotic leakage, as well as the reoperation rate and mortality. However, a stoma diversion may cause many inconveniences to patients. Garfinkle et al. (31) reported that 8% of patients had complications such as intestinal obstruction after loop ileostomy closure. Song et al. (32) reported that in 520 cases of loop ileostomy closure, 9.8% of patients underwent restoma due to postoperative complications. The reasons may include anastomosis-related complications, local recurrence, and loss of anal sphincter function. In this study, 15 patients (2.3%) underwent prophylactic ileostomy. Stoma diversion showed more complications after surgery but was not an independent risk factor. Who would benefit from a

TABLE 4 | Risk factors associated with anastomosis leakage.

Clinical factors	Cases	Leakage cases (%)	Univariate analysis		Multivariate analysis	
			OR value (95% *CI*)	P-value	OR value (95% *CI*)	P-value
Gender			2.101 (1.018–4.329)	0.044*	2.247 (1.126–4.902)	0.023*
Female	238	10(4.2%)				
Male	403	34 (11.3%)				
Age			1.160 (0.614–2.191)	0.647		
≥65	254	16(6.3%)				
<65	387	28(7.2%)				
BMI(kg/m^2)			1.161 (0.608–2.217)	0.651		
≥25	199	15(7.5%)				
<25	442	29(6.6%)				
ASA score			1.058 (0.620–1.804)	0.837		
I–II	588	40 (6.8%)				
III	53	4 (7.5%)				
Diabetes			1.082 (0.443–2.646)	0.862		
yes	82	6(7.3%)				
no	559	38(6.8%)				
Hb(g/L)			0.765 (0.266–2.204)	0.620		
<110	73	4(5.5%)				
≥110	528	40(7.6%)				
ALB(g/L)			1.496 (0.789–2.837)	0.217		
<40	181	16(8.8%)				
≥40	460	28(6.1%)				
CEA (ng/ml)			0.866 (0.449–1.670)	0.668		
<5	418	30(7.2%)				
≥5	223	14(6.3%)				
Tumor location from anus(cm)			2.183 (1.174–4.049)	0.014*	2.242 (1.197–4.202)	0.012*
>5	456	24(5.3%)				
≤5	185	20(10.8%)				
Tumor size(cm)			0.782 (0.414–1.477)	0.449		
>5	268	16(6.0%)				
≤5	373	28(7.5%)				
preoperative radiotherapy			1.106 (0.420–2.911)	0.838		
yes	67	5(7.4%)				
no	574	39(6.8%)				
Operation			1.066 (0.499–2.280)	0.869		
NOSES	125	9(7.2%)				
AR or LAR	516	35(6.8%)				
Diverting stoma			0.968 (0.124–7.540)	0.976		
yes	15	1(6.6%)				
no	626	43(6.9%)				
Estimated blood loss(ml)			1.702 (0.864–3.354)	0.124		
≥100	131	13(9.9%)				
<100	510	31(6.1%)				
Operation time(min)			1.992 (1.073–3.704)	0.029*	2.114 (1.127–3.968)	0.020*
<180	445	24(5.4%)				
≥180	196	20 (10.2%)				
Pathological type			1.181 (0.513–2.719)	0.696		
adenocarcinoma	525	37(7.0%)				
Mucinous adenocarcinoma	116	7(6.0%)				
Differentiation			0.957 (0.704–1.300)	0.779		
I–II	322	23(7.1%)				
III–IV	319	21(6.6%)				
Vascular invasion			0.787 (0.370–1.676)	0.535		
yes	156	9(5.8%)				
no	485	35(7.2%)				
Perineural invasion			1.321 (0.691–2.526)	0.400		
yes	183	15(8.2%)				
no	458	29(6.3%)				
N stage			0.772 (0.409–1.457)	0.424		
yes	270	16(5.9%)				
no	371	28(7.5%)				

(Continued)

TABLE 4 | Continued

Clinical factors	Cases	Leakage cases (%)	Univariate analysis		Multivariate analysis	
			OR value (95% *CI*)	P-value	OR value (95% *CI*)	P-value
T stage			0.842 (0.618–1.148)	0.276		
T_{1-2}	228	19(8.3%)				
T_{3-4}	413	24(5.8%)				

BMI, body mass index; ALB, albumin; ASA, American Society of Anesthesiologists; AR, anterior resection; LAR, low anterior resection; NOSES, natural orifice specimen extraction surgery.
**P < 0.05.*

stoma diversion is still a question. In Shimizu's study (33), ileostomy diversion following laparoscopic LAR decreased the risk of anastomotic leakage, especially in male patients with malnutrition, and due to ileostomy diversion-related morbidity, the procedure was not recommended in female patients. Kim et al. (34) reported that ileostomy diversion could increase the risk of anastomotic stricture. Anastomotic stenosis more easily occurs in patients with stoma diversion. Regular expansion and functional exercise of the anus is recommended after the anastomosis is healed.

Pinar et al. (35) reported that robotic surgery was equivalent to conventional laparoscopy in rectal cancer patients. The 3-year DFS and OS in our cohort were 87.1% and 93.7%, respectively, which were similar to other studies evaluating laparoscopic surgery for mid and low rectal cancer (36). Complications and anastomotic leakage showed no significant influences on the long-term outcomes, which was similar to some reports (4). There seemed to be a negative trend with complication in the long-term results in our study, but the difference was not significant. Thus, further research is needed. Care should be taken to reduce the instance of complications, including anastomotic leakage and surgical duration, by optimizing the operating team (37).

Limitations: Single-institution experiences with no direct comparison to a laparoscopic or open group are not adequate to make universal conclusions, which is the major limitation of our study. In addition, as this is a single-center, retrospective study, the surgeon's background may affect the results to some extent. There is the possibility that the patients may have been a highly selected group with good clinical status. Therefore, we must consider that selection bias may have played a role in our results. Furthermore, it is possible that longer surgical times and more blood loss are simply markers of surgical difficulty.

CONCLUSION

Robotic rectal resection was safe and adequate in treating mid and low rectal tumors in our study. Being male, having a lower tumor location, and having a prolonged operation time were independent risk factors for complication and anastomotic leakage in mid and low rectal cancer. The complication and anastomotic leakage might have no long-term impact on oncological outcomes for mid and low rectal cancer with robotic surgery.

ETHICS STATEMENT

The studies involving human participants were reviewed and approved by The Fudan University Ethics Committee. The patients/participants provided their written informed consent to participate in this study.

AUTHOR CONTRIBUTIONS

JC, ZZ, WC, and TY contributed equally to this work data collection and analysis. QF and DZ helped data collection. YW and GH guided the study. All authors contributed to the article and approved the submitted version.

REFERENCES

1. Dekker E, Tanis PJ, Vleugels JLA, Kasi PM, Wallace MB. Colorectal cancer. *Lancet (London England)* (2019) 394:1467–80. doi: 10.1016/S0140-6736(19)32319-0
2. Mari G, Maggioni D, Costanzi A, Miranda A, Rigamonti L, Crippa J, et al. "High or low Inferior Mesenteric Artery ligation in Laparoscopic low Anterior Resection: study protocol for a randomized controlled trial" (HIGHLOW trial). *Trials* (2015) 16:21. doi: 10.1186/s13063-014-0537-5
3. Ha GW, Kim JH, Lee MR. Oncologic Impact of Anastomotic Leakage Following Colorectal Cancer Surgery: A Systematic Review and Meta-Analysis. *Ann Surg Oncol* (2017) 24:3289–99. doi: 10.1245/s10434-017-5881-8
4. Jang JH, Kim HC, Huh JW, Park YA, Cho YB, Yun SH, et al. Anastomotic Leak Does Not Impact Oncologic Outcomes After Preoperative Chemoradiotherapy and Resection for Rectal Cancer. *Ann Surg* (2019) 269:678–85. doi: 10.1097/SLA.0000000000002582
5. Mazeh H, Samet Y, Abu-Wasel B, Beglaibter N, Grinbaum R, Cohen T, et al. Application of a novel severity grading system for surgical complications after

colorectal resection. *J Am Coll Surg* (2009) 208:355–61. doi: 10.1016/j.jamcollsurg.2008.12.008

6. Rahbari NN, Weitz J, Hohenberger W, Heald RJ, Moran B, Ulrich A, et al. Definition and grading of anastomotic leakage following anterior resection of the rectum: a proposal by the International Study Group of Rectal Cancer. *Surgery* (2010) 147:339–51. doi: 10.1016/j.surg.2009.10.012
7. Brown SR, Mathew R, Keding A, Marshall HC, Brown JM, Jayne DG. The impact of postoperative complications on long-term quality of life after curative colorectal cancer surgery. *Ann Surg* (2014) 259:916–23. doi: 10.1097/SLA.0000000000000407
8. Stevenson ARL, Solomon MJ, Lumley JW, Hewett P, Clouston AD, Gebski VJ, et al. Effect of Laparoscopic-Assisted Resection vs Open Resection on Pathological Outcomes in Rectal Cancer. *JAMA* (2015) 314:1356. doi: 10.1001/jama.2015.12009
9. Jayne D, Pigazzi A, Marshall H, Croft J, Corrigan N, Copeland J, et al. Effect of Robotic-Assisted vs Conventional Laparoscopic Surgery on Risk of Conversion to Open Laparotomy Among Patients Undergoing Resection for Rectal Cancer: The ROLARR Randomized Clinical Trial. *JAMA* (2017) 318:1569–80. doi: 10.1001/jama.2017.7219
10. Chang W, Wei Y, Ren L, Jian M, Chen Y, Chen J, et al. Short-term and long-term outcomes of robotic rectal surgery-from the real word data of 1145 consecutive cases in China. *Surg Endosc* (2000) 34:4079–88. doi: 10.1007/s00464-019-07170-6
11. Fukada M, Matsuhashi N, Takahashi T, Imai H, Tanaka Y, Yamaguchi K, et al. Risk and early predictive factors of anastomotic leakage in laparoscopic low anterior resection for rectal cancer. *World J Surg Oncol* (2019) 17:178. doi: 10.1186/s12957-019-1716-3
12. Frasson M, Flor-Lorente B, Rodríguez JLR, Granero-Castro P, Hervás D, Alvarez Rico MA, et al. Risk Factors for Anastomotic Leak After Colon Resection for Cancer: Multivariate Analysis and Nomogram From a Multicentric, Prospective, National Study With 3193 Patients. *Ann Surg* (2015) 262:321–30. doi: 10.1097/SLA.0000000000000973
13. Parthasarathy M, Greensmith M, Bowers D, Groot-Wassink T. Risk factors for anastomotic leakage after colorectal resection: a retrospective analysis of 17 518 patients. *Colorectal Dis* (2017) 19:288–98. doi: 10.1111/codi.13476
14. Frouws MA, Snijders HS, Malm SH, Liefers G-J, Van de Velde CJH, Neijenhuis PA, et al. Clinical Relevance of a Grading System for Anastomotic Leakage After Low Anterior Resection: Analysis From a National Cohort Database. *Dis Colon Rectum* (2017) 60:706–13. doi: 10.1097/DCR.0000000000000800
15. Yasui M, Takemasa I, Miyake Y, Hata T, Ikeda M, Miyake Y, et al. Tumor Size as an Independent Risk Factor for Postoperative Complications in Laparoscopic Low Anterior Resection for Advanced Rectal Cancer: A Multicenter Japanese Study. *Surg Laparosc Endosc Percutan Tech* (2017) 27:98–103. doi: 10.1097/SLE.0000000000000377
16. Simillis C, Lal N, Thoukididou SN, Kontovounisios C, Smith JJ, Hompes R, et al. Open Versus Laparoscopic Versus Robotic Versus Transanal Mesorectal Excision for Rectal Cancer: A Systematic Review and Network Meta-analysis. *Ann Surg* (2019) 270:59–68. doi: 10.1097/SLA.0000000000003227
17. Leichtle SW, Mouawad NJ, Welch KB, Lampman RM, Cleary RK. Risk factors for anastomotic leakage after colectomy. *Dis Colon Rectum* (2012) 55:569–75. doi: 10.1097/DCR.0b013e3182423c0d
18. Schiffmann L, Wedermann N, Schwandner F, Gock M, Klar E, Kühn F. Neoadjuvant radio-chemotherapy prolongs healing of anastomotic leakage after rectal resection treated with endoscopic vacuum therapy. *Therap Adv Gastroenterol* (2019) 12:1756284819877606. doi: 10.1177/1756284819877606
19. Borstlap WAA, Westerduin E, Aukema TS, Bemelman WA, Tanis PJDutch Snapshot Research Group. Anastomotic Leakage and Chronic Presacral Sinus Formation After Low Anterior Resection: Results From a Large Cross-sectional Study. *Ann Surg* (2017) 266:870–7. doi: 10.1097/SLA.0000000000002429
20. Sebag-Montefiore D, Stephens RJ, Steele R, Monson J, Grieve R, Khanna S, et al. Preoperative radiotherapy versus selective postoperative chemoradiotherapy in patients with rectal cancer (MRC CR07 and NCIC-CTG C016): a multicentre, randomised trial. *Lancet (London England)* (2009) 373:811–20. doi: 10.1016/S0140-6736(09)60484-0
21. Salmenkylä S, Kouri M, Österlund P, Pukkala E, Luukkonen P, Hyöty M, et al. Does preoperative radiotherapy with postoperative chemotherapy increase acute side-effects and postoperative complications of total mesorectal excision? Report of the randomized Finnish rectal cancer trial. *Scand J Surg* (2012) 101:275–82. doi: 10.1177/145749691210100410
22. Guan X, Liu Z, Parvaiz A, Longo A, Saklani A, Shafik AA, et al. International consensus on natural orifice specimen extraction surgery (NOSES) for gastric cancer (2019). *Gastroenterol Rep* (2020) 8:5–10. doi: 10.1093/gastro/goz067
23. Liu D, Luo R, Wan Z, Zhu W, He P, Ye S, et al. Clinical outcomes and prognostic factors of robotic assisted rectal cancer resection alone versus robotic rectal cancer resection with natural orifice extraction: a matched analysis. *Sci Rep* (2020) 10:12848. doi: 10.1038/s41598-020-69830-1
24. Ding Y, Li Z, Gao H, Cao Y, Jin W. Comparison of efficacy between natural orifice specimen extraction without abdominal incision and conventional laparoscopic surgery in the treatment of sigmoid colon cancer and upper rectal cancer. *J BUON* (2019) 24:1817–23.
25. Liu Z, Efetov S, Guan X, Zhou H, Tulina I, Wang G, et al. A Multicenter Study Evaluating Natural Orifice Specimen Extraction Surgery for Rectal Cancer. *J Surg Res* (2019) 243:236–41. doi: 10.1016/j.jss.2019.05.034
26. Sciuto A, Merola G, De Palma GD, Sodo M, Pirozzi F, Bracale UM, et al. Predictive factors for anastomotic leakage after laparoscopic colorectal surgery. *World J Gastroenterol* (2018) 24:2247–60. doi: 10.3748/wjg.v24.i21.2247
27. Maeda K, Nagahara H, Shibutani M, Ohtani H, Sakurai K, Toyokawa T, et al. Efficacy of intracorporeal reinforcing sutures for anastomotic leakage after laparoscopic surgery for rectal cancer. *Surg Endosc* (2015) 29:3535–42. doi: 10.1007/s00464-015-4104-2
28. Roumen RM, Rahusen FT, Wijnen MH, Croiset van Uchelen FA. "Dog ear" formation after double-stapled low anterior resection as a risk factor for anastomotic disruption. *Dis Colon Rectum* (2000) 43:522–5. doi: 10.1007/BF02237198
29. Lee S, Ahn B, Lee S. The Relationship Between the Number of Intersections of Staple Lines and Anastomotic Leakage After the Use of a Double Stapling Technique in Laparoscopic Colorectal Surgery. *Surg Laparosc Endosc Percutan Tech* (2017) 27:273–81. doi: 10.1097/SLE.0000000000000422
30. Gu W, Wu S. Meta-analysis of defunctioning stoma in low anterior resection with total mesorectal excision for rectal cancer: evidence based on thirteen studies. *World J Surg Oncol* (2015) 13:9. doi: 10.1186/s12957-014-0417-1
31. Garfinkle R, Savage P, Boutros M, Landry T, Reynier P, Morin N, et al. Incidence and predictors of postoperative ileus after loop ileostomy closure: a systematic review and meta-analysis. *Surg Endosc* (2019) 33:2430–43. doi: 10.1007/s00464-019-06794-y
32. Song O, Kim KH, Lee SY, Kim CH, Kim YJ, Kim HR. Risk factors of stoma re-creation after closure of diverting ileostomy in patients with rectal cancer who underwent low anterior resection or intersphincteric resection with loop ileostomy. *Ann Surg Treat Res* (2018) 94:203–8. doi: 10.4174/astr.2018.94.4.203
33. Shimizu H, Yamaguchi S, Ishii T, Kondo H, Hara K, Takemoto K, et al. Who needs diverting ileostomy following laparoscopic low anterior resection in rectal cancer patients? Analysis of 417 patients in a single institute. *Surg Endosc* (2000) 34:839–46. doi: 10.1007/s00464-019-06837-4
34. Kim MJ, Kim YS, Park SC, Sohn DK, Kim DY, Chang HJ, et al. Risk factors for permanent stoma after rectal cancer surgery with temporary ileostomy. *Surgery* (2016) 159:721–7. doi: 10.1016/j.surg.2015.09.011
35. Pinar I, Fransgaard T, Thygesen LC, Gögenur I. Long-Term Outcomes of Robot-Assisted Surgery in Patients with Colorectal Cancer. *Ann Surg Oncol* (2018) 25:3906–12. doi: 10.1245/s10434-018-6862-2
36. Watanabe J, Ishibe A, Suwa Y, Ozawa M, Nakagawa K, Suwa H, et al. Short- and long-term outcomes of laparoscopic versus open lateral lymph node dissection for locally advanced middle/lower rectal cancer using a propensity score-matched analysis. *Surg Endosc* (2020). doi: 10.1007/s00464-020-07943-4
37. van Rooijen SJ, Huisman D, Stuijvenberg M, Stens J, Roumen RMH, Daams F, et al. Intraoperative modifiable risk factors of colorectal anastomotic leakage: Why surgeons and anesthesiologists should act together. *Int J Surg* (2016) 36:183–200. doi: 10.1016/j.ijsu.2016.09.098

26

Plasma N-Acetylaspartate is Related to Age, Obesity and Glucose Metabolism: Effects of Antidiabetic Treatment and Bariatric Surgery

Giuseppe Daniele[1], Beatrice Campi[2], Alessandro Saba[3,4], Simone Codini[1], Annamaria Ciccarone[1], Laura Giusti[1], Stefano Del Prato[1], Russel L. Esterline[5] and Ele Ferrannini[2]*

[1] Department of Clinical and Experimental Medicine, University of Pisa, Pisa, Italy, [2] C.N.R. Institute of Clinical Physiology, Pisa, Italy, [3] Department of Surgical, Medical and Molecular Pathology and Critical Care Medicine, University of Pisa, Pisa, Italy, [4] Laboratory of Clinical Pathology, St. Chiara University Hospital, Pisa, Italy, [5] AstraZeneca Pharmaceutical, Gaithersburg, MD, United States

***Correspondence:**
Ele Ferrannini
ferranni@ifc.cnr.it

Background: N-acetylaspartate (NAA) is synthesized only by neurons and is involved in neuronal metabolism and axonal myelination. NAA is the strongest signal on brain magnetic resonance spectroscopy, and its concentration have been associated with cognitive dysfunction in neurodegenerative diseases, obesity, and type 2 diabetes (T2D).

Materials and Methods: We explored the impact of obesity and T2D on circulating NAA as well as the impact of bariatric surgery and antidiabetic treatments. We developed an LC-MS method for the accurate measurements of fasting plasma NAA levels in 505 subjects (156 subjects with normal glucose tolerance, 24 subjects with impaired glucose tolerance, and 325 patients with T2D) to examine the associations of NAA with obesity and dysglycemia. To validate cross-sectional findings, plasma NAA was measured 6 months after Roux-en-Y Gastric Bypass (RYGB) in 55 morbidly obese subjects, and after 1 year of antidiabetic treatment (with dapagliflozin, exenatide, or dapagliflozin plus exenatide) in 192 T2D patients.

Results: In the whole population, NAA was associated with age ($r = 0.31$, $p < 0.0001$) and BMI ($r = -0.20$, $p < 0.0001$). Independently of age and BMI, NAA was reciprocally related to HbA1c and fasting plasma glucose (partial $r = -0.13$, both $p = 0.01$). Surgically-induced weight loss raised NAA (by 18 nmol/L on average, $p < 0.02$). Glucose lowering treatment increased NAA in proportion to the drop in HbA1c ($r = 0.31$, $p < 0.0001$) regardless of the agent used.

Conclusions: Circulating NAA concentrations are modulated by age, obesity, and glycemic control. Whether they may mark for the corresponding metabolic effects on brain function remains to be established by joint measurements of spectroscopic signal and cognitive function.

Keywords: N-acetylaspartate, neuronal function, type 2 diabetes, obesity, dapagliflozin, exenatide, bariatric surgery, glucose metabolism

INTRODUCTION

Type 2 diabetes (T2D) and obesity increase the risk of serious complications in multiple organs, including the brain (1). Obesity and T2D are associated with a higher prevalence of cognitive dysfunction, dementia, and neurodegenerative diseases, including Alzheimer and Parkinson diseases (2–5). Microvascular disease induced by hyperglycemia is responsible for disruption of the blood-brain barrier (BBB) through pericyte depletion, possibly caused by excess superoxide produced during enhanced mitochondrial respiration (6, 7). Loss of the BBB ability to protect the brain from circulating substances results in neurotoxicity and neuronal cell death (8). Neuroimaging has documented several structural and functional alterations in numerous brain regions of patients with T2D (9–11). Magnetic resonance spectroscopy (MRS) has provided details regarding metabolite changes in the brain that might be related to functional and structural alterations. Recent MRS-based analyses carried out in humans have suggested that N-acetylaspartate (NAA), the most concentrated metabolite in the brain (~10 mM) (12–14), is significantly reduced in several diseases including Alzheimer (15, 16), Huntington disease (17), bipolar disorder (18), schizophrenia (19), multiple sclerosis (20), and T2D (21–25).

NAA is reputed to be a marker of neuronal number and viability (26) but its role in brain metabolism and function in humans is far from being fully elucidated. NAA is synthesized in neuronal mitochondria and then transported by a sodium/dicarboxylate symporter (27) to aspartoacylase-containing oligodendrocytes (28) and astrocytes. NAA has two primary roles, as a facilitator of energy metabolism in neuronal mitochondria (29) and a source of acetate for fatty acid and steroid synthesis necessary for axonal myelination by oligodendrocytes (30, 31). Astrocytes, which represent the main cell type within the BBB structure, play a role in the removal of NAA from the extracellular space; a continuous NAA efflux from the brain to the circulation has been proposed (32). Therefore, plasma NAA levels might be used as a marker of central NAA alterations in neurodegenerative diseases and T2D-related brain damage. One difficulty is that the few studies measuring circulating NAA concentrations report widely different values even in healthy controls, ranging from a mean 0.11 mmol/L (33) to 0.44 µmol/L (34), very likely due to assay differences.

To the best of our knowledge, the impact of obesity and T2D on circulating NAA has not been previously explored. We therefore set forth to measure plasma NAA in non-diabetic obese and T2D subjects and the effect of treatment on plasma NAA.

Abbreviations: NAA, N-acetylaspartate; T2DM, type 2 diabetes; IGT, impaired glucose tolerance; NGT, normal glucose tolerance; RYGB, Roux-en-Y Gastric Bypass; FPG, Fasting plasma glucose; MRS, magnetic resonance spectroscopy; BBB, blood-brain barrier; GLP-1RAs, GLP-1 receptor agonists/analogs; Dapa+Plb, dapagliflozin + placebo; EQW, exenatide once weekly; EQW+Dapa, exenatide-dapagliflozin combination.

MATERIALS AND METHODS

Study Subjects

This was a data pooling project of different cohort studies. A total of 505 study subjects included patients with T2D or impaired glucose tolerance (IGT) and non-diabetic obese subjects. Two subgroups of participants were studied: (i) to assess the impact of major weight loss on circulating NAA levels, we included obese subjects undergoing Roux-en-Y Gastric Bypass (RYGB) between 2015 and 2018; (ii) to evaluate the effect of glycemic control, we included T2D patients from the DURATION-8 study (NCT02229396), which was a 52-week, multicenter, double-blind, randomized, active-controlled phase 3 trial. In DURATION-8, participants were randomly assigned to receive once-weekly exenatide (2 mg) by subcutaneous injection plus once-daily dapagliflozin (10 mg) (EQW+Dapa), exenatide with dapagliflozin-matched oral placebo (EQW), or dapagliflozin with exenatide-matched placebo injections (Dapa+Plb) (35). Lean healthy subjects with normal glucose tolerance (NGT) were included as control group. Exclusion criteria were: type 1 diabetes, psychiatric disorders, severe cognitive impairment, neurodegenerative diseases, epilepsy, depression treatment, traumatic brain injury over the preceding months, liver function enzymes higher more than two times the upper limit, heart failure (NYHA III-IV), GFR <60 ml/min/1.73 m^2, diabetes treatment other than metformin, or sulphonylureas. The ethical committee approvals refers to specific ethical approval of each study included in the pooled analysis. All procedure performed were in accordance with the Helsinki Declaration of 1975 as revised 1983.

All plasma samples were obtained in the overnight fasted [10–14 h) state, and stored at −80°C for NAA analysis. Baseline and post-treatment samples were assayed in the same run to reduce within-subject variability.

Reagents and Materials

NAA and internal standard *N*-Acetyl-L-aspartic acid-1,2,3,4-$^{13}C_4$ (IS, $^{13}C_4$-NAA) as well as acetonitrile (LC-MS grade), ultra-pure water (LC-MS grade), formic acid (MS grade), and 3N hydrochloric acid in butan-1-ol were provided by Sigma-Aldrich (Saint Louis, MO, USA).

Equipments and Analytical Method

An Agilent 1290 Infinity UHPLC system (Santa Clara, CA, USA), including binary pump, autosampler, and column oven, fitted with a Kinetex C18 (100Å, 2.6 µm, 50 × 2.10 mm ID) HPLC column (Phenomenex, Torrance, CA, USA), protected by a KrudKatcher Ultra HPLC in-line filter (0.5 µm depth × 0.004 in ID), was used for sample injection and chromatographic separation. This latter was carried out under the gradient conditions at a flow rate of 400 µL/min, by using H_2O + 0.1% formic acid (FA) as an aqueous solvent and ACN + 20% MeOH + 0.1% FA as an organic solvent. The injection volume of samples was 5 µL.

Mass spectrometry runs were carried out by an AB Sciex API 4000 triple quadrupole mass spectrometer (Concord, ON, Canada), equipped with an electrospray (ESI) Turbo-V ion source. The MS method was based on positive ion mode selected reaction monitoring (SRM) and made use of parameters optimized in order to get the best possible sensitivity and selectivity. In particular, SRM acquisitions were based on transitions 288.2 → 143.9 Da (quantifier, Q) and 288.2 → 186.1 Da (qualifier, q) for NAA and 292 → 146.9 Da (Q), 292 → 189.1 Da (q) for $^{13}C_4$-NAA.

Sample preparation was carried out as follows: plasma samples were thawed at room temperature, vortexed (15 min), and a 100 μL aliquot was added with 300 μL of acetonitrile, formic acid 1% (V%), and internal standard. The obtained suspensions were vortexed (15 min) and centrifuged (18,620 × g, 15 min). Then, 300 μL of supernatants were collected and dried under stream of N_2 at 40°C. The samples were derivatized to butyl esters (Fischer esterification reaction) by adding 100 μL 3N 1-butanol/ HCl, vortexing (15 min), heating at 60°C for 40 min. The reaction products were dried under a gentle stream of nitrogen and the dry residues were reconstituted with 100 μL ACN/H_2O (20/80; V/V), vortexed (15 min), and 5 μL of the obtained solutions were injected into the LC-MS-MS system.

The analytical method, which is not the main subject of this paper and that will be extensively described in a paper under preparation, was validated in compliance with EMA guidelines (36) for sample stability, linearity, lower limits of detection and quantitation (LLOD and LLOQ), matrix effect, recovery, selectivity, precision, and accuracy.

Statistical Analysis

Data are given as mean ± SD. Because of their skewed distribution, plasma NAA concentrations were summarized as median [interquartile range, IQR], and logarithmically transformed for use in parametric statistical tests. Group values were compared by the Mann-Whitney *U*-test, paired values by the Wilkinson signed-rank test. Change by treatment were analyzed by MANOVA for repeated measures. Univariate and multivariate linear regressions were carried out by standard methods. Data analyses were performed using JMP® 7.0 (SAS Institute Inc., 2007); $p \leq 0.05$ was considered statistically significant.

RESULTS

In the study population (259 women, 246 men), 156 subjects had normal glucose tolerance (NGT), 325 had T2D, and 24 had IGT; age ranged from 23 to 78 years, and BMI ranged from 20.1 to 57.9 kg/m^2 (**Figure 1**). In the whole data set, fasting plasma NAA concentrations ranged from 94 to 567 nmol/L, with a significantly ($p < 0.0001$) skewed distribution. Compared to NGT, T2D/IGT subjects were older ($p < 0.0001$) and more often men ($p = 0.002$) (**Table 1**). Plasma NAA concentrations were higher in men than women ($p < 0.02$), were positively associated with age, and negatively related to BMI (**Figure 2**). In the 63 NGT, normal-weight (i.e., BMI≤25 kg/m^2) subjects aged <65 years (42 women, 21 men), plasma NAA ranged 143–407 nmol/L (median 204, IQR 110 nmol/L) in men and 101–378 nmol/L (median 239, IQR 95) in women. By adjusting the entire data set for gender, age, and BMI, plasma NAA levels were inversely related to both

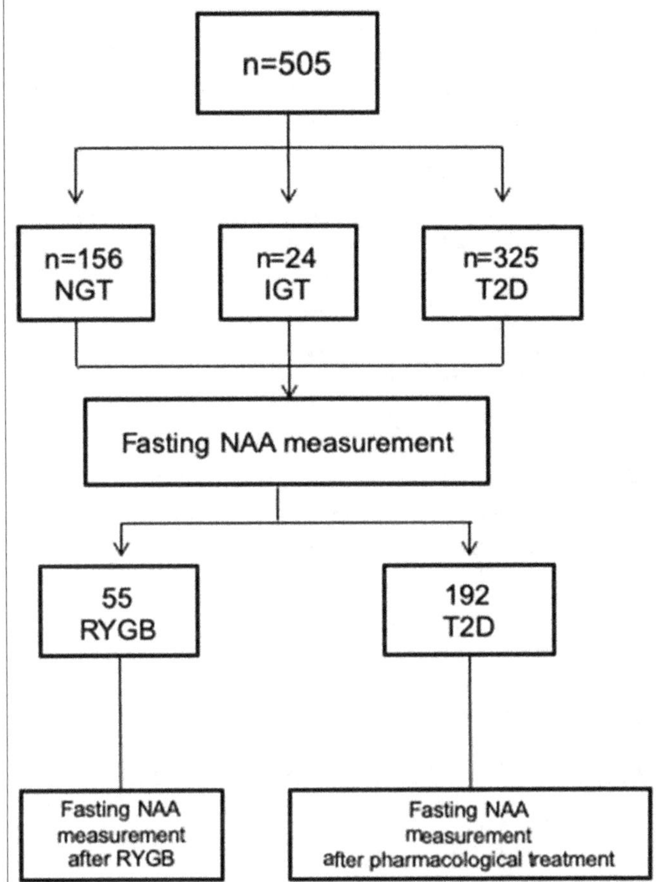

FIGURE 1 | Participants flow chart. NGT, normal glucose tolerance; IGT, Impaired glucose regulation; T2D; type 2 diabetes.

FPG and HbA_{1c} (**Figure 3**); in this model, age was still a positive ($p < 0.0001$), and BMI a negative ($p = 0.044$), covariate. To characterize the clinical phenotype of subjects with low plasma NAA levels, we split the NAA distribution into quartiles. In the lower quartile of plasma NAA levels there were more women, a younger age and higher BMI, and a worse glycemic control (**Table 2**).

In the 55 subjects (45 NGT and 10 T2D) who underwent bariatric surgery, the change in BMI at 6 months post-surgery averaged −11.5 ± 3.6 kg/m^2 ($p < 0.0001$), and was similar in NGT and T2D. Fasting plasma glucose dropped by 10 ± 16 mg/dL in NGT and by 95 ± 77 mg/dL in T2D ($p < 0.0001$ for both), and plasma NAA increased by 18 (37) μmol/L ($p < 0.02$).

Out of the 265 T2D patients, 192 individuals were randomized to receive dapagliflozin + placebo (Dapa+Plb), exenatide once weekly (EQW), or the combination (EQW+Dapa) in a 1:1:1 ratio for 1 year. At 52 weeks, NAA values were higher than at baseline [248 [94] vs. 239 [83] nmol/L, delta = 13 (38), $p = 0.0013$] across treatment. Each treatment resulted in significant reductions in BMI, fasting glucose, and HbA_{1c}, and an increase in plasma NAA; the changes were (for BMI, FPG, and NAA) or tended to be (for HbA_{1c}) accentuated with the combination as compared to

TABLE 1 | Characteristics of the study subjects*.

	NGT		T2D/IGT	
	Men	**Women**	**Men**	**Women**
N	60	96	186	163
Age (years)	50 ± 12	45 ± 12	58 ± 9	55 ± 10
BMI (kg/m^2)	29.5 ± 8.8	37 ± 11.1	32.0 ± 5.3	33.5 ± 6.0
HbA_{1c} (%)	5.9 ± 1.7	5.7 ± 0.6	8.2 ± 1.4	8.6 ± 1.5
FPG (mg/dL)	93 ± 19	92 ± 17	158 ± 49	171 ± 61
NAA (nmol/L)	249 [113]	227 [88]	249 [67]	239 [75]

**entries are mean ± SD or median [interquartile range]; BMI, body mass index; FPG, fasting plasma glucose; NAA, N-acetylaspartate.*

either agent alone (**Table 3**). In the pooled data from all treatment arms, the changes in plasma NAA were inversely related to the concomitant changes in both HbA_{1c} (**Figure 4**). The regression predicts a mean NAA increase of 16 nmol/L for a 2% decrement in HbA_{1c}.

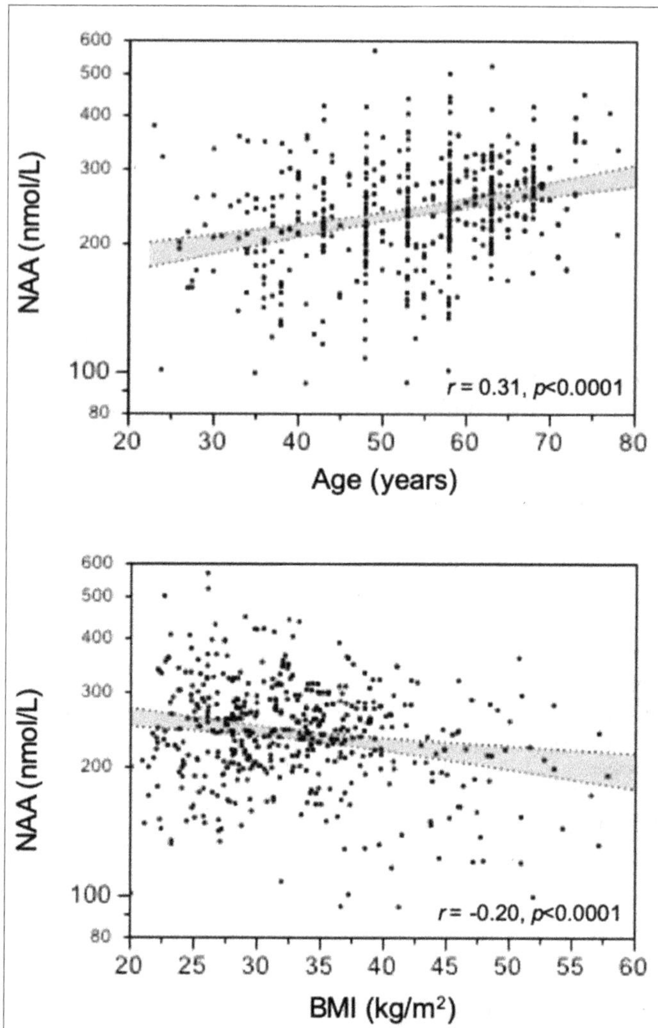

FIGURE 2 | Association of plasma N-acetylaspartate (NAA) concentrations with age and BMI.

DISCUSSION

The data of this study allowed us to establish normative circulating NAA metrics, namely, median fasting concentrations of 230 nmol/L in non-obese, non-diabetic subjects below 65 years of age, and consistent, if not large, deviations with age and obesity (in opposite direction). Additionally, we report for the first time an inverse relation of plasma NAA to glycemic indices—HbA_{1c} and fasting glucose—even after controlling for sex, age, and BMI. The intervention protocols provided a prospective confirmation of this relationship by showing a consistent increase in plasma NAA concentrations following antidiabetic treatment (**Figure 3**).

It should be emphasized that no information is available on the acute changes in circulating NAA following physiological stimuli, e.g., a meal or a bout of physical exercise. More importantly, changes in plasma levels could reflect changes in NAA production/spillover from the brain into the bloodstream or changes in NAA removal from the plasma (or a combination thereof) (26). Thus, dysfunctional neurons might synthetize less NAA and/or the activity of the NAA-cleaving enzyme in glial cells [but also in brown adipocytes (39) and enterocytes (40)] might be increased: either process would reduce circulating NAA concentrations. The resulting clinical phenotype would resemble that profiled in subjects with lower NAA concentration (**Table 3**).

With regard to the effect of age, our finding of an independent, direct relationship between plasma NAA and age conflicts with two studies from the same group showing an age-related decline in serum NAA levels (41, 42). In the latter studies, however, the measured NAA concentrations were in the millimolar range, whereas reported values—including ours—are in the nanomolar range (34). Therefore, rather than a reflection of increased neuronal mass/function [i.e., an implausible correlate of aging (43)], our finding may suggest an age-related decrease in aspartoacylase, resulting in higher NAA levels. The extreme of this phenomenon would be Canavan disease, an autosomal-recessive mutation of the aspartoacylase gene associated with severe neurodegeneration (44).

The current finding of decreasing plasma NAA levels with increasing BMI is in line with the suggested role of obesity in NAA metabolism. By magnetic resonance spectroscopy (MRS), a higher BMI is associated with lower concentrations of NAA in brain frontal, parietal, and temporal white matter as well as in frontal gray matter and hippocampus (45, 46), and with progressive neuronal impairment and loss. Obesity can lead to astrogliosis, which is characterized by an increase in the number of primary astrocytic processes as well as in the length of these processes, leading to a more extensive contact between these cells and the local vasculature (47, 48). Astrocytes can be activated early after high-fat intake (49, 50) as a neuroprotective response to the rise in the concentration of fatty acids reaching the brain via the BBB (51–53). These structural changes could modify the ability of astrocytes to transport substances from the brain to the circulation, including a reduced release of

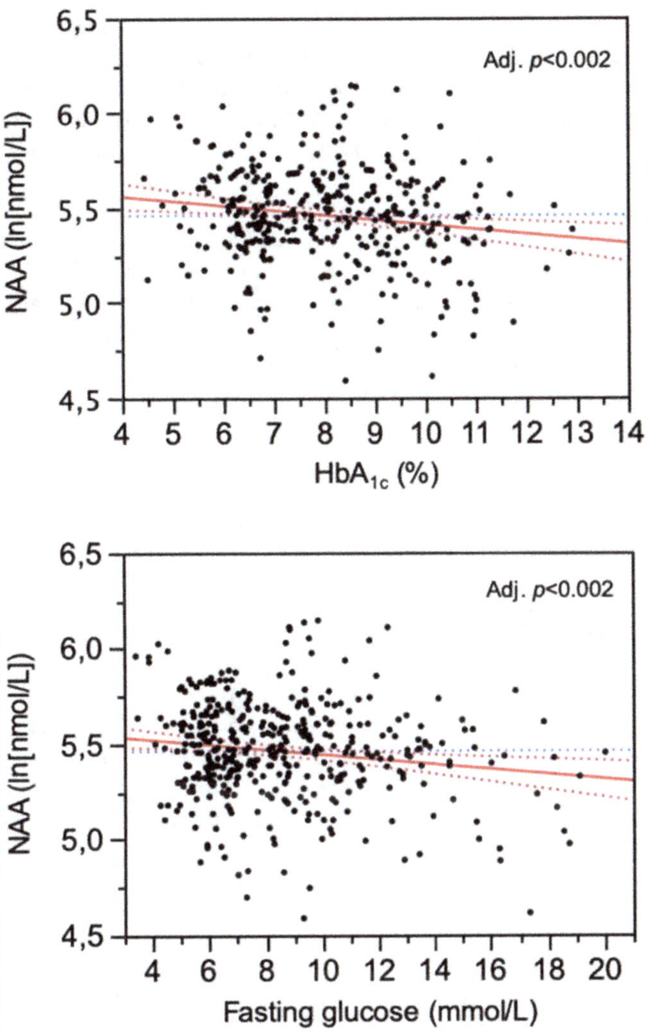

FIGURE 3 | Association of plasma N-acetylaspartate (NAA) concentrations with HbA_{1c} and fasting glucose levels. The plots are for logNAA residuals after controlling for gender, age, and BMI.

TABLE 2 | Clinical phenotype of subjects by quartile of NAA distribution*.

	Plasma NAA distribution		
	Bottom 25%	**Upper 75%**	***p***
NAA (nmol/L)	129 [41]	260 [66]	<0.0001
Women (%)	61	48	0.0138
Age (years)	48 ± 11	56 ± 11	<0.0001
BMI (kg/m^2)	34.2 ± 9.3	32.5 ± 6.6	0.07
HbA_{1c} (%)	8.2 ± 2.1	7.7 ± 1.6	0.0366
FPG (mg/dL)	158 ± 69	146 ± 53	0.09

**entries are mean ± SD or median [interquartile range]; BMI, body mass index; FPG, fasting plasma glucose; NAA, N-acetylaspartate.*

TABLE 3 | Variables by time and treatment#.

	Baseline	**1 year**	***p1***	***p2***	***p3***
Fasting glucose (mg/dL)			<0.0001	0.374	0.0214
Dapa + Plb (*n* = 70)	190 ± 42	145 ± 44			
EQW + Plb (*n* = 62)	190 ± 53	138 ± 37			
EQW + Dapa (*n* = 60)	194 ± 60	123 ± 32			
BMI (kg/m^2)			*<0.0001*	0.412	0.0004
Dapa + Plb	33.1 ± 6.1	32.3 ± 5.9			
EQW + Plb	31.6 ± 5.4	31.5 ± 5.5			
EQW + Dapa	33.6 ± 6.4	32.1 ± 6.0			
HbA1c (%)			*<0.0001*	0.249	0.084
Dapa + Plb	9.3 ± 1.0	7.7 ± 1.1			
EQW + Plb	9.3 ± 1.0	7.6 ± 1.3			
EQW + Dapa	9.3 ± 1.1	7.2 ± 1.3			
NAA (nmol/L)			*0.0005*	0.539	0.035
Dapa + Plb	242 [97]	245 [100]			
EQW + Plb	236 [82]	248 [73]			
EQW + Dapa	238 [88]	248 [110]			

#values are mean ± SD or median [IQR]; p^1 = time, p^2 = treatment, p^3 = time x treatment by MANOVA for repeated measures.

NAA (54). Several studies have documented changes in urinary NAA excretion or expression of NAA producing enzymes in association with obesity and/or diabetes (39, 40, 55–57). In the present study, the body weight reduction induced by bariatric surgery was associated to a significant increase in circulating NAA. One can therefore speculate that weight loss might have had multiple favorable consequences on central and peripheral NAA metabolism, including the reduction of brain astrogliosis.

Hyperglycemia dramatically increases neuronal glucose levels, which leads to neuronal damage, a phenomenon known as glucose neurotoxicity (58). Several mechanisms have been proposed for glucose neurotoxicity, including glucose-driven oxidative stress, and protein glycation. In line with this *in vitro* evidence, it has been shown that NAA/creatine ratio is decreased in the frontal brain cortex in diabetic patients with poor glycemic control (25). High glucose has a dramatic impact on astrocyte phenotype by inhibiting its proliferation and disrupting its energy flow (59, 60). Moreover, high glucose is associated with an increased expression and secretion of inflammatory cytokines (interleukin-6 and interleukin-8) by astrocytes (61). These hyperglycemia-induced abnormalities of astrocyte-neuron coupling may underlie the reduced central NAA concentrations and NAA spill-over into the peripheral circulation.

Although peripheral NAA levels alone cannot be taken to reflect spill-over or astrocyte-neuron coupling, our finding of consensual changes in glycemic indices and plasma NAA (**Figure 3**) does lend support to the possibility that long-term changes in circulating NAA may be markers for brain dysfunction. Clearly, simultaneous measurements of plasma NAA, brain NAA signal in relevant areas, and cognitive function before and after antihyperglycemic treatment would conclusively establish origin and value of peripheral NAA assessment.

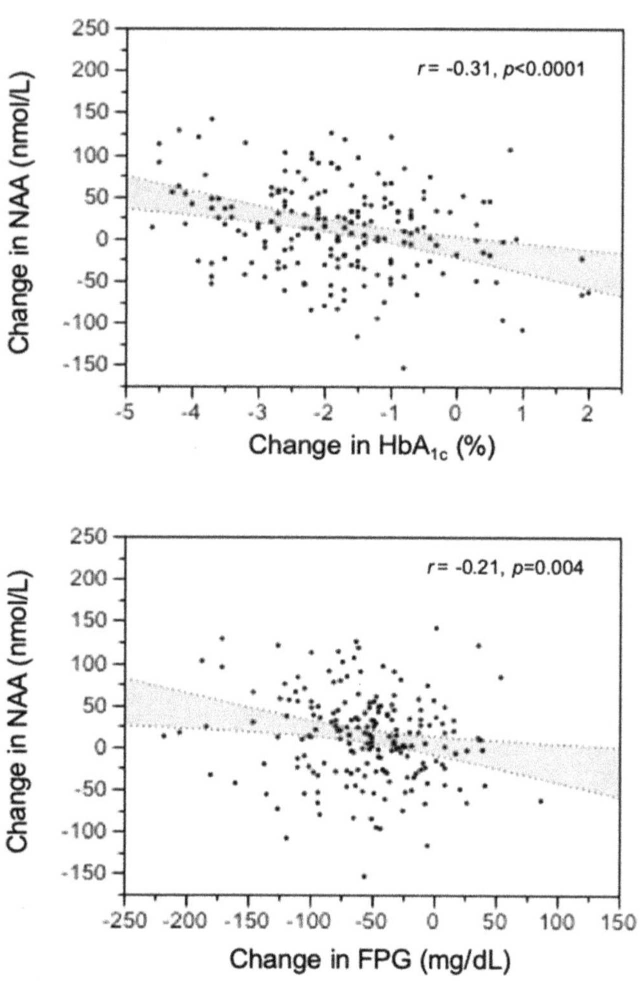

FIGURE 4 | Relation of treatment-induced changes in plasma N-acetylaspartate (NAA) concentrations to the corresponding changes in HbA_{1c} and fasting glucose levels at 1-year post-treatment.

Of note is that glucagon-like peptide 1 (GLP-1) receptors are expressed in neurons, in particular pyramidal neurons in the hippocampus and neocortex, which suggests that they may play a role in neuronal activity and synaptic transmission (62–64). Glia cells also express the receptor (65). GLP-1 analogs have demonstrated an impressive range of protective effects on neurogenesis, synaptogenesis, cell repair, and reduced inflammation, which is consistent with the profile of growth factor activity (37, 66–70). In this context, it is intriguing that patients in either EQW treatment arm showed a significantly greater change in plasma NAA than patients in the Dapa+placebo arm (**Table 2**), suggesting a potential effect of GLP-1 receptor agonists/analogs independently of the glucose lowering effect (38, 71).

The strength of the study is based on a large population including subjects with a wide range of age and body weight, and well-characterized in terms of glucose metabolism and comorbidity. In both T2D and morbidly obese groups, psychiatric disorders, intellectual disability, severe cognitive impairment, neurodegenerative diseases, epilepsy, depression treatment, and traumatic brain injury over the preceding months were exclusion criteria, which reduced the chances of NAA alterations being due to specific brain abnormalities.

The main limitation of the present study is its retrospective nature. Consequently, the NAA associations we describe, whether cross-sectional or longitudinal, do not necessarily intimate a causative role of glucose metabolism for plasma NAA or a direct relation of plasma NAA to brain NAA metabolism. The results of the study provide preliminary, inferential evidence, which remains to be confirmed by multilevel prospective studies.

ETHICS STATEMENT

The studies involving human participants were reviewed and approved by University of Pisa. The patients/participants provided their written informed consent to participate in this study. Written informed consent was obtained from the individual(s) for the publication of any potentially identifiable images or data included in this article.

AUTHOR CONTRIBUTIONS

EF and GD conceived the experimental design, analyzed the data, wrote and edited the manuscript. AS developed the tandem mass spectrometry-based assay and directed its validation. BC and SC performed LC-MS. AC and LG provided clinical samples. SD and RE provided feedback and contributed to the write-up and review of the manuscript. EF directed the study and is the guarantor of this work and, as such, had full access to all the data in the study and takes responsibility for the integrity of the data and accuracy of the data analysis. All authors read and approved the final manuscript.

ACKNOWLEDGMENTS

We thank Simona Baldi for assisting in the lab work.

REFERENCES

1. Klein JP, Waxman SG. The brain in diabetes: molecular changes in neurons and their implications for end-organ damage. *Lancet Neurol.* (2003) 2:548–54. doi: 10.1016/S1474-4422(03)00503-9
2. Biessels GJ, Staekenborg S, Brunner E, Brayne C, Scheltens P. Risk of dementia in diabetes mellitus: a systematic review. *Lancet Neurol.* (2006) 5:64–74. doi: 10.1016/S1474-4422(05)70284-2
3. Gustafson D, Rothenberg E, Blennow K, Steen B, Skoog I. An 18-year follow-up of overweight and risk of Alzheimer disease. *Arch Intern Med.* (2003) 163:1524–8. doi: 10.1001/archinte.163.13.1524
4. Whitmer RA, Gunderson EP, Barrett-Connor E, Quesenberry CP Jr, Yaffe K. Obesity in middle age and future risk of dementia: a 27-year longitudinal population based study. *BMJ.* (2005) 330:1360. doi: 10.1136/bmj.38446.466238.E0
5. Xu WL, Atti AR, Gatz M, Pedersen NL, Johansson B, Fratiglioni L. Midlife overweight and obesity increase late-life dementia risk: a population-based twin study. *Neurology.* (2011) 76:1568–74. doi: 10.1212/WNL.0b013e3182190d09
6. Shah GN, Morofuji Y, Banks WA, Price TO. High glucose-induced mitochondrial respiration and reactive oxygen species in mouse cerebral pericytes is reversed by pharmacological inhibition of mitochondrial carbonic anhydrases: implications for cerebral microvascular disease in diabetes. *Biochem Biophys Res Commun.* (2013) 440:354–8. doi: 10.1016/j.bbrc.2013.09.086
7. Liu Y, Fiskum G, Schubert D. Generation of reactive oxygen species by the mitochondrial electron transport chain. *J Neurochem.* (2002) 80:780–7. doi: 10.1046/j.0022-3042.2002.00744.x
8. Huber JD, VanGilder RL, Houser KA. Streptozotocin-induced diabetes progressively increases blood-brain barrier permeability in specific brain regions in rats. *Am J Physiol Heart Circ Physiol.* (2006) 291:H2660–8. doi: 10.1152/ajpheart.00489.2006
9. Musen G, Jacobson AM, Bolo NR, Simonson DC, Shenton ME, McCartney RL, et al. Resting-state brain functional connectivity is altered in type 2 diabetes. *Diabetes.* (2012) 61:2375–9. doi: 10.2337/db11-1669
10. Climie RE, Moran C, Callisaya M, Blizzard L, Sharman JE, Venn A, et al. Abdominal obesity and brain atrophy in type 2 diabetes mellitus. *PLoS ONE.* (2015) 10:e0142589. doi: 10.1371/journal.pone.0142589
11. Zhang Y, Lu S, Liu C, Zhang H, Zhou X, Ni C, et al. Altered brain activation and functional connectivity in working memory related networks in patients with type 2 diabetes: an ICA- based analysis. *Sci Rep.* (2016) 6:23767. doi: 10.1038/srep23767
12. Tallan HH. Studies on the distribution of N-acetyl-L-aspartic acid in brain. *J Biol Chem.* (1957) 224:41–5.
13. Tallan HH, Moore S, Stein WH. N-Acetyl-L-aspartic acid in brain. *J Biol Chem.* (1956) 219:257–64.
14. Miyake M, Kakimoto Y, Sorimachi M. A gas chromatographic method for the determination of N-acetyl-L-aspartic acid, N-acetyl-aspartylglutamic acid and beta-citryl-L-glutamic acid and their distributions in the brain and other organs of various species of animals. *J Neurochem.* (1981) 36:804–10. doi: 10.1111/j.1471-4159.1981.tb01665.x
15. Kwo-On-Yuen PF, Newmark RD, Budinger TF, Kaye JA, Ball MJ, Jagust WJ. BrainN-acetyl-L-aspartic acid in Alzheimer's disease: a proton magnetic resonance spectroscopy study. *Brain Res.* (1994) 667: 167–74. doi: 10.1016/0006-8993(94)91494-X
16. Zhu X, Schuff N, Kornak J, Soher B, Yaffe K, Kramer JH, et al. Previous magnetic resonance (MR) spectroscopy studies of Alzheimer disease (AD) reporting reduced N-acetyl aspartate (NAA), Alzheimer disease. *Assoc Disord.* (2006) 20:77–85. doi: 10.1097/01.wad.0000213809.12553.fc
17. Tsai G, Coyle JT. N-acetylaspartate in neuropsychiatric disorders, *Prog Neurobiol.* (1995) 46:531–40 doi: 10.1016/0301-0082(95)00014-M
18. Winsberg ME, Sachs N, Tate DL, Adalsteinsson E, Spielman D, Ketter TA. Decreased dorsolateral prefrontal N-acetyl aspartate in bipolar disorder. *Biol Psychiatry.* (2000) 47:475–81. doi: 10.1016/S0006-3223(99)00183-3
19. Molina V, Sánchez J, Reig S, Sanz J, Benito C, Santamarta C, et al. N-acetyl-aspartate levels in the dorsolateral prefrontal cortex in the early years of schizophrenia are inversely related to disease duration. *Schizophr Res.* (2005) 73:209–19. doi: 10.1016/j.schres.2004.02.001
20. Teunissen CE, Iacobaeus E, Khademi M, Brundin L, Norgren N, Koel-Simmelink MJA, et al. Combination of CSF N-acetylaspartate and neurofilaments in multiple sclerosis. *Neurology.* (2009) 72: 1322–9. doi: 10.1212/WNL.0b013e3181a0fe3f
21. Sinha S, Ekka M, Sharma U, Raghunandan P, Pandey RM, Jagannathan NR. Assessment of 17 changes in brain metabolites in Indian patients with type-2 diabetes mellitus 18 using proton magnetic resonance spectroscopy. *BMC Res Notes.* (2014) 7:41. doi: 10.1186/1756-0500-7-41
22. Lin Y, Zhou J, Sha L, Li Y, Qu X, Liu L, et al. Metabolite differences in the lenticular nucleus in type 2 diabetes mellitus 22 shown by proton MR spectroscopy. *AJNR Am J Neuroradiol.* (2013) 34:1692–6. doi: 10.3174/ajnr.A3492
23. Duarte JM. Metabolic alterations associated to brain dysfunction in diabetes. *Aging Dis.* (2015) 6:304–21. doi: 10.14336/AD.2014.1104
24. Duarte JM. Metabolism in the diabetic brain neurochemical profiling by 1H magnetic resonance spectroscopy. *J Diabetes Metab Disord.* (2016) 3:011. doi: 10.24966/DMD-201X/100011
25. Sahin I, Alkan A, Keskin L, Cikim A, Karakas HM, Firat AK, et al. Evaluation of in vivo cerebral metabolism on proton magnetic resonance spectroscopy in patients with impaired glucose tolerance and type 2 diabetes mellitus. *J Diabetes Complicat.* (2008) 22:254–60. doi: 10.1016/j.jdiacomp.2007.03.007
26. John R, Moffett JR, Brian Ross B, Peethambaran Arun P, Chikkathur N, Madhavarao CN, et al. N-Acetylaspartate in the CNS: from neurodiagnostics to neurobiology. *Progr Neurobiol.* (2007) 81:89–131. doi: 10.1016/j.pneurobio.2006.12.003
27. Fujita T, Katsukawa H, Yodoya E, Wada M, Shimada A, Okada N, et al. Transport characteristics of N-acetyl-L-aspartate in rat astrocytes: involvement of sodium-coupled high-affinity carboxylate transporter NaC3/ NaDC3-mediated transport system. *J Neurochem.* (2005) 93:706–14. doi: 10.1111/j.1471-4159.2005.03067.x
28. Madhavarao CN, Moffett JR, Moore RA, Viola RE, Namboodiri MA, Jacobowitz DM. Immunohistochemical localization of aspartoacylase in the rat central nervous system. *J Comp Neurol.* (2004) 472:318–29. doi: 10.1002/cne.20080
29. Clark, JB. N-acetyl aspartate: a marker for neuronal loss or mitochondrial dysfunction. *Dev Neurosci.* (1998) 20:271–6. doi: 10.1159/000017321
30. Chakraborty G, Mekala P, Yahya D, Wu G, Ledeen RW. Intraneuronal N-acetylaspartate supplies acetyl groups for myelin lipid synthesis: evidence for myelin-associated aspartoacylase. *J. Neurochem.* (2001) 78:736–45. doi: 10.1046/j.1471-4159.2001.00456.x
31. D'Adamo AF Jr, Yatsu, FM. Acetate metabolism in the nervous system. N-acetyl-L-aspartic acid and the biosynthesis of brain lipids. *J Neurochem.* (1966) 13:961–5. doi: 10.1111/j.1471-4159.1966.tb10292.x
32. Kelley RI, Stamas JN. Quantification of N-acetyl-L-aspartic acid in urine by isotope dilution gas chromatography-mass spectrometry. *J Inherit Metab Dis.* (1992) 15:97–104. doi: 10.1007/BF01800351
33. Tortorella C, Ruggieri M, Di Monte E, Ceci E, Iaffaldano P, Direnzo V, et al. Serum and CSF N-acetyl aspartate levels differ in multiple sclerosis

and neuromyelitis optica. *J Neurol Neurosurg Psychiatry.* (2011) 82:1355–9. doi: 10.1136/jnnp.2011.241836

34. Jakobs C, Brink HJ, Langelaar SA, Zee T, Stellaard F, Macek M, et al. Stable isotope dilution analysis of N-acetylaspartic acid in CSF, blood, urine and amniotic fluid: accurate postnatal diagnosis and the potential for prenatal diagnosis of canavan disease. *J Inherit Metab Dis.* (1991) 14:653–60. doi: 10.1007/BF01799929
35. Frías JP, Guja C, Hardy E, Ahmed A, Dong F, Öhman P, et al. Exenatide once weekly plus dapagliflozin once daily versus exenatide or dapagliflozin alone in patients with type 2 diabetes inadequately controlled with metformin monotherapy (DURATION-8): a 28 week, multicentre, double-blind, phase 3, randomised controlled trial. *Lancet Diabetes Endocrinol.* (2016) 4:1004–16. doi: 10.1016/S2213-8587(16)30267-4
36. European Medicines Agency. *Guidelines on Bioanalytical Method Validation.* Available online at: http://www.ema.europa.eu/docs/en_GB/document_library/Scientific_guideline/2011/08/WC500109686.pdf (accessed 1 October, 2011).
37. McClean PL, Gault VA, Harriott P, Hölscher C. Glucagon-like peptide-1 analogues enhance synaptic plasticity in the brain: a link between diabetes and Alzheimer's disease. *Eur J Pharmacol.* (2010) 630:158–62. doi: 10.1016/j.ejphar.2009.12.023
38. Gejl M, Gjedde A, Egefjord L, Moller A, Hansen SB, Vang K, et al. In Alzheimer's disease, 6-month treatment with GLP-1 analog prevents decline of brain glucose metabolism: randomized, placebo-controlled, double-blind clinical trial. *Front Aging Neurosci.* (2016) 8:108. doi: 10.3389/fnagi.2016.00108
39. Pessentheiner AR, Pelzmann HJ, Walenta E, Schweiger M, Groschner LN, Graier WF, et al. NAT8L (N-acetyltransferase 8-like) accelerates lipid turnover and increases energy expenditure in brown adipocytes. *J Biol Chem.* (2013) 288:36040–51. doi: 10.1074/jbc.M113.491324
40. Surendran S, Matalon R, Tyring SK. Upregulation of aspartoacylase activity in the duodenum of obesity induced diabetes mouse: implications on diabetic neuropathy. *Biochem Biophys Res Commun.* (2006) 345:973–5. doi: 10.1016/j.bbrc.2006.04.179
41. Ruggieri M, Tortorella C, Ceci E, Paolicelli D, Solfrizzi V, Di Bitonto G, et al. Age-related changes of serum N-acetyl-aspartate in healthy controls. *Age Ageing.* (2011) 40:391–5. doi: 10.1093/ageing/afr021
42. Simone IL, Ruggieri M, Tortelli R, Ceci E, D'Errico E, Leo A, et al. Serum N-acetylaspartate level in amyotrophic lateral sclerosis. *Arch Neurol.* (2011) 68:1308–12. doi: 10.1001/archneurol.2011.217
43. Arai H, Satake S, Kozaki K. Cognitive frailty in geriatrics. *Clin Geriatr Med.* (2018) 34:667–75. doi: 10.1016/j.cger.2018.06.011
44. Namboodiri AM, Peethambaran A, Mathew R, Sambhu PA, Hershfield J, Moffett JR, et al. Canavan disease and the role of N-acetylaspartate in myelin synthesis. *Mol Cell Endocrinol.* (2006) 252:216–23. doi: 10.1016/j.mce.2006.03.016
45. Gazdzinski S Kornak J, Weiner MW, Meyerhoff DJ. Body mass index and magnetic resonance markers of brain integrity in adults. *Ann Neurol.* (2008) 63:652–7. doi: 10.1002/ana.21377
46. Coplan JD, Fathy HM, Abdallah CG, Ragab SA, Kral JG, Mao X, et al. Reduced hippocampal N-acetyl-aspartate (NAA) as a biomarker for overweight. *Neuroimage Clin.* (2014) 4:326–35. doi: 10.1016/j.nicl.2013.12.014
47. Thaler JP, Yi CX, Schur EA, Guyenet SJ, Hwang BH, Dietrich MO, et al. Obesity is associated with hypothalamic injury in rodents and humans. *J Clin Invest.* (2012) 122:153–62. doi: 10.1172/JCI59660
48. Buckman LB, Thompson MM, Lippert RN, Blackwell TS, Yull FE, Ellacott KLJ. Evidence for a novel funcional role of astrocytes in the acute homeostatic response to HFD. *Mol Metab.* (2014) 4:58–63. doi: 10.1016/j.molmet.2014.10.001
49. Garcia-Caceres C, Fuente-Martin E, Burgos-Ramos E, Granado M, Frago LM, Barrios V, et al. Differential acute and chronic effects of leptin on hypothalamic astrocyte morphology and synaptic protein levels. *Endocrinology.* (2011) 152:1809–18. doi: 10.1210/en.2010-1252
50. Fuente-Martin E, Garcia-Caceres C, Granado M, De Ceballos ML, Sanchez-Garrido MA, Sarman B, et al. Leptin regulates glutamate and glucose transporters in hypothalamic astrocytes. *J Clin Invest.* (2012) 122:3900–13. doi: 10.1172/JCI64102
51. Dhopeshwarkar GA, Mead JF. Uptake and transport of fatty acids into the brain and the role of the blood-brain barrier system. *Adv Lipid Res.* (1973) 11:109–42. doi: 10.1016/B978-0-12-024911-4.50010-6
52. Miller JC, Gnaedinger JM, Rapoport SI. Utilization of plasma fatty acid in rat brain: distribution of [14C] palmitate between oxidative and synthetic pathways. *J Neurochem.* (1987) 49:1507–14. doi: 10.1111/j.1471-4159.1987.tb01021.x
53. Smith QR, Nagura H. Fatty acid uptake and incorporation in brain: studies with the perfusion model. *J Mol Neurosci.* (2001) 16:167–72. doi: 10.1385/JMN:16:2-3:167
54. Horvath TL, Sarman B, Garcia-Caceres C, Enriori PJ, Sotonyi P, Shanabrough M, et al. Synaptic input organization of the melanocortin system predicts diet- induced hypothalamic reactive gliosis and obesity. *Proc Natl Acad Sci USA.* (2010) 107:14875–80. doi: 10.1073/pnas.1004282107
55. Won EY, Yoon MK, Kim SW, Jung Y, Bae HW, Lee D, et al. Gender-specific metabolomic profiling of obesity in leptin-deficient ob/ob mice by 1H NMR spectroscopy. *PLoS ONE.* (2013) 8:e75998. doi: 10.1371/journal.pone.0075998
56. Hardy OT, Perugini RA, Nicoloro SM, Gallagher-Dorval K, Puri V, Straubhaar J, et al. Body mass index-independent inflammation in omental adipose tissue associated with insulin resistance in morbid obesity. *Surg Obes Relat Dis.* (2011) 7:60–7. doi: 10.1016/j.soard.2010.05.013
57. Salek RM, Maguire ML, Bentley E, Rubtsov DV, Hough T, Cheeseman M, et al. A metabolomic comparison of urinary changes in type 2 diabetes in mouse, rat, and human. *Physiol Genomics.* (2007) 29:99–108. doi: 10.1152/physiolgenomics.00194.2006
58. Tomlinson DR, Gardiner NJ. Glucose neurotoxicity. *Nat Rev Neurosci.* (2008) 9:36–45. doi: 10.1038/nrn2294
59. Jacob RJ, Fan X, Evans ML, Dziura J, Sherwin RS. Brain glucose levels are elevated in chronically hyperglycemic diabetic rats: no evidence for protective adaptation by the blood brain barrier. *Metabolism.* (2002) 51:1522–4. doi: 10.1053/meta.2002.36347
60. Salceda R, Vilchis C, Coffe V, Hernandez-Munoz R. Changes in the redox state in the retina and brain during the onset of diabetes in rats. *Neurochem Res.* (1998) 23:893–7. doi: 10.1023/A:1022467230259
61. Bahniwal M, Little JP, Klegeris A. High glucose enhances neurotoxicity and inflammatory cytokine secretion by stimulated human astrocytes. *Curr Alzheimer Res.* (2017) 14:731–41. doi: 10.2174/1567205014666170117104053
62. During MJ, Cao L, Zuzga DS, Francis JS, Fitzsimons HL, Jiao X, et al. Glucagon-likepeptide-1 receptor is involved in learning and neuroprotection. *Nat Med.* (2003) 9:1173–9. doi: 10.1038/nm919
63. Perry T, Holloway HW, Weerasuriya A, Mouton PR, Duffy K, Mattison JA, et al. Evidence of GLP-1-mediated neuroprotection in an animal model of pyridoxine-induced peripheral sensory neuropathy. *Exp Neurol.* (2007) 203:293–301. doi: 10.1016/j.expneurol.2006.09.028
64. Hamilton A, Holscher C. Receptors for the insulin-like peptide GLP-1 are expressed on neurons in the CNS. *Neuroreport.* (2009) 20:1161–6. doi: 10.1097/WNR.0b013e32832fbf14
65. Iwai T, Ito S, Tanimitsu K, Udagawa S, Oka J. Glucagon-like peptide-1 inhibits LPS-induced IL-1beta production in cultured rat astrocytes. *Neurosci Res.* (2006) 55:352–60. doi: 10.1016/j.neures.2006.04.008
66. Gengler S, McClean P, McCurtin R, Gault VA, Hölscher C. Val(8)GLP-1 rescues synaptic plasticity and reduces dense core plaques in APP/PS1 mice. *Neurobiol Aging.* (2012) 33:265–76. doi: 10.1016/j.neurobiolaging.2010.02.014

67. Wang XH, Li L, Holscher C, Pan YF, Chen XR, QI JS. Val8-glucagon-like pep- tide-1 protects against Aβ 1-40-induced impairment of hippocampal late-phase long-term potentiation and spatial learning in rats. *Neuroscience.* (2010) 170:1239–48. doi: 10.1016/j.neuroscience.2010.08.028

68. Han W-N, Holscher C, Yuan L, Yang W, Wang XH, Wu MN, et al. Liraglutide protects against amyloid-β protein-induced impairment of spatial learning and memory in rats. *Neurobiol Aging.* (2012) 34:576-88. doi: 10.1016/j.neurobiolaging.2012.04.009

69. Perry T, Haughey NJ, Mattson MP, Egan JM, Greig NH. Protection and reversal of excitotoxic neuronal damage by glucagon-like peptide-1 and exendin-4. *J Pharmacol Exp Ther.* (2002) 302:881–8. doi: 10.1124/jpet.102.037481

70. Perry T, Lahiri DK, Sambamurti K, Chen D, Mattson MP, Egan JM, et al. Glucagon-like peptide-1 decreases endogenous amyloid-beta peptide (Abeta) levels and protects hippocampal neurons from death induced by Abeta and iron. *J Neurosci Res.* (2003) 72:603–12. doi: 10.1002/jnr.10611

71. Egefjord L, Gejl M, Moller A, Braendgaard H, Gottrup H, Antropova O, et al. Effects of liraglutide on neurodegeneration, blood flow and cognition in Alzheimer s disease-protocol for a controlled, randomized double-blinded trial. *Dan Med J.* (2012) 59:A4519.

27

Controversial Role of Robot in Primary and Revisional Bariatric Surgery Procedures: Review of the Literature and Personal Experience

Giovanni Fantola[1], Enrico Moroni[1], Matteo Runfola[2], Emanuele Lai[1], Stefano Pintus[1], Pierpaolo Gallucci[3], Francesco Pennestrì[4] and Marco Raffaelli[4]*

[1]Obesity Surgery Unit, Department of Surgery, ARNAS G. Brotzu, Cagliari, Italy, [2]Emergency Surgery Unit, Department of Surgery, ARNAS G. Brotzu, Cagliari, Italy, [3]Division of Endocrine and Metabolic Surgery, Fondazione Policlinico Universitario Agostino Gemelli IRCCS, Rome, Italy, [4]Division of Endocrine and Metabolic Surgery, Fondazione Policlinico Universitario Agostino Gemelli IRCCS, Università Cattolica del Sacro Cuore, Rome, Italy

***Correspondence:**
Giovanni Fantola
giovannifantola@aob.it

Laparoscopy is the surgical standard of care for bariatric procedures; however, during the last two decades, the robotic approach has gained increasing interest. It is currently considered a safe and effective alternative to laparoscopy. This literature review investigates the role of the robotic approach for primary and revisional bariatric procedures, with the particular aim of comparing this technique with the standard-of-care laparoscopic approach. The feasibility of robotic dissection and suturing could have potential advantages: robotics may prevent the risk of leak and bleeding and other surgical complications, determining potential benefits in terms of operative time, length of hospital stay, and learning curve. Considering primary procedures, the literature reveals no advantages in robotic versus the laparoscopic approach for adjustable gastric banding and sleeve gastrectomy. Robotic Roux-en-Y gastric bypass is associated with a longer operative time and a shorter hospital length of stay than laparoscopy. The robotic approach in revisional surgery has been proven to be safe and effective. Despite the longer operative time, the robotic platform could achieve a lower bleeding rate compared with laparoscopy. The surgeon's selection criteria related to referrals to the robotic approach of difficult-perceived cases could represent a bias. In conclusion, robotic surgery can be considered a safe and effective approach in both primary and revisional bariatric surgery, despite the lack of evidence to support its routine use in primary bariatric surgery. However, in revisional bariatric surgery and in surgical complex procedures, the robotic approach could have potential benefits in terms of surgical complications and learning curves.

Keywords: robotic surgery, daVinci, revisional surgery, gastric bypass, SADIS

INTRODUCTION

Bariatric surgery has emerged as a safe and effective treatment (1) for morbid obesity, defined as BMI ≥ 40 or BMI ≥ 35 associated with obesity-related diseases. In 2019, 256,000 bariatric surgery operations have been performed in the USA (2), and in 2021, 22,469 bariatric surgery operations have been performed in Italy (3).

Minimally invasive bariatric surgical procedures have been associated with improved early postoperative outcomes in comparison with open approaches, with very low mortality and low morbidity rates (4).

Laparoscopic surgery is currently considered the standard of care in the bariatric surgery approach, as open surgery remains only as a rescue operation or in case of contraindications to laparoscopy. However, advanced laparoscopic skills are required to achieve adequate surgical outcomes after laparoscopic bariatric procedures (5). In some conditions, such as patients with prior abdominal surgery or in complex bariatric procedures, like biliopancreatic diversion with duodenal switch (BPDDS), the laparoscopic approach can be challenging. With this background, the use of the robotic platform in bariatric surgery has been growing over the last two decades (6).

The aim of this review is to assess the current literature about the advantages and disadvantages of primary and revisional robot-assisted bariatric procedures in comparison with the standard-of-care laparoscopic approach.

MATERIALS AND METHODS

A systematic literature search was performed on PubMed and Google Scholar. Searched terms included keywords [robotic] [bariatric] [surgery] [davinci] [rygb] [sleeve gastrectomy] [sadi-s] [revisional] [primary]. All titles and abstracts were assessed to select those focusing on robotic bariatric surgery. Subsequently, the full text of the selected trials was independently screened by the authors for eligibility. Inclusion criteria were comparative and non-comparative studies, including patients who underwent primary and revisional robotic bariatric surgery.

ROBOTIC SURGERY

For two decades, the robotic platform has offered surgeons better instruments for performing minimally invasive procedures, allowing more difficult procedures to be performed, from esophageal to rectal resections, including bariatric surgery. Technical advantages include tridimensional viewing with a binocular camera, wristed graspers, dissectors, and staplers, providing both improved articulation and rotation, tremor filtering for more precise handling (7), allowing hand-sewn anastomosis (8), resulting in reduced fatigue (9), and improved surgical abilities (10) compared with laparoscopic surgery.

On the other hand, robotic surgery is still a subject of debate because of its longer learning curve, increased costs, and consequently reduced cost-effectiveness.

Indeed, cost is an important drawback in robotic surgery. Costs include robotic platform purchase, instruments with a limited life span, and annual service maintenance (20% of total cost/year). Overall, the DaVinci Robotic Surgical System with dual console and fourth arm costs about 4.5 million Euros on a 7-year pay-off period. Consequently, direct procedural costs are generally higher for robotic bariatric procedures in comparison with conventional laparoscopy. This overcost is on average about 2.3 times more expensive per patient (11). There are several factors that could reduce the cost per patient and improve cost-effectiveness. The number of robotic procedures per year using a specific robotic system may reduce the costs of initial purchase and annual maintenance. It is generally estimated that less than 250 procedures/year is not sufficient for a medical center to rationalize robotic overcosts. Decreasing the length of hospital and ICU stay could also be used to balance the overcosts in comparison with laparoscopic procedures. However, this remains to be proven using clear comparative data, because Bertoni et al. recently demonstrated that robotic surgery is only non-inferior to laparoscopic surgery (12).

PRIMARY PROCEDURES

Sleeve Gastrectomy

In 2000, Sudan et al. described the first case of robotic Sleeve Gastrectomy (SG) as the first part of robotic BPDDS (13). Current data have shown no clear postoperative improvements in comparison with the conventional laparoscopic approach. In this review, we only selected studies including more than 50 patients (**Table 1**). Romero et al. compared 134 patients who underwent a robotic SG with a systematic review of 3,148 patients after conventional laparoscopic sleeve (14). Sixty-three cases of anastomotic leaks (1.97%), 12 gastric strictures (0.43%), and 34 bleedings (1.21%) in the laparoscopic group were observed. No leak, no stricture, and only one bleeding (0.7%) were observed in the robotic group. The mean surgical time was longer in the robotic group (106 versus 94.5 min). However, the mean hospital stay was significantly shorter in

TABLE 1 | Literature review of robotic Sleeve Gastrectomy.

Study	N	Type	Operative time (min)	Major morbidity (%)	Conversion (%)	Los (day)
Romero (1)	134	CCT	106.6	3	0	2.2
Vilallonga (2)	100	CCT	108.18	5	0	4.3
Kannan (3)	103	CCT	110	0	0	4.2
Nasser (4) *(Revisional)*	1,077	RS	145.2	6.7%	0.3%	1.9

CCT, clinical controlled trial; RS, retrospective study; NA, not available.

the robotic group (2.2 versus 3.3 days). This study concluded that similar perioperative outcomes were observed in both approaches, although the robotic platform could provide a more comfortable environment for the operating surgeon.

Another comparative study analyzed 100 robotic versus 100 laparoscopic SG (15). It reported three leaks in the robotic group (3%) and four in the laparoscopic group (4%). The mean hospital stay was similar in both groups ranging from 3 to 4 days. This study concluded that the robotic approach was feasible, but cost issues and mean operative times may need to be improved. Kannan et al. (16) reported 108 patients (62 laparoscopic versus 46 robotic SG). This study showed no difference in terms of postoperative complication rates and mean operating time.

Gastric By-Pass

In this literature review, we selected six clinical controlled trials, three case series, one systematic review, and one meta-analysis (**Table 2**). Only published series including more than 50 patients were considered. Ayloo et al. (17) reported a total of 135 RYGB (Roux-en-Y gastric bypass). Among them, 45 RYGB were performed laparoscopically and 90 were robot-assisted. This study showed no difference in terms of postoperative morbidity rates. Intraoperative data also showed a shorter operative time in robotic group patients (207 versus 227 min). Hagen et al. (18) reported 990 patients who underwent a gastric bypass from June 1997 to July 2010. There were 524 open, 323 laparoscopic, and 143 robotic cases. This study concluded that significantly fewer anastomotic complications were observed after open and robotic RYGB (0%) in comparison with laparoscopic RYGB (4.1%). However, this study is associated with potential bias due to its long inclusion period spanning over 13 years.

A review including a total of 18 studies was published by Fourman et al. (19). A total of 1,750 patients was included with a mean operative time of 192 min in robotic versus 173 min in laparoscopic group patients. The postoperative complication rate was similar in both groups (7.9% versus 8.6%). This review concluded that robotic group patients had fewer anastomotic leaks (4 versus 21 patients) and fewer anastomotic strictures (17 versus 40 patients).

In 2013, Benizri et al. (20) reported 200 RYGB performed by two experienced bariatric surgeons (100 robotic versus 100 conventional laparoscopic RYGB). This study showed a significantly higher postoperative morbidity rate in robotic group patients regarding surgical complications (13% versus 1%; $p = 0.001$). Consequently, more patients had a reoperation (9% versus 1%). However, intraoperative data showed a shorter mean operative time in the robotic group (130 versus 147 min). Overall, the mean hospital stay was longer in the robotic group (9.3 versus 6.7 days, $p = 0.001$). Later, Ahmad et al. (21) reported 173 laparoscopic versus 172 robotic RYGB procedures. No difference was observed in terms of intraoperative events, conversions to open procedures, leaks, strictures, returns to the operating room within 30 days, and mortality. Smeenk et al. (22) reported 100 laparoscopic versus 100 robotic RYGB procedures. The morbidity rate was 5% in both groups and major morbidity rates (Clavien-Dindo class 3–4) were similar (3% versus 1%; $p = 0.62$), and there was no mortality. The mean operative room time was 117 min in robotic versus 66 min in laparoscopic group patients ($p < 0.05$).

Non-comparative series was also used to evaluate robotic RYGB. Tieu et al. (23) included 1,100 patients with robotic RYGB from two high-volume medical centers. The ninety-day major complication rate was 4.09% (45 patients). Fantola et al. analyzed 302 consecutive robotic RYGB. In this study, the 60-day major complication rate (Clavien-Dindo score 3 or 4) and reoperation rate were 12.2% and 10.2%, respectively. Fourteen patients (4.6%) had a postoperative anastomotic leak requiring specific surgical management (24).

SADI-S

Single Anastomosis Duodenal-ileostomy with Sleeve gastrectomy (SADI-S) is a novel surgical technique, emerging

TABLE 2 | Literature review of robotic Roux-en-Y Gastric Bypass.

Study	N	Type	Operative time (min)	Overall morbidity (%)	Major morbidity (%)	Conversion (%)	Los (day)
Sanchez (5)	50	RCT	130.8	0	0	1	2.72
Ayloo (6)	90	CCT	207	2.2	1.1	0	2
Fourman (7)	1,750	Systematic review	192	7.9	NA	NA	2.72–3
Hagen (8)	143	CCT	NA	16.1	NA	1.4	7.4
Tieu (9)	1,100	Case series	155	14	4.09	0	NA
Renaud (10)	154	Case series	141	33.1	11	2.6	NA
Ahmad (10)	172	CCT	155	NA	0	0	2.4
Smeenk (11)	100	CCT	117	5	3	0	2
Economopoulos (12)	5,155	Meta-analysis	NA	NA	NA	NA	NA
Myers (13)	100	CCT	144	NA	12	NA	2.1
Benizri (14)	100	CCT	130	24	13	0	9.3
Nasser (4) (Revisional)	1,230	RS	196.7	9.3%	NA	0.7	2.4

RCT, randomized controlled trial; CCT, clinical controlled trial; RS, retrospective study; NA, not available.

from the BDPDDS legacy, aiming to reduce BPDDS risks, while maintaining its efficacy as one of the most effective interventions. It is considered a valid alternative to BPDDS, associated with a lower complication rate (25). It has also usually been considered an alternative to one-anastomosis gastric bypass (OAGB), more challenging from a technical point of view, but associated with a lower risk of complications.

Very few studies reported data from robotic SADI-S procedures. Nelson et al. reported a case series of robotic procedures (also including 10 laparoscopic procedures) and demonstrated that the robotic approach is safe and effective with an acceptable risk–benefit ratio but does not offer a comparison with the laparoscopic or open approach.

REVISIONAL SURGERY

In the last few years, the number of reoperative procedures is rapidly increasing, as every year, more and more primary bariatric procedures are performed.

Reoperative bariatric surgery has been classified by Brethauer et al. (26) into the following:

- Conversion: procedures that change from an index procedure to a different type of procedure.
- Corrective: procedures addressing complications or incomplete treatment effect of a previous bariatric operation.
- Reversal: procedures that restore original anatomy.

Insufficient weight loss or weight regain, initial defect or late-surgical complication (e.g., GERD (27)), excessive weight loss, and malnutrition are an indication for revisional bariatric surgery (28) that must be taken into account in a multidisciplinary setting that includes surgical, nutritional, and psychological risks and benefits (29).

Revisional surgery has been associated with poorer outcomes in both RYGB (30), with increased intraoperative blood loss, longer operative time, longer adhesiolysis, longer hospital length of stay, higher rate of splenic injury, anastomotic leakage, and surgical site infections in comparison with primary RYGB, and in revisional SG compared with primary SG (31), with longer operative time, higher complication rate, and anastomotic leakage rate.

Due to increased operative difficulty, because revisional surgery is more challenging and requires a higher level of technical skills, the robotic platform may be considered for better visualization, dissection, and a wider range of movement provided by robotic instruments that could provide a better outcome to bariatric revisional procedures (32).

Clapp et al. (33) systematically analyzed revisional weight loss robotic surgery from the MBSAQIP database spanning from 2015 to 2016 and compared them with laparoscopic revisional procedures. One thousand nine hundred twenty-nine robotic procedures and 35,998 laparoscopic revisional procedures were found. Statistical analysis showed a longer operative time, prolonged hospital length of stay, and higher ICU admission rate in the robotic group than in the laparoscopic group. Other parameters taken into account showed no differences, which led the authors to state that no difference exists in postoperative complications. As a higher number of anastomosis revisions were done in the robotic group, the authors hypothesized that a selection bias could exist, with surgeons preferring robotic surgery in high-difficulty-perceived procedures.

A comparative analysis from Nasser et al. (34) (**Tables 1, 2**) taking into account procedures from the MBSAQIP database performed between 2015 and 2017 analyzed a series of revisional procedures, comparing the laparoscopic and robotic approaches.

As for revisional SG, 15,935 procedures were laparoscopic and 1,077 were robotic. Demographic characteristics were homogeneous in the two groups, and the authors found differences in terms of longer operative time in the robotic group, higher incidence of intraoperative adhesiolysis in the robotic group, higher incidence of overall morbidity in the robotic group, and higher incidence of ICU admission, sepsis, and organ-space SSI in the robotic group. No differences were found in terms of other parameters.

As for revisional RYGB, 11,212 procedures were laparoscopic and 1,230 were robotic. Demographic characteristics were homogeneous, a higher rate of drainage placement was found in the laparoscopic group, the operative time was longer in the robotic group, respiratory complications, postoperative pneumonia, and superficial SSI were higher in the laparoscopic group, and the incidence of bleeding requiring transfusion was higher in the laparoscopic group. No differences were found in terms of other parameters. Study limitation embraced a possible surgeon's selection bias, as challenging cases might have been purposely selected for the robotic or laparoscopic group, and the MBSAQIP database provides postoperative data only up to 30 days, from a variety of heterogeneous centers.

Vilallonga et al. (35) presented a 3-case report of robotic revisional SADI-S (36) secondary to SG. In this study (35), the authors conclude the feasibility of robotic revisional SADI-S and its advantages over RYGB, as the Billroth-2 style duodenal-ileal-anastomosis might reduce operative time and postoperative complications.

A single-center study from King et al. (37) including 167 revisional procedures (115 laparoscopic, 52 robotic) demonstrated a reduced major complication rate in the robotic group than in the laparoscopic group (1 [1.9%] versus 6 [5.2%], $p > 0.05$) and a shorter hospital length of stay in the robotic group than in the other group (40.2 versus 62.6 h, respectively, $p < 0.05$), with no differences in minor complications, blood loss, and readmission rates.

Rebecchi et al. (38), reporting their results from a single-center study, performed a cost-related analysis of revisional robotic RYGB performed with the DaVinci Robotic Surgical System. The mean cost was found to be 14,334.70€ ± 2,920.40€, but they demonstrated that specific-robot expenses decreased in the last 10 cases of the study (9,708.50€ ± 515.70€) compared with the first 30 cases (12,168.70€ ± 1,438.40€), as the total cost for a laparoscopy procedure was 3,176.50€ ± 850.50€.

The increased costs of the robotic procedure have to be addressed in specific semidisposable instruments and robotic maintenance fees, even though the clinical benefits could overcome increased costs.

AUTHORS' PERSONAL EXPERIENCE

Between the period January 2013 and March 2022, over 3,659 bariatric procedures (403—11.6% revisional ones) were performed at the Division of Endocrine and Metabolic Surgery (Fondazione Policlinico Universitario Agostino Gemelli IRCCS, Rome, Italy). Sixty-seven (1.8%) patients were scheduled for a robotic approach. Specifically, 37 RYGB, 23 SADI-S, 6 OAGB, and one BPD were performed.

The first robotic procedure, an RYGB, was performed in January 2013, while the first robotic SADI-S was performed in July 2016. However, the robotic approach was implemented starting from 2019, with a relative reduction in the number of performed procedures during the first phases of the COVID-19 pandemic (2020–2021).

As previously reported, 37 robotic-assisted RYGBs were performed. The median operative time was 201 min. We experienced only one postoperative surgical complication, a gastroenteric anastomotic leak, in a super-super-obese patient (BMI $\geq$ 60 kg/m^2), which required surgical exploration (Clavien-Dindo IIIb). The subsequent postoperative course was uneventful, and the patient was discharged after 14 days.

In addition, 23 SADI-S were performed, in 22 cases as a primary procedure and in 1 case as a revisional operation. Recently, we reported our personal experience (currently under peer review) comparing the robotic and laparoscopic approaches in SADI-S, using propensity score matching analysis to avoid potential bias selection. The median operative time for robotic SADI-S was 191.5 min with the docking step requiring approximately 10 min. Using the CUSUM method to analyze the learning curves of the different approaches (laparoscopic versus robotic) for SADI-S, we observed a significant reduction in operating time after the first seven cases for the robotic SADI-S and after the first 47 cases for the laparoscopic approach. Thus, the use of the robotic platform reduces the time required to complete the learning curve for these challenging procedures. In addition, our analysis highlights that the laparoscopic and robotic approaches for SADI-S are comparable in terms of safety for reoperative and postoperative complications.

Furthermore, we performed six OAGBs (five primary procedures and one revisional) with a median operative time of 191 min. We chose this procedure at the beginning of our experience with the robotic platform in obese patients before the introduction of SADI-S in our clinical practice. For the same reason, we also performed a DPD with an operative time of 240 min.

From July 2021, the Obesity Surgery Unit (ARNAS G. Brotzu, Cagliari, Italy) started a robotic bariatric program. Eight robotic-assisted RYGB were performed. The median operative time was 240 min, with an improvement after the first five cases. One patient was reoperated because of alimentary limb occlusion due to jejuno-jejunal kinking.

Overall, after combining both series, no intraoperative deaths occurred in our robotic experience. No conversion was necessary, either to open or laparoscopic surgery. No 30-day mortality was recorded.

In our experience, the main indications for the robotic approach are challenging for bariatric patients. "Challenging cases" are a clinical characteristic that cannot be assessed by a single parameter but is determined by the presence of one or more of these conditions: patients with a BMI $\geq$ 50 kg/m^2, especially if they are male and/or with a previous major abdominal surgery. Furthermore, according to other authors, we trust that the robotic platform can add value to these patients by reducing the number of two-stage procedures.

DISCUSSION

Laparoscopy has been the standard of care in choosing a surgical approach in bariatric surgery since the last two decades and has contributed to the large diffusion of bariatric procedures worldwide. In this context, robotic surgery remains controversial.

In our review, we analyzed some of the most performed procedures, considering both primary and revisional procedures, and we observed that in primary surgery, robotic surgery is safe and effective but offers no advantages in perioperative care compared with laparoscopic surgery. However, in revisional surgery, which has a higher rate of postoperative complications due to adhesions and altered anatomy and, therefore, requiring higher laparoscopic skills, the robotic approach could have a primary role. This was proved by Nasser et al. (34), who demonstrated a reduced complication rate in revisional robotic RYGB compared with the laparoscopic approach.

It must also be considered that in most studies taken into account, there was no patient randomization, and patients who were perceived more challenging by the surgeon were assigned to robotic surgery, with a clear selection bias. These obviously included superobese patients (BMI > 50 kg/m^2) in whom fine dissection and, especially, suturing could be particularly challenging without the robotic platform. Further studies comparing a similar group of patients, eventually by randomization, are, thus, necessary in order to draw a definitive conclusion in this regard.

On the other hand, as most of the bariatric procedures are performed on a single abdominal quadrant, robotic platform benefits could be less emphasized compared with other surgical fields and have a longer learning curve and longer operative time than laparoscopy (39). However, the authors' personal experience has demonstrated that the robotic platform is able to reduce the learning curve for a single, complex procedure, as SADI-S does.

Cost-effectiveness has been, since its adoption, one of the main drawbacks in robotic surgery, as DRG reimburses might be insufficient to cover robotic extra costs (40). A cost analysis by Khorgami et al. (41) demonstrated that robotic surgery is the factor associated with the highest impact on extra costs in bariatric surgery.

However, as Hagen et al. (42) demonstrated that laparoscopic staplers might reduce robotic costs compared with robotic staplers, robotic costs can be further mitigated with avoidance of staplers with handsewn anastomosis, which showed a reduced complication rate compared with laparoscopic-stapled anastomosis (18) and, therefore, a further cost mitigation. Moreover, as a robotic platform enhances the surgeon's ability in sewing compared with laparoscopy, further studies are needed to compare handsewn anastomosis and stapled mechanical anastomosis, considering that handsewn anastomosis is tailored, is opposed to standardized staplers, and the anastomotic stricture rate tends to be lower with a handsewn technique (43), and that could be most useful in complex procedures (i.e., SADI-S).

Most studies found in the current literature were based on the DaVinci Robotic Surgical System, while no data were found in regard to other robotic platforms.

More studies are, however, necessary to address the efficacy and sustainability of the robotic approach, as most studies to date have lacked randomization and, therefore, have a selection bias that has prevented a proper data evaluation. It should also be noted that a fully trained surgeon in robotic bariatric surgery, and, therefore, able to deal with challenging cases intended for robotic surgery, has to complete a learning curve that, especially in the initial stages, cannot be based on challenging cases and, therefore, includes primary bariatric procedures that currently, due to increased costs, are not routinely performed with the robotic platform but with laparoscopy instead.

CONCLUSION

Robotic surgery remains a valid surgical approach in treating morbid obesity, but, because of its inflated costs, it cannot be a first-choice option as its advantages over laparoscopy are restricted to surgeon ergonomics and not to patient perioperative care and, therefore, it is not financially sustainable. However, in selected cases, including revisional cases and superobese patients, robotic surgery could have a potential role in reducing postoperative complications and improving perioperative care, and, therefore, it also could be economically sustainable.

AUTHOR CONTRIBUTIONS

GF contributed to primary procedures, EL, MR, SP, EM, FP, and PG contributed to introduction, revisional procedures, and discussion, and MR reviewed the manuscript.

REFERENCES

1. Arterburn DE, Telem DA, Kushner RF, Courcoulas AP. Benefits and risks of bariatric surgery in adults: a review. *JAMA.* (2020) 324:879–87. doi: 10.1001/jama.2020.12567
2. Estimate of Bariatric Surgery Numbers, 2011–2019. *American Society for Metabolic and Bariatric Surgery* (2021). Available from: https://asmbs.org/resources/estimate-of-bariatric-surgery-numbers (Accessed December 29, 2021).
3. SICOB. Indagine conoscitiva anno 2021. *Soc Ital Chir Dell Obesità* (2022). Available from: https://www.sicob.org/00_allegati_news/indagine_2021.pdf (Accessed February 16, 2022).
4. DeMaria EJ, Pate V, Warthen M, Winegar DA. Baseline data from American society for metabolic and bariatric surgery-designated bariatric surgery centers of excellence using the bariatric outcomes longitudinal database. *Surg Obes Relat Dis Off J Am Soc Bariatr Surg.* (2010) 6:347–55. doi: 10.1016/j.soard.2009.11.015
5. Wilson EB, Sudan R. The evolution of robotic bariatric surgery. *World J Surg.* (2013) 37:2756–60. doi: 10.1007/s00268-013-2125-3
6. Antanavicius G, Mohammed R, Van Houtte O. Total robotic biliopancreatic diversion with duodenal switch technique. *Obes Surg.* (2017) 27:1104–8. doi: 10.1007/s11695-016-2513-5
7. Vining CC, Skowron KB, Hogg ME. Robotic gastrointestinal surgery: learning curve, educational programs and outcomes. *Updat Surg.* (2021) 73:799–814. doi: 10.1007/s13304-021-00973-0
8. Jiang H-P, Lin L-L, Jiang X, Qiao H-Q. Meta-analysis of hand-sewn versus mechanical gastrojejunal anastomosis during laparoscopic Roux-en-Y gastric bypass for morbid obesity. *Int J Surg.* (2016) 32:150–7. doi: 10.1016/j.ijsu.2016.04.024
9. Aitchison LP, Cui CK, Arnold A, Abbott J. The ergonomics of laparoscopic surgery in live surgical environments. *J Minim Invasive Gynecol.* (2015) 22:S105. doi: 10.1016/j.jmig.2015.08.283
10. Moorthy K, Munz Y, Dosis A, Hernandez J, Martin S, Bello F, et al. Dexterity enhancement with robotic surgery. *Surg Endosc Interv Tech.* (2004) 18:790–5. doi: 10.1007/s00464-003-8922-2
11. Myers SR, McGuirl J, Wang J. Robot-assisted versus laparoscopic gastric bypass: comparison of short-term outcomes. *Obes Surg.* (2013) 23:467–73. doi: 10.1007/s11695-012-0848-0
12. Bertoni MV, Marengo M, Garofalo F, Volontè F, La Regina D, Gass M, et al. Robotic-assisted versus laparoscopic revisional bariatric surgery: a systematic review and meta-analysis on perioperative outcomes. *Obes Surg.* (2021) 31:5022–33. doi: 10.1007/s11695-021-05668-4
13. Sudan R, Puri V, Sudan D. Robotically assisted biliary pancreatic diversion with a duodenal switch: a new technique. *Surg Endosc.* (2007) 21:729–33. doi: 10.1007/s00464-006-9171-y
14. Romero RJ, Kosanovic R, Rabaza JR, Seetharamaiah R, Donkor C, Gallas M, et al. Robotic sleeve gastrectomy: experience of 134 cases and comparison with a systematic review of the laparoscopic approach. *Obes Surg.* (2013) 23:1743–52. doi: 10.1007/s11695-013-1004-1
15. Vilallonga R, Fort JM, Caubet E, Gonzalez O, Armengol M. Robotic sleeve gastrectomy versus laparoscopic sleeve gastrectomy: a comparative study with 200 patients. *Obes Surg.* (2013) 23:1501–7. doi: 10.1007/s11695-013-1039-3
16. Kannan U, Ecker BL, Choudhury R, Dempsey DT, Williams NN, Dumon KR. Laparoscopic hand-assisted versus robotic-assisted laparoscopic sleeve gastrectomy: experience of 103 consecutive cases. *Surg Obes Relat Dis Off J Am Soc Bariatr Surg.* (2016) 12:94–9. doi: 10.1016/j.soard.2015.07.011
17. Ayloo SM, Addeo P, Buchs NC, Shah G, Giulianotti PC. Robot-assisted versus laparoscopic Roux-en-Y gastric bypass: is there a difference in outcomes? *World J Surg.* (2011) 35:637–42. doi: 10.1007/s00268-010-0938-x
18. Hagen ME, Pugin F, Chassot G, Huber O, Buchs N, Iranmanesh P, et al. Reducing cost of surgery by avoiding complications: the model of robotic roux-en-Y gastric bypass. *Obes Surg.* (2012) 22:52–61. doi: 10.1007/s11695-011-0422-1
19. Fourman MM, Saber AA. Robotic bariatric surgery: a systematic review. *Surg Obes Relat Dis Off J Am Soc Bariatr Surg.* (2012) 8:483–8. doi: 10.1016/j.soard.2012.02.012
20. Benizri EI, Renaud M, Reibel N, Germain A, Ziegler O, Zarnegar R, et al. Perioperative outcomes after totally robotic gastric bypass: a prospective nonrandomized controlled study. *Am J Surg.* (2013) 206:145–51. doi: 10.1016/j.amjsurg.2012.07.049

21. Ahmad A, Carleton JD, Ahmad ZF, Agarwala A. Laparoscopic versus robotic-assisted Roux-en-Y gastric bypass: a retrospective, single-center study of early perioperative outcomes at a community hospital. *Surg Endosc.* (2016) 30:3792–6. doi: 10.1007/s00464-015-4675-y
22. Smeenk RM, van 't Hof G, Elsten E, Feskens PGBM. The results of 100 robotic versus 100 laparoscopic gastric bypass procedures: a single high volume centre experience. *Obes Surg.* (2016) 26:1266–73. doi: 10.1007/s11695-015-1933-y
23. Tieu K, Allison N, Snyder B, Wilson T, Toder M, Wilson E. Robotic-assisted Roux-en-Y gastric bypass: update from 2 high-volume centers. *Surg Obes Relat Dis Off J Am Soc Bariatr Surg.* (2013) 9:284–8. doi: 10.1016/j.soard.2011.11.022
24. Fantola G, Nguyen-Thi PL, Reibel N, Sirveaux MA, Germain A, Ayav A, et al. Risk factors for postoperative morbidity after totally robotic gastric bypass in 302 consecutive patients. *Obes Surg.* (2015) 25:1229–38. doi: 10.1007/s11695-014-1530-5
25. Pennestrì F, Sessa L, Prioli F, Salvi G, Gallucci P, Ciccoritti L, et al. Single anastomosis duodenal-ileal bypass with sleeve gastrectomy (SADI-S): experience from a high-bariatric volume center. *Langenbecks Arch Surg.* (2022). doi: 10.1007/s00423-022-02501-z
26. Brethauer SA, Kothari S, Sudan R, Williams B, English WJ, Brengman M, et al. Systematic review on reoperative bariatric surgery: American society for metabolic and bariatric surgery revision task force. *Surg Obes Relat Dis.* (2014) 10:952–72. doi: 10.1016/j.soard.2014.02.014
27. Clapp B, Wynn M, Martyn C, Foster C, O'Dell M, Tyroch A. Long term (7 or more years) outcomes of the sleeve gastrectomy: a meta-analysis. *Surg Obes Relat Dis.* (2018) 14:741–7. doi: 10.1016/j.soard.2018.02.027
28. Bion AL, Le Roux Y, Alves A, Menahem B. Bariatric revisional surgery: what are the challenges for the patient and the practitioner? *J Visc Surg.* (2021) 158:38–50. doi: 10.1016/j.jviscsurg.2020.08.014
29. Vilallonga R, Fort JM, Rodríguez Luna MR, García Ruiz de Gordejuela A, Gonzalez O, Caubet E, et al. The panoramic view of revisional bariatric surgery. *J Laparoendosc Adv Surg Tech.* (2022) 32:6–11. doi: 10.1089/lap.2021.0506
30. Zhang L, Tan WH, Chang R, Eagon JC. Perioperative risk and complications of revisional bariatric surgery compared to primary Roux-en-Y gastric bypass. *Surg Endosc.* (2015) 29:1316–20. doi: 10.1007/s00464-014-3848-4
31. Mahawar KK, Graham Y, Carr WRJ, Jennings N, Schroeder N, Balupuri S, et al. Revisional roux-en-Y gastric bypass and sleeve gastrectomy: a systematic review of comparative outcomes with respective primary procedures. *Obes Surg.* (2015) 25:1271–80. doi: 10.1007/s11695-015-1670-2
32. Vilallonga R, Cirera de Tudela A, Möller EG, Piñeiro LV, Segura MB, Ferreruela MP, et al. Robotic revisional experience. single centre prospective cohort study and review of the literature. *Chir Buchar Rom 1990.* (2021) 116:7–15. doi: 10.21614/chirurgia.116.1.7
33. Clapp B, Liggett E, Jones R, Lodeiro C, Dodoo C, Tyroch A. Comparison of robotic revisional weight loss surgery and laparoscopic revisional weight loss surgery using the MBSAQIP database. *Surg Obes Relat Dis.* (2019) 15:909–19. doi: 10.1016/j.soard.2019.03.022
34. Nasser H, Munie S, Kindel TL, Gould JC, Higgins RM. Comparative analysis of robotic versus laparoscopic revisional bariatric surgery: perioperative outcomes from the MBSAQIP database. *Surg Obes Relat Dis.* (2020) 16:397–405. doi: 10.1016/j.soard.2019.11.018
35. Vilallonga R, Fort JM, Caubet E, Gonzalez O, Balibrea JM, Ciudin A, et al. Robotically assisted single anastomosis duodenoileal bypass after previous sleeve gastrectomy implementing high valuable technology for complex procedures. *J Obes.* (2015) 2015:1–6. doi: 10.1155/2015/586419
36. Sánchez-Pernaute A, Rubio Herrera MA, Pérez-Aguirre E, García Pérez JC, Cabrerizo L, Díez Valladares L, et al. Proximal duodenal–ileal end-to-side bypass with sleeve gastrectomy: proposed technique. *Obes Surg.* (2007) 17:1614–8. doi: 10.1007/s11695-007-9287-8
37. King K, Galvez A, Stoltzfus J, Claros L, El Chaar M. Robotic-assisted surgery results in a shorter hospital stay following revisional bariatric surgery. *Obes Surg.* (2021) 31:634–9. doi: 10.1007/s11695-020-05022-0
38. Rebecchi F, Ugliono E, Allaix ME, Toppino M, Borello A, Morino M. Robotic roux-en-Y gastric bypass as a revisional bariatric procedure: a single-center prospective cohort study. *Obes Surg.* (2020) 30:11–7. doi: 10.1007/s11695-019-04117-7
39. Addison P, Yoo A, Duarte-Ramos J, Addy J, Dechario S, Husk G, et al. Correlation between operative time and crowd-sourced skills assessment for robotic bariatric surgery. *Surg Endosc.* (2021) 35:5303–9. doi: 10.1007/s00464-020-08019-z
40. Mühlmann G, Klaus A, Kirchmayr W, Wykypiel H, Unger A, Höller E, et al. DaVinci robotic-assisted laparoscopic bariatric surgery: is it justified in a routine setting? *Obes Surg.* (2003) 13:848–54. doi: 10.1381/096089203322618632
41. Khorgami Z, Aminian A, Shoar S, Andalib A, Saber AA, Schauer PR, et al. Cost of bariatric surgery and factors associated with increased cost: an analysis of national inpatient sample. *Surg Obes Relat Dis.* (2017) 13:1284–9. doi: 10.1016/j.soard.2017.04.010
42. Hagen ME, Jung MK, Fakhro J, Buchs NC, Buehler L, Mendoza JM, et al. Robotic versus laparoscopic stapling during robotic Roux-en-Y gastric bypass surgery: a case-matched analysis of costs and clinical outcomes. *Surg Endosc.* (2018) 32:472–7. doi: 10.1007/s00464-017-5707-6
43. Kravetz AJ, Reddy S, Murtaza G, Yenumula P. A comparative study of handsewn versus stapled gastrojejunal anastomosis in laparoscopic Roux-en-Y gastric bypass. *Surg Endosc.* (2011) 25:1287–92. doi: 10.1007/s00464-010-1362-x

28

The Effect of Metabolic Surgery on the Complications of Diabetes: What are the Unanswered Questions?

Karl J. Neff[1*†] *and Carel W. Le Roux*[1,2†]

[1] *Diabetes Complications Research Centre, Conway Institute, University College Dublin, Dublin, Ireland,* [2] *Metabolic Medicine, Imperial College London, London, United Kingdom*

Correspondence:
Karl J. Neff
karl.neff@hse.ie

† These authors have contributed equally to this work

It is now established that metabolic surgery (also known as bariatric surgery or obesity surgery) is an effective treatment for type 2 diabetes. Data from several randomized controlled trials have shown that surgery, when used as an adjunct to best medical therapy, is superior to medical therapy alone in achieving glycaemic and metabolic treatment targets in diabetes care. This has resulting in metabolic surgery being recommended as a treatment option for obesity-associated type 2 diabetes in national and international diabetes care guidelines. While the superior glycaemic effect of surgery is clear, the effect of surgery on the complications of diabetes is not fully understood. There are observational and epidemiological data that indicate a preventative effect in cohorts who do not have complications at baseline, as well as a positive effect on those with established diabetic kidney disease. However, there is a dearth of randomized controlled studies that specifically examine the effect of surgery on the complications of diabetes. Therefore, we should remain cautious in some cases, especially in those with retinopathy or neuropathy, as there is potential for deterioration of disease post-operatively. Further study is needed on this important topic. A lot is known, but there remain several unanswered questions. This article summarizes what we know about the effect of metabolic surgery on the complications of diabetes, poses some unanswered questions, and suggests how we could answer them.

Keywords: metabolic surgery, diabetes, kidney disease, nephropathy, retinopathy, neuropathy

INTRODUCTION

Metabolic surgery (also referred to as bariatric surgery or obesity surgery) is now recommended as a mainstream treatment for type 2 diabetes in people who have both obesity and type 2 diabetes (1). This recommendation, supported by multiple international diabetes organizations including the American Diabetes Association and the International Diabetes Federation, is based on data from randomized controlled trials comparing surgical intervention to best medical therapy (2). In these trials, metabolic surgery has been proven to improve glycaemic control, in the short- and medium-term, to a greater extent than medical therapy alone (2). Surgery is particularly recommended for people with both obesity and type 2 diabetes in whom dietary and medical therapy has been unsuccessful in achieving diabetes treatment targets.

In many cases, the effect of surgery on type 2 diabetes can be so great as to induce remission of disease and normalization of glycaemia. It should be noted that this effect is often transient (3, 4). Therefore, surgery should not be offered as a "cure"' for diabetes, but rather as an effective treatment for type 2 diabetes. Approximately 50% of those who have metabolic surgery and achieve remission of their diabetes will have recurrence of diabetes within the subsequent 10 years (3). However, despite the recurrence of diabetes, these patients usually achieve much better glycaemic and metabolic control than they did before surgery, and so the beneficial glycaemic and metabolic effect of surgery, as compared to medical therapy alone, is retained (3).

However, it should be noted that surgical treatment of diabetes and obesity has associated complications (1, 2). The specific surgical complications are procedure dependent, but all surgical recipients will be at risk of hospitalization for treatment of complications of surgery, and will remain at high risk of micronutrient malnutrition, with the potential for associated anemia or neuropathy, for life (1). Surgery is not for everyone. An expert multidisciplinary assessment is needed for all surgical candidates to ensure that they are suitable and ready for surgery. Given the highly specialist nature of this work, surgery should only be performed in high volume centers by specialist surgeons who work within expert multidisciplinary teams (1).

The improved glycaemic control achieved with surgery could be expected to reduce the burden of microvascular complications in people with diabetes. However, there are not many randomized controlled trials specifically examining the effect of metabolic surgery on microvascular outcomes. There are experimental models, observational data, and one randomized controlled trial, that support the hypothesis that surgery could have a role in managing not only diabetes, but also its complications. However, many unanswered questions remain.

DIABETIC KIDNEY DISEASE

Diabetic Kidney Disease: What We Know

Type 2 diabetes and obesity often co-exist, and both can contribute to the development of renal dysfunction and disease (5–7). Obesity is associated with proteinuric renal disease even in the absence of diabetes (8). In cohorts with both diseases, there appears to be an additive effect. Having both obesity and diabetes increases the risk of developing renal disease, and a diagnosis of obesity is a key risk factor in the progression of diabetic kidney disease (DKD) (7, 9). Therefore, populations with both obesity and type 2 diabetes should be considered at elevated risk for the development of DKD. Given this pathological synergy, it seems sensible to suggest that in cohorts with both obesity and type 2 diabetes, treatment approaches should be simultaneously targeted at both diseases in order to prevent or treat any associated DKD.

In diabetic kidney disease (DKD), the first clinical manifestation is albuminuria. Metabolic surgery reduces the risk of developing albuminuria in the first instance (10–14). Surgery also results in reduced proteinuria, including albuminuria, even in cases of established disease (15, 16). This effect of surgery is seen within the first 12 months post-operatively, and lasts for at least five years (16–19). This effect is reported in cohorts with and without type 2 diabetes, and can lead to remission of established microalbuminuria in both cohorts (16, 18). A single randomized controlled trial has shown that Roux-en-Y gastric bypass is superior to best medical treatment in causing remission of albuminuria over 2 years, and thus inducing remission of early diabetic kidney disease (JAMA Surg; in press).

While the data for the effect of surgery on both preventing and remediating proteinuria are generally based on measured protein excretion, including 24 h urine collections, almost all of the data on the effect of metabolic surgery on renal function are based on estimated glomerular filtration rate (eGFR) rather than measured glomerular filtration rate (mGFR). It should be noted that in the context of significant weight loss, serum creatinine concentrations usually decrease, resulting in an apparent increase in eGFR (17, 20). Calculators for eGFR have not been validated for use in the context of significant and rapid weight loss, as occurs after metabolic surgery. Therefore, eGFR in this population should be interpreted with caution.

In general, there is no deleterious effect of surgery on eGFR in those with preserved renal function at the time of surgery (19). This seems to be the case for populations both with and without type 2 diabetes at baseline. There are data to suggest a potent renoprotective effect of surgery in people with type 2 diabetes and early DKD. In case-control data comparing metabolic surgery and medical therapy in people with type 2 diabetes, and albuminuria with preserved renal function, surgery was associated with stabilization of eGFR and remission of albuminuria over a 10 year follow-up period, as compared with a steady decline in renal function in the medical group (21).

While there are very few data on the effect of metabolic surgery on people with an eGFR of <60 ml/min/1.73 m^2 (stage 3–5 chronic kidney disease), the available data indicate potential benefit (17, 19, 22). When using eGFR, there seems to be a stablisation in renal function in recipients of metabolic surgery that can last up to 9 years post-operatively (19, 22–24). Notwithstanding the limitations of eGFR in this cohort, the renal data are reassuring. The maximal weight loss typically occurs within 2 years of surgery. After this point, weight loss stabilizes, and the eGFR calculators are presumably more robust (although this is not proven to be the case).

In clinical practice, metabolic surgery is offered to selected patients on dialysis who require transplantation, but who are excluded from transplant lists solely on the basis of their weight. While this cohort is understandably at high risk of peri-operative and post-operative morbidity and mortality, the benefits of surgery can exceed in the risks in some cases. For selected cohorts, surgery can be risk-acceptable and effective, resulting in successful renal transplantation (25). In some series of patients with end-stage renal disease who have surgery, cases of recovery of renal function in dialysis-dependent patients have been reported (26, 27). In these cases, histological markers of renal disease improved after surgery in parallel with the improvements in renal function.

The mechanisms for the above-described improvement in renal function and prevention of renal disease are not fully understood. Metabolic surgery reduces weight, improves hypertension and ameliorates hyperglycaemia, which can explain some of the effect on eGFR (3, 14, 19, 22, 28, 29). However, other mechanisms, such as resolution of pro-inflammatory pathways, may also contribute to the improvement in markers of renal disease (30, 31). The interplay between obesity and diabetes is difficult to tease out in human studies, but in animal models of DKD the inflammatory effect of obesity seems to be only partially responsible for improvements in proteinuria (30). Therefore, it seems that several mechanisms work together to produce the renal benefits seen in recipients of metabolic surgery.

Glomerular hyperfiltration is a phenomenon seen in obesity related renal disease, with or without co-morbid type 2 diabetes. Hyperfiltration results in glomerular hypertrophy, and the increased rate of filtration is associated with oxidative stress and activation of pro-inflammatory pathways. In some cases, the end-point of chronic hyperftltration is focal segmental glomerulosclerosis, with an associated clinical presentation of proteinuric renal disease termed obesity related glomerulopathy, which is similar in clinical presentation to diabetic kidney disease, but which can occur in the absence of diabetes or hyperglycaemia (8). This condition can result in end stage renal failure.

Obesity related glomerulopathy is a result of a confluence of pro-inflammatory pathways, ectopic lipid accumulation within the kidney, and podocyte dysfunction in the context of insulin resistance and oxidative stress (8). As it can occur in the absence of diabetes and hypertension, it is a clear demonstration of the importance of multiple non-glucocentric mechanisms that are involved in the onset and progression of diabetic kidney disease in those with type 2 diabetes and obesity (8). As is the case in diabetic kidney disease, metabolic and bariatric surgery can ameliorate obesity related glomerulopathy by remediating inflammation and reducing hyperfiltration (8).

Unanswered Questions in Diabetic Kidney Disease

GFR Accuracy—Do the Estimates Measure Up?

An essential question to answer is whether the estimated GFR calculators can be relied upon after metabolic surgery. Measured GFR before and after surgery appears stable when corrected for body surface area (17, 20, 32–36). However, in these studies there were very few participants with diabetes, and follow-up was less then 24 months in almost all cases.

This is problematic as we are basing our current ideas around the use of metabolic surgery in DKD on the effect of eGFR [usually estimated with the Modification of Diet in Renal Disease (MDRD) formula] in long-term epidemiological and cohort studies. The MDRD formula has been shown to be inaccurate in cohorts with type 2 diabetes and obesity (37, 38). Part of the problem is the presumption of a body surface area of 1.73 m^2, which is an underestimate in many people with obesity (38). However, even in longitudinal studies of measured GFR, concerns around eGFR calculators exist with respect to their validity in people with type 2 diabetes (39).

This issue is compounded by the changes in muscle mass that occurs after metabolic surgery (40). Serum creatinine is primarily derived from muscle mass, and so calculators based on serum creatinine may be prone to error if we compare eGFR before and after significant weight loss. The loss of muscle mass only appears to be significant in the first year after surgery, with apparent stabilization of muscle mass from the end of the first post-operative year (40). While the studies of measured GFR completed in the first year post operatively have been reassuring, very few participants were followed beyond the weight loss phase (17, 20–22). Therefore, it is unknown if the current creatinine based calculators for eGFR are valid in people with type 2 diabetes following metabolic surgery.

Calculators for eGFR other than MDRD can be used, although none appear to be as accurate as we would like (33). This is especially true in the weight loss phase in the first year after bariatric or metabolic surgery (33, 34, 37). Of the currently available calculators, CKD-EPI is the most accurate (33). CKD-EPI can underestimate GFR in people with obesity before surgery, and overestimate it in the post-operative phase, but the use of Cystatin C as a marker of filtration can enhance the accuracy of CKD-EPI (33, 34). However, Cystatin C is not widely available for use, and remains outside of standard clinical practice at present. While the estimated values may not be entirely accurate in any of the calculators, the trends over time do parallel, and so whatever calculator is used at the onset, should be consistently used over time to detect any significant changes in eGFR (22).

Given the above, in our opinion, it seems that that new studies are needed. These should be validation studies of eGFR calculators in populations with type 2 diabetes and obesity. Two cohorts are needed in these studies; a post-operative population who had metabolic surgery over 2 years before entry into the study, and a cohort matched for age, weight, and relevant comorbidities and medication use. It should be noted that given the dynamic physiological changes associated with surgery, eGFR calculation may not be able to achieve acceptably accurate results. Direct measurement of GFR is the only way to really gauge the effect of metabolic and bariatric surgery on renal function and disease. While the complexity of the measurement process means that measured GFR remains inaccessible for standard clinical care, the use of simplified direct measurement of GFR may prove to be the future of renal surveillance in this cohort.

Is Metabolic Surgery Better Than Medical Management for Treating People With DKD and an eGFR of <60 ml/min/1.73 m^2?

There is abundant evidence that metabolic surgery is more effective than medical therapy alone in treating type 2 diabetes. There is also evidence that it can treat hypertension more effectively than with medication alone, although this evidence base is not as well-developed (3, 41). Given that these two major risk factors are well-treated by metabolic surgery, it seems logical to presume that surgery would be more effective than medical therapy in treating established DKD.

However, it remains the case that we still do not have any randomized controlled data from trials specifically powered to detect treatment effect differences between surgery and medical therapy in DKD with an eGFR <60 ml/min/1.73 kg/m^2. This is particularly important in the longer-term in people with renal impairment at baseline. While glycaemic control and blood pressure improve shortly after surgery, and remain improved in the medium to long-term, there is an increased risk of nephrolithiasis in surgical recipients (42). Oxalate nephropathy may develop after metabolic surgery, predisposing to nephrolithiasis and chronic renal disease (43). This risk appears to be procedure dependent, but is not well-quantified. However, it may be that in people with eGFRs of <60 ml/min/1.73 kg/m^2 the risk/benefit balance is not that strongly in favor of surgical treatment.

On balance, it seems likely that the potential renal benefits would exceed the risks. However, this needs to be specifically studied. Randomized controlled trials of surgery and best medical therapy are needed in people with established DKD and eGFR of <60 ml/min/1.73 m^2. These studies should incorporate a treat-to-target protocol, so that the medical arms achieve equivalent glycaemic and blood pressure targets. Best medical therapy should include renin-angiotensin-aldosterone system inhibitor or blockade, and sodium glucose co-transporter 2 inhibitor therapy. They should also include longer-term follow-up and measurement of urinary markers of nephrolithiasis.

DIABETIC RETINOPATHY

Diabetic Retinopathy: What We Know

There is little evidence to inform us on the effect of metabolic surgery on diabetic retinopathy. From the existing data, it seems that most people who do not have retinopathy pre-operatively, do not go on to develop it post-operatively (44–46). For those with pre-existing retinopathy, most either remain stable, or improve, in disease severity (44–46). However, some do deteriorate and develop more severe, and potentially sight-threatening, disease (44, 45, 47).

The existing longitudinal data on microvascular outcomes suggest that in most people surgery prevents the development or progression of diabetic retinopathy (11, 13, 14, 29). While none of these studies were specifically powered to examine the effect of surgery on retinopathy, these long-term real-world data are reassuring as they show that surgery is associated with significant reductions in the risk of developing retinopathy without a strong signal for significant deterioration of disease at population level (11, 13, 29).

This makes physiological sense, as surgery is proven to be more effective that medical therapy alone in helping people with type 2 diabetes meet glycaemic treatment targets (28, 48, 49). Hyperglycaemia is the major risk factor for the development and progression of retinopathy (50). Therefore, ameliorating hyperglycaemia with surgery would be expected to be protective against retinopathy.

However, while the long-term effect may be expected to be protective, the immediate post-operative period should be considered to be a time when the individual is at elevated risk of disease progression. This is due to the rapid improvement in glycaemic control seen after surgery. Rapid improvement in hyperglycaemia has long been associated with progression of retinopathy (51). Metabolic surgery results in an improvement in hyperglycaemia in the immediate post-operative period, with significant changes in HbA1c within months of treatment (48). This rapid improvement should be expected to put the surgical recipient at risk of progression of disease.

The existing evidence base is almost exclusively limited to cohort studies and uncontrolled case series. The populations studied are heterogenous with varying degrees of pre-operative disease and post-operative follow-up. There are very few randomized controlled data available on retinopathy. In the STAMPEDE trial, where 150 participants were randomized to sleeve gastrectomy, Roux-en-Y gastric bypass, or best medical therapy, formal scoring of retinopathy was not published, but it was reported that there was no significant change in retinopathy disease severity in any of the treatment groups (28).

However, the concern about the immediate post-operative effect of surgery on retinopathy is borne out in some of the published case series documenting the effect of surgery on retinopathy (44, 45, 47). In these series, many cases of disease progression have been described. Given the design of these studies, we cannot be clear as to the major risk factors for progression of disease, but it does seem that pre-operative hyperglycaemia is likely to be a major risk factor. In one study, the authors noted a difference in pre-operative HbA1c of over 11 mmol/mol (1%) between those who had progression of disease post-operatively and those who did not (47). The mean change in HbA1c was comparable between groups, but pre-operative HbA1c concentrations were higher in those who had post-operative progression of retinopathy (47).

In some cases, progression of disease can be sight threatening. From the reported cases, it appears to be a combination of pre-operative HbA1c, magnitude of change in HbA1c concentration post-operatively, and presence of pre-existing retinal disease, that is most important in determining the risk of progression to sight-threatening disease following surgery (44, 47, 52). Therefore, while in general surgery could be expected to prevent the development or progression of retinopathy, caution must be taken in candidates for surgery who have pre-existing retinopathy, especially if they are significantly off glycaemic targets pre-operatively.

Unanswered Questions in Retinopathy

What Is the Effect of Metabolic Surgery on Retinopathy?

The case series and cohort data outlined above suggest a rate of post-operative deterioration in retinopathy of between 1 and 45%. (46, 47, 52–56). This wide range is likely explained by the heterogeneity of the cohorts, both in terms of clinical characteristics and size. Different grading systems were also used across studies, which critically limits comparison between study cohorts.

This illustrates the need for robust prospective large-scale cohort studies examining the effect of surgery on retinopathy specifically. Any such study should include people with type 2 diabetes, both those with and without retinopathy, who are followed up after surgery with a robust validated grading system to determine if there is any change before and after surgery. In order to control for background rates of progression of retinopathy, the surgical cohort should be matched with a control cohort. Adequate matching will require a cohort with similar glycaemic control at baseline, comparable retinal grading at baseline, and equivalent duration of diabetes.

Follow-up for any study of retinopathy needs to be up to 5 years at least, as there can be changes in retinal scores for up to 4 years post-operatively (47). Therefore, even in those who achieve treatment targets, or even remission of diabetes, after surgery, a risk of progression of disease may exist. In the absence of definitive evidence, caution is best, and so in current practice, retinal screening should continue in those who have had surgery for at least 4 years. A longer-term study would inform us to the need for such an approach.

Are There Risk Factors for Development or Progression of Retinopathy After Metabolic Surgery?

There are signals in the existing cohort studies that pre-operative HbA1c concentrations, and grading of pre-existing retinopathy, are both important risk factors for progression of disease post-operatively. However, this needs to be proven and defined. What are the risk factors that are important in predicting progression? And what are the thresholds that define high-risk from normal risk? A well-designed prospective case control study could answer these questions.

In most studies, higher pre-operative HbA1c concentrations are associated with a higher rate of post-operative progression of retinopathy (47, 52, 54). The HbA1c threshold at which retinal risk really accelerates is not known, but in the cohort study with the highest rate of deterioration in retinopathy after surgery (9 people out of 20), the mean pre-operative HbA1c was 81 mmol/mol (9.5%) (54). In one study, the authors defined an increased risk of higher grades of post-operative retinopathy with every 1 mmol/mol increase in pre-operative HbA1c (47). This needs to be verified in a larger study.

As well as baseline HbA1c, the rapid change in HbA1c concentrations that often occur after surgery may be associated with progression of retinopathy. In this case, the cohort data have shown conflicting results. In some cohorts, there is a clear trend for deterioration in those who achieve the greatest improvement in HbA1c (52). In others, there is no such trend (47). However, the differing design of the studies, and differences in baseline characteristics between cohorts, explain this conflict. Based on the evidence for retinal disease progression with rapid improvements in glycemic control in other settings, it seems very likely that rapid changes in glycaemic control will prove to be a risk factor for progression of retinopathy. However, this remains to be proven. Theoretically, this risk factor could be modified with anti-diabetes medical therapy prior to surgery, in an effort to reduce HbA1c pre-operatively, thus reducing the rapid slope of change immediately after surgery.

There is no clear threshold for risk of post-operative progression of retinopathy. While baseline hyperglycaemia is clearly important, rapid improvement of hyperglycaemia is also important (51). Given what we know so far a pre-operative HbA1c of over 75 mmol/mol (9%) and a change in HbA1c of over 11 mmol/mol (1%) before and after surgery, seems reasonable as markers of risk (47, 52, 54). However, further study is needed to clearly define these glycaemic risk thresholds.

Recent data have suggested there are many phenotypes of type 2 diabetes that could be mapped genetically, and potentially via proteomic or metabolomics profiles (57). It is known that likelihood of remission of type 2 diabetes can be partially predicted by pre-operative factors including HbA1c and C-peptide concentrations (58). Using these parameters with other biochemical, metabolic, and anthropometric factors in multivariate models may be able to predict those who will have a rapid glycaemic response to surgery (59).

The other likely risk marker of post-operative deterioration in retinopathy is pre-operative grade of disease. It seems that any grade of retinopathy, no matter how early, increases the likelihood of higher grades post-operatively (47, 52). Most people who do not have retinopathy pre-operatively remain disease free after surgery (44–46). In those who do have deterioration of disease, there is no clear relationship between grade for pre-operative disease and eventual post-operative grading. Cases of severe and potentially sight-threatening disease have been described in people with minimal retinal disease pre-operatively (44, 45, 47). These cases are confounded by other changes in characteristics, predominantly glycaemic change, over time, and so the importance of the grade of retinal disease itself as a risk factor remains unclear.

Therefore, a large long-term case control study is needed, where people who go on to have metabolic surgery are well-characterized at baseline and then followed over at least 5 years. The surgical cohort should be matched to a control cohort for all relevant risk factors. Given the likely confounding effect of improvement in glycaemic control, statistical input should be sought as how to delineate the glycaemic effects from the effect of pre-existing grade of retinal disease and other potential risk factors.

While awaiting the results of any future study on retinopathy, it is best to be cautious. Therefore, we recommend pre-operative retinal assessment for all patients with type 2 diabetes who go on to have bariatric or metabolic surgery. Reassessment should be scheduled post-operatively. If there is any retinopathy, then reassessment should occur within three to 6 months post-operatively. If pre-proliferative retinopathy, or any maculopathy, is detected, then specialist ophthalmology advice should be sought to determine if pre-operative treatment is needed.

DIABETIC NEUROPATHY

Diabetic Neuropathy: What We Know

There are even fewer data on the effect of metabolic surgery on diabetic neuropathy than there are on the effect of surgery on retinopathy. However, the data that do exist demonstrate that metabolic surgery is associated with a reduced risk of developing diabetic neuropathy (13, 14, 28, 29, 60). These data were all derived from subjective reporting of neuropathy, either by patients themselves or from healthcare providers. In a small study using nerve conduction studies, there was no change in electrophysiological markers of neuropathy before and after surgery (46).

It is reasonable to expect that neuropathy would be less likely to occur after surgery given the significant improvement in glycaemic control induced by metabolic surgery. Therefore, the available data agree with expectation. However, there are very few people included in these studies with pre-existing neuropathy or diabetic foot disease. There is some cause for concern that surgery may result in treatment-induced neuropathy given the rapid rate of improvement in glycaemic control (61, 62).

Unanswered Questions in Neuropathy and Diabetic Foot Disease

Metabolic surgery can result in neuropathy, even in the absence of diabetes (63). The etiology of neuropathy after surgery varies, but can be related to deficiencies in micronutrients such as vitamin B12. While there is no evidence that treatment induced neuropathy is a common phenomenon after metabolic surgery, cases of serious diabetic neuropathy and arthropathy have been described in the context of rapid improvements in glycaemic control and weight (61, 62). Therefore, it will be necessary to study the effect of metabolic surgery on neuropathy, especially in people with pre-operative disease, in order to quantify the risk of post-operative deterioration.

As well as quantifying the effect of surgery on neuropathy, prospective cohort studies are needed to delineate the important mechanisms that could be associated with post-operative neuropathy. There are multiple potential insults associated with surgery. The rapid improvement in glycaemic control may induce a treatment-induced neuritis. Micronutrient deficiencies can also produce neuropathy. Anecdotal evidence would suggest that those that present with late onset of neuropathy, often many years after surgery, are those who are not taking regular comprehensive micronutrient supplementation. Specifically, deficiencies in B vitamins may be critical factors in the development of neuropathy. Therefore, any such study must be designed to comprehensively gather all the relevant data to allow a full analysis of all potential risk factors.

Diabetic foot disease is a source of major morbidity in people with type 2 diabetes. Neuropathy is a major contributor to diabetic foot disease. Therefore, if there was a risk of deterioration in neuropathy post-operatively, this may worsen existing diabetic foot disease or increase the risk of developing diabetic foot disease. There are no studies on this topic, but given the risk of harm in people with active diabetic foot disease (ulceration or arthropathy), there is an urgent need to investigate the effect of surgery on nerve function, both in those without neuropathy at baseline, and those with active diabetic foot disease.

CARDIOVASCULAR DISEASE

Cardiovascular Disease: What We Know

Metabolic surgery significantly improves blood pressure and cholesterol concentrations in tandem with improved glycaemic control in type 2 diabetes. Therefore, is it not surprising to note that surgery is consistently associated with reduced rates of myocardial infarction and stroke (4, 14, 64). This reduces the cardiovascular mortality rate in these cohorts by ~50%.

While the observational and epidemiological evidence are very convincing, it is not conclusively proven that surgery would be more effective than medical therapy in reducing cardiovascular mortality. There are no randomized controlled trials of surgery and best medical care where cardiovascular morbidity or mortality are primary outcomes. These studies remain to be completed, and should be focused on those with increased cardiovascular risk in the first instance.

Unanswered Questions in Cardiovascular Disease

Can We Determine Who Is Likely to Benefit Most From Metabolic Surgery?

It may be that there are certain cohorts who would benefit more from surgery than others. Those with existing cardiovascular disease may not be good surgical candidates. However, if metabolic surgery was being considered in order to reduce cardiovascular risk, it would be useful to know who would be most likely to benefit from intervention.

As mentioned above, there are different clinical phenotypes of type 2 diabetes that can be mapped to genotypes (57). It may be that some of these phenotypes would be more likely than others to respond to surgery in terms of weight loss or improved glycaemic control. However, it may also be the case that there are certain genotypes that would respond better than others in terms of improvements in cardiovascular risk factors. Multivariate models including phenotypic, genotypic, and proteomic parameters may be able to predict those who will have a good response to surgery (59).

Therefore, large-scale population studies are needed. People who go on to have surgery should be characterized genotypically and phenotypically. Samples for proteomic and metabolomics profiles should be taken. Then, as the population ages, and cardiovascular disease becomes apparent, modeling for identifiable risk markers should be completed. This would need to be a longer-term project if completed prospectively, but use of existing bariatric registries could make such a project more feasible (presuming that they included the relevant data).

Do Patients With Obesity and Type 2 Diabetes Have a Greater Health Economic Benefit From Surgery With Respect to Cardiovascular Disease?

Metabolic surgery is associated with reduced cardiovascular morbidity and mortality, including reduced rates of hospital admission for cardiovascular disease and heart failure (4, 64, 65). It is clear that in general metabolic surgery is cost-saving not just cost-effective (66). However, this is when people both with and without diabetes are included. A large proportion of the cost-saving is due to prevention of chronic disease, including diabetes and cardiovascular disease, and therefore reduced costs of treatment.

It would be reasonable to expect that there would be a greater cost saving associated with type 2 diabetes given the reduced medication and insulin use that generally occurs post-operatively (28). However, the health economic data are not entirely clear. Some studies indicate a greater cost benefit in people with type 2 diabetes, but others do not find a cost benefit (67, 68). This is likely due to differences in analysis. The lack of cost benefit is due to a greater number of hospital presentations for both routine follow-up care and emergency care (68). However, this is only a cost issue in the first 2 years post-operatively (68). In longer-term follow up, cost savings may be greater.

In cardiovascular disease and diabetes, it may be that there is a major cost saving. In addition to preventing primary events, metabolic surgery can offer secondary prevention and reduce costs associated with coronary artery disease treatment (69). This is not fully defined, and therefore a cost-analysis of people with both diabetes and cardiovascular disease at baseline is needed. It may be that due to a reduced number of secondary events and reduced medication use, people with both type 2 diabetes and cardiovascular disease offer greater health economic benefit to a healthcare system.

CONCLUSIONS

Metabolic surgery is an effective treatment for type 2 diabetes, and given the data available to date, is effective at preventing the development of diabetic complications. However, there is a lack of specific randomized controlled studies on the effect of surgery on the complications of diabetes. These are urgently needed. While waiting for these data, we should exercise care in people with retinopathy, neuropathy and diabetic foot disease, as there is potential for deterioration of disease post-operatively.

As well as physiological and clinical effects, more study is needed on the health economic effects of surgery. It seems logical to assume that people with type 2 diabetes and complications such as diabetic kidney disease or cardiovascular disease would be likely to offer greater cost savings to healthcare systems. Further studies are needed to determine if this is the case.

AUTHOR CONTRIBUTIONS

KN and CL both contributed to the literature review and the drafting of this article.

REFERENCES

1. Rubino F, Nathan DM, Eckel RH, Schauer PR, Alberti KG, Zimmet PZ, et al. Metabolic surgery in the treatment algorithm for type 2 diabetes: a joint statement by international diabetes organizations. *Diabetes Care.* (2016) 39:861–77. doi: 10.2337/dc16-0236
2. Park CH, Nam SJ, Choi HS, Kim KO, Kim DH, Kim JW, et al. Comparative efficacy of bariatric surgery in the treatment of morbid obesity and diabetes mellitus: a systematic review and network meta-analysis. *Obes Surg.* (2019) 29:2180–90. doi: 10.1007/s11695-019-03831-6
3. Sjostrom L, Lindroos AK, Peltonen M, Torgerson J, Bouchard C, Carlsson B, et al. Lifestyle, diabetes, and cardiovascular risk factors 10 years after bariatric surgery. *N Engl J Med.* (2004) 351:2683–93. doi: 10.1056/NEJMoa035622
4. Sjostrom L, Peltonen M, Jacobson P, Sjostrom CD, Karason K, Wedel H, et al. Bariatric surgery and long-term cardiovascular events. *JAMA.* (2012) 307:56–65. doi: 10.1001/jama.2011.1914
5. Wang Y, Chen X, Song Y, Caballero B, Cheskin LJ. Association between obesity and kidney disease: a systematic review and meta-analysis. *Kidney Int.* (2008) 73:19–33. doi: 10.1038/sj.ki.5002586
6. Kramer H, Reboussin D, Bertoni AG, Marcovina S, Lipkin E, Greenway FL III, et al. Obesity and albuminuria among adults with type 2 diabetes: the look AHEAD (Action for Health in Diabetes) study. *Diabetes Care.* (2009) 32:851–3. doi: 10.2337/dc08-2059
7. Go AS, Chertow GM, Fan D, McCulloch CE, Hsu CY. Chronic kidney disease and the risks of death, cardiovascular events, and hospitalization. *N Engl J Med.* (2004) 351:1296–305. doi: 10.1056/NEJMoa041031
8. D'Agati VD, Chagnac A, de Vries AP, Levi M, Porrini E, Herman-Edelstein M, et al. Obesity-related glomerulopathy: clinical and pathologic characteristics and pathogenesis. *Nat Rev Nephrol.* (2016) 12:453–71. doi: 10.1038/nrneph.2016.75
9. Collins AJ, Foley RN, Chavers B, Gilbertson D, Herzog C, Johansen K, et al. United States renal data system 2011 annual data report: atlas of chronic kidney disease & end-stage renal disease in the united states. *Am J Kidney Dis.* (2012) 59(1 Suppl 1):A7–e1–420. doi: 10.1053/j.ajkd.2011.11.015
10. Carlsson LM, Romeo S, Jacobson P, Burza MA, Maglio C, Sjöholm K, et al. The incidence of albuminuria after bariatric surgery and usual care in Swedish Obese Subjects (SOS): a prospective controlled intervention trial. *Int J Obes.* (2015) 39:169–75. doi: 10.1038/ijo.2014.72
11. Carlsson LMS, Sjoholm K, Karlsson C, Jacobson P, Andersson-Assarsson JC, Svensson PA, et al. Long-term incidence of microvascular disease after bariatric surgery or usual care in patients with obesity, stratified by baseline glycaemic status: a post-hoc analysis of participants from the Swedish Obese Subjects study. *lancet Diabetes Endocrinol.* (2017) 5:271–9. doi: 10.1016/S2213-858730061-X
12. Coleman KJ, Haneuse S, Johnson E, Bogart A, Fisher D, O'Connor PJ, et al. Long-term microvascular disease outcomes in patients with type 2 diabetes after bariatric surgery: evidence for the legacy effect of surgery. *Diabetes Care.* (2016) 39:1400–7. doi: 10.2337/dc16-0194
13. O'Brien R, Johnson E, Haneuse S, Coleman KJ, O'Connor PJ, Fisher DP, et al. Microvascular outcomes in patients with diabetes after bariatric surgery versus usual care: a matched cohort study. *Ann Intern Med.* (2018) 169:300–10. doi: 10.7326/M17-2383
14. Sjostrom L, Peltonen M, Jacobson P, Ahlin S, Andersson-Assarsson J, Anveden A, et al. Association of bariatric surgery with long-term remission of type 2 diabetes and with microvascular and macrovascular complications. *JAMA.* (2014) 311:2297–304. doi: 10.1001/jama.2014.5988
15. Afshinnia F, Wilt TJ, Duval S, Esmaeili A, Ibrahim HN. Weight loss and proteinuria: systematic review of clinical trials and comparative cohorts. *Nephrol Dial Transplant.* (2010) 25:1173–83. doi: 10.1093/ndt/gfp640
16. *Agrawal V, Khan I, Rai B, Krause KR, Chengelis DL, Zalesin KC*, et al. The effect of weight loss after bariatric surgery on albuminuria. *Clin Nephrol.* (2008) 70:194–202. doi: 10.5414/CNP70194
17. Navarro-Diaz M, Serra A, Romero R, Bonet J, Bayes B, Homs M, et al. Effect of drastic weight loss after bariatric surgery on renal parameters in extremely obese patients: long-term follow-up. *J Am Soc Nephrol.* (2006) 17(12 Suppl 3):S213–7. doi: 10.1681/ASN.2006080917
18. Heneghan HM, Cetin D, Navaneethan SD, Orzech N, Brethauer SA, Schauer PR. Effects of bariatric surgery on diabetic nephropathy after 5 years of follow-up. *Surg Obes Relat Dis.* (2013) 9:7–14. doi: 10.1016/j.soard.2012.08.016
19. Navaneethan SD, Yehnert H, Moustarah F, Schreiber MJ, Schauer PR, Beddhu S. Weight loss interventions in chronic kidney disease: a systematic review and meta-analysis. *Clin J Am Soc Nephrol.* (2009) 4:1565–74. doi: 10.2215/CJN.02250409
20. Chagnac A, Weinstein T, Herman M, Hirsh J, Gafter U, Ori Y. The effects of weight loss on renal function in patients with severe obesity. *J Am Soc Nephrol.* (2003) 14:1480–6. doi: 10.1097/01.ASN.0000068462.38661.89
21. Iaconelli A, Panunzi S, De Gaetano A, Manco M, Guidone C, Leccesi L, et al. Effects of bilio-pancreatic diversion on diabetic complications: a 10-year follow-up. *Diabetes Care.* (2011) 34:561–7. doi: 10.2337/dc10-1761
22. Neff KJ, Baud G, Raverdy V, Caiazzo R, Verkindt H, Noel C, et al. renal function and remission of hypertension after bariatric surgery: a 5-year prospective cohort study. *Obes Surg.* (2017) 27:613–9. doi: 10.1007/s11695-016-2333-7
23. Imam TH, Fischer H, Jing B, Burchette R, Henry S, DeRose SF, et al. Estimated GFR before and after bariatric surgery in CKD. *Am J Kidney Dis.* (2017) 69:380–8. doi: 10.1053/j.ajkd.2016.09.020

24. Chang AR, Chen Y, Still C, Wood GC, Kirchner HL, Lewis M, et al. Bariatric surgery is associated with improvement in kidney outcomes. *Kidney Int.* (2016) 90:164–71. doi: 10.1016/j.kint.2016.02.039
25. Freeman CM, Woodle ES, Shi J, Alexander JW, Leggett PL, Shah SA, et al. Addressing morbid obesity as a barrier to renal transplantation with laparoscopic sleeve gastrectomy. *Am J Transpl.* (2015) 15:1360–8. doi: 10.1111/ajt.13116
26. Alexander JW, Goodman HR, Hawver LR, Cardi MA. Improvement and stabilization of chronic kidney disease after gastric bypass. *Surg Obe Relat Dis.* (2009) 5:237–41. doi: 10.1016/j.soard.2008.08.016
27. Huan Y, Tomaszewski JE, Cohen DL. Resolution of nephrotic syndrome after successful bariatric surgery in patient with biopsy-proven FSGS. *Clin Nephrol.* (2009) 71:69–73. doi: 10.5414/CNP71069
28. Schauer PR, Bhatt DL, Kirwan JP, Wolski K, Aminian A, Brethauer SA, et al. Bariatric surgery versus intensive medical therapy for diabetes - 5-year outcomes. *N Engl J Med.* (2017) 376:641–51. doi: 10.1056/NEJMoa1600869
29. Johnson BL, Blackhurst DW, Latham BB, Cull DL, Bour ES, Oliver TL, et al. Bariatric surgery is associated with a reduction in major macrovascular and microvascular complications in moderately to severely obese patients with type 2 diabetes mellitus. *J Am Coll Surg.* (2013) 216:545–56. doi: 10.1016/j.jamcollsurg.2012.12.019
30. Neff KJ, Elliott JA, Corteville C, Abegg K, Boza C, Lutz TA, et al. Effect of roux-en-y gastric bypass and diet-induced weight loss on diabetic kidney disease in the zucker diabetic fatty rat. *Surg O Relat Dis.* (2017) 13:21–7. doi: 10.1016/j.soard.2016.08.026
31. Fenske WK, Dubb S, Bueter M, Seyfried F, Patel K, Tam FW, et al. Effect of bariatric surgery-induced weight loss on renal and systemic inflammation and blood pressure: a 12-month prospective study. *Surg Obes Relat Dis.* (2013) 9:559–68. doi: 10.1016/j.soard.2012.03.009
32. Brochner-Mortensen J, Rickers H, Balslev I. Renal function and body composition before and after intestinal bypass operation in obese patients. *Scand J Clin Lab Invest.* (1980) 40:695–702. doi: 10.3109/003655180090 95584
33. Friedman AN, Moe S, Fadel WF, Inman M, Mattar SG, Shihabi Z, et al. Predicting the glomerular filtration rate in bariatric surgery patients. *Am J Nephrol.* (2014) 39:8–15. doi: 10.1159/000357231
34. Lieske JC, Collazo-Clavell ML, Sarr MG, Rule AD, Bergstralh EJ, Kumar R. Gastric bypass surgery and measured and estimated GFR in women. *Am J Kidney Dis.* (2014) 64:663–5. doi: 10.1053/j.ajkd.2014.06.016
35. Saliba J, Kasim NR, Tamboli RA, Isbell JM, Marks P, Feurer ID, et al. Roux-en-Y gastric bypass reverses renal glomerular but not tubular abnormalities in excessively obese diabetics. *Surgery.* (2010) 147:282–7. doi: 10.1016/j.surg.2009.09.017
36. Serpa Neto A, Bianco Rossi FM, Dal Moro Amarante R, Alves Buriti N, Cunha Barbosa Saheb G, Rossi M. Effect of weight loss after Roux-en-Y gastric bypass, on renal function and blood pressure in morbidly obese patients. *J Nephrol.* (2009) 22:637–46. doi: 10.13712Fjournal.pone.0163907
37. Chudleigh RA, Dunseath G, Peter R, Harvey JN, Ollerton RL, Luzio S, et al. Influence of body weight on the performance of glomerular filtration rate estimators in subjects with type 2 diabetes. *Diabetes Care.* (2008) 31:47–9. doi: 10.2337/dc07-1335
38. Nair S, Mishra V, Hayden K, Lisboa PJ, Pandya B, Vinjamuri S, et al. The four-variable modification of diet in renal disease formula underestimates glomerular filtration rate in obese type 2 diabetic individuals with chronic kidney disease. *Diabetologia.* (2011) 54:1304–7. doi: 10.1007/s00125-011-2085-9
39. Gaspari F, Ruggenenti P, Porrini E, Motterlini N, Cannata A, Carrara F, et al. The GFR and GFR decline cannot be accurately estimated in type 2 diabetics. *Kidney Int.* (2013) 84:164–73. doi: 10.1038/ki.2013.47
40. Davidson LE, Yu W, Goodpaster BH, DeLany JP, Widen E, Lemos T, et al. Fat-free mass and skeletal muscle mass five years after bariatric surgery. *Obesity.* (2018) 26:1130–6. doi: 10.1002/oby.22190
41. Schiavon CA, Bersch-Ferreira AC, Santucci EV, Oliveira JD, Torreglosa CR, Bueno PT, et al. Effects of bariatric surgery in obese patients with hypertension: the GATEWAY randomized trial (Gastric bypass to treat obese patients with steady hypertension). *Circulation.* (2018) 137:1132–42. doi: 10.1161/CIRCULATIONAHA.117.032130
42. Lieske JC, Mehta RA, Milliner DS, Rule AD, Bergstralh EJ, Sarr MG. Kidney stones are common after bariatric surgery. *Kidney Int.* (2015) 87:839–45. doi: 10.1038/ki.2014.352
43. Nasr SH, D'Agati VD, Said SM, Stokes MB, Largoza MV, Radhakrishnan J, et al. Oxalate nephropathy complicating Roux-en-Y gastric Bypass: an underrecognized cause of irreversible renal failure. *Clini J Am Soc Nephrol.* (2008) 3:1676–83. doi: 10.2215/CJN.02940608
44. Cheung D, Switzer NJ, Ehmann D, Rudnisky C, Shi X, Karmali S. The impact of bariatric surgery on diabetic retinopathy: a systematic review and meta-analysis. *Obes Surg.* (2015) 25:1604–9. doi: 10.1007/s11695-014-1539-9
45. Merlotti C, Ceriani V, Morabito A, Pontiroli AE. Bariatric surgery and diabetic retinopathy: a systematic review and meta-analysis of controlled clinical studies. *Obes Rev.* (2017) 18:309–16. doi: 10.1111/obr.12490
46. Miras AD, Chuah LL, Khalil N, Nicotra A, Vusirikala A, Baqai N, et al. Type 2 diabetes mellitus and microvascular complications 1 year after Roux-en-Y gastric bypass: a case-control study. *Diabetologia.* (2015) 58:1443–7. doi: 10.1007/s00125-015-3595-7
47. Chen Y, Laybourne JP, Sandinha MT, de Alwis NMW, Avery P, Steel DH, et al. Does bariatric surgery prevent progression of diabetic retinopathy? *Eye.* (2017) 31:1131–9. doi: 10.1038/eye.2017.119
48. Buchwald H, Estok R, Fahrbach K, Banel D, Jensen MD, Pories WJ, et al. Weight and type 2 diabetes after bariatric surgery: systematic review and meta-analysis. *Am J Med.* (2009) 122:248–56.e5. doi: 10.1016/j.amjmed.2008.09.041
49. Mingrone G, Panunzi S, De Gaetano A, Guidone C, Iaconelli A, Nanni G, et al. Bariatric-metabolic surgery versus conventional medical treatment in obese patients with type 2 diabetes:5 year follow–up of an open–label, single–centre, randomised controlled trial. *Lancet.* (2015) 386:964–73. doi: 10.1016/S0140-6736(15)00075-6
50. UK Prospective Diabetes Study (UKPDS) Group. Intensive blood-glucose control with sulphonylureas or insulin compared with conventional treatment risk of complications in patients with type 2 diabetes (UKPDS 33) UK Prospective Diabetes Study (UKPDS) Group. *Lancet.* (1998) 352:837–53. doi: 10.1016/S0140-6736(98)07019-6
51. Diabetes C, Complications Trial Research G, Nathan DM, Genuth S, Lachin J, Cleary P, et al. The effect of intensive treatment of diabetes on the development and progression of long-term complications in insulin-dependent diabetes mellitus. *N Engl J Med.* (1993) 329:977–86. doi: 10.1056/NEJM199309303291401
52. Murphy R, Jiang Y, Booth M, Babor R, MacCormick A, Hammodat H, et al. Progression of diabetic retinopathy after bariatric surgery. *Diabet Med.* (2015) 32:1212–20. doi: 10.1111/dme.12727
53. Brynskov T, Laugesen CS, Svenningsen AL, Floyd AK, Sorensen TL. Monitoring of diabetic retinopathy in relation to bariatric surgery: a prospective observational study. *Obes Surg.* (2016) 26:1279–86. doi: 10.1007/s11695-015-1936-8
54. Kim YJ, Seo du R, Kim MJ, Lee SJ, Hur KY, Choi KS. Clinical course of diabetic retinopathy in korean type 2 diabetes after bariatric surgery: a pilot study. *Retina.* (2015) 35:935–43. doi: 10.1097/IAE.0000000000000412
55. Thomas RL, Prior SL, Barry JD, Luzio SD, Eyre N, Caplin S, et al. Does bariatric surgery adversely impact on diabetic retinopathy in persons with morbid obesity and type 2 diabetes? A pilot study. *J Diabetes Compl.* (2014) 28:191–5. doi: 10.1016/j.jdiacomp.2013.10.006
56. Varadhan L, Humphreys T, Walker AB, Cheruvu CV, Varughese GI. Bariatric surgery and diabetic retinopathy: a pilot analysis. *Obes Surg.* (2012) 22:515–6. doi: 10.1007/s11695-012-0600-9
57. Ahlqvist E, Storm P, Karajamaki A, Martinell M, Dorkhan M, Carlsson A, et al. Novel subgroups of adult-onset diabetes and their association with outcomes: a data-driven cluster analysis of six variables. *lancet Diabetes Endocrinol.* (2018) 6:361–9. doi: 10.1016/S2213-8587(18)30051-2
58. Dixon JB, Chuang LM, Chong K, Chen SC, Lambert GW, Straznicky NE, et al. Predicting the glycemic response to gastric bypass surgery in patients with type 2 diabetes. *Diabetes Care.* (2013) 36:20–6. doi: 10.2337/dc12-0779
59. Szczerbinski L, Taylor MA, Citko A, Gorska M, Larsen S, Hady HR, et al. Clusters of glycemic response to oral glucose tolerance tests explain multivariate metabolic and anthropometric outcomes of bariatric surgery in obese patients. *J Clin Med.* (2019) 8:1091. doi: 10.3390/jcm8081091
60. Muller-Stich BP, Fischer L, Kenngott HG, Gondan M, Senft J, Clemens G, et al. Gastric bypass leads to improvement of diabetic neuropathy

independent of glucose normalization–results of a prospective cohort study (DiaSurg 1 study). *Ann Surg.* (2013) 258:760–5. doi: 10.1097/SLA.0b013e3182a618b2
61. Murchison R, Gooday C, Dhatariya K. The development of a charcot foot after significant weight loss in people with diabetes: three cautionary tales. *J Am Podiatr Med Assoc.* (2014) 104:522–5. doi: 10.7547/0003-0538-104.5.522
62. Gibbons CH, Freeman R. Treatment-induced neuropathy of diabetes: an acute, iatrogenic complication of diabetes. *Brain.* (2015) 138(Pt 1):43–52. doi: 10.1093/brain/awu307
63. Aghili R, Malek M, Tanha K, Mottaghi A. The effect of bariatric surgery on peripheral polyneuropathy: a systematic review and meta-analysis. *Obes Surg.* (2019) 29:3010–20. doi: 10.1007/s11695-019-04004-1
64. Adams TD, Gress RE, Smith SC, Halverson RC, Simper SC, Rosamond WD, et al. Long-term mortality after gastric bypass surgery. *N Engl J Med.* (2007) 357:753–61. doi: 10.1056/NEJMoa066603
65. Aleassa EM, Khorgami Z, Kindel TL, Tu C, Tang WHW, Schauer PR, et al. Impact of bariatric surgery on heart failure mortality. *Surg Obes Relat Dis.* (2019) 15:1189–96. doi: 10.1016/j.soard.2019.03.021
66. Borisenko O, Lukyanov V, Ahmed AR. Cost-utility analysis of bariatric surgery. *Br J Surgery.* (2018) 105:1328–37. doi: 10.1002/bjs.10857
67. James R, Salton RI, Byrnes JM, Scuffham PA. Cost-utility analysis for bariatric surgery compared with usual care for the treatment of obesity in Australia. *Surg Obes Relat Dis.* (2017) 13:2012–20. doi: 10.1016/j.soard.2016.12.016
68. Banerjee S, Garrison LP Jr, Flum DR, Arterburn DE. Cost and health care utilization implications of bariatric surgery versus intensive lifestyle and medical intervention for type 2 diabetes. *Obesity.* (2017) 25:1499–508. doi: 10.1002/oby.21927
69. Baimas-George M, Hennings DL, Al-Qurayshi Z, Emad K, DuCoin C. No more broken hearts: weight loss after bariatric surgery returns patients' postoperative risk to baseline following coronary surgery. *Surg Obes Relat Dis.* (2017) 13:1010–5. doi: 10.1016/j.soard.2016.12.008

Clinical Insights to Complete and Incomplete Surgical Revascularization in Atrial Fibrillation and Multivessel Coronary Disease

Michal Pasierski[1,2†], Jakub Staromłyński[1,2†], Janina Finke[1], Radoslaw Litwinowicz[2,3], Grzegorz Filip[3], Adam Kowalówka[4,5], Wojciech Wańha[2,6], Michalina Kołodziejczak[2,7,8], Natalia Piekuś-Słomka[9], Andrzej Łoś[10], Sebastian Stefaniak[11], Wojciech Wojakowski[6], Marek Jemielity[11], Jan Rogowski[10], Marek Deja[4,5], Dariusz Jagielak[10], Krzysztof Bartus[3], Silvia Mariani[12], Tong Li[13], Matteo Matteucci[2,14], Daniele Ronco[2,14], Federica Jiritano[2,15], Dario Fina[2,16], Gennaro Martucci[2,17], Paolo Meani[2,16], Giuseppe Maria Raffa[2,18], Artur Słomka[2,19], Pietro Giorgio Malvidni[20], Roberto Lorusso[12], Michal Zembala[21], Piotr Suwalski[1] and Mariusz Kowalewski[1,2,12] on behalf of Thoracic Research Centre*

[1] Department of Cardiac Surgery, Central Clinical Hospital of the Ministry of Interior, Centre of Postgraduate Medical Education, Warsaw, Poland, [2] Thoracic Research Centre, Innovative Medical Forum, Collegium Medicum Nicolaus Copernicus University, Bydgoszcz, Poland, [3] Department of Cardiovascular Surgery and Transplantology, Jagiellonian University Medical College, John Paul II Hospital, Kraków, Poland, [4] Department of Cardiac Surgery, School of Medicine in Katowice, Medical University of Silesia, Katowice, Poland, [5] Department of Cardiac Surgery, Upper-Silesian Heart Center, Katowice, Poland, [6] Department of Cardiology and Structural Heart Diseases, Medical University of Silesia, Katowice, Poland, [7] Department of Anaesthesiology and Intensive Care, Antoni Jurasz University Hospital No. 1, Collegium Medicum Nicolaus Copernicus University, Bydgoszcz, Poland, [8] Division of Cardiology, Yale School of Medicine, New Haven, CT, United States, [9] Department of Inorganic and Analytical Chemistry, Ludwik Rydygier Collegium Medicum in Bydgoszcz, Nicolaus Copernicus University, Toruń, Poland, [10] Department of Cardiac and Vascular Surgery, Medical University of Gdańsk, Gdańsk, Poland, [11] Department of Cardiac Surgery and Transplantology, Poznań University of Medical Sciences, Poznań, Poland, [12] Cardio-Thoracic Surgery Department, Heart and Vascular Centre, Maastricht University Medical Centre, Cardiovascular Research Institute Maastricht, Maastricht, Netherlands, [13] Department of Cardiac Surgery, University Hospital Düesseldorf, Düesseldorf, Germany, [14] Department of Cardiac Surgery, Circolo Hospital, University of Insubria, Varese, Italy, [15] Department of Cardiac Surgery, University Magna Græcia of Catanzaro, Catanzaro, Italy, [16] Department of Cardiothoracic and Vascular Anesthesia and Intensive Care Unit (ICU), Istituto di Ricovero e Cura a Carattere Scientifico (IRCCS) Policlinico San Donato, Milan, Italy, [17] Anesthesia and Intensive Care Department, Istituto di Ricovero e Cura a Carattere Scientifico (IRCCS)-Istituto Mediterraneo per i Trapianti e Terapie ad Alta Specializzazione (ISMETT), Palermo, Italy, [18] Cardiac Surgery Unit, Istituto di Ricovero e Cura a Carattere Scientifico (IRCCS)-Istituto Mediterraneo per i Trapianti e Terapie ad Alta Specializzazione (ISMETT), Palermo, Italy, [19] Department of Pathophysiology, Ludwik Rydygier Collegium Medicum Bydgoszcz, Nicolaus Copernicus University, Toruń, Poland, [20] Cardiac Surgery Unit, Lancisi Cardiovascular Center, Polytechnic University of Marche, Ancona, Italy, [21] Department of Cardiac, Vascular and Endovascular Surgery and Transplantology, Silesian Center for Heart Diseases, Zabrze, Poland

Specialty section:
This article was submitted to Heart Surgery, a section of the journal Frontiers in Cardiovascular Medicine

Objectives: Although endorsed by international guidelines, complete revascularization (CR) with Coronary Artery Bypass Grafting (CABG) remains underused. In higher-risk patients such as those with pre-operative atrial fibrillation (AF), the effects of CR are not well studied.

Methods: We analyzed patients' data from the HEIST (HEart surgery In AF and Supraventricular Tachycardia) registry. Between 2012 and 2020 we identified 4770 patients with pre-operative AF and multivessel coronary artery disease who underwent isolated CABG. We divided the cohort according to the completeness of the revascularization and used propensity score matching (PSM) to minimize differences between baseline characteristics. The primary endpoint was all-cause mortality.

Results: Median follow-up was 4.7 years [interquartile range (IQR) 2.3–6.9]. PSM resulted in 1,009 pairs of complete and incomplete revascularization. Number of distal anastomoses varied, accounting for 3.0 + –0.6 vs. 1.7 + –0.6, respectively. Although early (< 24 h) and 30-day post-operative mortalities were not statistically different between non-CR and CR patients [Odds Ratio (OR) and 95% Confidence Intervals (CIs): 1.34 (0.46–3.86); P = 0.593, Hazard Ratio (HR) and 95% CIs: 0.88 (0.59–1.32); P = 0.542, respectively] the long term mortality was nearly 20% lower in the CR cohort [HR (95% CIs) 0.83 (0.71–0.96); P = 0.011]. This benefit was sustained throughout subgroup analyses, yet most accentuated in low-risk patients (younger i.e., < 70 year old, with a EuroSCORE II < 2%, non-diabetic) and when off-pump CABG was performed.

Conclusion: Complete revascularization in patients with pre-operative AF is safe and associated with improved survival. Particular survival benefit with CR was observed in low-risk patients undergoing off-pump CABG.

Keywords: atrial fibrillation, CABG, complete revascularization, survival, long-term

INTRODUCTION

Although never compared directly in a randomized controlled trial (RCT), complete revascularization (CR) during coronary artery bypass grafting (CABG) is considered to be superior to incomplete revascularization (ICR) in multi-vessel coronary artery disease (MV-CAD). The benefit is thought to originate from reduced risk of future cardiovascular events, namely periprocedural myocardial infarction (MI) and repeat revascularization (RR). Many observational studies, as well as insights from subgroup analysis of RCTs reinforced this notion (1–3). Several RCTs which investigated CR in the context of percutaneous intervention (PCI) for ST-elevation myocardial infarction (STEMI) have shown the benefit of complete, compared to ICR for MV-CAD (4–6). However, surgical revascularization is still the first-choice procedure in high-risk non-acute MI patients, specifically those with diabetes (7) and intermediate-to-high anatomical complexity coronary disease (8).

The 2018 ESC/EACTS guidelines on myocardial revascularization emphasized that the expected highest completeness of revascularization should guide the choice of treatment strategy (9). The question arises if surgeons should attempt CR at all costs and, if not, what type of risk factors may discourage them from pursuing one. Atrial fibrillation (AF) is an independent predictor of mortality and morbidity after CABG (10, 11). Apart from an increased risk of stroke, AF is also associated with an over a fourfold increased risk of developing heart failure (12). Moreover, an impaired graft flow in AF CABG patients was observed (13). Most reports estimate the pre-op AF prevalence in CABG patients at 6–10%, but in some reports, it was as high as 20% (14). Because of aging of the society, the prevalence of AF is likely to rise.

The disparity in reported results of CR in CABG, and the shortage of evidence in high-risk patients, requires further investigation (15, 16). The current study aimed to address whether there exists a survival benefit with CR in MV-CAD and underlying AF.

PATIENTS AND METHODS

Study Population and Clinical Variables

Because of the retrospective nature of the study, the ethics committee approval was waived. Our investigation was a part of the HEIST (Heart Surgery In atrial fibrillation and Supraventricular tachycardia) Registry (NCT04860882). We included consecutive AF patients, over 18 year old, admitted to 8 tertiary centers in Poland, Netherlands, and Italy between January 2012 and December 2020 who had isolated CABG for MV-CAD performed (**Supplementary Figure 1**). Patients who (1) had no diagnosis of AF; (2) had CABG with concomitant valvular or aortic procedures, were not included in the study. Similarly, (3) patients with single-vessel CAD or (4) patients in whom the number of distal anastomoses and/or type of graft material used could not be determined were excluded from the analyses. (5) Patients undergoing hybrid revascularization by intention-to-treat protocol, or who were admitted for (6) staged revascularization strategy or (7) re-do surgery were not included.

Endpoints and Definitions

The primary endpoint was all-cause mortality following complete vs. incomplete surgical revascularization for MV-CAD. We defined CR as grafting two significantly stenotic lesions in two-vessel disease and three lesions in three-vessel disease of different territories: right coronary artery (RCA), left anterior descending- (LAD), and circumflex- (Cx) artery. Additional grafts to the diseased systems were encouraged and when the number of grafts was greater than the number required for CR, the approach was considered as "supracomplete" revascularization (SCR). Only the coronary vessels with significant stenosis were bypassed. We defined ICR as failure to graft two significantly

TABLE 1 | Pre-operative characteristics after PS-matching.

	Total (2018)	Non-CR (1009)	CR (1009)	*P*-value
Baseline characteristics				
Age years [median (IQR)]	70 (64–76)	70 (64–76)	70 (64–76)	0.792
Male gender	1589 (78.7)	795 (78.8)	794 (78.7)	0.99
EuroSCORE II	1.91 (1.21,3.19)	1.92 (1.22, 3.19)	1.90 (1.18, 3.19)	0.760
Diabetes	899 (44.5)	457 (45.3)	442 (43.8)	0.531
Insulin ± oral hypoglycemic drugs	372 (18.4)	186 (18.4)	186 (18.4)	0.99
Smoking	1247 (61.8)	628 (62.2)	619 (61.3)	0.714
Hypertension	1829 (90.6)	917 (90.9)	912 (90.4)	0.760
Hyperlipidemia	1293 (64.1)	656 (65.0)	637 (63.1)	0.404
BMI [median (IQR)]	28.69 (25.78–31.70)	28.70 (25.65, 31.71)	28.69 (25.95, 31.67)	0.815
Pulmonary hypertension[a]	154 (7.6)	86 (8.5)	68 (6.7)	0.154
Renal impairment	1128 (55.9)	570 (56.5)	558 (55.3)	0.622
Dialysis (regardless of CC)	26 (1.3)	13 (1.3)	13 (1.3)	0.99
Peripheral artery disease	515 (25.5)	263 (26.1)	252 (25.0)	0.610
Cerebrovascular disease	162 (8)	75 (7.4)	87 (8.6)	0.368
History of stroke	73 (3.6)	34 (3.4)	39 (3.9)	0.634
History of TIA/RIND	72 (3.6)	28 (2.8)	44 (4.4)	0.071
chronic lung disease	111 (5.5)	56 (5.6)	55 (5.5)	0.99
LVEF (%) [median (IQR)][a]	50 (40–55)	50 (40–55)	49 (40–55)	0.527
3 vessel CAD	1609 (79.7)	813 (80.6)	796 (78.9)	0.376
Previous MI	1076 (53.3)	517 (51.2)	559 (55.4)	0.067
Previous PCI	304 (15.1)	152 (15.1)	152 (15.1)	0.99
NYHA IV	31 (1.5)	14 (1.4)	17 (1.7)	0.718
CCS 4	194 (9.6)	93 (9.2)	101 (10.0)	0.597
ACS	95 (4.7)	47 (4.7)	48 (4.8)	0.99

[a]*Missing data.*

PS, propensity score; IQR, interquartile range; BMI, body mass index; PA, pulmonary artery; CC, creatinine clearance; TIA, transient ischemic attack; LVEF, left ventricle ejection fraction; CAD, coronary artery disease; VD, vessel disease; MI, myocardial infarction; PCI, percutaneous coronary intervention; NYHA, New York Heart Association; CCS, Canadian Cardiovascular Society; ACS, Acute Coronary Syndrome.

stenotic lesions in two-vessel disease and three lesions in three-vessel disease of different territories for whatever reason (15). Each distal anastomosis was counted as a separate graft, e.g., sequential conduit was counted as more than one graft. Whenever the territory that sequential graft supplied couldn't be determined from the registry or this data was missing, it was not taken into consideration when assessing the completeness of revascularization. We report data on early post-operative (< 24 h) mortality rates, in-hospital complications, lengths of stay in the intensive care unit (ICU) and in the hospital (HLoS).

Statistical Analyses

Continuous variables were summarized as mean with standard deviation if normally distributed; non-normal distributions were summarized as median with IQR and compared with the Mann–Whitney U test or standard *t*-test, as appropriate. Categorical variables [number (%)] were compared with the Fisher exact test. Propensity matching was generated for each patient from a non-parsimonious multivariable logistic regression model that was based on baseline characteristics (age, number of vessels diseased, comorbidities, EuroSCORE II, LVEF, CCS, NYHA, and others listed in **Table 1**) and procedural [concomitant ablation, type of surgery (Off-Pump, On-Pump), procedure urgency] covariates as independent variables with treatment type (CR vs. non-CR) as a dependent variable. We used and opt-match and matchIt packages, 1-to-1 pairing, without replacement within a specific caliper width of 0.2 standard deviation of the propensity score. We computed standardized mean differences (SMDs) to verify the balance between CR versus non-CR groups after matching (**Supplementary Figure 2**). Risk Ratios (RRs) were used for in-hospital outcomes, whereas Cox proportional-hazards models were used to determine factors related to the event-free survival at long-term follow-up. We calculated Hazard Ratios (HRs) point estimate and 95% confidence intervals (95% CIs) with ensuing statistical models. Mortality was assessed with Kaplan–Meier survival curves fitted after PS matching. As a further sensitivity analysis, defined subgroup analyses were performed to assess the mortality in different scenarios. STATA MP v13.0 software (StataCorp, College Station, TX, United States) and R (with Rcmdr package and EZR software) were used for computations.

RESULTS

We identified 4,770 patients with pre-operative AF undergoing CABG; of those, in 3,193 (66.9%) patients, CR according to predefined criteria was achieved. During the 9-year follow-up, there were no marked differences in the proportion of complete vs. ICR, nor there were

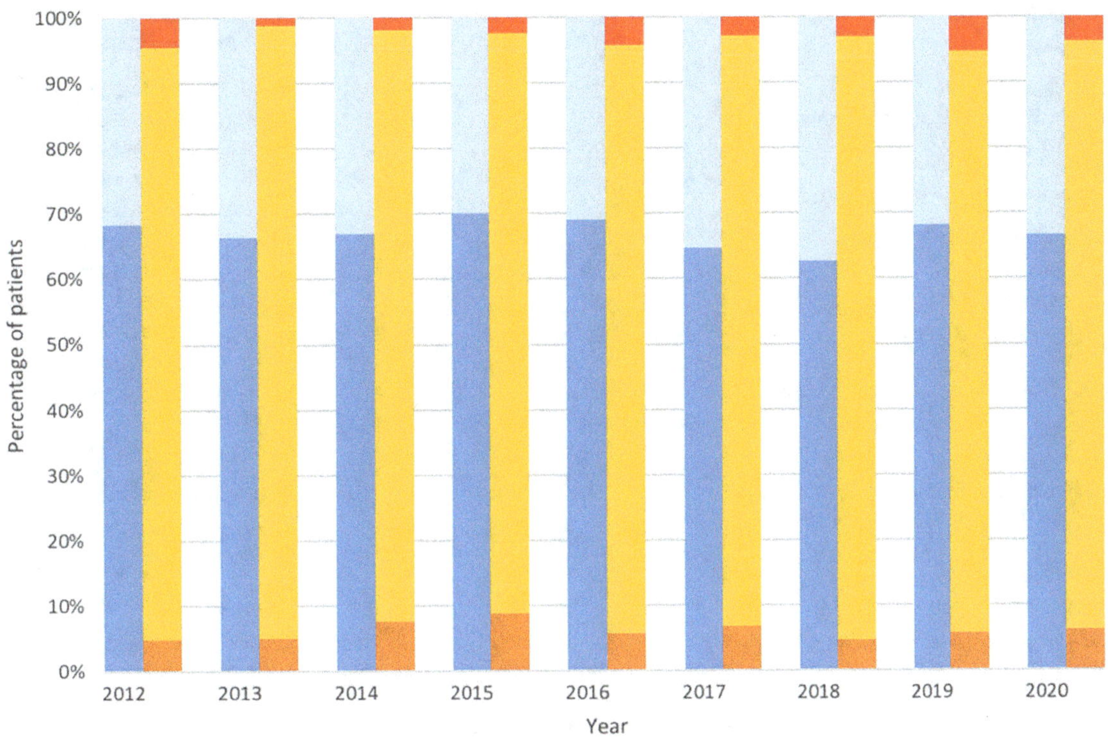

FIGURE 1 | Temporal trends in completeness of revascularization and utilization of arterial grafting. Complete revascularization (dark blue), non-complete revascularization (light blue), multiple arterial grafting (orange), single arterial grafting (yellow), total arterial revascularization (red).

any differences in the adoption of multi-arterial grafting (MAG) (**Figure 1**). Using the propensity score matching (PSM) model, two groups of 1,009 patients each were determined, by pairing non-CR patients with CR controls to achieve similar baseline (**Table 1**) and surgical (**Table 2**) characteristics. We report details on matching quality in **Supplementary Figure 2**.

TABLE 2 | Operative characteristics after PS-matching.

	Total (2018)	Non-CR (1009)	CR (1009)	*P*-value
Procedural characteristics				
Critical pre-operative state	43 (2.1)	22 (2.2)	21 (2.1)	0.99
IABP	8 (0.4)	4 (0.4)	4 (0.4)	0.99
iv. inotropes	35 (1.7)	19 (1.9)	16 (1.6)	0.734
Mechanical vent	8 (0.4)	5 (0.5)	3 (0.3)	0.726
Emergency surgery	74 (3.7)	37 (3.7)	37 (3.7)	0.99
OPCAB	1031 (51.1)	531 (52.6)	500 (49.6)	0.182
CPB (min)[a]	74 (55–95)	60 (45–74)	90 (71–109)	< 0.001
X-clamp (min)[a]	41 (29–54)	32 (24–41)	50 (40–61)	< 0.001
Conversion to ONCAB	17 (0.8%)	11 (1.1)	6 (0.6)	0.330
Concomitant ablation	79 (3.9)	41 (4.1)	38 (3.8)	0.819

[a]*Missing data.*
PS, propensity score; CPR, cardiopulmonary resuscitation; IABP, intra-aortic balloon pump; iv, intravenous; OPCAB, Off-Pump Coronary Artery Bypass; ONCAB, On-Pump Coronary Artery Bypass; CPB, cardiopulmonary bypass; LAAO, left atrial appendage occlusion; ±; SD, Standard Deviation.

Baseline and Surgical Characteristics

Baseline characteristics were balanced between groups, with similar EUROSCORE values [median (IQR): 1.92 (1.22–3.19) and 1.90 (1.18–3.19), respectively in patients with incomplete and CR]. The median age was identical in both groups – 70 years (64–76). Of included patients, 78.8% (non-CR) vs. 78.7% (CR) were men, 80.6% of non-CR patients in comparison with 78.9% in the CR group had a 3-vessel coronary artery disease ($p = 0.376$). Concomitant ablation was performed in 4.1% of non-CR and 3.8% of the CR group; 531 (52.6%) non-CR and

TABLE 3 | Grafts and anastomoses after PS-matching.

	Total (2018)	Non-CR (1009)	CR (1009)
LIMA	1860 (92.2)	914 (90.5)	950 (94.2)
RIMA	83 (4.1)	35 (3.5)	48 (4.8)
BIMA	77 (3.8)	34 (3.4)	43 (4.3)
Pedicled IMA[a]	619 (30.7)	295 (34.6)	324 (38.0)
Skeletonized IMA[a]	1085 (53.8)	557 (65.4)	528 (62.0)
Radial artery	44 (2.2)	25 (2.5)	19 (1.9)
Multiple arterial grafts	203 (10.1)	82 (8.1)	121 (12.0)
Total Arterial Revascularization	42 (2.1)	0 (0.0)	42 (4.2)
Number of anastomoses (Mean + –SD)		2 (1–2)	3 (3–3)

[a]*Missing data.*
LIMA/RIMA/BIMA, Left/Right/Bilateral Internal Mammary Artery; RA, Radial Artery. ±; SD, Standard Deviation.

TABLE 4 | In-hospital outcomes after PS-matching.

	Non-CR (1009)	CR (1009)	Risk ratio (95% CIs)	*P*-value
Early post-operative mortality (< 24 h)	7 (0.7)	8 (0.8)	1.14 (0.42–3.14)	0.288
Cardiac tamponade and/or rethoracotomy for bleeding	31 (3.1)	51 (5.1)	1.65 (1.06–2.55)	0.032
Respiratory failure	60 (5.9)	74 (7.3)	1.23 (0.89–1.71)	0.245
Neurologic complications	25 (2.5)	21 (2.1)	0.84 (0.47–1.49)	0.655
Multiorgan failure	21 (2.1)	21 (2.1)	1.00 (0.55–1.82)	1.000
Gastrointestinal complications	13 (1.3)	16 (1.6)	1.23 (0.6–2.55)	0.709
Acute kidney failure and/or dialysis	32 (3.2)	34 (3.4)	1.06 (0.66–1.71)	0.901
Superficial sternal wound infection	19 (1.9)	21 (2.1)	1.11 (0.60–2.04)	0.873
Deep sternal wound infection	18 (1.8)	14 (1.4)	0.78 (0.39–1.56)	0.594
Mediastinitis	4 (0.4)	6 (0.6)	1.50 (0.42–5.3)	0.753
PPI	4 (0.4)	4 (0.4)	1.00 (0.25–3.99)	1.000
ECMO	1 (0%)	1 (0%)	1.00 (0.06–15.97)	1.000
IABP	18 (1.8%)	21 (2.1%)	1.17 (0.63–2.18)	0.628

PS, propensity score; CIs, confidence intervals; MI, myocardial infarction; ICU, intensive care unit; PPI, permanent pacemaker implantation; ECMO, extracorporeal membrane oxygenation; IABP, intra-aortic balloon pump.

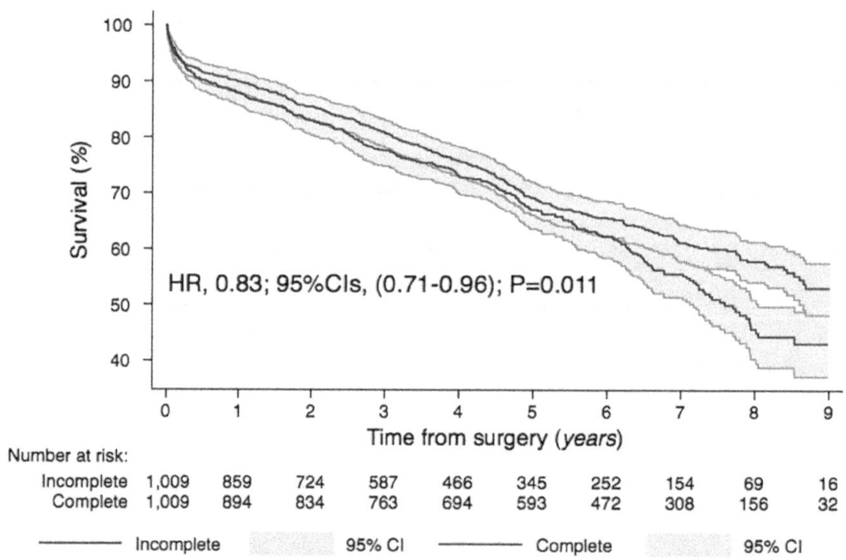

FIGURE 2 | Long-term mortality, propensity matched Kaplan–Meier survival curves between the two groups: CR vs. non-CR CABG for the analysis of long-term survival. Hazard Ratios and respective 95% Confidence Intervals.

500 (49.6%) CR patients were operated on without the use of cardio-pulmonary bypass ($p = 0.182$). As expected, the number of distal anastomoses varied between groups (1.7 ± 0.6 non-CR vs. 3.0 ± 0.6 CR, $P < 0.001$). **Table 3** lists information regarding grafts and anastomoses.

Clinical Outcomes

In-hospital outcomes and post-operative complications were consistent between groups (**Table 4**). Early mortality (24 h) and 30-day mortality were unaffected by CR [Odds Ratio (OR) and 95% Confidence Intervals (CIs): 1.34 (0.46–3.86), $P = 0.593$, Hazard Ratio (HR) and 95% CIs: 0.88 (0.59–1.32), $P = 0.542$, respectively]. Cardiac tamponade and/or re-thoracotomy for bleeding occurred in 3.1 vs. 5.1% and was statistically more frequent in the CR group [Risk Ratio (RR) and 95% CIs, 1.65 (1.06–2.55), $P = 0.032$]. Cardiopulmonary bypass (CBP) and aortic X-clamp times were significantly longer in the CR group: the median of CBP time was 65 vs. 79 min ($P \leq 0.001$) in the CR and non-CR group and respectively 34 vs. 40 min ($P \leq 0.001$) of aortic X-clamp time. In the long-term follow-up [As stated in the abstract median follow up was 4.7 years (2.3–6.9)], CR was associated with significantly lower mortality [HR (95% CIs) 0.83 (0.71–0.96), $P = 0.011$] (**Figure 2**).

The CR group was further divided into patients who underwent complete- and "supracomplete" revascularization. The latter was associated with an even greater reduction in mortality HR (95% CIs) 0.76 (0.59–0.97), $P = 0.023$ (for SCR vs. ICR). Between ICR, CR, and SCR we observed a significant trend toward lower mortality (log rank $P = 0.032$, **Figure 3**).

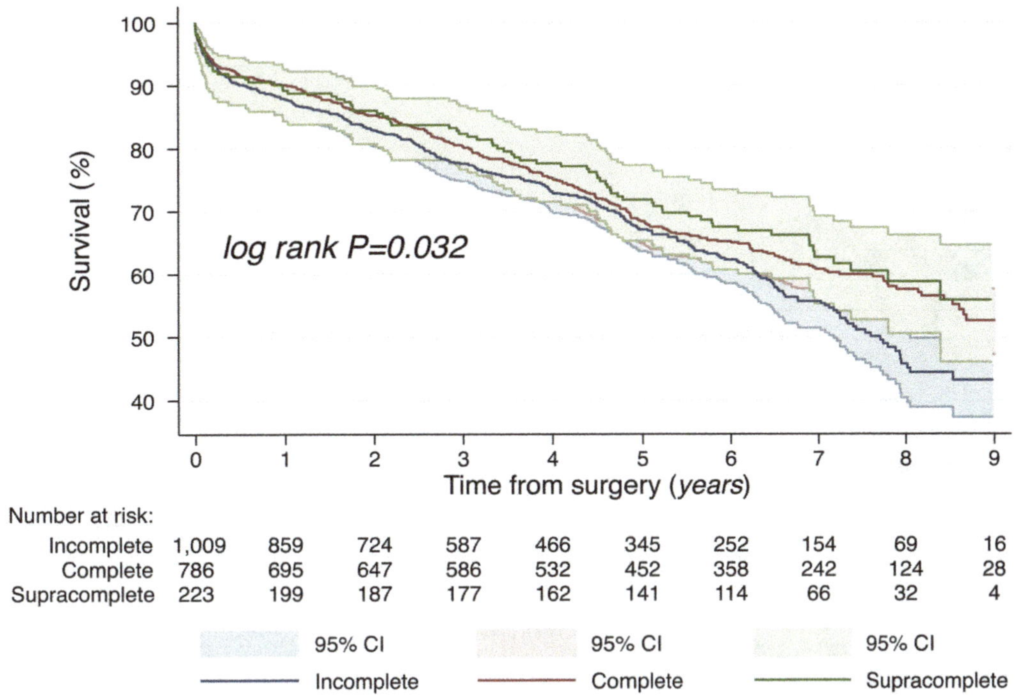

FIGURE 3 | Long-term mortality, propensity matched Kaplan–Meier survival curves between three groups: CR, non-CR, SCR CABG. Logrank test for differences in survival between groups. CR, complete revascularization; SCR, "supracomplete" revascularization.

In subgroup analyses, the benefit of improved long-term survival was sustained across diverse patient populations. Especially beneficent were younger (< 70 years old.) patients [HR (95% CIs) 0.67 (0.53–0.85), P = 0.001 for < 70 year old Vs. HR (95% CIs) 0.94 (0.78–1.13), P = 0.497 for ≥ 70 year old; P interaction = 0.027]. The effect was also more pronounced in patients with lower EuroSCORE II, without diabetes and when off-pump CABG was performed. Further details on the subgroup analyses are shown in **Figure 4**.

DISCUSSION

The current analysis is the first to focus on the long-term results of complete and incomplete surgical revascularization for MV-CAD in patients with pre-existing AF. Its main findings are as follows; (1) there was a high rate of ICR; (2) long-term benefit of CR; (3) even greater benefit with a higher number of additional grafts; (4) low prevalence of MAG and TAR in the population of AF patients, without significant temporal trends.

Complete revascularization, especially achieved through CABG, is characterized by improved long-term survival and a lower rate of reinterventions compared with ICR (1–3). It remains to be established whether this distinction is specifically because of ICR as a surgical method, deficiency, or anatomical obstacles during CABG or, whether the ICR is only a marker of more advanced and progressive coronary disease. The ICR usually indicates complex coronary pathology, with unfavorable outcomes originating from the patient's baseline risk profile. In reality, even though ICR may contrarily influence long-term results (17), it may be the most appropriate treatment method in a specific subset of prohibitive-risk patients. When the risks of surgery must be minimized to reduce perioperative mortality and complications, target vessel revascularization represents possibly the best feasible course of action (6).

Patients presenting with AF are at markedly elevated, yet non-prohibitive, operative risk, nor is AF itself accounted for in prognostic scores (e.g., EuroSCORE II). Although, the prevalence of AF in patients undergoing CABG is much lower than in patients undergoing mitral valve surgery (18, 19), up to 20% of patients presenting for coronary surgical procedures may have preoperative AF (14, 20), which is often used as a marker for high-risk patients (10, 11, 21). This percentage rises with age and decreased left ventricular function, which is seen in an increasing number of patients referred for CABG surgery. Although no data exists on performing CR in this population, because of their high-risk nature, surgeons may be reluctant to aim for CR as it is associated with longer operative time. Until now, no single study has focused on a comparison of CR/ICR in the AF population undergoing CABG.

One subgroup analysis of the Atrial Fibrillation undergoing Coronary Artery Stenting (AFCAS) registry focusing on the impact of ICR, has shown that of 445 (46.8%) PCI subjects in whom physicians opted for ICR, at 1-year follow-up, had a higher rate of the composite endpoint of acute MI, stent thrombosis and RR, compared to patients with CR (13.9% vs. 9.4%, p = 0.003) (22). In an adjusted multivariable analysis, only creatinine clearance (inverse relationship) and ICR were

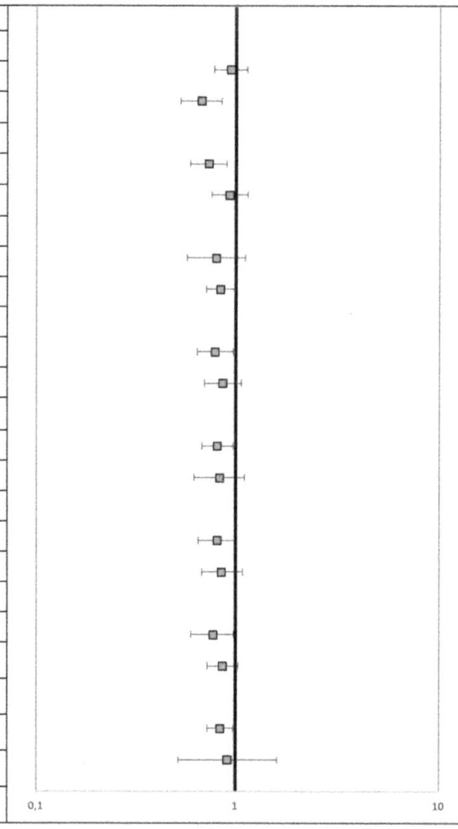

	Hazard Ratio (95%CIs)	P_{value}	$P_{interaction}$
Age ≥ 70 yrs			
Yes	0.94 (0.78 – 1.13)	0.497	0.027
No	0.67 (0.53 – 0.85)	0.001	
Type of surgery			
Off-pump	0.73 (0.59 – 0.90)	0.004	0.105
On-pump	0.93 (0.76 - 1.14)	0.475	
Coronary Artery Disease			
2-VD	0.80 (0.57 - 1.11)	0.176	0.797
3-VD	0.84 (0.71 - 0.99)	0.036	
Diabetes			
Yes	0.79 (0.64 - 0.97)	0.028	0.571
No	0.86 (0.70 - 1.06)	0.157	
LVEF ≤ 50%			
Yes	0.81 (0.68 - 0.97)	0.018	0.887
No	0.83 (0.62 - 1.10)	0.194	
Previous MI			
Yes	0.81 (0.65 - 1.00)	0.053	0.765
No	0.85 (0.68 - 1.08)	0.186	
Euroscore			
< 2%	0.77 (0.60 - 0.98)	0.031	0.476
≥2%	0.86 (0.72 - 1.03)	0.105	
Type of conduits			
SAG	0.84 (0.72-0.97)	0.021	0.786
MAG	0.91 (0.52-1.59)	0.740	

CIs. confidence intervals; LVEF. left ventricle ejection fraction MI. myocardial infarction; SAG, single arterial grafting; MAG, multiple arterial grafting

FIGURE 4 | Subgroup Analysis, Hazard Ratios and 95% Confidence Intervals (Cis) for death from any cause in CR as compared to non-CR according to selected characteristics; CR, complete revascularization; VD, vessel disease; LVEF, left ventricle ejection fraction; MI, myocardial infarction.

independently associated with a higher risk of the composite endpoint [HR (95% CIs) 1.66, (1.10–2.50), $p = 0.013$] (22).

The latest reports and registries analyses present data on safety and efficacy of surgical CR in AF. In a study of 900 patients with end-stage renal disease, where 14.1% of all patients had pre-existing AF, emergency surgery, diabetes mellitus, the number of vein grafts and age were identified as risk factors for mortality (23). CR, the use of an internal thoracic artery and the sinus rhythm pre-op were recognized as beneficial factors for long-term survival (23). Although AF was not identified as an independent risk factor for perioperative mortality ($p = 0.59$), it was an independent predictor for late mortality ($p < 0.001$) (23). In an analysis of the KROK registry Off-Pump CABG offered a 30-day survival benefit to patients undergoing CABG surgery and presenting with underlying AF (24). On-Pump CABG, on the other hand, was associated with significantly improved long-term survival. CR was possible in 67.5% of patients and was significantly higher, by 10%, in patients undergoing On-Pump CABG (73.3 vs. 62.6%; $P < 0.001$) (24).

One finding of the preset report requires special attention; it was demonstrated that "supra-complete" revascularization, may further improve survival in AF patients undergoing CABG. A study by Schwann et al. investigated the effects of SCR in SAG and MAG and concluded that it conveyed a survival benefit in patients with 3-VD in a single arterial grafting group (which is the majority in our study) (25). Conversely, Chu et al. observed no survival benefit with multiple grafts to each myocardial territory (26). Supra-complete revascularization could be beneficial in several ways, by securing the vulnerable myocardium during the early phase post-op, particularly prone to arrhythmias and disturbances in blood flow, or protecting distal coronary arteries from MI in long-term when functionally non-significant and non-revascularized lesions become significant (27). However, aiming for SCR must increase operative times and since its benefit is not well established the surgeons face a difficult decision. Our results suggest that preoperative AF, although a poor prognostic factor in general, should not be deemed prohibitive while considering additional grafts to each coronary territory.

Several factors, beyond the completeness of the revascularization, can influence the outcome in the AF population. Analysis of the KROK registry (28) showed a significant survival benefit associated with concomitant surgical ablation (SA) in the setting of CABG. The same analysis showed that it remains severely underused, as it was performed only in 4.4%. Recent guidelines give a recommendation to concomitant SA during CABG surgery. Considering that both CR and SA prolong operative times, surgeons might decide to choose SA over the additional graft that would ensure completeness of the revascularization. Our results suggest that in non-prohibitive risk patients, both SA and CR should be aimed for. Another analysis of the KROK registry showed that patients undergoing multiple arterial grafting have survival benefits at long-term follow-up (13 years post-op) as compared to single arterial grafting (29). This benefit was further sustained in subgroup analyses, yet most appraised in low risk patients (< 70-year-old; EuroSCORE < 2; no diabetes) and when CR was achieved ($P = 0.009$). Some studies suggest that benefit with the CR may be conferred to SAG patients, wheares when multiple arterial grafts are used their superior patency could neutralize survival benefit associated with completeness of revascularization (30). Indeed, in our sensitivity analysis the benefit in MAG group was non-significant, although it has to be noted that the number of MAG patients was low.

LIMITATIONS

Our study has several limitations. First, only all-cause mortality assessment is possible; the information regarding the cause of death, reinterventions, MIs, heart failure hospitalizations, adherence to anticoagulation therapy, or angiographic patency follow-up is not recorded in the registry. Second, although we addressed a potential selection bias, with propensity score matching according to baseline clinical variables, several confounders could prevail, an important of which is the lack of coronary angiograms that would allow us to access the percentage of chronic total occlusions. Additionally, we did not include the grafting choice (arterial vs. venous grafting) and patient allocation in the propensity score model. Third, detailed anatomy of coronary vessels is not available and therefore the feasibility of CR in each case could not be assessed. Finally, our data regarding coronary revascularization concerns CABG surgery only. Perhaps, some patients, in whom CR during surgery was deemed infeasible, could benefit from a staged hybrid revascularization with PCI as a second stage. Unfortunately, the registry at that time did not gather data regarding subsequent interventions.

CONCLUSION

In this multicenter retrospective propensity-matched study of patients with preoperative AF, CR during CABG was associated with improved long-term survival. The particular benefit was observed in lower-risk patients. A significant trend was observed toward lower mortality with "supracomplete" revascularization.

ETHICS STATEMENT

Ethical review and approval was not required for the study on human participants in accordance with the local legislation and institutional requirements. Written informed consent for participation was not required for this study in accordance with the national legislation and the institutional requirements.

AUTHOR CONTRIBUTIONS

MP, JS, JF, and MKow: conception and design. PS, RLo, MD, WWo, JR, MJ, MZ, and KB: administrative support. JS, RLi, GF, AK, WWa, AŁ, SS, DJ, FJ, MM, GM, and GR: provision of study materials or patients. NP-S, SM, TL, DR, and AS: collection and assembly of data. MP, MKow, MKoł, PGM, PM, and DF: data analysis and interpretation. MP, JS, JF, MKow, MKoł, and SM: manuscript writing. All authors approved the final manuscript.

REFERENCES

1. Garcia S, Sandoval Y, Roukoz H, Adabag S, Canoniero M, Yannopoulos D, et al. Outcomes after complete versus incomplete revascularization of patients with multivessel coronary artery disease: a meta-analysis of 89,883 patients enrolled in randomized clinical trials and observational studies. *J Am Coll Cardiol.* (2013) 62:1421–31. doi: 10.1016/j.jacc.2013.05.033
2. Zimarino M, Ricci F, Romanello M, Di Nicola M, Corazzini A, De Caterina R. Complete myocardial revascularization confers a larger clinical benefit when performed with state-of-the-art techniques in high-risk patients with multivessel coronary artery disease: a meta-analysis of randomized and observational studies. *Catheter Cardiovasc Interv.* (2016) 87:3–12. doi: 10.1002/ccd.25923
3. Takahashi K, Serruys PW, Gao C, Ono M, Wang R, Thuijs DJFM, et al. Ten-year all-cause death according to completeness of revascularization in patients with three-vessel disease or left main coronary artery disease: insights from the SYNTAX extended survival study. *Circulation.* (2021) 144:96–109. doi: 10.1161/CIRCULATIONAHA.120.046289
4. Mehta SR, Wood DA, Storey RF, Mehran R, Bainey KR, Nguyen H, et al. Complete Revascularization with multivessel PCI for myocardial infarction. *N Engl J Med.* (2019) 381:1411–21.
5. Engstrøm T, Kelbæk H, Helqvist S, Høfsten DE, Kløvgaard L, Holmvang L, et al. Complete revascularisation versus treatment of the culprit lesion only in patients with ST-segment elevation myocardial infarction and multivessel disease (DANAMI-3—PRIMULTI): an open-label, randomised controlled trial. *Lancet.* (2015) 386:665–71. doi: 10.1016/s0140-6736(15)60648-1
6. Kowalewski M, Schulze V, Berti S, Waksman R, Kubica J, Kołodziejczak M, et al. Complete revascularisation in ST-elevation myocardial infarction and multivessel disease: meta-analysis of randomised controlled trials. *Heart.* (2015) 101:1309–17. doi: 10.1136/heartjnl-2014-307293
7. Farkouh ME, Domanski M, Sleeper LA, Siami FS, Dangas G, Mack M, et al. Strategies for multivessel revascularization in patients with diabetes. *N Engl J Med.* (2012) 367:2375–84.
8. Serruys PW, Morice MC, Kappetein AP, Colombo A, Holmes DR, Mack MJ, et al. Percutaneous coronary intervention versus coronary-artery bypass grafting for severe coronary artery disease. *N Engl J Med.* (2009) 360:961–72.

9. Neumann FJ, Sousa-Uva M, Ahlsson A, Alfonso F, Banning AP, Benedetto U, et al. 2018 ESC/EACTS guidelines on myocardial revascularization. *Eur Heart J.* (2019) 40:87–165.
10. Batra G, Ahlsson A, Lindahl B, Lindhagen L, Wickbom A, Oldgren J. Atrial fibrillation in patients undergoing coronary artery surgery is associated with adverse outcome. *Ups J Med Sci.* (2019) 124:70–7. doi: 10.1080/03009734.2018.1504148
11. Böning A, Diegeler A, Hilker M, Zacher M, Reents W, Faerber G, et al. Preoperative atrial fibrillation and outcome in patients undergoing on-pump or off-pump coronary bypass surgery: lessons learned from the GOPCABE trial. *Interact Cardiovasc Thorac Surg.* (2015) 20:74–8. doi: 10.1093/icvts/ivu331
12. Ruddox V, Sandven I, Munkhaugen J, Skattebu J, Edvardsen T, Otterstad JE. Atrial fibrillation and the risk for myocardial infarction, all-cause mortality and heart failure: a systematic review and meta-analysis. *Eur J Prev Cardiol.* (2017) 24:1555–66. doi: 10.1177/2047487317715769
13. Shin H, Hashizume K, Iino Y, Koizumi K, Matayoshi T, Yozu R. Effects of atrial fibrillation on coronary artery bypass graft flow. *Eur J Cardiothorac Surg.* (2003) 23:175–8. doi: 10.1016/s1010-7940(02)00730-3
14. McCarthy PM, Davidson CJ, Kruse J, Lerner DJ, Braid-Forbes MJ, McCrea MM, et al. Prevalence of atrial fibrillation before cardiac surgery and factors associated with concomitant ablation. *J Thorac Cardiovasc Surg.* (2020) 159:2245–2253.e15. doi: 10.1016/j.jtcvs.2019.06.062
15. Schaefer A, Conradi L, Schneeberger Y, Reichenspurner H, Sandner S, Tebbe U, et al. Clinical outcomes of complete versus incomplete revascularization in patients treated with coronary artery bypass grafting: insights from the TiCAB trial. *Eur J Cardiothorac Surg.* (2020) 59:417–25. doi: 10.1093/ejcts/ezaa330
16. Vander Salm TJ, Kip KE, Jones RH, Schaff HV, Shemin RJ, Aldea GS, et al. What constitutes optimal surgical revascularization? Answers from the bypass angioplasty revascularization investigation (BARI). *J Am Coll Cardiol.* (2002) 39:565–72. doi: 10.1016/s0735-1097(01)01806-x
17. Mocanu V, Buth KJ, Kelly R, Légaré JF. Incomplete revascularization after coronary artery bypass graft operations is independently associated with worse long-term survival. *Ann Thorac Surg.* (2014) 98:549–55. doi: 10.1016/j.athoracsur.2014.02.090
18. Suwalski P, Kowalewski M, Jasiński M, Staromłyński J, Zembala M, Widenka K, et al. Survival after surgical ablation for atrial fibrillation in mitral valve surgery: analysis from the polish national registry of cardiac surgery procedures (KROK). *J Thorac Cardiovasc Surg.* (2019) 157:1007–1018.e4. doi: 10.1016/j.jtcvs.2018.07.099
19. Rankin JS, He X, O'Brien SM, Jacobs JP, Welke KF, Filardo G, et al. The Society of Thoracic Surgeons risk model for operative mortality after multiple valve surgery. *Ann Thorac Surg.* (2013) 95:1484–90. doi: 10.1016/j.athoracsur.2012.11.077
20. Malaisrie SC, McCarthy PM, Kruse J, Matsouaka RA, Churyla A, Grau-Sepulveda MV, et al. Ablation of atrial fibrillation during coronary artery bypass grafting: late outcomes in a Medicare population. *J Thorac Cardiovasc Surg.* (2021) 161:1251–61. doi: 10.1016/j.jtcvs.2019.10.159
21. Ad N, Barnett SD, Haan CK, O'Brien SM, Milford-Beland S, Speir AM. Does preoperative atrial fibrillation increase the risk for mortality and morbidity after coronary artery bypass grafting? *J Thorac Cardiovasc Surg.* (2009) 137:901–6. doi: 10.1016/j.jtcvs.2008.09.050
22. Proietti M, Airaksinen KEJ, Rubboli A, Schlitt A, Kiviniemi T, Karjalainen PP, et al. P1177 Impact of incomplete revascularization in atrial fibrillation patients undergoing percutaneous coronary intervention: the afcas registry. *EP Europace.* (2018) 20:i227. doi: 10.1093/europace/euy015.662
23. Schönburg M, Ziegelhoeffer T, Weinbrenner F, Bechtel M, Detter C, Krabatsch T, et al. Preexisting atrial fibrillation as predictor for late-time mortality in patients with end-stage renal disease undergoing cardiac surgery–a multicenter study. *Thorac Cardiovasc Surg.* (2008) 56:128–32. doi: 10.1055/s-2007-989432
24. Kowalewski M, Jasiński M, Staromłyński J, Zembala M, Widenka K, Brykczyński M, et al. On-Pump vs Off-Pump coronary artery bypass surgery in atrial fibrillation. Analysis from the polish national registry of cardiac surgery procedures (KROK). *PLoS One.* (2020) 15:e0231950. doi: 10.1371/journal.pone.0231950
25. Schwann TA, Yammine MB, El-Hage-Sleiman AM, Engoren MC, Bonnell MR, Habib RH. The effect of completeness of revascularization during CABG with single versus multiple arterial grafts. *J Card Surg.* (2018) 33:620–8. doi: 10.1111/jocs.13810
26. Chu D, Bakaeen FG, Wang XL, Coselli JS, LeMaire SA, Huh J. The impact of placing multiple grafts to each myocardial territory on longterm survival after coronary artery bypass grafting. *J Thorac Cardiovasc Surg.* (2009) 137:60–4. doi: 10.1016/j.jtcvs.2008.09.018
27. Thuesen AL, Riber LP, Veien KT, Christiansen EH, Jensen SE, Modrau I, et al. Fractional flow reserve versus angiographically-guided coronary artery bypass grafting. *J Am Coll Cardiol.* (2018) 72:2732–43. doi: 10.1016/j.jacc.2018.09.043
28. Suwalski P, Kowalewski M, Jasiński M, Staromłyński J, Zembala M, Widenka K, et al. Surgical ablation for atrial fibrillation during isolated coronary artery bypass surgery. *Eur J Cardiothorac Surg.* (2020) 57:691–7.
29. Kowalewski M, Pasierski M, Litwinowicz R, Zembala M, Piekuś-Słomka N, Tobota Z, et al. Multiple versus single arterial coronary arterial bypass grafting surgery for multivessel disease in atrial fibrillation. *Semin Thorac Cardiovasc Surg.* (2021) 33:974–83. doi: 10.1053/j.semtcvs.2020.11.015
30. Rosenblum JM, Binongo J, Wei J, Liu Y, Leshnower BG, Chen EP, et al. Priorities in coronary artery bypass grafting: is midterm survival more dependent on completeness of revascularization or multiple arterial grafts? *J Thorac Cardiovasc Surg.* (2021) 161:2070–8. doi: 10.1016/j.jtcvs.2019.11.125

30

Septal Thickness does not Impact Outcome After Hypertrophic Obstructive Cardiomyopathy Surgery (Septal Myectomy and Subvalvular Mitral Apparatus Remodeling): A 15-Years of Experience

Giuseppe M. Raffa[1], Eluisa La Franca[1], Carlo Lachina[1], Andrea Palmeri[1], Mariusz Kowalewski[2,3], Steven Lebowitz[4], Alessandro Ricasoli[1], Matteo Greco[1], Sergio Sciacca[1], Marco Turrisi[1], Marco Morsolini[1], Vincenzo Stringi[1], Gabriella Mattiucci[1] and Michele Pilato[1]*

[1] Department for the Treatment and Study of Cardiothoracic Diseases and Cardiothoracic Transplantation, IRCCS-ISMETT (Istituto Mediterraneo per i Trapianti e Terapie ad Alta Specializzazione), Palermo, Italy, [2] Department of Cardiac Surgery, Central Clinical Hospital of the Ministry of Interior, Center of Postgraduate Medical Education, Warsaw, Poland, [3] Innovative Medical Forum, Thoracic Research Center, Collegium Medicum, Nicolaus Copernicus University, Bydgoszcz, Poland, [4] The University of Pittsburgh School of Medicine, Pittsburgh, PA, United States

***Correspondence:**
Giuseppe M. Raffa
giuseppe.raffa78@gmail.com

Background: The aim of this study was to assess the impact of septal thickness on long-term outcomes of surgical treatment for hypertrophic obstructive cardiomyopathy (HOCM) and correction of mitral subvalvular anomalies.

Methods: Sixty-six consecutive patients (58 $\pm$ 12 years, 56% female) undergoing extended septal myectomy and subvalvular mitral apparatus remodeling from 2007 to 2021 were retrospectively reviewed. Patients were divided into 2 groups according to septal thickness: moderate [$<$ 18 mm, 29 patients (44%)] and severe [$\geq$ 18 mm, 37 patients (56%)]. End points included survival, symptom improvement, reduction of left ventricle outflow tract (LVOT) gradient, resolution of mitral regurgitation (MR), and reoperation.

Results: The mean interventricular septal thickness was 19 $\pm$ 3 mm, 15.8 $\pm$ 0.8 mm in patients with moderate and 21.4 $\pm$ 3.2 mm in those with severe hypertrophy. Preoperative data, intraoperative variables, postoperative complication rates, pre-discharge echocardiographic and clinical parameters did not differ between the two study groups [except for procedures involving the posterior mitral leaflet (p = 0.033) and septal thickness after myectomy (p = 0.0001)]. Subvalvular apparatus remodeling (secondary chordae of mitral valve resection and papillary muscle and muscularis trabecula procedures including resection, splitting, and elongation) was invariably added to septal myectomy (100%). Four (6%) procedures involved the posterior mitral leaflets. Mitral valve replacement was carried out in two patients (3%, p = 0.4). Reoperation for persistent MR was necessary in one patient (1%, $p = 0.4$). Neither iatrogenic ventricular septal defect nor in-hospital mortality occurred. During follow-up (mean 4.8 ± 3.8 years), two deaths occurred. NYHA class was reduced from 2.9 ± 0.7 to 1.6 ± 0.6 ($p < 0.0001$), the LVOT gradient from 89.7 ± 34.5 to 16.3 ± 8.8 mmHg ($p < 0.0001$), mitral valve regurgitation grade from 2.5 ± 1 to 1.2 ± 0.5 ($p < 0.0001$), and septal thickness from 18.9 ± 3.7 to 13.9 ± 2.7 mm ($p < 0.0001$).

Conclusions: Regardless of septal thickness, subvalvular apparatus remodeling with concomitant septal myectomy can provide satisfactory long-term outcomes in terms of symptom improvement, LVOT obstruction relief, and MR resolution (without mitral valve replacement in most cases) in patients with HOCM.

Keywords: hypertrophic obstructive cardiomyopathy, mitral valve repair, mitral approach, systolic anterior motion, extensive myectomy

INTRODUCTION

Transaortic surgical septal myectomy (1) for the treatment of hypertrophic obstructive cardiomyopathy (HOCM) is associated with low operative morbidity and mortality, and reduction of the outflow gradient (2, 3). Systolic anterior motion (SAM) of the anterior mitral leaflet (AML) as a contributor to the pathophysiology of left ventricle outflow tract (LVOT) obstruction has been addressed (4–6) and in patients without severe hypertrophy (7, 8), SAM and mitral abnormalities (e.g., leaflet elongation and a wide array of malformations of the papillary muscles (PM) and chordae) may influence the dynamic obstruction of LVOT. In this context, the correction of subvalvular mitral apparatus abnormalities in addition to septal myectomy has been advocated (6, 8, 9) in order to abolish the LVOT gradient and to restore mitral competence. Although a matter of debate (10), these procedures include secondary chordae cutting (11), anterior leaflet plication (12) or extension (13), reorientation of PM (14), edge-to-edge repair (15), and mitral valve (MV) surgery (6, 7, 9, 16). MV replacement has been also reported (7, 16) if SAM and severe mitral regurgitation (MR) are challenging to manage.

The role of septal thickness in long-term outcomes of correction of subvalvular mitral apparatus abnormalities during myectomy is an under-studied matter of debate.

In this study we sought to assess the implications of septal thickness in long-term clinical and echocardiographic outcomes of patients requiring subvalvular MV remodeling (6, 9) in addition to extended septal myectomy.

MATERIALS AND METHODS

This retrospective and monocentric study was approved by the ethics committee of our institute (IRRB/35/16) and individual consent was obtained from each patient.

Study Population

The study included 66 consecutive adult patients with HOCM treated surgically by extended septal myectomy and subvalvular MV remodeling between March 2007 and September 2021 at our institution. The patients had peak LVOT gradients ≥ 50 mmHg at rest or during stress and drug-refractory disabling symptoms (17) and were divided in 2 groups according to the septal thickness: moderate [< 18 mm, 29 patients (44%)] and severe [≥ 18 mm, 37 patients (56%)]. The cutoff of 18 mm was decided according to data available in the literature (7, 8). The 66 patients operated on represent 37% of 178 patients referred to our dedicated hypertrophic obstructive cardiomyopathy out-patient clinic who underwent surgery. Exclusion criteria were: history of mitral operation (including Mitraclip). Emergency operations and patients having undergone previous surgical myectomy or alcoholization were included.

Review of hospital records and analysis of preoperative history and reports, operative notes, and postoperative and follow-up echocardiography reports were carried out using a dedicated database.

Diagnosis

All patients underwent preoperative Doppler transthoracic echocardiogram examination. Measurements of septal thickness were performed at end-diastole, in short-axis views from the mitral and mid left ventricle levels. Resting LVOT velocity was measured by continuous-wave Doppler of the outflow tract from an apical window. In HOCM patients who had a resting LVOT gradient < 30 mmHg but manifested drug refractory symptoms, provocative maneuvers such as the Valsalva were used during examination. Less symptomatic patients with LVOT gradient > 50 mmHg at rest underwent stress-echocardiogram. MV anatomy and function were evaluated by transthoracic and transesophageal echocardiogram (TEE) using an interactive approach. The degree of MR was measured by Doppler color flow imaging and quantitatively graded as mild (1 + /4 +), moderate (2 + /4 +), moderate-to-severe (3 + /4 +) and severe (4 + /4 +). A thorough analysis of the mitral subvalvular anomalies, including fibrotic and retracted secondary chordae inserted on the AML, abnormal chordae tendineae attached to the ventricular septum or free wall, and PM abnormalities was performed (6, 18). Cardiovascular magnetic resonance imaging providing detailed information on cardiac morphology, ventricular function, and myocardial tissue characteristics was not routinely performed. Most patients underwent pre-operative genetic and electrophysiology consults. Coronary anatomy was evaluated by angiograms and computed tomography scans. Intraoperative specimens were evaluated by pathologists.

Surgical Technique

Complete surgical details have been reported previously (6), **Figure 1**. The operations were guided by TEE with particular attention paid to the septal anatomy and thickness, and MV apparatus. Briefly, all operations were performed through a full sternotomy, with aorta and right atrial cannulation and intermittent antegrade cold blood cardioplegia, and with mild hypothermia (34°C). Transaortic myectomy was performed in all patients starting at nadir of the right coronary sinus, and extended apically to achieve exposure of the PM bases. Muscular resection was extended toward the lateral ventricular wall up to the left trigone. The PM were carefully inspected to detect any hypertrophy, fusion, displacement, anomalies, or aberrances (e.g., bifurcation and fibrosis). Subvalvular mitral apparatus remodeling included (1) resection of all anomalous muscular trabecula and accessory PM; (2) resection of fibrotic, thickened, and agglutinated secondary chordae tendineae from the tip of the PM to the ventricular surface of the anterior mitral leaflet; and (3) splitting of hypertrophied and thickened PM. In cases of mitral leaflet repair, bicaval cannulation and a left or right atrial approach was used. The leaflet repair was done after myectomy and after the complete "release" of the AML obtained by the resection of diseased secondary chordae "anchoring" the leaflet itself to the PM and the septum. Further procedures on cardiopulmonary bypass were performed if necessary. After weaning from cardiopulmonary bypass and before protamine administration, a pharmacological stress test with adrenaline (from 5 to 10 mcg) was performed to assess for any residual LVOT gradient, SAM, and MR by the induction of tachycardia and systemic hypertension.

Outcomes

Primary outcomes of the study were survival, symptom improvement [decrease in New York Heart Association (NYHA) functional class], reduction of LVOT gradient, and resolution of MR. Secondary outcomes included postoperative complications and reoperation for recurrence of LVOT obstruction and severe MR.

Follow-Up Data

Yearly patient follow-up included physical examination, chest X-ray, electrocardiogram, transthoracic echocardiogram, and blood tests, and was performed in our dedicated outpatient clinic or by telephone interview. At September 1, 2021, the follow-up was 100% complete. The longest follow-up time was 14.6 years.

Statistical Analysis

Continuous variables were expressed as mean, standard deviation, and range. Categorical variables were expressed as absolute value and percentage. The comparison between (1) patients with septal thickness < 18 mm and ≥ 18 mm; (2) NYHA, LVOT gradient, septum thickness, and residual MR before and after surgery were assessed by Chi-Square test, Fisher's exact test, and logistic regression. Linear regression analysis was also applied to assess association with outcomes with septal thickness considered as a continuous predictor. Freedom from events at follow-up was assessed with Kaplan–Meier estimator and log-Rank test. Data management and analysis were done with SAS version 9.4. All p-values of < 0.05 were considered statistically significant.

RESULTS

Patient Characteristics

The preoperative characteristics of the patients are depicted in **Table 1**. No major differences were observed between the two groups. The mean age was 58 ± 12 years, with 29 males and 37 females. Although patients were treated medically with β-blockers and/or calcium-channel blockers, all were symptomatic in NYHA class I-II ($n = 15$), III ($n = 40$), or IV ($n = 11$). Nine patients (13%) had a history of acute pulmonary edema and one (1%) was hospitalized at our institute due to cardiogenic shock. One patient underwent a second reoperation because of failure of previous surgeries performed elsewhere. History of previous alcoholization was recorded in one patient.

The mean interventricular septal thickness was 19 ± 3 mm, 15.8 ± 0.8 mm in patients with moderate and 21.4 ± 3.2 mm in those with severe hypertrophy. Six (9%) patients had an extreme septal thickness (≥ 26 mm). Intraventricular peak gradient was 89 ± 34 mmHg. MR was graded 1 + and 2 + /4 + in 29 patients, 3 + /4 + in 25 patients, and 4 + /4 + in 12 patients. The average length of the AML and posterior mitral leaflet were 26 ± 3 mm and 16 ± 3 mm, respectively. A significant difference in neither preoperative clinical characteristics nor in echocardiographic data were detected between patients with moderate and severe septal thickness.

Perioperative Outcomes

Surgical data and postoperative outcomes are summarized in **Table 2**. Intraoperative data, postoperative complication rate, and pre-discharge echocardiographic and clinical parameters did not differ between the two study groups [except for procedures involving the posterior mitral leaflet ($p = 0.033$) and septal thickness after myectomy ($p = 0.0001$)]. The analysis of the LVOT demonstrated thickened secondary chordae tendineae tractioning the AML to the interventricular septum in 64 patients (97%) and PM malformations in 55 patients (83%) including PMs hypertrophy (25 patients, 37%), accessory PMs (17 patients, 25%) and PMs fusion (13 patients, 20%). Surgical myectomy was performed in all patients (100%). Subvalvular mitral apparatus remodeling by means of secondary MV chordae resection (97%) and PM procedures (resection, splitting, and elongation; 83%) was added to myectomy where indicated. The mean number of resected secondary chordae was 3 ± 1.

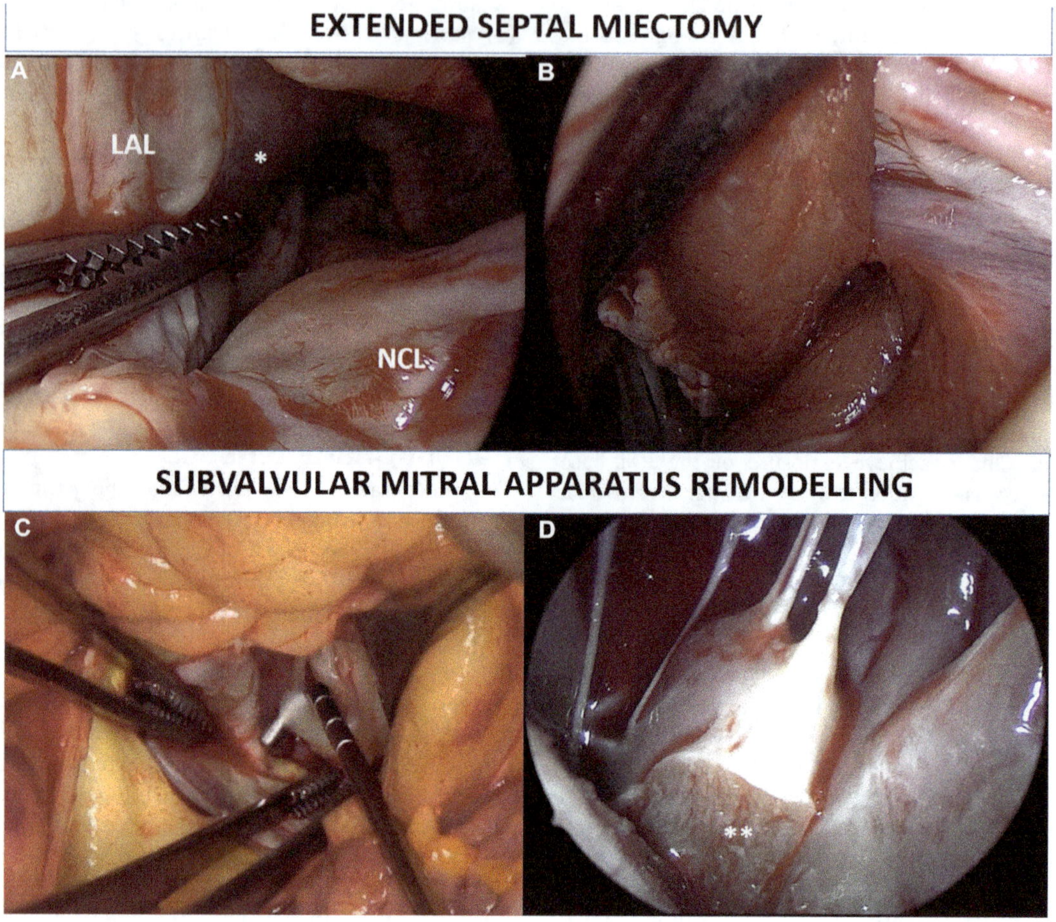

FIGURE 1 | Extended septal myectomy. Surgical view of the left ventricle outflow tract before the procedure is depicted in panel **(A)**. Transaortic myectomy was performed in all patients starting at nadir of the right coronary sinus, and extended apically to achieve exposure of the papillary muscles bases. Muscular resection was extended toward the lateral ventricular wall up to the left trigone **(B)**. Subvalvular mitral apparatus remodeling included (1) resection of fibrotic, thickened, and agglutinated secondary chordae tendineae from the tip of the papillary muscles to the ventricular surface of the anterior mitral leaflet **(C)**; (2) resection of all anomalous muscular trabecula and splitting (**) of hypertrophied and thickened papillary muscles **(D)**. LAL, left aortic leaflet; NCL, non-coronary leaflet. *Interventricular septum bulging.

In 4 patients, due to redundancy and excessive tissue of the posterior mitral leaflet, resection and shortening of the leaflet itself was performed. Of note, all four of these patients were in the moderate septal thickness group. Intuitively, the septal thickness reduction was greater in the group with septal thickness less than 18 mm (12.7 ± 1.4 mm vs. 15 ± 2.9 mm, $p = 0.0001$). Two patients required valve replacement due to persistent severe MR after LVOT obstruction resolution. One patient, at the beginning of our experience in 2007, underwent early reoperation (during the same hospitalization) after a complicated postoperative course. A mechanical mitral prosthesis for recurrent SAM and severe MR was implanted on postoperative day 55 and the patient was discharged on post-operative day 6. In a 58-year-old female patient, a mechanical prosthesis was necessary after 3 failed attempts (including posterior leaflet shortening) to correct severe MR, although complete LVOT obstruction and SAM resolution were obtained. In this case, the AML was dysplastic and retracted. Aortic valve replacement (6 patients) and coronary artery bypass (2 patients) were also performed. No iatrogenic ventricular septal defect occurred. Intraoperative, in-hospital, and 30-day mortality were 0%. No patients developed complete atrioventricular block, but 3 patients (4%) required pacemaker implantation because of tachy-brady syndrome. Pre-discharge pharmacological treatment included b-blockers (56 patients, 85%), diuretics (52 patients, 79%), renin-angiotensin-aldosterone system inhibitors (23 patients, 35%) and calcium channel blockers (4 patients, 6%).

Follow-Up Results

The mean follow-up time was 4.8 ± 3.8 years (range 0–14.5). Two deaths occurred, one at 83 days after surgery due to gastrointestinal bleeding and cardiogenic shock. The same patient was admitted in cardiogenic shock before HOCM surgery and a postmortem autopsy showed severe myocardial fibrosis, suggesting irreversible diastolic dysfunction. A late death

TABLE 1 | Baseline characteristics.

	All, $n = 66$	Septal thickness < 18 mm ($n = 29$)	Septal thickness ≥ 18 mm ($n = 37$)	*P*-value
Female sex	37 (56)	20 (54)	17 (46)	0.08
Age (years)	58.4 ± 12.5 (26–80)	59.5 ± 11.7 (36–80)	57.5 ± 13.2 (26–75)	0.5
BMI (kg/m^2)	27.6 ± 3.4 (20–39)	26.8 ± 3.1 (20–35)	28.3 ± 3.4 (21–39)	0.07
Family history for HOCM	22 (33)	9 (13)	13 (20)	0.7
Family history for SCD	23 (34)	9 (13)	14 (21)	0.6
Previous alcoholization	1 (1)	1 (1)	0 (0)	0.4
Syncope/lipothimia	15 (22)	6 (9)	9 (13)	0.7
Angina	33 (50)	12 (18)	21 (32)	0.3
Acute pulmonary edema	9 (13)	4 (6)	5 (7)	1
Pre-operative NYHA functional class	2.9 ± 0.7 (1–4)			0.6
I–II, n (%)	15 (22)	6 (9)	9 (13)	
III, n (%)	40 (61)	18 (28)	22 (33)	
IV, n (%)	11 (17)	5 (7)	6 (10)	
Pre-operative atrial fibrillation	37 (56)	13 (19)	24 (37)	0.1
Pre-operative SAM	53 (80)	22 (41)	31 (59)	0.5
Pre-operative ICD	13 (19)	3 (4)	10 (15)	0.1
Pre-operative LVEF (%)	64.2 ± 7.1 (40–83)	63.9 ± 5.3 (55–75)	64.5 ± 8.3 (40–83)	0.7
Pre-operative SPAP (mmHg)	27.4 ± 11.1 (19–70)	28.8 ± 12.8 (19–70)	26.4 ± 9.6 (20–58)	0.3
Pre-operative LVOT gradient* (mmHg)	89.7 ± 34.5 (28–174)	95.5 ± 35.6 (28–174)	85.1 ± 33.4 (40–165)	0.2
Pre-operative septal thickness (mm)	18.9 ± 3.7 (14–29)	15.8 ± 0.8 (14–17)	21.4 ± 3.2 (19–29)	0.7
Pre-operative MR grade	2.5 ± 1 (0–4)			0.4
1 + and 2 + /4 +	29 (43)	14 (21)	15 (22)	
3 + /4 +	25 (39)	9 (13)	16 (26)	
4 + /4 +	12 (18)	6 (9)	6 (9)	
Anterior mitral leaflet length (mm)	26.5 ± 3.8 (18–35)	26.2 ± 3.5 (21–32)	26.7 ± 4 (18–35)	0.6
Posterior mitral leaflet length (mm)	16.6 ± 3.7 (8–24)	17.5 ± 2.8 (11–22)	16 ± 4.2 (8–24)	0.1

BMI, body mass index; HOCM, Hypertrophic obstructive cardiomyopathy; SCD, sudden cardiac death; NYHA, New York Heart Association; SAM, systolic anterior motion; ICD, implantable cardioverter defibrillator; LVEF, left ventricular ejection fraction; SPAP, systolic pulmonary artery pressure; LVOT, left ventricle outflow tract; MR, mitral regurgitation.
**Peak gradient at rest.*
Continuous variables were expressed as mean, standard deviation and range.
Categorical variables were expressed as absolute value and percentage.

occurred in one patient due to pneumonia 717 days after surgery. This patient underwent reoperation 97 days after HOCM surgery because of endocarditis of the aortic prosthesis and pacemaker lead. Follow-up data are available in **Table 2**. Recurrence of SAM was detected in 7 patients without significant obstruction. Severe MR occurred in one patient who is currently under close follow-up for asymptomatic MR. Two patients with obesity had NYHA III symptoms at follow-up.

At the last available follow-up, the survival and freedom from reoperation was 96%. NYHA class was reduced from 2.9 ± 0.7 to 1.6 ± 0.6 ($p < 0.0001$), the LVOT gradient from 89.7 ± 34.5 to 16.3 ± 8.8 mmHg ($p < 0.0001$), MV regurgitation grade from 2.5 ± 1 to 1.2 ± 0.5 ($p < 0.0001$), and septal thickness from 18.9 ± 3.7 to 13.9 ± 2.7 mm ($p < 0.0001$), **Figure 2**. Freedom from composite end points at follow-up by means of recurrent LVOT obstruction (peak gradient ≥ 20 mmHg), MR ≥ 3 + /4 + , and NYHA ≥ 3 are depicted in **Figure 3**. Seven patients (10%) showed a mean LVOT peak gradient of 35.8 ± 2.6 mmHg and a mean NYHA class 2.2 ± 0.4 (in two patients were detected a 2 + /4 + grade of MV regurgitation. All these patients are medically treated and strictly followed at out outpatients clinic. Details of these patients are depicted in **Supplementary Table 1**.

Further linear regression analysis of LVOT obstruction ($p = 0.2232$), SAM ($p = 0.2982$), and MR ($p = 0.6468$) recurrence with septal thickness as the continuous variable did not show any statistical relationship.

DISCUSSION

This study reports the long-term clinical and echocardiographic outcomes of subvalvular mitral anomalies correction with concomitant extended septal myectomy in HOCM patients with moderate (< 18 mm) and severe (≥ 18 mm) inteventricular septal thickness.

Our 15-year experience demonstrates that (1) HOCM is a wide spectrum of disease in which both septal hypertrophy and the MV apparatus invariably contribute to dynamic LVOT obstruction; (2) the subvalvular mitral apparatus (chordae and PM) promote SAM and contribute to obstruction; (3) regardless of septal thickness, subvalvular apparatus remodeling

TABLE 2 | Intraoperative results, early and long term outcomes.

	All, $n = 66$	Septal thickness < 18 mm ($n = 29$)	Septal thickness ≥ 18 mm ($n = 37$)	P-value
Aortic cross-clamp (min)	41.4 ± 10.6 (20–80)	41.9 ± 10.9 (20–65)	41.1 ± 10.6 (24–80)	0.7
Cardiopulmonary bypass (min)	56.5 ± 12.7 (25–105)	56.8 ± 13.7 (25–88)	56.2 ± 12.1 (38–105)	0.8
Resected cords (n)	3.5 ± 1.6 (0–8)	3.5 ± 1.6 (0–8)	3.5 ± 1.6 (0–7)	0.9
Procedures on papillary muscles (n)	1.3 ± 0.8 (0–3)	1.4 ± 0.9 (0–3)	1.2 ± 0.8 (0–2)	0.4
Mitral valve replacement	2 (3)	0	2 (3)	0.4
Intraoperative mitral valve replacement for MR	1 (1)	0	1 (1)	0.4
Posterior mitral leaflet shortening	4 (6)	4 (6)	0 (0)	**0.033**
Other procedures	6 (9)	4 (6)	2 (3)	0.3
Blood transfusion	37 (56)	17 (25)	20 (30)	0.8
Re-exploration	1 (1)	1 (1)	0 (0)	0.4
Low cardiac output syndrome	2 (3)	1 (1)	1 (1)	1
Sepsis	3 (4)	1 (1)	2 (3)	1
Post-operative atrial fibrillation	33 (50)	11 (16)	22 (34)	0.1
Post-operative PM implantation	3 (4)	2 (3)	1 (1)	0.5
Post-operative Complete AV block	0			
Iatrogenic ventricular septal defect	0			
Length of stay (days)	10.6 ± 8.3 (5–62)	10.1 ± 6 (5–33)	10.9 ± 9.8 (5–62)	1
Pre-discharge SAM	2 (3)	1 (1)	1 (1)	1
Pre-discharge				
LVOT gradient* (mmHg)	15.4 ± 8.5 (0–33)	14.7 ± 8 (0–30)	16 ± 8.8 (0–33)	0.5
Septal thickness (mm)	14 ± 2.6 (7–16)	12.7 ± 1.4 (10–16)	15 ± 2.9 (7–16)	**0.0001**
NYHA functional class	1.3 ± 0.5 (1–3)			0.7
I–II	63 (95)	27 (41)	36 (55)	0.7
III	3 (5)	2 (3)	1 (1)	
MR grade	1.2 ± 0.6 (0–3)			0.2
≤ 1 + /4 +	50 (75)	25 (37.5)	25 (37.5)	
2 + /4 +	15 (22)	4 (6)	11 (16)	
3 + /4 +	1 (3)	0	1 (3)	
Hospital mortality	0			
Follow-up				
SAM	7 (11)	2 (3)	5 (8)	0.5
LVOT gradient* (mmHg)	16.3 ± 8.8 (6–40)	18.2 ± 9.2 (6–40)	14.8 ± 8.2 (8–39)	0.1
Septal thickness (mm)	13.9 ± 2.7 (9–16)	12.9 ± 1.9 (10–18)	14.8 ± 3 (9–16)	**0.0068**
NYHA functional class	1.6 ± 0.6 (1–3)			0.9
I	27 (43)	11 (17)	16 (25)	
II	35 (54)	16 (25)	19 (29)	
III	2 (3)	1 (1)	1 (1)	
MR grade	1.2 ± 0.5 (0–4)			0.6
≤ 2 + /4 +	62 (98)	28 (44)	34 (54)	
4 + /4 +	1 (2)	0	1 (1)	
Reoperation at follow-up for MR	0			
Exitus at follow-up	2 (3)	1 (1.5)	1 (1.5)	1

MR, mitral regurgitation; PM, pacemaker; AV, atrio-ventricular; SAM, systolic anterior motion. LVOT, left ventricle outflow tract; NYHA, New York Heart Association.
**Peak gradient at rest.*
Continuous variables were expressed as mean, standard deviation and range.
Categorical variables were expressed as absolute value and percentage.
Bold values are referred to the significative p value.

added to septal myectomy can provide satisfactory early- and long-term outcomes in terms of symptom improvement, LVOT obstruction, and MR resolution; (4) conservative procedures on the subvalvular mitral apparatus ("remodeling") can correct SAM and MR and avoid, in most cases, MV replacement; (5) surgical remodeling of the subvalvular apparatus does not impair MV function at long-term follow-up; and (6) a dedicated HOCM team (dedicated clinical

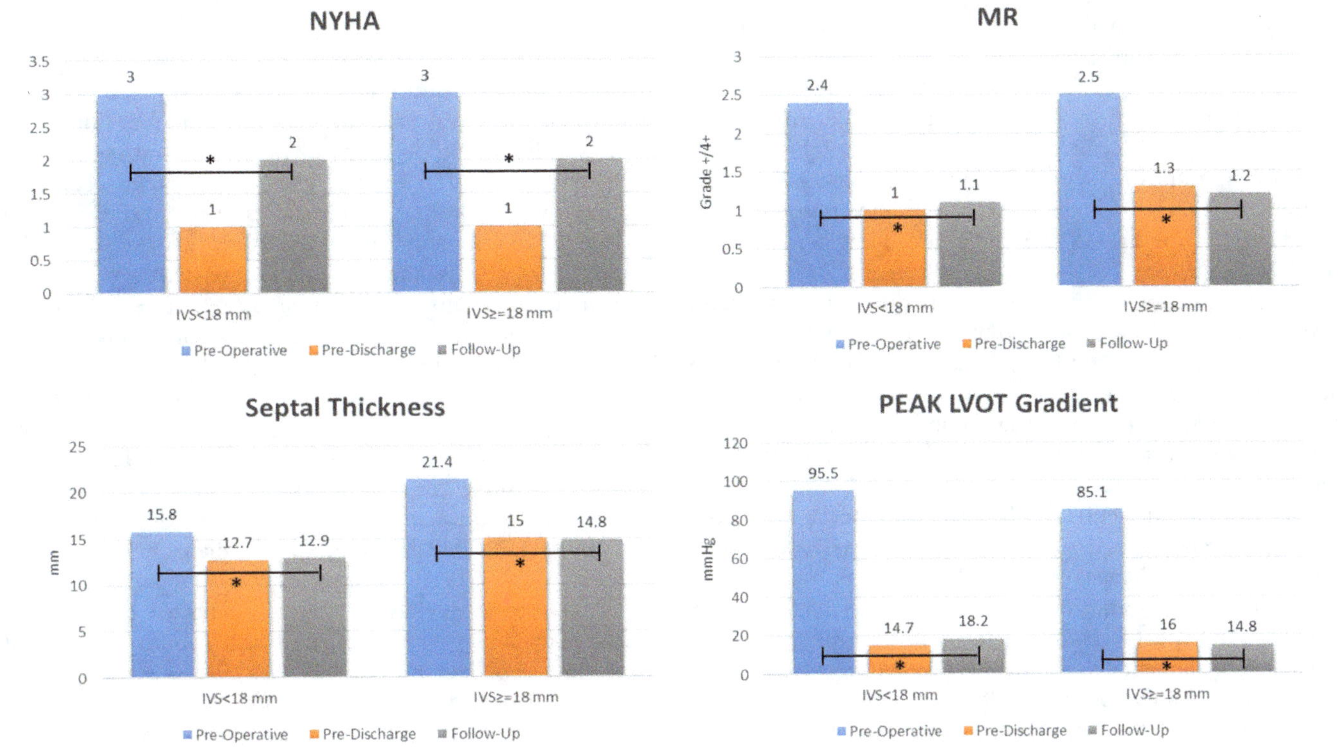

FIGURE 2 | Early and long term outcome after extended septal myectomy and subvalvular mitral apparatus remodeling. NYHA: New York Heart Association; MR: mitral regurgitation; LVOT: left ventricle outflow tract; IVS: interventricular septum. "*" explains the events.

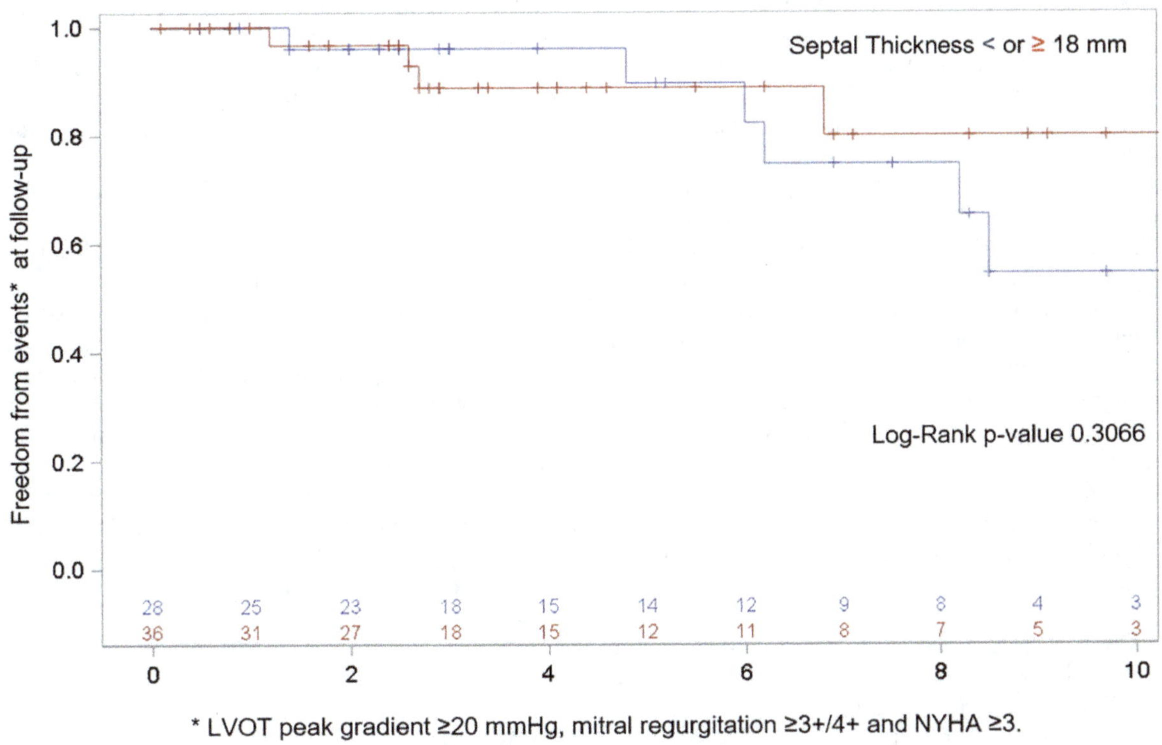

FIGURE 3 | Freedom from composite end points at follow-up by means of recurrent LVOT obstruction (peak gradient $\geq$ 20 mmHg), MR $\geq 3+/4+$ and NYHA $\geq$ 3. *$p = 0.0001$.

and interventional cardiologists, radiologists, surgeons, pathologists, and geneticists) is crucial to assess patients with hypertrophic cardiomyopathy and for planning the most appropriate treatment.

In our series, septal myectomy was performed in all cases, confirming the well-defined role of this technique for the relief of drug-refractory symptoms in patients with LV outflow obstruction (1–3, 17). Presently, the mortality rate after this procedure is below 1% (19, 20) and approaching zero in some series (21).

Concerns surround managing patients with moderate hypertrophy (7, 8, 11) in which the role of the MV in LVOT obstruction is predominant (4–6). Isolated myectomy should be considered cautiously because of iatrogenic ventricular septal defect occurrence and the insignificant relief of symptoms and LVOT obstruction (22). In fact, less marked septal basal hypertrophy may not be the sole cause of LVOT obstruction (8) and this clinical picture has been reported to be associated with mitral valvular and subvalvular anomalies (7, 8). These variants include changes in the MV leaflets (elongation, laxity, calcifications) and, more often, aberrancies of PM and secondary chordae (4, 5). We defined the complex anatomy of the LVOT in patients with HOCM as a "crowded" LVOT (18) in which, historically, replacement of the MV and subvalvular apparatus resection was the only viable option to treat the SAM-mediated obstruction and MR (22). In 2019, The Society of Thoracic Surgeons reported results of septal myectomy in the United States from a national database of more than 2,300 patients (16). About 1/3 of septal myectomy cases required MV operation (n = 801), including mitral repair (62%) and replacement (38%). Replacement compared to repair was associated with an increased risk of in-hospital mortality (4.4% vs. 1.9%) and MV surgery in addition to isolated septal myectomy (mortality 1.6%) was associated with an increased composite risk [OR 1.81, 95% confidence interval (CI): 1.39 to 2.36, $p < 0.0001$]. In the series by Lapenna et al. (7) the long-term mortality was higher in 23 patients with moderate septal thickness that required MV replacement plus septal myectomy compared to those with septal myectomy alone (n = 41) or septal myectomy plus MV repair (n = 12). In a prospective clinical trial (NCT02054221), 88 patients were randomized to MV replacement or repair during myectomy. At 2-year follow-up, the rates of overall survival, freedom from sudden cardiac death, and freedom from thromboembolic events were significantly higher in the repair group (23). Finally, the same group conducted a meta-analysis of over 2,762 patients with HOCM and MR (24) reporting a strong clinical benefit of MV repair compared to replacement in adult patients with HOCM.

The superiority of MV repair is well established for degenerative MV disease (25) and all efforts should be made to preserve the MV in patients with HOCM.

There is debate whether myectomy alone is enough to achieve the best outcome even in patients with moderate septal thickness. A dedicated high-volume center (10) reported on 1,486 surgical HOCM patients stratified by basal septal thickness (< 18 mm, n = 369; 18–21 mm, n = 612; and > 21 mm, n = 505). All patients underwent septal myectomy alone, regardless of septal thickness and degree of SAM-related MR. Concomitant MV procedures were performed for patients with intrinsic MV disease (66%) or insufficient intraoperative results in terms of residual mitral regurgitation (30%) and gradient (2%) after extended septal myectomy. In the group with septum < 18 mm, at early postoperative follow-up, moderate/severe mitral regurgitation was documented in only 2% of patients and SAM in 27.5%, with no difference compared to patients with a baseline septum ≥ 18 mm. The lack of long-term follow-up echocardiographic data is the major limitation of this study.

On the other hand, subvalvular mitral procedures are routinely performed at other dedicated HOCM centers with excellent results (6, 9, 11–13). For instance, the role of diseased secondary chordae in obstruction, especially in cases of a relatively thin septum, has been demonstrated by Ferrazzi et al. (11) Anomalous chordae resection (median of 3, range 1–8) associated with a shallow myectomy in 39 patients (with a ventricular septal thickness ≤ 19 mm) showed better clinical and hemodynamic results compared with a control group (only myectomy, 29 patients).

Our series provides long-term clinical and echocardiographic outcomes of procedures involving the subvalvular mitral apparatus during HOCM surgery. Release of the AML achieved by the technique described allows for coaptation of the mitral leaflet far from the septum and provides resolution of LVOT obstruction. Neither ventricular septal defect nor hospital mortality occurred. Intraoperative MV replacement because of a failed procedure due to severe MR recurrence was necessary in one patient. Pacemaker implantation rate was consistent with data from another single-center report (16). Our research highlights the complex anatomic interactions among the basal septal hypertrophy, mitral valvular and subvalvular abnormalities and SAM-in HOCM moreover when the septal thickness is less marked (91% of patients showed a septal thickness ≤ 24 mm), and contributes further data to the debate over surgical myectomy or alcoholization, though the use of the latter has increased in Europe in recent decades (25). This study also reports the definitive benefits of subvalvular mitral apparatus procedures added to septal myectomy in experienced centers. Preoperative planning, based on individual anatomic findings, and tailored surgical treatment resulted in excellent outcomes.

This is a single-center series of consecutive patients retrospectively reviewed. The small sample size and the lack of certain data (e.g., type of HOCM and hypertrophy localization, weight of the resected muscle, histopathologic analysis and cardiac magnetic resonance findings) should be considered its major limitations.

CONCLUSION

Subvalvular apparatus remodeling added to septal myectomy can provide satisfactory early and long-term outcomes in terms of symptom improvement, LVOT obstruction relief, and MR resolution in patients with HOCM regardless of septal thickness.

ETHICS STATEMENT

The studies involving human participants were reviewed and approved by IRCCS-ISMETT. The patients/participants provided their written informed consent to participate in this study. Written informed consent was obtained from the individual(s) for the publication of any potentially identifiable images or data included in this article.

AUTHOR CONTRIBUTIONS

GR: conceptualization, formal analysis, methodology, supervision, validation, and writing—original draft. EF, CL, AP, AR, and MG: data curation and validation. MK and SL: methodology and writing—review and editing. SS, MT, VS, MM, and GM: data curation and supervision. MP: conceptualization, supervision, and validation. All authors contributed to the article and approved the submitted version.

REFERENCES

1. Morrow AG, Brockenbrough EC. Surgical treatment of idiopathic hypertrophic subaortic stenosis: technic and hemodynamic results of subaortic ventriculomyotomy. *Ann Surg.* (1961) 154:181–9. doi: 10.1097/00000658-196108000-00003
2. Ommen SR, Maron BJ, Olivotto I, Maron MS, Cecchi F, Betocchi S, et al. Long-term effects of surgical septal myectomy on survival in patients with obstructive hypertrophic cardiomyopathy. *J Am Coll Cardiol.* (2005) 46:470–6. doi: 10.1016/j.jacc.2005.02.090
3. Smedira NG, Lytle BW, Lever HM, Rajeswaran J, Krishnaswamy G, Kaple RK, et al. Current effectiveness and risks of isolated septal myectomy for hypertrophic obstructive cardiomyopathy. *Ann Thorac Surg.* (2008) 85:127–33. doi: 10.1016/j.athoracsur.2007.07.063
4. Sherrid MV, Balaram S, Kim B, Axel L, Swistel DG. The mitral valve in obstructive hypertrophic cardiomyopathy: a test in context. *J Am Coll Cardiol.* (2016) 67:1846–58. doi: 10.1016/j.jacc.2016.01.071
5. Silbiger JJ. Abnormalities of the mitral apparatus in hypertrophic cardiomyopathy: echocardiographic, pathophysiologic, and surgical insights. *J Am Soc Echocardiogr.* (2016) 29:622–39. doi: 10.1016/j.echo.2016.03.003
6. Raffa GM, Romano G, Turrisi M, Morsolini M, Gentile G, Sciacca S, et al. Pathoanatomic findings and treatment during hypertrophic obstructive cardiomyopathy surgery: the role of mitral valve. *Heart Lung Circ.* (2019) 28:477–85.
7. Lapenna E, Nisi T, Carino D, Bargagna M, Ruggeri S, Zancanaro E, et al. Hypertrophic cardiomyopathy with moderate septal thickness and mitral regurgitation: long-term surgical results. *Eur J Cardiothorac Surg.* (2021) 60:244–51. doi: 10.1093/ejcts/ezab097
8. Patel P, Dhillon A, Popovic ZB, Smedira NG, Rizzo J, Thamilarasan M, et al. Left ventricular outflow tract obstruction in hypertrophic cardiomyopathy patients without severe septal hypertrophy: implications of mitral valve and papillary muscle abnormalities assessed using cardiac magnetic resonance and echocardiography. *Circ Cardiovasc Imaging.* (2015) 8:e003132. doi: 10.1161/CIRCIMAGING.115.003132
9. Raffa GM, Pilato M. Hypertrophic obstructive cardiomyopathy and subvalvular mitral apparatus remodeling. *Ann Thorac Surg.* (2019) 108:964. doi: 10.1016/j.athoracsur.2019.01.056
10. Nguyen A, Schaff HV, Nishimura RA, Dearani JA, Geske JB, Lahr BD, et al. Does septal thickness influence outcome of myectomy for hypertrophic obstructive cardiomyopathy? *Eur J Cardiothorac Surg.* (2018) 53:582–9. doi: 10.1093/ejcts/ezx398
11. Ferrazzi P, Spirito P, Iacovoni A, Calabrese A, Migliorati K, Simon C, et al. Transaortic chordal cutting: mitral valve repair for obstructive hypertrophic cardiomyopathy with mild septal hypertrophy. *J Am Coll Cardiol.* (2015) 66:1687–96. doi: 10.1016/j.jacc.2015.07.069
12. Vriesendorp PA, Schinkel AF, Soliman OI, Kofflard MJ, de Jong PL, van Herwerden LA, et al. Long-term benefit of myectomy and anterior mitral leaflet extension in obstructive hypertrophic cardiomyopathy. *Am J Cardiol.* (2015) 115:670–5. doi: 10.1016/j.amjcard.2014.12.017
13. Dulguerov F, Marcacci C, Alexandrescu C, Chan KM, Dreyfus GD. Hypertrophic obstructive cardiomyopathy: the mitral valve could be the key. *Eur J Cardiothorac Surg.* (2016) 50:61–5. doi: 10.1093/ejcts/ezv473
14. Kwon DH, Smedira NG, Thamilarasan M, Lytle BW, Lever H, Desai MY. Characteristics and surgical outcomes of symptomatic patients with hypertrophic cardiomyopathy with abnormal papillary muscle morphology undergoing papillary muscle reorientation. *J Thorac Cardiovasc Surg.* (2010) 140:317–24. doi: 10.1016/j.jtcvs.2009.10.045
15. Lapenna E, Nisi T, Ruggeri S, Trumello C, Del Forno B, Schiavi D, et al. Edge-to-edge mitral repair associated with septal myectomy in hypertrophic obstructive cardiomyopathy. *Ann Thorac Surg.* (2020) 110:783–9. doi: 10.1016/j.athoracsur.2020.03.095
16. Wei LM, Thibault DP, Rankin JS, Alkhouli M, Roberts HG, Vemulapalli S, et al. Contemporary surgical management of hypertrophic cardiomyopathy in the United States. *Ann Thorac Surg.* (2019) 107:460–6. doi: 10.1016/j.athoracsur.2018.08.068
17. Ommen SR, Mital S, Burke MA, Day SM, Deswal A, Elliott P, et al. 2020 AHA/ACC guideline for the diagnosis and treatment of patients with hypertrophic cardiomyopathy: a report of the American college of cardiology/American heart association joint committee on clinical practice guidelines. *J Am Coll Cardiol.* (2020) 76:e159–240.
18. Raffa GM, Pilato M. Letter to the editor: hypertrophic obstructive cardiomyopathy and a "crowded" left ventricular outflow tract (response to the letter of Professor Ismail Yurekli, et al.). *Heart Lung Circ.* (2021) 30:e45–6. doi: 10.1016/j.hlc.2020.06.013
19. Iacovoni A, Spirito P, Simon C, Iascone M, Di Dedda G, De Filippo P, et al. A contemporary European experience with surgical septal myectomy in hypertrophic cardiomyopathy. *Eur Heart J.* (2012) 33:2080–7. doi: 10.1093/eurheartj/ehs064
20. Maron BJ, Dearani JA, Ommen SR, Maron MS, Schaff HV, Nishimura RA, et al. Low operative mortality achieved with surgical septal myectomy: role of dedicated hypertrophic cardiomyopathy centers in the management of dynamic subaortic obstruction. *J Am Coll Cardiol.* (2015) 66:1307–8. doi: 10.1016/j.jacc.2015.06.1333
21. Ji Q, Wang Y, Liu F, Yang Y, Xia L, Ding W, et al. Hypertrophic cardiomyopathy with latent obstruction: clinical characteristics and surgical results. *J Cardiol.* (2021) 79:42–9. doi: 10.1016/j.jjcc.2021.09.002
22. McIntosh CL, Maron BJ. Current operative treatment of obstructive hypertrophic cardiomyopathy. *Circulation.* (1988) 78:487–95. doi: 10.1161/01.cir.78.3.487
23. Bogachev-Prokophiev A, Afanasyev A, Zheleznev S, Fomenko M, Sharifulin R, Kretov E, et al. Mitral valve repair or replacement in hypertrophic obstructive

cardiomyopathy: a prospective randomized study. *Interact Cardiovasc Thorac Surg.* (2017) 25:356–62. doi: 10.1093/icvts/ivx152

24. Afanasyev A, Bogachev-Prokophiev A, Lenko E, Sharifulin R, Ovcharov M, Kozmin D, et al. Myectomy with mitral valve repair versus replacement in adult patients with hypertrophic obstructive cardiomyopathy: a systematic review and meta-analysis. *Interact Cardiovasc Thorac Surg.* (2019) 28:465–72. doi: 10.1093/icvts/ivy269
25. Falk V, Baumgartner H, Bax JJ, De Bonis M, Hamm C, Holm PJ, et al. 2017 ESC/EACTS guidelines for the management of valvular heart disease. *Eur J Cardiothorac Surg.* (2017) 52:616–64.

Permissions

All chapters in this book were first published by Frontiers; hereby published with permission under the Creative Commons Attribution License or equivalent. Every chapter published in this book has been scrutinized by our experts. Their significance has been extensively debated. The topics covered herein carry significant findings which will fuel the growth of the discipline. They may even be implemented as practical applications or may be referred to as a beginning point for another development.

The contributors of this book come from diverse backgrounds, making this book a truly international effort. This book will bring forth new frontiers with its revolutionizing research information and detailed analysis of the nascent developments around the world.

We would like to thank all the contributing authors for lending their expertise to make the book truly unique. They have played a crucial role in the development of this book. Without their invaluable contributions this book wouldn't have been possible. They have made vital efforts to compile up to date information on the varied aspects of this subject to make this book a valuable addition to the collection of many professionals and students.

This book was conceptualized with the vision of imparting up-to-date information and advanced data in this field. To ensure the same, a matchless editorial board was set up. Every individual on the board went through rigorous rounds of assessment to prove their worth. After which they invested a large part of their time researching and compiling the most relevant data for our readers.

The editorial board has been involved in producing this book since its inception. They have spent rigorous hours researching and exploring the diverse topics which have resulted in the successful publishing of this book. They have passed on their knowledge of decades through this book. To expedite this challenging task, the publisher supported the team at every step. A small team of assistant editors was also appointed to further simplify the editing procedure and attain best results for the readers.

Apart from the editorial board, the designing team has also invested a significant amount of their time in understanding the subject and creating the most relevant covers. They scrutinized every image to scout for the most suitable representation of the subject and create an appropriate cover for the book.

The publishing team has been an ardent support to the editorial, designing and production team. Their endless efforts to recruit the best for this project, has resulted in the accomplishment of this book. They are a veteran in the field of academics and their pool of knowledge is as vast as their experience in printing. Their expertise and guidance has proved useful at every step. Their uncompromising quality standards have made this book an exceptional effort. Their encouragement from time to time has been an inspiration for everyone.

The publisher and the editorial board hope that this book will prove to be a valuable piece of knowledge for researchers, students, practitioners and scholars across the globe.

List of Contributors

Francesco Santullo, Carlo Abatini, Miriam Attalla El Halabieh, Claudio Lodoli and Andrea Di Giorgio
Surgical Unit of Peritoneum and Retroperitoneum, Fondazione Policlinico Universitario A. Gemelli IRCCS, Rome, Italy

Francesco Giovinazzo
General Surgery and Liver Transplant Unit, Fondazione Policlinico Universitario A. Gemelli IRCCS, Rome, Italy

Federica Ferracci and Lorenzo Barberis
Dipartimento di Medicina e Chirurgia Traslazionale, Università Cattolica del Sacro Cuore, Rome, Italy

Fabio Pacelli
Surgical Unit of Peritoneum and Retroperitoneum, Fondazione Policlinico Universitario A. Gemelli IRCCS, Rome, Italy
Dipartimento di Medicina e Chirurgia Traslazionale, Università Cattolica del Sacro Cuore, Rome, Italy

Atanas G. Sivevski, Dafina Karadjova and Emilija Ivanov
Department of Anaesthesia, Clinical Center Mother Teresa, University Clinic for Gynecology and Obstetrics, Skopje, Macedonia

Andrijan Kartalov
Clinical Center Mother Teresa, University Clinic for TOARILUC, Skopje, Macedonia

Situ Xiong, Ming Jiang, Bing Hu, Ru Chen, Zhijun Yao, Wen Deng and Bin Fu
Department of Urology, The First Affiliated Hospital of Nanchang University, Nanchang, China
Jiangxi Institute of Urology, Nanchang, China

Xiaoqiang Liu and Luyao Chen
Department of Urology, The First Affiliated Hospital of Nanchang University, Nanchang, China

Yi Jiang
Jiangxi Institute of Urology, Nanchang, China
Department of Urology, The Second Affiliated Hospital of Nanchang University, Nanchang, China

Xianwen Wan
Department of Anesthesiology, The First Affiliated Hospital of Nanchang University, Nanchang, China

Borislava Pujic
Clinical Center Vojvodina, Obstetrics and Gynecology Hospital, Novi Sad, Serbia

Mirjana Kendrisic
General Hospital, Sremska Mitrovica, Serbia

Matthew Shotwell and Yaping Shi
Department of Biostatistics, School of Medicine, Vanderbilt University, Nashville, TN, United States

Curtis L. Baysinger
Department of Anesthesiology, School of Medicine, Vanderbilt University, Nashville, TN, United States

YouYuan Bao, YouQing Yang, Lin Zhou, ShenHao Xie, Xiao Wu, Han Ding, Jie Wu, Limin Xiao, Le Yang, Bin Tang and Tao Hong
Department of Neurosurgery, The First Affiliated Hospital of Nanchang University, Nanchang, China

Gordana Jovanovic
University of Novi Sad, Faculty of Medicine, Department of Anesthesia and Perioperative Medicine, Novi Sad, Serbia
Clinic for Anesthesia and Intensive Care Therapy, Clinical Center of Vojvodina, Novi Sad, Serbia
University of Novi Sad, Faculty of Medicine, Department of Physiology and Sports Medicine, Novi Sad, Serbia

Mirka Lukic-Šarkanovic
Clinic for Anesthesia and Intensive Care Therapy, Clinical Center of Vojvodina, Novi Sad, Serbia

Dea Karaba Jakovljevic
University of Novi Sad, Faculty of Medicine, Department of Physiology and Sports Medicine, Novi Sad, Serbia

Meng Wei, Yize Liang, Zhibo Yan, Danping Sun, Yadi Huang, Xin Zhong, Peng Liu and Wenbin Yu
Department of Gastrointestinal Surgery, General Surgery, Qilu Hospital, Cheeloo College of Medicine, Shandong University, Jinan, China

Limei Wang and Zhen Li
Department of Gastroenterology, Qilu Hospital, Cheeloo College of Medicine, Shandong University, Jinan, China

Yuanyuan Chen
Nursing Department, Qilu Hospital, Cheeloo College of Medicine, Shandong University, Jinan, China

Zorana Stanković, Irena Simić and Ivana Petrov
Department of Anesthesiology and Intensive Care, University Children's Hospital, Belgrade, Belgrade, Serbia

Dušica Simić and Marija Stević
Department of Anesthesiology and Intensive Care, University Children's Hospital, Belgrade, Belgrade, Serbia
Medical Faculty University of Belgrade, Belgrade, Serbia

Siniša Dučić
Department of Anesthesiology and Intensive Care, University Children's Hospital, Belgrade, Belgrade, Serbia
Department of Orthopedic Surgery, University Children's Hospital, Belgrade, Belgrade, Serbia

Miodrag Milenović
Medical Faculty University of Belgrade, Belgrade, Serbia
Department of Anesthesiology and Intensive Care, Clinical Center of Serbia, Belgrade, Serbia

Hiroshi Ishikawa and Makio Shozu
Department of Reproductive Medicine, Graduate School of Medicine, Chiba University, Chiba, Japan

Michael Akerman
Weill Cornell Medical College, Cornell University, New York City, NY, United States

Nada Pejčić
General Hospital Leskovac, Leskovac, Serbia

Ivan Veličković
SUNY Downstate Medical Center, Brooklyn, NY, United States

Shiyi Peng, Ying Zheng, Fan Yang, Kana Wang and Sijing Chen
Department of Gynecology, West China Second Hospital, Sichuan University, Chengdu, China
Key Laboratory of Obstetrics, Gynecologic and Pediatric Diseases and Birth Defects of Ministry of Education, West China Second Hospital, Sichuan University, Chengdu, China

Yawen Wang
Department of Obstetrics and Gynecology, Shanxi Bethune Hospital, Taiyuan, China

Mingjie Zhang
Department of Surgery, Shengjing Hospital of China Medical University, Shenyang, China

Xiaoxue Wang and Xueting Chen
Department of Health Management, Shengjing Hospital of China Medical University, Shenyang, China

Zixuan Song, Yuting Wang, Yangzi Zhou and Dandan Zhang
Department of Obstetrics and Gynecology, Shengjing Hospital of China Medical University, Shenyang, China

Darko Aleksa Golic, Dragan Svraka, Nataša Keleman and Snjezana Petrovic
Medical Faculty of Banja Luka, University Clinical Center of Republic of Srpska, University Banja Luka, Banjaluka, Bosnia and Herzegovina

Peng-yue Zhao and Xiao-hui Du
Department of General Surgery, First Medical Center of the Chinese PLA General Hospital, Beijing, China

Ke Han
Department of Gastroenterology, First Medical Center of the Chinese PLA General Hospital, Beijing, China

Ren-qi Yao
Translational Medicine Research Center, Medical Innovation Research Division and Fourth Medical Center of the Chinese PLA General Hospital, Beijing, China

Chao Ren
Department of Pulmonary and Critical Care Medicine, Beijing Chaoyang Hospital, Capital Medical University, Beijing, China

Milena Dragisa Stojanovic, Danica Markovic, Vladan Cvetanovic and Anita Zoran Vukovic
Center for Anesthesiology and Reanimatology, Clinical Center of Niš, Niš, Serbia

Radmilo J. Jankovic
Center for Anesthesiology and Reanimatology, Clinical Center of Niš, Niš, Serbia
School of Medicine, University of Niš, Niš, Serbia

Qingshun Zhu, Lei Yu and Bowen Li
Department of Clinical Medical College, Weifang Medical University, Weifang, China

Guangxu Zhu, Xuguang Jiao and Jianjun Qu
Department of General Surgery, The First Affiliated Hospital of Weifang Medical College, Weifang People's Hospital, Weifang, China

Stefano Cianci
Unit of Gynecology, Department of Human Pathology of Adult and Childood 'G. Barresi', University of Messina, Messina, Italy

Vito Andrea Capozzi
Department of Medicine and Surgery, University Hospital of Parma, Parma, Italy

Andrea Rosati, Valerio Rumolo, Giacomo Corrado, Salvatore Gueli Alletti and Anna Fagotti
Dipartimento Scienze Della Salute Della Donna e del Bambino, Fondazione Policlinico Universitario A. Gemelli IRCCS, Rome, Italy

Stefano Uccella
Department of Obstetrics and Gynecology, AOUI Verona, University of Verona, Verona, Italy

Matteo Riccò
Department of Public Health, Service for Health and Safety in the Workplace, Reggio Emilia, Italy

Francesco Cosentino
Department of Medicine and Health Science, "V.Tiberio" Università Degli Studi del Molise, Campobasso, Italy
Department of Gynecologic Onocology, Gemelli Molise SpA, Campobasso, Italy

Natalija Vukovic
Anesthesiology and Reanimation Center, Clinical Center Nis, Nis, Serbia

Ljubomir Dinic
Urology Clinic, Clinical Center Nis, Nis, Serbia

Jiao Wang, Qing Yang, Dandan Wang, Mengyuan Li and Ningning Zhang
Department of Obstetrics and Gynecology, Shengjing Hospital of China Medical University, Shenyang, China

Huimin Tang, Zhiyong Dong, Zhenyue Qin, Shoufeng Zhang, Huihui Wang, Weiwei Wei, Ruxia Shi and Jiming Chen
Department of Gynecology, The Affiliated Changzhou No. 2 People's Hospital of Nanjing Medical University, Changzhou, China

Bairong Xia
Department of Gynecology, The First Affiliated Hospital of USTC, Division of Life Sciences and Medicine, University of Science and Technology of China, Hefei, China

Milena D. Stojanovic, Danica Z. Markovic, Anita Z. Vukovic, Vesna D. Dinic, Aleksandar N. Nikolic and Tijana G. Maricic
Center for Anesthesiology, Reanimatology and Intensive Care, Clinical Center Nis, Nis, Serbia

Radmilo J. Janković
Center for Anesthesiology, Reanimatology and Intensive Care, Clinical Center Nis, Nis, Serbia
School of Medicine, University of Nis, Nis, Serbia

Guozheng Li, Xingda Zhang, Xin Ma, Hui Li, Yihai Chen, Lei Zhang, Xin Zhang, Jiale Wu, Xinheng Wang and Shouping Xu
Department ofs Breast Surgery, Harbin Medical University Cancer Hospital, Harbin, China

Jiyun Zhao and Yan Zhang
School of Life Science and Technology, Computational Biology Research Center, Harbin Institute of Technology, Harbin, China

Giuseppe Campagna, Lorenzo Vacca, Giovanni Panico, Daniela Caramazza and Monia Marturano
Department of Woman, Child, and Public Health, Fondazione Policlinico Universitario A. Gemelli Istituto di Ricovero e Cura a Carattere Scientifico (IRCCS), Rome, Italy

Giuseppe Vizzielli
Department of Medicinal Area (DAME) Clinic of Obstetrics and Gynecology, Santa Maria della Misericordia Hospital, Azienda Sanitaria Universitaria Friuli Centrale, Udine, Italy

Riccardo Zaccoletti
Obstetrics and Gynecology Unit, P. Pederzoli Hospital, Peschiera del Garda, Verona, Italy

Roberta Granese and Martina Arcieri
Department of Biomedical, Dental, Morphological and Functional Imaging Science, University of Messina, Messina, Italy

Alfredo Ercoli
Department of Human Pathology in Adult and Childhood "G. Barresi," University of Messina, Messina, Italy

Giovanni Scambia
Department of Woman, Child, and Public Health, Fondazione Policlinico Universitario A. Gemelli Istituto di Ricovero e Cura a Carattere Scientifico (IRCCS), Rome, Italy
Department of Woman, Child and Public Health, Catholic University of Sacred Heart, Rome, Italy
Dipartimento Scienze Della Salute Della Donna e del Bambino, Fondazione Policlinico Universitario A. Gemelli IRCCS, Rome, Italy

Andrea Balla, Diletta Corallino, Silvia Quaresima, Livia Palmieri, Francesca Meoli, Ingrid Cordova Herencia and Alessandro M. Paganini
Department of General Surgery and Surgical Specialties "Paride Stefanini", Sapienza University of Rome, Rome, Italy

Jingwen Chen, Zhiyuan Zhang, Wenju Chang, Tuo Yi, Qingyang Feng, Dexiang Zhu, Guodong He and Ye Wei
Department of General Surgery, Zhongshan Hospital, Fudan University, Shanghai, China

Giuseppe Daniele, Simone Codini, Annamaria Ciccarone, Laura Giusti and Stefano Del Prato
Department of Clinical and Experimental Medicine, University of Pisa, Pisa, Italy

Beatrice Campi and Ele Ferrannini
C.N.R. Institute of Clinical Physiology, Pisa, Italy

Alessandro Saba
Department of Surgical, Medical and Molecular Pathology and Critical Care Medicine, University of Pisa, Pisa, Italy
Laboratory of Clinical Pathology, St. Chiara University Hospital, Pisa, Italy

Russel L. Esterline
AstraZeneca Pharmaceutical, Gaithersburg, MD, United States

Giovanni Fantola, Enrico Moroni, Emanuele Lai and Stefano Pintus
Obesity Surgery Unit, Department of Surgery, ARNAS G. Brotzu, Cagliari, Italy

Matteo Runfola
Emergency Surgery Unit, Department of Surgery, ARNAS G. Brotzu, Cagliari, Italy

Pierpaolo Gallucci
Division of Endocrine and Metabolic Surgery, Fondazione Policlinico Universitario Agostino Gemelli IRCCS, Rome, Italy

Francesco Pennestrì and Marco Raffaelli
Division of Endocrine and Metabolic Surgery, Fondazione Policlinico Universitario Agostino Gemelli IRCCS, Università Cattolica del Sacro Cuore, Rome, Italy

Karl J. Neff
Diabetes Complications Research Centre, Conway Institute, University College Dublin, Dublin, Ireland

Carel W. Le Roux
Diabetes Complications Research Centre, Conway Institute, University College Dublin, Dublin, Ireland
Metabolic Medicine, Imperial College London, London, United Kingdom

Michal Pasierski and Jakub Staromłyński
Department of Cardiac Surgery, Central Clinical Hospital of the Ministry of Interior, Centre of Postgraduate Medical Education, Warsaw, Poland
Thoracic Research Centre, Innovative Medical Forum, Collegium Medicum Nicolaus Copernicus University, Bydgoszcz, Poland

Janina Finke and Piotr Suwalski
Department of Cardiac Surgery, Central Clinical Hospital of the Ministry of Interior, Centre of Postgraduate Medical Education, Warsaw, Poland

Mariusz Kowalewski
Department of Cardiac Surgery, Central Clinical Hospital of the Ministry of Interior, Centre of Postgraduate Medical Education, Warsaw, Poland
Thoracic Research Centre, Innovative Medical Forum, Collegium Medicum Nicolaus Copernicus University, Bydgoszcz, Poland
Cardio-Thoracic Surgery Department, Heart and Vascular Centre, Maastricht University Medical Centre, Cardiovascular Research Institute Maastricht, Maastricht, Netherlands

Radoslaw Litwinowicz
Thoracic Research Centre, Innovative Medical Forum, Collegium Medicum Nicolaus Copernicus University, Bydgoszcz, Poland
Department of Cardiovascular Surgery and Transplantology, Jagiellonian University Medical College, John Paul II Hospital, Kraków, Poland

Grzegorz Filip and Krzysztof Bartus
Department of Cardiovascular Surgery and Transplantology, Jagiellonian University Medical College, John Paul II Hospital, Kraków, Poland

Adam Kowalówka and Marek Deja
Department of Cardiac Surgery, School of Medicine in Katowice, Medical University of Silesia, Katowice, Poland
Department of Cardiac Surgery, Upper-Silesian Heart Center, Katowice, Poland

Wojciech Wańha
Department of Cardiology and Structural Heart Diseases, Medical University of Silesia, Katowice, Poland
Thoracic Research Centre, Innovative Medical Forum, Collegium Medicum Nicolaus Copernicus University, Bydgoszcz, Poland

Wojciech Wojakowski
Department of Cardiology and Structural Heart Diseases, Medical University of Silesia, Katowice, Poland

Michalina Kołodziejczak
Thoracic Research Centre, Innovative Medical Forum, Collegium Medicum Nicolaus Copernicus University, Bydgoszcz, Poland
Department of Anaesthesiology and Intensive Care, Antoni Jurasz University Hospital No. 1, Collegium Medicum Nicolaus Copernicus University, Bydgoszcz, Poland
Division of Cardiology, Yale School of Medicine, New Haven, CT, United States

Natalia Piekuś -Słomka
Department of Inorganic and Analytical Chemistry, Ludwik Rydygier Collegium Medicum in Bydgoszcz, Nicolaus Copernicus University, Toruń, Poland

Andrzej Łoś, Jan Rogowski and Dariusz Jagielak
Department of Cardiac and Vascular Surgery, Medical University of Gdańsk, Gdańsk, Poland

Sebastian Stefaniak and Marek Jemielity
Department of Cardiac Surgery and Transplantology, PoznańUniversity of Medical Sciences, Poznań, Poland

Silvia Mariani and Roberto Lorusso
Cardio-Thoracic Surgery Department, Heart and Vascular Centre, Maastricht University Medical Centre, Cardiovascular Research Institute Maastricht, Maastricht, Netherlands

Tong Li
Department of Cardiac Surgery, University Hospital Düesseldorf, Düesseldorf, Germany

Matteo Matteucci and Daniele Ronco
Thoracic Research Centre, Innovative Medical Forum, Collegium Medicum Nicolaus Copernicus University, Bydgoszcz, Poland
Department of Cardiac Surgery, Circolo Hospital, University of Insubria, Varese, Italy

Federica Jiritano
Thoracic Research Centre, Innovative Medical Forum, Collegium Medicum Nicolaus Copernicus University, Bydgoszcz, Poland
Department of Cardiac Surgery, University Magna Græcia of Catanzaro, Catanzaro, Italy

Dario Fina and Paolo Meani
Thoracic Research Centre, Innovative Medical Forum, Collegium Medicum Nicolaus Copernicus University, Bydgoszcz, Poland
Department of Cardiothoracic and Vascular Anesthesia and Intensive Care Unit (ICU), Istituto di Ricovero e Cura a Carattere Scientifico (IRCCS) Policlinico San Donato, Milan, Italy

Gennaro Martucci
Thoracic Research Centre, Innovative Medical Forum, Collegium Medicum Nicolaus Copernicus University, Bydgoszcz, Poland
Anesthesia and Intensive Care Department, Istituto di Ricovero e Cura a Carattere Scientifico (IRCCS)-Istituto Mediterraneo per i Trapianti e Terapie ad Alta Specializzazione (ISMETT), Palermo, Italy

Giuseppe Maria Raffa
Thoracic Research Centre, Innovative Medical Forum, Collegium Medicum Nicolaus Copernicus University, Bydgoszcz, Poland
Cardiac Surgery Unit, Istituto di Ricovero e Cura a Carattere Scientifico (IRCCS)-Istituto Mediterraneo per i Trapianti e Terapie ad Alta Specializzazione (ISMETT), Palermo, Italy

Artur Słomka
Thoracic Research Centre, Innovative Medical Forum, Collegium Medicum Nicolaus Copernicus University, Bydgoszcz, Poland
Department of Pathophysiology, Ludwik Rydygier Collegium Medicum Bydgoszcz, Nicolaus Copernicus University, Toruń, Poland

Pietro Giorgio Malvidni
Cardiac Surgery Unit, Lancisi Cardiovascular Center, Polytechnic University of Marche, Ancona, Italy

Michal Zembala
Department of Cardiac, Vascular and Endovascular Surgery and Transplantology, Silesian Center for Heart Diseases, Zabrze, Poland

Giuseppe M. Raffa, Eluisa La Franca, Carlo Lachina, Andrea Palmeri, Alessandro Ricasoli, Matteo Greco, Sergio Sciacca, Marco Turrisi, Marco Morsolini, Vincenzo Stringi, Gabriella Mattiucci and Michele Pilato
Department for the Treatment and Study of Cardiothoracic Diseases and Cardiothoracic Transplantation, IRCCS-ISMETT (Istituto Mediterraneo per i Trapianti e Terapie ad Alta Specializzazione), Palermo, Italy

Steven Lebowitz
The University of Pittsburgh School of Medicine, Pittsburgh, PA, United States

Index

www.ingramcontent.com/pod-product-compliance
Lightning Source LLC
LaVergne TN
LVHW080929210926
848485LV00004B/757
* 9 7 8 1 6 4 6 4 6 5 5 3 8 *